TEACHING
IN NURSING

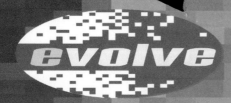

The Latest *Evolution* in Learning.

Evolve provides online access to free learning resources and activities designed specifically for the textbook you are using in your class. The resources will provide you with information that enhances the material covered in the book and much more.

Visit the Web address listed below to start your learning evolution today!

▶▶ *LOGIN: http://evolve.elsevier.com/Billings/teaching/*

Evolve Learning Resources to accompany Teaching in Nursing:
A Guide for Faculty, 2nd Edition offers the following features:

- **WebLinks**
  An exciting resource that lets you link to hundreds of websites carefully chosen to supplement the content of the textbook. The WebLinks are regularly updated, with new ones added as they develop.

Think outside the book...evolve.

TEACHING IN NURSING

A Guide for Faculty

Second Edition

Diane M. Billings, EdD, RN, FAAN
Chancellor's Professor
Professor of Nursing and Associate Dean, Teaching, Learning,
    and Information Resources
Center for Teaching and Lifelong Learning
Indiana University School of Nursing
Indianapolis, Indiana

Judith A. Halstead, DNS, RN
Professor of Nursing
Director, Undergraduate Nursing Program
University of Southern Indiana School of Nursing and
    Health Professions
Evansville, Indiana

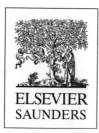

ELSEVIER
SAUNDERS

ELSEVIER
SAUNDERS

11830 Westline Industrial Drive
St Louis, Missouri 63146

Library of Congress Cataloging in Publication Data

Teaching in nursing: a guide for faculty/[edited by] Diane M. Billings, Judith A. Halstead—2nd ed.
     p.; cm.
   Includes bibliographical references and index.
   ISBN 0-7216-0377-7 (alk. paper)
     1. Nursing—Study and teaching. I. Billings, Diane McGovern. II. Halstead, Judith A.
     [DNLM: 1. Education, Nursing—methods. 2. Faculty, Nursing. 3. Teaching—methods.
WY 18 T25175 2004]
RT71.T336 2005
610.73'071—dc22   2004046663

Senior Editor: Tom Wilhelm
Associate Developmental Editor: Jennifer Anderson
Publishing Services Manager: Deborah L. Vogel
Design Manager: Bill Drone

Printed in the United States of America

Last digit is the print number: 9 8 7 6 5 4 3 2 1

To our students and colleagues from whom we continually learn.

CONTRIBUTORS

Donna L. Boland, PhD, RN

Associate Professor and Associate Dean for Undergraduate Programs, Indiana
University School of Nursing, Indianapolis, Indiana
*Curriculum Designs; Developing Curriculum: Frameworks, Outcomes, and
Competencies*

Wanda Bonnel, PhD, RN

Associate Professor, University of Kansas, Kansas City, Kansas
Clinical Performance Evaluation

Mary P. Bourke, PhD(c), RN

Assistant Professor, Ivy Tech State College, Indianapolis, Indiana
The Evaluation Process: An Overview

Charlene E. Clark, MEd, RN, FAAN

Associate Dean for Instructional Resources and Extended College Activities,
Washington State University College of Nursing/Intercollegiate College of
Nursing, Spokane, Washington
Teaching and Learning at a Distance

Judie Csokasy, PhD, RN

Organizational Effectiveness Consultant, The DJC Group, Cincinnati, Ohio
Philosophical Foundations of the Curriculum

Diann DeWitt-Weaver, DNS, RN

St. John's College, Springfield, Illinois
Strategies for Evaluating Learning Outcomes

Nancy Dillard, DNS, RN, CS, ANP

Assistant Professor, Ball State University, School of Nursing, Muncie, Indiana
Curriculum Development: An Overview

Linda Finke, PhD, RN

Director, Professional Development Center, Sigma Theta Tau International,
Indianapolis, Indiana
Teaching in Nursing: The Faculty Role; Curriculum Designs

Betsy Frank, PhD, RN

Professor, Indiana State University School of Nursing, Terre Haute, Indiana
Teaching Students with Disabilities

Kay E. Hodson-Carlton, EdD, RN, FAAN

Professor and Coordinator, Education Resources and Extended Education,
Ball State University, Muncie, Indiana
The Learning Resource Center

Barbara A. Ihrke, PhD, RN

Associate Professor, Indiana Wesleyan University, Marion, Indiana
The Evaluation Process: An Overview

Pamela R. Jeffries, DNS, RN

Associate Professor, Indiana University School of Nursing, Indianapolis,
Indiana
Selecting Learning Experiences to Achieve Curriculum Outcomes

Elizabeth G. Johnson, DSN, RN

Associate Professor of Nursing, School of Nursing and Health Professions,
University of Southern Indiana, Evansville, Indiana
The Academic Performance of Students: Legal and Ethical Issues

Jane M. Kirkpatrick, MSN, RN

Associate Professor, Purdue University School of Nursing, West Lafayette,
Indiana
Strategies for Evaluating Learning Outcomes

Gail Kost, MSN, RN

Clinical Lecturer, Indiana University, Indianapolis, Indiana
Teaching in the Clinical Setting

Carla Mueller, PhD, RN

Associate Professor, Director of Educational Innovation, University of Saint
Francis, Fort Wayne, Indiana
Service Learning: Developing Values and Social Responsibility

Roy W. Ramsey, EdD, MEd, BA

Manager of Educational Technology, Intercollegiate College of Nursing,
Washington State University College of Nursing, Spokane, Washington
Teaching and Learning at a Distance

Virginia Richardson, DNS, RN, CPNP

Assistant Dean for Student Affairs and Associate Professor, Indiana University
School of Nursing, Indianapolis, Indiana
The Diverse Learning Needs of Students

Connie J. Rowles, DSN, RN, CNAA

Clinical Associate Professor, Indiana University School of Nursing, Indianapolis, Indiana

Strategies to Promote Critical Thinking and Active Learning; Improving Teaching and Learning: Classroom Assessment Techniques

Marcia K. Sauter, DNS, RN

Vice President for Academic Affairs, University of Saint Francis, Fort Wayne, Indiana

Educational Program Evaluation

Linda Siktberg, PhD, RN

Director, Ball State University, School of Nursing, Muncie, Indiana

Curriculum Development: An Overview

Lillian Stokes, PhD, RN

Associate Professor and Director, Diversity and Enhancement, Indiana University School of Nursing, Indianapolis Indiana

Teaching in the Clinical Setting

Prudence Twigg, PhD(c), APRN-BC

Part-time Lecturer, Indiana University, Indianapolis, Indiana

Developing and Using Classroom Tests

Melissa Vandeveer, PhD, RN, PNP

Associate Professor, Sonoma State University, Rohnert Park, California

From Teaching to Learning: Theoretical Foundations

Joanne Rains Warner, DNS, RN

Associate Dean for Graduate Programs, Indiana University School of Nursing, Indianapolis, Indiana

Forces and Issues Influencing Curriculum Development

Pamela J. Worrell-Carlisle, PhD, RN

Assistant Professor, Ball State University, Muncie Indiana

The Learning Resource Center

Lillian Yeager, EdD, RN

Dean and Associate Professor of Nursing, Indiana University Southeast, New Albany, Indiana

Strategies for Evaluating Learning Outcomes

Enid Errante Zwirn, PhD, MPH, RN

Associate Professor, Indiana University School of Nursing, Indianapolis, Indiana

Using Media, Multimedia, and Technology-Rich Learning Environments

REVIEWERS

Wanda Bonnel, PhD, RN, ANCC

Clinical Associate Professor
School of Nursing
University of Kansas
Kansas City, Kansas

Norma G. Cuellar, DSN, RN, CCRN

Assistant Professor
College of Nursing
University of Southern Mississippi
Hattiesburg, Mississippi

Carol Heinrich, PhD, MA

Associate Professor
Department of Nursing
East Stroudsburg University
East Stroudsburg, Pennsylvania

Nancy Kramer, EdD, CPNP, MSN, ARNP

Professor
BSN Program Chair
Allen College
Waterloo, Iowa

Josie Lu O'Quinn, PhD, RN

Assistant Dean and Assistant Professor
School of Nursing
University of Texas at Arlington
Arlington, Texas

Kathleen Deska Pagana, PhD

Professor of Nursing
Department of Nursing
Lycoming College
Williamsport, Pennsylvania

Debra P. Shelton, MSN, RN, CAN, OCN
Assistant Professor
College of Nursing
Northwestern State University
Shreveport, Louisiana

Karen Gahan Tarnow, PhD, RN
Clinical Assistant Professor
Director, Learning Laboratory
School of Nursing
University of Kansas
Kansas City, Kansas

Ann B. Tritak, EdD, RN
Associate Professor
Fairleigh Dickinson University
Teaneck, New Jersey

Jean T. Walker, PhD, RN
Assistant Professor
School of Nursing
University of Mississippi Medical Center
Jackson, Mississippi

PREFACE

When we wrote the first edition of this book in 1998, we stated that the nursing profession was facing some of the greatest challenges in its history. In the few short years since that time, the challenges that face the nursing profession and nurse educators have become increasingly complex. The increasing diversity of students, the restructuring of institutions of higher education, the diminishing fiscal resources, the redesigning of health care delivery systems, and the continuing explosion of the use of information technologies in education and practice are just a few of the issues that nursing faculty must consider when designing curricula. The shortage of nurses and nurse educators is an additional challenge that must be addressed by the nursing profession. Nursing faculty, charged with the responsibility of preparing practitioners who represent the future of our profession, are stepping forward to meet these challenges, and others that await them on college campuses and in varied practice settings.

These are issues that require nursing faculty to reexamine, within the context of relevance and readiness for the demands of the twenty-first century, the mission of their schools, the purpose and design of the curricula of their programs, and the very nature of their role as educators. Faculty, whether they be novices or experts, must be prepared to embrace new ways of teaching in classroom and clinical settings. For example:

- Faculty must be prepared to teach in an environment that offers new roles and rewards. Although maintaining clinical competence and serving as professional role models continue to be at the core of the faculty role, faculty also need to develop skills as "learning mentors" and instructional designers, and learn to integrate the use of technology effectively into the learning environment. The focus of the educational process has shifted from primarily faculty-driven models, where students await the direction of the faculty, to student-driven models, where the faculty guides the individual development of students as needed. Curricula must be dynamic, with learning experiences designed as modules that can be customized and individualized. Designing flexible, contemporary curricula that meet the learning needs of students and impart the values of the nursing profession is essential, as is faculty collaboration with students to develop relevant learning experiences.
- Teaching continues to be, more than ever, a public endeavor that must meet the public's demands for accountability of outcomes. Teaching is a scholarly endeavor with the accompanying requirements that teaching

efforts be evidence based, peer reviewed, and evaluated to ensure quality and accountability and to maintain the public trust.

- Faculty must be prepared to teach with a focus on learning outcomes and accountability for student learning and program effectiveness. Faculty must be able to use an array of models and tools for assessing, evaluating, and certifying learning. Teaching becomes a process of continuous improvement as the faculty assess classroom and learning outcomes to ensure quality. Faculty rewards will accrue based on the success of the students.

- Faculty members must be prepared to teach students with diverse backgrounds and diverse learning needs. The nursing profession is emphasizing the need to prepare a diverse workforce, one that reflects the society within which we live. Schools of nursing and their universities are actively recruiting students representative of the community in which they will work. These students draw on a rich cultural heritage and a diversity of life experiences; have multiple work and family responsibilities; and require learning experiences that are relevant, accessible, and convenient. To effectively teach these students, faculty must be prepared to design curricula and delivery systems that acknowledge and meet the needs of this diverse population.

- The faculty must be prepared to design learning architectures that are student focused, interdisciplinary, and community based. Increasingly, the curriculum will be developed and implemented as a partnership with other health care facilities, health professionals, or commercial education providers. Clinical experts who work in collaboration with faculty will more frequently be used to teach students in practice settings. The faculty must be able to establish curriculum structures and processes that can accommodate rapid changes and responses to meet health care delivery needs, and faculty must develop effective collaborative partnerships with care providers that facilitate student learning in practice settings.

- Faculty must be prepared to teach in learning communities where the emphasis is on learning, not teaching. The main faculty teaching roles are to assist students in the development of individualized learning plans and to establish environments where students construct their own knowledge. Teaching and learning are increasingly occurring in networked and distributed environments, and at a distance—often asynchronously. Therefore faculty members must be prepared to effectively use information technologies and learning resources that create and support these learning communities.

This guide to teaching in nursing has been written for nurse educators preparing to teach in these learning communities. This book is for nurses who recently have become faculty members and who are searching for answers to the daily challenges presented in their role as educators, and for experienced faculty members who are transforming teaching practices for the future. This book is also written for nurses who are combining clinical practice and teaching as preceptors or part-time or adjunct faculty, and for graduate students or teaching assistants who ultimately aspire to assume a faculty teaching role.

Because many of the nursing profession's expert educators contemplate retirement within the next decade, it is crucial that faculty begin preparing and mentoring future nursing faculty now. It is our hope that this book can help influence that preparation by providing guidance on the competencies essential to the effective implementation of the educator role.

We continue to consider this book to be a guide, bringing under one cover an overview of methods and strategies for working with students; developing curricula; designing learning experiences; using learning resources; and evaluating students, faculty, courses, and programs. Although the book is organized in five sections, teaching in nursing is an integrative process, and we encourage readers to select chapters as appropriate for their needs and teaching practice.

Since we wrote the first edition of this book, there has been a renewed interest in developing a science of nursing education. This edition integrates current evidence-based practices and also draws on the classics in nursing, education, and other fields. We have attempted to provide a balance of the practical and the theoretical. Because any one of the topics could be, and often is, a book within itself, we encourage readers to seek out other references to supplement the information contained within this book and to read the emerging literature for new evidence for the best practices in teaching and learning.

We suggest that readers use the book as a guide and resource but recognize that implementation must be adapted to the values and mission of the institutional settings and the personal style and philosophy of the faculty. We intend for this book to stimulate faculty to engage in the scholarship of teaching by reflecting on their own teaching practices, implementing and evaluating new approaches to creating an interactive learning community, and conducting their own educational research in classroom and clinical settings.

This is an exciting time to teach nursing—a time that is filled with many challenges, opportunities, and rewards for those who step forward to accept the responsibility. It is our hope that this book provides those who engage in the rewarding activity of teaching the future of our profession—our students— with a resource that will lead to a greater fulfillment of the teaching role.

Diane M. Billings
Judith A. Halstead

ACKNOWLEDGMENTS

Many individuals were involved in the publication of the second edition of this book. First, we thank the contributors, who shared their expertise and wisdom, as well as their enthusiasm about nursing education. They are truly master teachers who serve as role models for others. We also acknowledge the work of the contributors to the first edition of *Teaching in Nursing: A Guide for Faculty*: Juanita Laidig, EdD, RN, from the Indiana University School of Nursing, Indianapolis, Indiana; Carole Brigham, EdD, RN, from the Ball State University School of Nursing, Muncie, Indiana; Pamela J. Cole, MA, RN, CS, from Bullis Family Medicine, Muncie, Indiana; Lori Rasmussen, MSN, RN, from Marian College, Indianapolis, Indiana; Diana J. Speck, MSN, RN, from the J. Everett Light Career Center, Indianapolis, Indiana; Dorothy A. Gomez, MSN, RN, from Marian College, Indianapolis, Indiana; Stacy Lobodzinski, MSN, RN, from Methodist Hospital, Indianapolis, Indiana; Cora D. Hartwell West, MSN, RN, from Indiana University School of Nursing, and Staff Builders Home Health Care, Indianapolis, Indiana; Margaret H. Applegate, EdD, RN, FAAN, from the Indiana University School of Nursing, Indianapolis, Indiana.

We also thank those who served as reviewers of the book for their insightful comments and the many nurse educators who have used the book over the past few years and provided us with feedback on our efforts. We greatly appreciate your willingness to share your thoughts and suggestions with us.

Many thanks, as well, to the design and production staff who helped bring this book into existence: Debbie Vogel, Bill Drone, Kelley Barbarick, Ruth Kaufman, Warren Perkins, and Claire Kramer. We also wish to thank Jennifer Anderson at Elsevier who facilitated the development of the manuscript.

And always, we thank our families and colleagues for their continued support and encouragement throughout this project. We also offer a special thanks to our students, who continue to be our own guides to teaching in nursing.

Diane M. Billings
Judith A. Halstead

CONTENTS

TEACHING
IN NURSING

FACULTY AND STUDENTS

Teaching in Nursing

THE FACULTY ROLE

Linda M. Finke, PhD, RN

As the demands of society have changed, the faculty role in higher education has grown from the singular colonial unitarian mission of teaching to a multifaceted challenge of teaching, scholarship, and service. Over time, as nursing education has moved from the service sector to college and university campuses, the role of nursing faculty has evolved and become increasingly complex. As higher education and the science of nursing have developed, the impact on nursing education has been tremendous.

Today higher education and nursing education are poised on the brink of sweeping changes. The forces driving these changes are numerous and difficult to isolate: the increasing multiculturalism of society; finite financial resources in education and health care; expanding technology and the accompanying knowledge explosion; the need for lifelong learning; a shifting emphasis to learning, instead of teaching; and the increasing public demand for accountability of educational outcomes are just a few of the issues educators must consider as they fulfill the responsibilities of their role.

As faculty in higher education face these many challenges, they are finding that their role is undergoing exciting changes as well. Dolence and Norris (1996) stated, "Fresh vision is needed to create new delivery systems for learning, new paradigms for financing, and new models for higher education" (p. 7). The purpose of this chapter is to provide a brief historical perspective of the faculty role; identify faculty rights and responsibilities; and describe the process of faculty appointment, promotion, and tenure. In addition, faculty development of the competencies related to teaching as a scholarly endeavor is discussed and implications of change in the faculty role are addressed.

HISTORICAL PERSPECTIVE OF FACULTY ROLE IN HIGHER EDUCATION

The role of the faculty member in academe has developed through time as the role of higher education in America has changed. If one reviews the history of American higher education, three phases of overlapping development can be identified (Boyer, 1990).

The first phase of development occurred during colonial times. Heavily influenced by British tradition, the role of faculty in the colonial college was a singular one: that of teaching. The educational system "was expected to educate and morally uplift the coming generation" (Boyer, 1990, p. 4). Teaching was considered an honored vocation with the intended purpose of developing student character and preparing students for leadership in civic and religious roles. This focus on teaching as the central mission of the university continued well into the nineteenth century.

Gradually, however, the focus of education began to shift from the development of the individual to the development of a nation, signaling the beginning of the second phase of development within higher education. Legislation such as the Morrill Act of 1862 and the Hatch Act of 1887 helped to create public expectations that added the additional responsibility of service to the traditional faculty role of teaching. This legislation provided each state with land and funding to support the education of leaders for agriculture and industry. Universities and colleges took on the mission to educate for the common good (Boyer, 1990). Educational systems were expected to provide service to the states, businesses, and industries. It was in the 1870s that the first formal schools of nursing began to appear in the United States. Nursing programs were established in hospitals to help meet the service needs of the hospitals. Nursing faculty were expected to provide service to the institution and to teach new nurses along the way. Nursing students were expected to learn while they helped to staff the hospitals.

In the mid-nineteenth century, a commitment to the development of science began in many universities on the East Coast (Boyer, 1990), thus beginning the third phase of development in higher education. Scholarship through research was added as an expectation to the role of faculty. This emphasis on research was greatly enhanced in later years by federal support for academic research that began during World War II and continued after the war. Gradually, as expectations for faculty to conduct research spread throughout institutions across the nation, teaching and service began to be viewed with less importance as a measurement tool for academic prestige and productivity within institutions. Faculty found it increasingly difficult to achieve tenure without a record of research and publication, despite accomplishments in teaching and service. As nursing education entered the university setting, nursing faculty began to be held to the same standards of research productivity as faculty in other more traditionally academia-based disciplines. Because of the prominence of practice in nursing, the integration of scholarship into the role of nursing faculty initially came slowly. The emphasis on research in higher education as evidence of faculty productivity has continued to this day.

Currently a rapidly changing political environment and health care reform are having a dramatic effect on the role of nursing faculty. Universities are facing a "new and sometimes hostile world" (Association of Governing Boards of Universities and Colleges, 1996, p. 2). Diminishing resources and increasing public scrutiny and expectations place a heavy burden on faculty in higher education. Changes in health care demand that nursing faculty critically evaluate the design of curricula and the competencies of graduates. There is an increasing emphasis on the teaching role of faculty, with an accompanying expectation that outcomes of the educational process will be regularly assessed at the institutional and program levels. The balance among teaching, research, and service is being reexamined in many institutions for its congruence with the institution's mission.

Further changes in higher education include a revolution in teaching strategies. Sole reliance on the use of lecture is no longer an accepted teaching method. Instead, faculty are integrating the use of technology into their teaching and promoting the active involvement of students in the learning process. Computer-mediated courses are the future of higher education as movement is made away from the structured classroom to the much larger learning environments of home, community, and the clinical setting. Distance education strategies will play an increasingly important role in the education of learners.

Furthermore, nursing care delivery is changing to a community-based, consumer-driven system. The shift from acute care to the important role of primary care has had an impact on the curricula of undergraduate and graduate nursing education. There also remains the need for increased numbers of doctorally prepared nurses, not only to teach but also to collect and to analyze data necessary to evaluate the effectiveness of health care and to identify trends of future development. All of these issues provide new and exciting challenges for nursing faculty as they assume the responsibility for educating health care providers for the twenty-first century.

FACULTY RIGHTS AND RESPONSIBILITIES IN ACADEMIA

In the academic environment faculty have traditionally enjoyed a number of rights, including the right to self-governance within the university setting. Governance may include participation on department and university committees and "using . . . professional expertise to solve community problems" (Gaff & Lambert, 1996, p. 40). Self-governance includes developing policies for faculty behavior, student affairs, and curriculum; performing administrative activities; and providing advice to administrators or student groups. Serving on committees or task forces at the department, school, or university level is also an expectation of faculty (Tucker, 1992). Faculty, in cooperation with administrators, share in addressing the issues that face the university and the community that it serves.

As constituents place more and more expectations on faculty for productivity, faculty governance is not as highly valued by those outside of academia (Plater, 1995). However, the new environment for higher education demands new forms of governance, including representative forms. Methods must be instituted to maintain the participation of faculty in governance while allowing for less of a time commitment. The change that must permeate all other aspects of the role of twenty-first-century faculty must also permeate governance.

The core responsibility of faculty is the teaching and learning that takes place in the institution. Boards and administrators delegate decisions about most aspects of the teaching–learning process to faculty. This responsibility includes not only the delivery of content but also curriculum development and evaluation, development of student evaluation methods, and graduation requirements (Association of Governing Boards of Universities and Colleges, 1996).

Intellectual property, copyright, and fair use laws govern faculty and student use of works developed by faculty, students, and others. The easy online access of course content has added to this complicated issue. Most academic settings have policies that guide the development of "works for hire," which may include course content, written works, and products. Many institutions of higher learning now lay claim to works developed by faculty because the faculty member was hired to develop the content. A wise faculty member is well informed about these institutional policies so that there is no misunderstanding about ownership of course materials and other works developed by the faculty member.

Evaluation is a major responsibility of faculty. Faculty engage in the evaluation of students and of colleagues. Peer evaluation is a vital aspect of faculty development and is part of the documentation data considered in the decision-making process for promotion and tenure. Faculty are involved in the development of fair and equitable evaluation criteria on which to base these judgments.

Another responsibility of faculty is mentoring. Nursing faculty mentor not only nursing students but also other faculty members in their development as teachers and scholars. The mentoring of students may include not only formal academic advisement but also the coaching, supporting, and guiding of protégés through the academic system and into their professional career. The mentoring of faculty members also involves coaching, supporting, and guiding as they develop in their role as faculty. When starting at a new institution, even an experienced faculty member has some culture shock and requires mentoring (Lieb, 1995). Lieb's definition of mentoring is helping another to reach his or her potential.

The mentoring of new faculty members is an especially important responsibility because nurses are not usually prepared in graduate nursing programs for a role in academia. Faculty are dropped into an environment with unspoken rules and expectations that can be markedly different from those of their previous practice environment. Faculty know the role of student from experience but see the faculty role from a distance. Mentoring is needed to assist new faculty members as they learn to balance all aspects of their complex role.

The responsibilities of nursing faculty include teaching and scholarship, as well as service to the school, university, community, and the profession of nursing. Nursing faculty have the responsibility to expand their service beyond the university and local community to active participation in professional nursing organizations at local, regional, and national levels. Nursing faculty often provide the leadership for these organizations and set national public policy agendas. As a faculty member climbs the promotion and tenure ladder, service responsibilities increase and leadership at the national level is required.

True success as a faculty member is measured by the person's ability to juggle all aspects of the faculty role. Although some educational settings emphasize teaching, many require that faculty meet established criteria in all aspects of the role—teaching, research, and service. With careful planning and selection of activities, nursing faculty can integrate clinical interests into scholarship, service, and teaching, thus meeting the expectations of the role. On initial appointment to a faculty position, the faculty member will be well served by the development of a 5- to 6-year career plan designed to help ensure that he or she will meet the criteria for all aspects of the role.

Some faculty do work in a unionized environment. The American Association of University Professors (AAUP) is probably the best-known faculty union. Faculty can also be members of AAUP without belonging to a union. In a setting that has a union, faculty rights and responsibilities can be affected by the contracts negotiated.

Faculty Appointment, Promotion, and Tenure

Faculty are appointed by the governing body of the college or university and are responsible, in cooperation with the administration of the institution, for teaching, scholarship, and service (Association of Governing Boards of Universities and Colleges, 1996). Faculty are appointed to fulfill various responsibilities to meet the mission and goals of the college or university and the school of nursing and, according to their degrees and experience, are promoted and tenured on the basis of achievement of specified criteria (Sneed et al., 1995). Faculty may hold appointments in more than one unit of the institution, including other academic units or service units. Criteria for promotion and tenure are based on the institution's overall mission and thus vary among institutions.

Appointment

Faculty may be appointed to a variety of full-time and part-time positions. Faculty positions are described as tenured or tenure-probationary appointments or as nontenured, nonprobationary instructional appointments such as adjunct; distinguished; emeritus; and other part-time, temporary, or otherwise designated positions. Appointment in tenure tracks may lead to tenure and a permanent position at the school of nursing; other positions require reappointment at specific intervals (e.g., yearly or every 3 to 5 years). Reappointment and continued service in tenured positions is based on evaluation of teaching and other faculty activities, such as scholarship and service.

Ranks

Appointment ranks, or tracks, have been developed to specify the responsibilities of the faculty member in relation to teaching, scholarship, and service. The ranks may include tenure, clinical, or research scientist. Each rank has its own criteria for teaching, scholarship, and service and for promotion within the rank.

The *tenure* track is established for faculty whose primary responsibilities are teaching and research. There is expectation of a promise of excellence and the ability to be promoted to senior ranks. A doctoral degree is generally required for appointment to the tenure track at most schools of nursing. Faculty appointed to this rank are considered *tenure probationary* until they have obtained tenure.

The *clinical* track has been developed at some institutions for those faculty members whose primary responsibility is clinical supervision of students and/or clinical practice. The focus of this track is on health care delivery, and it is used to integrate faculty practice into the traditional university faculty structure (American Association of Colleges of Nursing, 1993; Sneed et al, 1995). This track may also be developed as an educator track, clinical educator track, or educator/practitioner track, depending on the primary focus of the responsibilities of the faculty appointed into this track. Appointment to this track is based on teaching and clinical skills. A doctoral degree may not be required for appointment to a clinical track.

The *research scientist* track is for faculty whose primary responsibilities are generating new knowledge and disseminating the findings. Although research scientists may have responsibilities for working with students; serving on dissertation committees; teaching in the area of their expertise; or providing service to the school, campus, or profession, their time is protected for research. Appointment is based on evidence of or promise of a program of research. A doctoral degree and at least beginning research experience are prerequisites for appointment to this track.

Within these ranks faculty are appointed at the levels of instructor (rarely used), assistant professor, associate professor, and professor. Each school of nursing defines the criteria for appointment and promotion to these levels. These criteria specify the responsibilities associated with teaching, scholarship and service, or other frameworks used to define the faculty role.

Schools of nursing may also develop temporary and other positions to which faculty can be appointed. *Visiting* positions may be held at any rank and designate someone who has a limited appointment (1 or 2 years), who is on leave from another institution, who is employed on a temporary basis, or who may be being considered for a permanent position within the school. The *lecturer* position is used for faculty who lack necessary credentials (usually degrees) for appointment to a tenure-track position. *Adjunct* faculty are courtesy appointments for individuals whose primary employment is outside the school of nursing but who have responsibility for teaching students or working with students on research projects.

Emeritus is a title that may be conferred on faculty who are retired. Faculty with emeritus status may be granted specific privileges, such as use of the library, use of computing services, and an office and secretarial support.

Students may also be employed in teaching positions. These appointments, such as *teaching assistant* and *associate instructor,* are temporary and usually part time. These students are responsible only for teaching or assisting faculty with teaching. They do not have the same level of responsibility as full-time faculty. Teaching assistants must be assigned to work with a faculty member who will assume responsibility for the quality of their work.

The Appointment Process

The appointment process in universities and schools of nursing is somewhat different from that for positions in nursing service, and nurses who are applying for teaching positions in schools of nursing should be cognizant of this. The interview is conducted by a search and screen committee appointed by the dean or other university administrator. Interested applicants submit an application and curriculum vitae that are screened by this committee. Potential candidates are invited for an interview with the search committee, faculty and administrators at the school of nursing, and others at the college or university as appropriate. Depending on the requirements of the position for which they are applying, applicants may be asked to make a presentation of their research or to demonstrate teaching skills. At the time of appointment to rank, the applicant's records are reviewed by the appointment, promotion, and tenure committee, or other appropriate committee, for recommendation to the dean about appointment.

Tenure and Promotion

Tenure

Tenure to the university is a reciprocal responsibility on the part of the university and faculty. The expectation is that the faculty member will remain competent and productive and maintain high standards of teaching, research, service, and professional conduct. Tenure also assumes that the faculty member is promotable, and typically promotion to the next level and tenure occur at the same time. Tenure, then, provides the faculty member protection of academic freedom. Academic freedom is the "freedom . . . to explore new ideas and theories unimpeded" (Whicker et al., 1993, p. 14). Academic freedom guarantees the protection of faculty against efforts by government, university administration, students, and even public opinion to influence their expression of opinions in class. On the other hand, academic freedom does not give faculty unbounded rights; for example, a faculty member does not have the right to alter the curriculum, sequence, or content of established courses, or to subject students to discussions that are irrelevant to the course. Tenure can be withdrawn for reasons of financial exigency on the part of the school or university and for behavior that is unprofessional. Finally, tenure does not mean not having to participate in performance review, and most institutions and their schools of nursing have instituted a posttenure review process (Suess, 1995).

Tenure is granted after a review by peers and administrators using published criteria of the evidence submitted by the faculty member (a curriculum vitae and dossier). This review is typically held in the faculty member's sixth year, with tenure granted in the seventh year. At appointment, faculty with a record of exceptional achievement may be granted a specific number of years toward tenure, thus shortening the time for the tenure review.

The tenure process is specific to each school of nursing, and faculty who are appointed to a tenure track should familiarize themselves with the criteria and process before appointment. Although the tenure and promotion process may seem mysterious, there are in fact clear and specified criteria. The current attitude is to employ faculty who show high promise for attaining tenure and being promoted and to provide support and mentoring that will facilitate their developing into successful and fully capable members of the academic community. Although at one time tenure was an unquestioned right of faculty, currently both prospective faculty and the academic community are questioning its true benefit, and some institutions of higher education have abandoned the notion altogether.

Promotion

Promotion refers to advancement in rank. As with the tenure review process, faculty must submit evidence of excellence in teaching, scholarship, and service, or other criteria established by the school and be judged by a committee of peers, school and university administrators, and governing bodies. Criteria and processes for promotion, like those for tenure, are established by faculty committees and are made public. In most schools of nursing, tenure-probationary faculty who are appointed as assistant professors are expected to be able to be promoted to the rank of associate professor at the time tenure is granted.

Faculty should familiarize themselves with promotion criteria and processes at the time of appointment and establish a relationship with the primary appointment, promotion, and tenure (APT) committee and the department chair, whose role it is to inform faculty about APT policies and procedures. As noted earlier, an expectation of senior faculty is to guide and mentor junior faculty through the tenure and promotion process. Some schools of nursing assign mentors at the time of appointment; if a mentor is not assigned, the newly appointed faculty member should seek one.

Teaching as a Scholarly Endeavor

Redefining the Faculty Role

As faculty face a redefining of their role for the twenty-first century, new definitions of the role are being proposed. For example, Dolence and Norris (1996) described numerous ways that the faculty role will change to meet the needs of the learners in the Information Age. They described the faculty role as one encompassing the synthesis of knowledge and a broader range of scholarship, with faculty assuming the role of "learning mentors" who guide learners through individualized programs of study and evaluate the mastery of learners. In such a role, faculty will need to develop expertise in flexible, fluid curricula design and outcome assessment. In the same vein, Barr and Tagg (1995) described a shift from a "teaching paradigm" to a "learning paradigm" to "create environments and experiences that allow students to discover and construct knowledge for themselves" (p. 15). Teaching, although always an important aspect of the faculty role, has assumed an even greater significance in recent years.

More than 10 years ago Boyer (1990) first proposed a new paradigm for scholarship that encompassed all aspects of the faculty role but placed a renewed emphasis on teaching as a scholarly endeavor. In *Scholarship Reconsidered: Priorities of the Professorate*, Boyer called for the development of a balance between research and teaching when measuring the faculty member's success in academe. He described four types of scholarship in which faculty engage: the scholarship of *discovery*, the scholarship of *integration*, the scholarship of *application*, and the scholarship of *teaching*. In these four types of scholarship the previously narrow view of scholarly productivity that rested only on the careful discovery of new knowledge through research has been greatly expanded. As Boyer stated:

> We believe the time has come to move beyond the tired old "teaching versus research" debate and give the familiar and honorable term "scholarship" a broader, more capacious meaning, one that brings legitimacy to the full scope of academic work. Surely, scholarship means engaging in original research. But the work of the scholar also means stepping back from one's investigation, looking for connections, building bridges between theory and practice, and communicating one's knowledge effectively to students. Specifically, we conclude that the work of the professorate might be thought of as having four separate, yet overlapping, functions. These are: the scholarship of discovery; the scholarship of integration; the scholarship of application; and the scholarship of teaching. (p. 16)

The Scholarship of Discovery. The scholarship of discovery is the traditional definition of original research or discovery of new knowledge (Boyer, 1990). The scholarship of discovery may be considered the foundation of the other three aspects of scholarship because new knowledge is generated for application and integration into the discipline, as well as for teaching (Brown et al., 1995).

It is through the scholarship of discovery that scientific methods are used to develop a strong knowledge base for the discipline. Most federal funding traditionally has been appropriated for the scholarship of discovery, and until recently tenure decisions in many universities have been based primarily on the faculty member's engagement in the generation of new knowledge. The scholarship of discovery remains a very important aspect of the role of many faculties, including nursing faculties. In nursing, the preparation of nurse researchers is the focus of almost all doctoral education. At the federal level research efforts in nursing are supported by the National Institute for Nursing Research.

The Scholarship of Integration. The scholarship of integration involves the interpretation and synthesis of knowledge across discipline boundaries in a manner that provides a larger context for the knowledge and the development of new insights (Boyer, 1990). The scholarship of integration requires communication among colleagues from various disciplines who work together to develop a more holistic view of a common concern. The combined expertise of all who are involved leads to a more comprehensive understanding of the issue and results in more thorough recommendations for solutions to the phenomena of concern.

Nursing faculty have long integrated knowledge from various disciplines into their practice (Brown et al., 1995) and have many competencies that enable them to be productive members of multidisciplinary teams studying a variety of health problems and issues. With the emphasis in today's world on the development of collaborative, team-building, and knowledge-sharing efforts across disciplines, the scholarship of integration assumes an ever increasing importance for faculty, who must remain at the forefront of the Information Age. This is especially true for health care professionals and faculty in this era of rapidly changing health care delivery systems and accompanying complex health care issues that require innovative solutions.

The Scholarship of Application. The scholarship of application, which connects theory and practice, is an area of scholarship in which nursing faculty should also excel. In the scholarship of application, faculty must ask themselves, "How can knowledge be responsibly applied to consequential problems?" (Boyer, 1990, p. 21). Service activities that are directly connected to a faculty member's areas of expertise warrant consideration as application scholarship. It is in the performance of service activities that practice and theory interact, thus leading to the potential development of new knowledge.

For example, in nursing, clinical practice and expertise that result in the development of examples of nursing interventions and positive patient care outcomes meet the definition of scholarship of application. Faculty practice in nursing centers is another example. Faculty should disseminate the knowledge gathered through practice and service activities by publishing in professional journals.

The scholarship of application, which includes service to the profession of nursing at the local, regional, national, and international levels, also involves developing policies and practices for nursing and health care. Nursing faculty often provide leadership in professional organizations and community or national panels and boards.

The Scholarship of Teaching. The heart of the faculty role can be found in the scholarship of teaching. An important attribute of any scholar is having the ability to effectively communicate the knowledge he or she possesses to students. Boyer's (1990) definition of scholarship provides a model through which the special competencies and skills that are an integral part of the scholarly endeavor of teaching are acknowledged. Developing innovative curricula, using a variety of teaching methods that actively involve students in the learning process, collaborating with students on learning projects, and exploring the most effective means of meeting the learning needs of diverse populations of students are all examples of the scholarship of teaching.

The scholarship of teaching requires *evidence* of effective teaching and dissemination of the knowledge that is acquired as a result of teaching. Faculty should share their teaching expertise with their colleagues through publication and presentation of their innovative teaching methods and the outcomes of their working with students.

The scholarship of teaching brings many exciting opportunities for nursing faculty in classroom and clinical settings. It is based on the scholarship of discovery, integration, and practice (Shoffner et al., 1994). At a time of rapidly changing health care practice arenas, newly emerging curriculum models designed to meet the needs of a global society, increasing use of technology in education, and changing perspectives on teaching and learning, the scholarship of teaching provides nursing faculty with the opportunity to demonstrate their innovation and creativity. It also provides a means for recognizing the effort spent preparing students to be competent health care providers for the future.

Summary

Although the role of the faculty member remains complex, Boyer's (1990) broad description of scholarship provides a model that legitimizes all aspects of the faculty role. Boyer has given credibility to aspects of the faculty role that extend beyond the creation of new knowledge through research to include teaching and service to the university, community, and profession. Teaching, as a scholarly endeavor, is the synthesis of all types of scholarship described by Boyer. Faculty can combine the role of researcher with the integration, application, and dissemination of knowledge. The ability to teach is an important criterion for the evaluation of faculty at most universities (Gaff & Lambert, 1996). Boyer has provided a model for nursing faculty to use to develop their expertise in teaching as a scholarly endeavor (Shoffner et al., 1994). Nursing education has moved from the notion that there is only one way to do something to a broader perspective that recognizes the creativity and uniqueness of each student. The teacher is no longer the only expert but instead is someone who joins with the student in the learning process.

Faculty Development for the Teaching Role

Teaching in nursing is a complex activity that integrates the art and science of nursing and clinical practice into the teaching–learning process. Specifically, teaching involves a set of skills, or competencies, that are essential to facilitating student learning outcomes. These competencies can be developed through educational preparation, faculty orientation programs, and faculty development opportunities.

Teaching Competencies

Teaching competencies are the knowledge, skills, and values that are critical to the fulfillment of the teaching component of the faculty role. Several authors have identified general competencies for teaching in nursing (Billings, 1995; Choudhry, 1992; Davis et al., 1992), and Kirschling et al. (1995) have identified domains of teaching effectiveness that can be used as standards for evaluating teaching competence. Promotion and tenure criteria articulate specific expectations of teaching competence and excellence at each school of nursing. Teaching and related role competencies include the following.

Competencies Related to Curriculum Development; Teaching; Using Teaching, Learning, and Information Resources; and Evaluating Student Outcomes. These competencies include being knowledgeable about the content area; setting learning objectives; designing learning activities; being well organized in the selection and presentation of learning experiences; selecting and using appropriate learning strategies; understanding and using theories of teaching and learning; teaching in the clinical setting; communicating expectations clearly; providing helpful and timely feedback; assisting students to develop critical thinking skills; using information technologies such as databases, spreadsheets, statistical software, electronic communications (e-mail), presentation systems, test-authoring programs, and videoconferencing applications; developing appropriate evaluation measures; and evaluating fairly (Billings, 1995; Choudhry, 1992; Davis et al., 1992; Kirschling et al., 1995).

Competencies Related to Professional Practice. Competencies related to professional practice include being knowledgeable about the content area and clinical practice, having the ability to influence change in nursing and health care by selecting appropriate strategies, and facilitating relationships with clinical agencies to benefit students (Choudhry, 1992; Kirschling et al., 1995).

Competencies Related to Relationships with Students and Colleagues. Competencies in this area include being an advocate for students; advising and counseling students; accepting student diversity; showing consideration for students; having a sense of humor; conveying a sense of caring to students; serving as a mentor and role model; facilitating student development; and developing collaborative, collegial relationships with students characterized by mutual respect (Choudhry, 1992; Halstead, 1996; Kirschling et al., 1995). Competence as a colleague means serving as a mentor to junior faculty, assisting colleagues with professional duties, conducting one's professional life without prejudice toward others, and respecting the views of others (Balsmeyer et al., 1996).

Competencies Related to Service and Faculty Governance. Competencies related to service and faculty governance include understanding institutional structure, policies, and procedures; understanding and assuming the rights and responsibilities of a faculty member; serving on committees and performing work necessary to the operation of the department; and serving on committees or providing leadership to the school, college or university, and profession (Balsmeyer et al., 1996; Choudhry, 1992; and Davis et al., 1992).

Competencies Related to Scholarship. Scholarship, a larger component of the faculty role, may or may not be a requirement of the teaching role depending on the position description. Competencies related to the scholarship of teaching include conducting research about teaching (and the area of content expertise), publishing about teaching and learning issues, presenting at national meetings, and consulting about teaching and learning issues (Choudhry, 1992; Davis et al., 1992).

More recently, the National League for Nursing (2004) has developed competencies for nurse educators. The competencies focus on eight areas: facilitating learning, facilitating learner development and socialization, using assessment and evaluation strategies, participating in curriculum design and evaluation of program outcomes, functioning as change agents and leaders, developing the educator role, engaging in scholarship, and functioning within the educational environment. A draft statement of the competencies can be found in Box 1-1. These competencies will be used to guide the development of graduate nursing programs that focus on the preparation of nurse educators, enhance recruitment and retention of nurse educators, influence public policy efforts affecting nurse educators and nursing education, and identify scholarship and research priorities related to the nurse educator role. A monograph reporting the final version of the competencies is scheduled to be published in fall 2004. Further information can be found on the NLN website at *http://www.nln.org*.

Preparation to Teach

Developing competent faculty requires an investment on the part of both the individual faculty member and the school of nursing. Preparation for teaching

Box 1-1
NATIONAL LEAGUE FOR NURSING NURSE EDUCATOR COMPETENCIES: FINAL DRAFT,
MARCH 2004

Competency 1: Facilitate Learning

To facilitate learning effectively the nurse educator:

- Implements a variety of teaching strategies appropriate to content, setting, learner's needs, and desired learner outcomes
- Grounds teaching strategies in a theoretical foundation and evidence-based practices
- Recognizes multicultural, gender, and experiential influences on teaching and learning
- Engages in self-reflection and continued learning to improve teaching practices and facilitate learning
- Uses information technologies skillfully to support the teaching-learning process
- Practices skilled oral, written, and electronic communication that reflects an awareness of self and relationships with others, along with an ability to convey ideas in a variety of contexts (for example: evaluation, collaboration, mentorship, and supervision)
- Models critical and reflective thinking practices and creates opportunities for learners that promote development of critical thinking
- Shows enthusiasm for teaching, learning, and the nursing profession that inspires and motivates students
- Demonstrates interest in and respect for learners and uses personal attributes that facilitate learning, including: caring, confidence, patience, integrity, and flexibility
- Develops collegial working relationships, including those with clinical agency personnel, to promote positive learning environments
- Maintains the professional practice knowledge base needed to instruct learners in contemporary nursing practice
- Serves as a role model of professional nursing in the practice setting

Competency 2: Facilitate Learner Development and Socialization

To facilitate learner development and socialization effectively the nurse educator:

- Identifies individual learning styles and unique learning needs of diverse learners, including but not limited to: international, adult, multicultural, educationally disadvantaged, physically challenged, at-risk, and second-degree learners
- Provides resources to meet the unique needs of diverse learners
- Advises and counsels learners to meet professional goals
- Creates learning environments that facilitate learners' self-reflection, personal goal setting, and experience in the role of the nurse
- Fosters the cognitive, psychomotor, and affective development of learners
- Recognizes the influence of teaching styles and interpersonal interactions on learner behaviors
- Assists learners to develop the ability to engage in thoughtful and constructive self and peer evaluation
- Models professional behaviors for learners including, but not limited to: involvement in professional organizations, engagement in lifelong learning activities, dissemination of information through publications and presentations, and political advocacy for health care policy changes

Competency 3: Use Assessment and Evaluation Strategies

To use assessment and evaluation strategies effectively the nurse educator:

- Demonstrates knowledge of current research related to assessment and evaluation practices
- Uses a variety of strategies to assess and evaluate learning in the cognitive, psychomotor, and affective domains
- Implements evidence-based assessment and evaluation strategies that are appropriate to the learner and learning situation
- Uses evidence-based criteria to analyze assessment and evaluation data

Continued

Box 1-1
NATIONAL LEAGUE FOR NURSING NURSE EDUCATOR COMPETENCIES: FINAL DRAFT, MARCH 2004—cont'd

- Uses assessment and evaluation data to enhance the teaching-learning process
- Provides timely, constructive, and thoughtful feedback to learners
- Demonstrates skill in the design and use of tools for assessing clinical behaviors and judgment

Competency 4: Participate in Curriculum Design and Evaluation of Program Outcomes

To participate effectively in curriculum design and evaluation of program outcomes the nurse educator:

- Ensures the curriculum reflects institutional philosophy and mission, current nursing and health care trends, and community and societal needs, so as to prepare graduates for practice in a complex, dynamic, multicultural health care environment
- Demonstrates knowledge of curriculum development including identifying program outcomes, developing competency statements, writing course objectives, and selecting appropriate learning activities and evaluation strategies
- Bases curriculum design and implementation decisions on sound educational principles, theory, and research
- Revises the curriculum based on assessment of program outcomes, learner needs, and societal trends
- Implements curricular revisions using appropriate change theories and strategies
- Collaborates with external constituencies, seeking input as appropriate, when engaged in curriculum change
- Designs and implements program assessment models that promote continuous quality improvement of all aspects of the program

Competency 5: Function as Change Agents and Leaders

To function effectively as a change agent and leader, the nurse educator:

- Models cultural sensitivity in activities relating to the diversity and complexity of factors that influence teaching and learning
- Integrates a long-term, innovative, and creative perspective into the nurse educator role
- Participates in interdisciplinary efforts to address health care and educational needs regionally, nationally, or internationally
- Evaluates organizational effectiveness in nursing education and implements strategies for organizational change
- Provides leadership in the parent institution as well as in the nursing program to enhance the visibility of nursing and its role in the academic community
- Promotes innovative practices in educational environments
- Develops leadership skills to shape and implement change

Competency 6: Develop Educator Role

To develop the educator role effectively, the nurse educator:

- Demonstrates commitment to lifelong learning
- Recognizes that career development needs change as experience is gained in the role
- Participates in professional development opportunities to increase effectiveness in the role
- Balances the teaching, scholarship, and service demands inherent in the role of the educator and institutional setting
- Uses feedback gained from self, peer, student, and administrative evaluation to improve role effectiveness
- Engages in activities that promote socialization to the role
- Uses knowledge of the legal and ethical issues relevant to higher education and nursing education in influencing, designing, and implementing policies and procedures
- Mentors and supports faculty colleagues

Box 1-1
**NATIONAL LEAGUE FOR NURSING NURSE EDUCATOR COMPETENCIES: FINAL DRAFT,
MARCH 2004—cont'd**

Competency 7: Engage in Scholarship

To engage effectively in scholarship, the nurse educator:

- Draws on evidence-based literature to improve and support teaching
- Exhibits a spirit of inquiry about teaching and learning
- Designs and implements scholarly activities in an established area of expertise
- Disseminates nursing and teaching expertise to a variety of audiences through various means
- Demonstrates skill in proposal writing for initiatives that include, but are not limited, to research, resource acquisition, program development, and policy development
- Demonstrates qualities of a scholar: integrity, courage, perseverance, vitality, and creativity

Competency 8: Function within the Educational Environment

To function effectively within the educational environment, the nurse educator:

- Uses knowledge of history and current trends and issues in higher education as rationale for actions
- Identifies how social, economic, political, and institutional forces influence nursing education
- Develops networks, collaborations, and partnerships to enhance the nursing profession's influence within the academic community
- Determines own professional goals within the context of academic nursing and the mission of the parent institution and nursing program
- Integrates the values of respect, collegiality, professionalism, and caring to build an organizational climate that fosters the development of students and teachers
- Incorporates the goals of the nursing program and the mission of the parent institution when proposing change or managing issues
- Assumes a leadership role in various levels of institutional governance
- Advocates for nursing and nursing education in the political arena

Included with the permission of the National League for Nursing, New York, NY.

---

requires participation in classroom and clinical experiences to acquire the competencies previously identified. These experiences may take place in teacher education courses or in focus areas in masters and doctoral degree programs in nursing schools or schools of education. Participating in orientation programs, teaching institutes, or continuing education offerings and working as a teaching assistant are other ways of preparing to teach. The mission of the particular college or university and its school of nursing determines the expectation of teaching experiences, competencies, and appointment, as well as how faculty prepare for these. Appointment in tenure-track and clinical positions requires proven teaching competencies and a commitment to teaching as a scholarly endeavor.

Orientation Programs and Faculty Development

Orientation to the teaching role and the school of nursing for newly appointed faculty, as well as ongoing faculty development for all faculty, is assuming renewed importance as rapid changes in higher education and health care and the use of information technologies are creating new environments for teaching and changes in the faculty role. Most schools of nursing have established orientation programs and instituted mechanisms for faculty development and renewal.

Orientation Programs. Comprehensive orientation programs are necessary to assist new faculty to acquire teaching competencies, facilitate socialization to the teaching role of the faculty, and support faculty members as they develop as fully participating members of the faculty (Genrich & Pappas, 1997; Norton & Spross, 1994; Sheehe & Schoener, 1994). Orientation programs should include information about the rights and responsibilities of the faculty and institution, information about school- and department-specific policies and procedures, an overview of the curriculum with an orientation to the instructional technologies and computer-mediated instruction used at the school, and orientation to teaching assignments and clinical facilities. Orientation is particularly important for part-time faculty members, who have fewer opportunities for contact with the school and faculty colleagues.

Orientation programs are most effective when they occur over time and provide for ongoing support (Genrich & Pappas, 1997). Some schools of nursing have school-, department-, or course-developed programs. Orientation to the teaching aspect of the faculty role also can be facilitated through a mentor relationship. Many schools of nursing have formal mentor programs in which each new faculty member is assigned to a senior faculty member, who guides the new faculty member. Other mentoring relationships can occur on an informal basis.

Faculty Development. Faculty development refers to a planned course of action to develop all faculty members, not only those newly appointed for current and future teaching positions. Faculty development is assuming new importance as faculty prepare for teaching in new and reformed health care environments and community-based settings, delivering instruction in new ways, and using new teaching and learning technologies (Riner & Billings, 1996).

Faculty development is a shared responsibility of the individual faculty members, the department chair and other academic officers, and the school of nursing. It may include the school's providing formal and informal workshops and sessions, credit courses, and informal "brown bag lunches" and encouraging faculty to attend local and national conferences related to teaching, as well as providing the financial support to do so. Because effective teaching also requires clinical competence, faculty are encouraged to maintain clinical expertise through faculty practice and by keeping abreast of changes in the field through literature review and attending professional meetings related to the practice area. Sabbatical leaves provide another opportunity for faculty renewal.

Evaluation of Teaching Performance

To ensure competent teaching, the faculty members themselves, as well as administrators, peers, colleagues, and students, regularly review their teaching performance. Evaluation of teaching is a critical component of tenure (and posttenure) review. Results of this evaluation may also be used for making decisions about reappointment, merit raises, and awards that recognize and honor excellence in teaching.

Evidence for review of teaching effectiveness can be provided by a number of sources, including student evaluations of teaching, peer and colleague observations of teaching and teaching products (e.g., syllabi, case studies, publications, videotapes, computer-mediated lessons, Internet-based courses, study guides), letters from former students, success of graduates in employment, publications of students, teaching awards, administrative review, and self-evaluation (Kirschling et al., 1995; Lashley, 1993; Melland & Volden, 1996; Suess, 1995). Methods for gathering data for evaluation include promotion and tenure review, peer and colleague review, posttenure review, and the use of a teaching portfolio or dossier. These methods are explained in Chapter 24.

SUMMARY

Because of the various aspects of the faculty role, the demands of a career in academia can be challenging. To be successful, individuals aspiring to the role of a faculty member must be clear about the expectations of the role. This chapter describes the various competencies expected of faculty members, as well as their rights and responsibilities.

Many nursing faculty members have found that the rewards of the role well outweigh the demands and expectations. The challenges of the role provide many creative and innovative opportunities for faculty, leading to a career filled with diversity and productivity. Whether it be through teaching a new generation of nurses the art and science of nursing; providing service and consultation to constituents within a local, regional, national, or even international community; or generating new knowledge that has an impact on the delivery of quality patient care, being a member of the academic community provides faculty with stimulation and the opportunity to debate and collaborate with colleagues from their own discipline and others. Faculty are given a "laboratory" to explore new technology and solutions to the problems found in society and health care, while meeting an important societal need. In what other role could a nurse touch the lives of patients and future generations of nurses while developing a knowledge base that will assist in the further evolution of nursing and health care? The career of a faculty member is indeed a rewarding one.

REFERENCES

American Association of Colleges of Nursing. (1993). *Nursing education's agenda for the 21st century*. New York: Author.

Association of Governing Boards of Universities and Colleges. (1996). *Renewing the academic presidency*. Washington, DC: Author.

Balsmeyer, B., Haubrich, K., & Quinn, C. (1996). Defining collegiality within the academic setting. *Journal of Nursing Education, 35*(6), 264-267.

Barr, R. B., & Tagg, J. (1995). From teaching to learning: A new paradigm for undergraduate education. *Change, 27*(6), 13-25.

Billings, D. M. (1995). Preparing nursing faculty for information-age teaching and learning. *Computers in Nursing, 13*(6), 264, 268-269.

Boyer, E. (1990). *Scholarship reconsidered: Priorities of the professorate*. Princeton, NJ: The Carnegie Foundation for the Advancement of Teaching.

Brown, S. A., Cohen, S. M., Kaeser, L., Levine, C., Littleton, L. Y., Meininger, J. C., Otto, D. A., & Rickman, K. J. (1995). Nursing perspective of Boyer's scholarship paradigm. *Nurse Educator, 20*(5), 26-30.

Choudhry, U. K. (1992). New nurse faculty: Core competencies for role development. *Journal of Nursing Education, 31*(6), 265-272.

Davis, D. C., Dearman, C., Schwab, C., & Kitchens, E. (1992). Competencies of novice nurse educators. *Journal of Nursing Education, 31*(4), 159-164.

Dolence, M. G., & Norris, D. M. (1996). *Transforming higher education: A vision for learning in the 21st century.* Ann Arbor, MI: Society for College and University Planning.

Gaff, J., & Lambert, L. (1996). Socializing future faculty to the values of undergraduate education. *Change, 28*(4), 38-45.

Genrich, S. J., & Pappas, A. (1997). Retooling faculty orientation. *Journal of Professional Nursing, 13*(2), 84-89.

Halstead, J. A. (1996). The significance of student-faculty interactions. In K. Stevens (Ed.), *Review of research in nursing education: Vol. VII* (pp. 67-90). New York: National League for Nursing.

Kirschling, J., Fields, J., Imle, M., Mowery, M., Tanner, C., Perrin, N., & Stewart, B. (1995). Evaluating teaching effectiveness. *Journal of Nursing Education, 34*(9), 401-410.

Lashley, M. E. (1993). Faculty evaluation for professional growth. *Nurse Educator, 18*(4), 26-29.

Lieb, M. (1995). Mentoring: Making a difference in nursing education. In P. Bayles & J. Parks-Doyle (Eds.), *The web of inclusion: Faculty helping faculty.* New York: National League for Nursing.

Melland, H. I., & Volden, C. M. (1996). Teaching portfolios for faculty evaluation. *Nurse Educator, 21*(2), 35-38.

National League for Nursing Task Group on Nurse Educator Competencies (2004). *Competencies for nurse educators.* New York: Author.

Norton, S. F., & Spross, J. (1994). From advanced practice to academia: Developmental tasks and strategies for role socialization. *Journal of Professional Nursing, 33*(8), 373-375.

Plater, W. (1995). Future work: Faculty time in the 21st century. *Change, 27*(3), 23-33.

Riner, M. E., & Billings, D. M. (1996). Faculty development for teaching in a changing health care environment: A statewide needs assessment. Unpublished manuscript, Indiana University School of Nursing.

Sheehe, J. B., & Schoener, L. (1994). Risk and reality for nurse educators. *Holistic Nursing Practice, 8*(2), 53-58.

Shoffner, D. H., Davis, M. W., & Bowen, S. M. (1994). A model for clinical teaching as a scholarly endeavor. *IMAGE: Journal of Nursing Scholarship, 26*(3), 181-184.

Sneed, N. V., Edlund, B. J., Allred, C. A., Hickey, M., Heriot, C. S., Haight, B., & Hoffman, S. (1995). Appointment, promotion, and tenure criteria to meet changing perspectives in healthcare. *Nurse Educator, 20*(2), 23-28.

Suess, L. R. (1995). Attitudes of nurse-faculty toward post-tenure performance evaluations. *Journal of Nursing Education, 34*(1), 25-30.

Tucker, A. (1992). *Chairing the academic department: Leadership among peers* (3rd ed.). New York: American Council on Education/Macmillan.

Whicker, M., Kronenfield, J., & Strickland, R. (1993). *Getting tenure.* Newbury Park, CA: Sage Publications.

2

THE DIVERSE LEARNING NEEDS OF STUDENTS

Virginia Richardson, DNS, RN, CPNP

Students in today's college classrooms represent a wide array of diversity in learning needs and expectations. It is common to find "traditional" college-aged students and "nontraditional" adult learners intermingled in the same classroom setting. The enrollment of those students not coming directly from high school, especially among women, has increased by 13% in recent years (U.S. Department of Education, 2001). The projection is for a rise of 21% in those younger than 25 years and 14% in those older than 25 years. This delay of entry into college has resulted in an older nursing student population. The mean age of baccalaureate nursing graduates is 27 years in 2003, whereas the mean age of associate degree nursing graduates has increased from 28 years in 1988 to 32 years in 2003 (National Council of State Boards of Nursing, personal communication, February 10, 2003). The college student population is also becoming more representative of the increasing cultural diversity present in America's society. Of all college students, 28% are African-American, Hispanic, Asian-American, or Native American (U.S. Department of Education, 2001).

Nursing faculty are faced with the challenges of teaching students from varying backgrounds and life experiences. The purpose of this chapter is to present a brief profile of today's nursing students and provide assessment information that can help faculty in their efforts to meet the diverse learning needs of students. Information that specifically relates to assessing the learning styles, critical thinking skills, and cognitive abilities of students is covered. The special needs of the culturally diverse student are also addressed. Specific teaching strategies related to student characteristics are presented to enable faculty to provide effective learning experiences for all students.

PROFILE OF THE NURSING STUDENT IN THE NEW MILLENNIUM

The profile of nursing students in the new millenium is markedly different from that of the past. Gone are the days of a nursing profession that is dominated by single women in their early 20s. Instead, recent trends have indicated that it is likely that nursing students will be increasingly older, more culturally diverse, married with families, and geographically removed from educational institutions and that they will have prior educational experience (Halstead & Billings, 1998). An increasingly diverse population of nursing students has implications for faculty as they contemplate the development of future curricula and determine the resources necessary to support the academic performance of students.

Those born between 1961 and 1981 have been called *Generation Xers* ("Gen Xers") and account for a large number of those in college classrooms. This group of college students is like no other. They were the first to pass through metal detectors to enter school, grew up with television, more than half have divorced parents and grew up with a working mother, and they were the first generation of "latchkey" kids. More than one third were physically, mentally, or sexually abused, often by a stepparent. Many were left alone as their parents pursued their careers and so became very independent and developed strong problem-solving skills. Gen Xers have a lower standard of living than their parents, the Baby Boomers, and the lowest set of job skills in recent years (Mahedy & Bernardi, 1994). They are eager to make lasting contributions but need to feel that what they have to offer is valued. They like to learn, and how they learn has been shaped by technology (Tulgan, 2000). Gen Xers view their work as a job, not a career; tend to be blunt in conversations; mistrust business practices; are self-reliant; seek a balance in their lives; are task and results oriented; and are unfazed by authority and authority figures (Raines & Hunt, 2000; Sacks, 1996). See Box 2-1 for other characteristics of Gen Xers.

Generation Y, known as *Millennials* or *Echo Boomers*, are those born between 1981 and 2003. They outnumber any previous generation. Millennials were very wanted babies more so than previous generations, and as a result have received lots of attention from caring adults. Millennials characteristically have good relationships with their parents and families and share interests in music and travel with their parents. Millennial teens are much more involved than Gen Xers with service activities because their parents value giving back to the community. Parents of Millennials are involving their children in academic and sports activities at younger and younger ages to prepare them for success. Millennials are used to living highly structured lives planned by their parents and have had very little free time. By the time they reach

---

Box 2-1
CHARACTERISTICS OF GENERATION XERS

- Can multitask well
- Flexible
- Independent
- Intolerant of busy work
- Pessimistic
- Prefer to work alone
- Self-reliant
- Used to change
- Want to get the job done

college they have learned how to work with others and be a member of a team. Group grades for projects and assignments are something they are used to and expect. Technology is a part of their life, and they spend much of their time online staying connected. They think of technology as another way to communicate (Strauss & Howe, 2000). See Box 2-2 for other characteristics of Millennials.

Generation Y is a much more diverse group than previous generations: 34% are Hispanic, Asian, African-American, or Native American. The parents of this generation expect that their children's schools and universities will reflect diversity and thus provide a richer experience.

As stated earlier, the new RNs of today are older, married, likely to have children, and more likely than nursing students of the past to have had educational experiences before nursing school (Rosenfeld, 1994). The age of new nursing graduates has remained static for the past several years. In a 2003 survey of new RNs, it was noted that their average age was 31 years, compared with 31.3 years in 1990 and 28.8 years in 1988 (National Council of State Boards of Nursing, personal communication, February 10, 2003).

The implications of such demographic trends are significant to nursing faculty and the profession as a whole. Older students who are returning to school with multiple role responsibilities may require support resources such as tutoring, remediation, and the opportunity for part-time study (Swail, 2002). The provision of on-campus childcare is also becoming more of an issue for institutions of higher education. Schools of nursing must prepare for an increasingly diverse student body by closely examining the changing demographics of their student body, the adequacy of support services for the adult learner in their institution, and the flexibility of nursing curricula in their program.

The enrollment of men in nursing programs is in a slight decline. In the 2002 to 2003 school year 8.3% of students enrolled in baccalaureate nursing programs were men, compared with 8.9% in the 2001 to 2002 school year. Men represented 10% of the new RN graduates in 1992 (Rosenfeld, 1994). In the 2002 to 2003 school year 9.5% of students enrolled in graduate nursing

---

Box 2-2
CHARACTERISTICS OF MILLENNIALS

- Accept authority
- Balance work and personal life
- Direct
- Optimistic
- Rule follower
- Self-confident
- Socially aware
- Socially involved
- Team player
- Vocal

programs were men (American Association of Colleges of Nursing [AACN], 2003).

Summary

Changes in student demographics and characteristics have had an impact on the educational environment of today's college campuses. Faculty need to accept that the characteristics of students enrolled in their nursing programs have changed and acknowledge that these changes have implications for curriculum development, teaching, and learning.

THE CULTURALLY DIVERSE STUDENT

The AACN issued a position paper in 1997 stating that because the population of the United States is increasingly diverse, cultural diversity needed to be included in nursing education, and a greater number of culturally diverse students should be recruited into schools of nursing (AACN, 1997). Despite this emphasis on recruitment of culturally diverse students, there continues to be an underrepresentation of minorities in schools of nursing and in the profession (Campbell & Davis, 1996). In nursing schools the proportion of students from racial or ethnic minority groups has remained stable for the past 2 years, with 17% of basic baccalaureate students identifying themselves as African-American, Hispanic, Asian-American, or Native American. Hispanic students represent 5.6% of all baccalaureate nursing students; African-American students, 11%; Asian-American students, 5%; and nonresident aliens, 1% (AACN, 2003). Less than 10% of nursing school faculty members identify themselves as a minority (Berlin et al., 2003).

Students with a culturally diverse background can face a number of barriers that hamper their ability to be successful in college. The most common barriers are the lack of ethnically diverse faculty, finances, and academics (Dowell, 1996; Martin-Holland et al., 2003).

Faculty commitment is crucial to the success of minority students. Minority students need a student–faculty relationship with a faculty member who is not responsible for assigning a grade to them. These students need someone to talk with about their feelings and experiences as they progress through the program. It is important to have appropriate faculty role models, but in many institutions there are too few minority faculty members available. It is essential for all faculty members and administrators to develop sensitivity with regard to the diversity of the students on their campus and an awareness of the needs of these students. Faculty commitment to student success results in more successful students.

Financial problems are a major stressor for minority students. Rising tuition costs and other fees, coupled with a reduction in government support for higher education, affect all students but may be particularly difficult for minority students. Minority students are often the first in their family to seek higher education. They often come from low-income households and therefore their families may lack the necessary financial resources to support their education. Financial aid in the form of loans or scholarships is becoming more competitive, and less money is available (Brown et al., 2003).

Insufficient academic preparation and lack of support can also prevent students from completing their program of study. Many Latino youth are in schools with few academic and physical resources and are thus not prepared for the academic challenges of a nursing program (Brown et al., 2003). Many colleges offer special programs to help students achieve basic academic skills, as well as adjust to the college learning environment. Through academic advisement, skills assessment, and assistance with developing study skills, students can be helped to achieve a better academic record. Mount Carmel's Learning Trail helps current students by providing mentoring, tutoring, counseling, and follow-up. More than 80% of the students in the program graduate (Martinez & Martinez, 2003).

Stewart and Cleveland (2003) described a program to introduce middle and high school students to college and nursing. The Wisconsin Youth in Nursing (WYN) program recruited minority youth with a high grade point average and the motivation to complete the program. Twenty-three students participated in the 2-week summer residential program on a college campus. The program included general education and nursing courses, and the students were in class all day 5 days a week. The nursing segment included classes on careers in nursing, introduction to nursing, pathophysiology, and case studies. Students also worked on computers and were taught some nursing skills, including physical assessment skills. Students evaluated the program as being very successful. Faculty will follow the participants to determine how many were successful in gaining admission to a nursing school.

Interventions to Increase the Success of Culturally Diverse Students

Role Models. Although the recruitment and retention of culturally diverse students into the nursing profession is an important issue, currently little research is available on the effectiveness of various recruitment and retention efforts directed toward minority students (Dowell, 1996; Villarruel et al., 2001). However, nursing students have identified that the lack of minority role models is a problem affecting retention (Yoder, 1996). Minority role models are needed to provide students with opportunities to see minority faculty functioning successfully in a variety of leadership positions in the university setting. Observing a competent role model can help increase students' self-confidence and motivation to pursue career goals (Campbell & Davis, 1996). Practicing minority nurses can be encouraged to function as a role model and mentor. Many nursing students plan to practice in a hospital or community setting after graduation, and matching them with a practicing nurse is a way to show them that they can be successful. Nursing school faculty could work with their school's alumni association and with minority nursing groups to provide role models for students.

Majority faculty members can also assist in the recruitment and retention of culturally diverse students by modeling a commitment to developing cultural competence. Cultural aspects of care are included in theory and clinical courses in nursing programs at all levels. The proliferation of study abroad programs and programs where students provide nursing care to those in developing countries is a testament to the interest of both students and faculty in learning more about people of other cultures. It is important for faculty to acknowledge cultural assumptions that they may hold and carefully consider how these assumptions can affect their interactions with minority students. Faculty can also advocate for policies and procedures and support services that assist minority students and support an institutional faculty "mix" that is culturally diverse. Majority faculty members need to remember that many minority students feel isolated in their educational experience and therefore faculty may need to be more assertive in establishing and maintaining open lines of communication with minority students. Helping students to access campus support services will help students feel more connected to the institution.

Support Services. Participating in special support programs can increase the chance of academic success for culturally diverse students. The Minority Academic Advising Program (MAAP) at a southern state health sciences university was developed to increase retention of African-American students in schools of nursing, dentistry, allied health, graduate studies, and medicine (Hesser et al., 1996). The school of nursing already provided help with study skills and academic counseling for minority students. MAAP services include a special orientation session for students, a training session for faculty and peer advisors, and referral to a study skills expert as needed. As a result of these efforts, African-American nursing students are retained at a higher rate (Hesser et al., 1996).

The Pathways Model (Rew, 1996) is an example of a faculty development program that focuses on developing positive faculty interactions with students who have diverse needs and are of varying backgrounds. The goal of the program is to increase faculty awareness of the implications of cultural diversity on teaching–learning strategies and to help faculty acquire the skills, values, and attitudes necessary for teaching culturally diverse students. The Pathways Model has been successful in making faculty more sensitive to cultural diversity and related issues (Rew). In this model faculty initially are oriented to multiculturalism and then meet monthly to discuss how to implement their newly gained knowledge about cultural diversity, report on literature reviews they have conducted, and identify the implications for teaching culturally diverse students. The faculty members each agree to mentor one student and share their experiences with their academic division within the school of nursing. The result is empowerment of both faculty and students.

Summary. The recruitment of academically qualified minority students has been a recent emphasis of many nursing schools. However, the data indicate that these recruitment efforts have been only marginally successful. It is a source of concern that minority students appear to be less successful than Caucasian students in graduating from nursing programs. It is important for nurse educators to reexamine their minority student recruitment efforts and also the support services that are available for these students. Developing a cultural sensitivity among faculty members is essential to the successful recruitment and retention of minority students.

ASSESSING LEARNING STYLE PREFERENCES

Students seeking educational degrees who are not coming directly from high school, such as nursing students, present a challenge for educational settings. Institutions of higher education have responded to the increased enrollment of older, nontraditional students by attempting to provide flexible educational offerings. A truly nontraditional approach to education involves responding to students' diverse needs and learning styles, emphasizing learner responsibility, providing experiential learning, and focusing on competence. *Learning style* refers to the unique way in which a person perceives, interacts with, and responds to a learning situation. Adult students need a variety of modes of delivery to meet their learning needs. They are nontraditional in many respects and benefit from a flexible and multifaceted program.

Distance learning can increase access to education for working adult students and can provide for the efficient use of nursing faculty. Online courses are convenient for those with a busy work schedule and enable students to work around their family's schedule. However, busy work schedules and families are also the reasons the attrition rate is so high for online courses (Carr, 2000). Younger students have grown up using computers and are very comfortable with online courses and navigating the Internet. They actually prefer to learn using this modality.

To be a successful "virtual" student, a person must have good computer skills and be comfortable communicating through text messages, not needing auditory or visual cues to aid in the communication process. Virtual students must be motivated and disciplined to keep up with the course, and it is important that they recognize when they do not understand a concept and take the initiative to contact the faculty immediately. Online courses require a significant time commitment, and students must be willing to put in this time to complete the course (Palloff & Pratt, 2003). More about online learning can be found in Chapter 19.

A student's learning style indicates the preferred educational conditions that will help that student to learn as much as possible. A variety of instruments have been developed to identify student learning styles. Knowles' principles of adult learning, which have been widely accepted; the Kolb Learning Style Inventory (LSI); and the Dunn, Dunn, and Price Productivity Environmental Preference Survey (PEPS) are discussed here.

Knowles' Principles of Adult Learning

Knowles (1970) realized that adults learn in a manner different from that of children. His ideas about adult education evolved mainly through observation of what worked best, what programs were the most productive as reported in the literature, and which teachers were the most successful. He viewed learning as an internal process, with the locus of control residing in the learner and being facilitated by outside helpers, such as teachers. Knowles (1978) stated that people learn best when treated as adults and that the ultimate purpose of all education is to help individuals develop the attitude that learning is a lifelong process. He described andragogy as the art and science of helping adults learn and viewed it as a separate and distinct theory of education. Additional discussion of Knowles' principles of adult learning can be found in Chapter 12.

To meet the needs of educating students as adults, nursing faculty must accept and internalize an andragogical orientation to education. In the andragogically oriented environment, the adult learner assumes responsibility for learning and the use of resources. By contrast, in the pedagogically oriented environment the teacher is the transmitter of knowledge, with the student assuming a more passive role (Knowles, 1970). Although older returning students are assumed to be adult learners, little is known about their attitudes toward education or whether they have an andragogical or pedagogical orientation to learning.

It was not until the 1970s and early 1980s that attempts were made to define, operationalize, and evaluate andragogy. One of the first questions concerned whether assumed learning differences between traditional and nontraditional students could be perceived and identified in an objective manner. The first area to be researched was that of measuring educational orientation on an andragogical–pedagogical scale. Beginning research on the andragogical–pedagogical orientation of adult educators indicated that andragogy could be operationalized. Research on the educational orientation of adult educators is of limited value if not used in conjunction with the educational orientation of students. More research needs to be conducted to determine whether educational orientation is affected by student characteristics and educational experiences.

Kolb's Model of Experiential Learning

Kolb (1976) envisioned learning as a four-stage cycle, with learning occurring as a person cycles from concrete experience, to reflective observation, to abstract conceptualization, to active experimentation. In Kolb's model two pairs of polar opposites comprise the four stages: concrete experience (feeling) versus abstract conceptualization (thinking) and active experimentation (doing) versus reflective observation (watching). A person emphasizes one of each of the two pairs of stages, and this combination indicates the person's preferred learning style. The four learning styles are accommodative, assimilative, divergent, and convergent.

1. Persons with the *accommodative style* prefer to learn through a combination of concrete experiences and active experimentation. They are good at completing tasks and are less concerned than others about the theories supporting their actions. They are risk takers and often solve problems through trial and error (Kolb, 1976).
2. Persons with the *assimilative style* prefer to learn through a combination of abstract conceptualization and reflective observation. They excel at assimilating diverse items into an integrated whole. They are much more concerned with abstract concepts than they are with people and the application of ideas (Kolb, 1976).
3. Persons with the *divergent style* prefer to learn through a combination of concrete experiences and reflective observations. They tend to be

imaginative, are good at generating ideas, are people oriented, and are emotional (Kolb, 1976).

4. Persons with the *convergent style* prefer to learn through a combination of abstract conceptualization and active experimentation. They like to deal with things, not people (Kolb, 1976).

Instrument

Kolb Learning Style Inventory. The Kolb Learning Style Inventory (LSI) has become the most commonly used instrument to measure nursing students' learning styles and is related to cognitive abilities students use in the classroom. The original LSI was a nine-item self-report questionnaire based on experiential learning theory. The student ranked four adjectives with regard to how well they described the student's learning style. The revised version (1985) has a 12-item sentence completion format and takes 15 to 20 minutes to complete. The student must rank four endings to best describe the student's learning style.

Use of the Kolb Learning Style Inventory in Nursing Education. King (1986) examined differences and similarities between RN and generic nursing students using the Kolb LSI. Results of the analyses revealed no difference between the RN students' and generic students' learning styles. The majority of students in both groups preferred the accommodative or divergent learning style. Booth's (1989) study compared 123 traditional and 29 nontraditional baccalaureate nursing students with regard to demographic variables, learning style using the Kolb LSI, and developmental stage. Booth found no difference in learning styles between RNs and traditional nursing students when using the Kolb LSI.

In a study by Staton-Cross (1988) with the Kolb LSI, 202 freshmen and sophomores in two associate degree nursing programs comprised the sample. Results revealed that most students in the sample population were concrete learners with accommodative or divergent learning styles. These same students preferred the lecture and discussion format and rejected the self-paced and self-study learning formats.

Laschinger and Boss (1989) studied 76 post-RN and 121 upper-level generic baccalaureate nursing students' attitudes toward theory-based nursing using the Kolb LSI, a measure of the perception of nursing learning environments, and a nursing theories questionnaire. Concrete learners and those subjects who perceived nursing environments to be predominantly concrete had a significantly more negative attitude toward theory-based nursing than did abstract learners. Learning style preference was not significantly related to preferred method of learning nursing theories.

The Kolb LSI was used by Morgan (1990) to reflect beliefs about how students learn best in the clinical setting. The subjects were 132 baccalaureate nursing students and 17 clinical instructors. Data analysis did not support experiential learning theory as a link between learning style, beliefs about learning style, perceptions of achievement, and effective clinical teaching.

Summary

The Kolb LSI is one of the most commonly used LSIs in nursing education, as well as in other disciplines. However, research has been inconclusive with regard to establishing significant relationships between learning style preferences and other student variables (DeCoux, 1990). Further research related to Kolb's model of experiential learning, as well as the LSI, is warranted.

Dunn, Dunn, and Price Productivity Environmental Preference Survey

The Dunn, Dunn, and Price Productivity Environmental Preference Survey (PEPS) (Dunn et al., 1986), a type of LSI, is derived from Price's (1986) learning style model. The model indicates that learning is influenced by student ability, learning style, delivery method, and attitude toward content.

Instrument

Productivity Environmental Preference Survey. The PEPS measures student preferences in four categories: environmental, sociological, physical, and emotional. The PEPS is a self-administered survey, takes 20 minutes to complete, and contains 100 Likert-type statements with a 5-point response scale indicating the extent to which the learner strongly agrees (1) to strongly disagrees (5) with the statement. The PEPS provides subscale summaries for 20 factors divided into the four categories, as follows:

1. *Environmental:* These statements measure whether the student prefers a quiet versus a noisy environment while learning; the student's temperature and lighting preferences; and the student's preference for formal versus informal design of the environment, such as sitting on a bed versus sitting in a chair while studying.
2. *Sociological:* These statements measure whether the student prefers to study alone or with others; prefers to have an authority available with special knowledge; or can learn in several ways (alone, with peers, and with an authority present) (Dunn et al., 1986).
3. *Physical:* The visual subscale indicates a learner's preference for reading to learn; the auditory subscale indicates a learner's preference for listening to a recording, lecture, discussion, or verbal instructions to learn; and the tactile subscale indicates a learner's preference for taking notes or underlining important information to learn (Dunn et al., 1986). Kinesthetic (tactile) learners prefer to use their whole body to learn; they retain information by practicing demonstrations or procedures. Preferences for time of day for studying, such as morning, afternoon, or evening; for taking frequent breaks versus working straight through an assignment; and for drinking or chewing while concentrating are also measured by these statements (Dunn et al., 1986).
4. *Emotional:* These statements measure a student's desire to do what is expected, desire to achieve academically (motivation), and need for direction to complete assignments (structure) (Dunn et al., 1986).

The reliability and validity of the PEPS instrument have been established for baccalaureate nursing students (LaMothe et al., 1991). A computer-administered version of PEPS is available (Billings, 1991).

Use of the Productivity Environmental Preference Survey in Nursing Education. LaMothe et al. (1991) studied 433 students in an upper division baccalaureate nursing program using the PEPS. In this study first semester junior students were found to need more structure than other class levels. In addition to needing more structure, these students had a stronger preference for working with an authority figure present than did first semester senior students.

Billings (1994) used the PEPS to identify the results of students' studying alone or in groups when using an interactive videodisc program. Students who used the videodisc in groups reported a greater comfort with using the technology, but they did not show greater gains in academic achievement on the posttest.

Performance on the National Council Licensure Examination for Registered Nurses (NCLEX-RN) has been examined as it relates to students' learning style preferences using the PEPS (Kizilay, 1991). Kizilay studied 158 senior nursing students and found differences between traditional students and adult learners. The adult learners preferred taking food breaks and having beverages at their desks. The traditional students preferred to be self-paced and to design creative activities. Students who preferred to work more closely with faculty (authority figures) and manipulate materials were more likely to be successful on the NCLEX-RN.

Summary

The PEPS instrument is easy to administer and has been found to be reliable and valid for use with baccalaureate nursing students. Although not as commonly used in nursing education as other LSIs, the PEPS is potentially useful for helping to determine students' learning preferences and responses to various learning experiences. Appropriate learning experiences can then be designed.

Using the Results of Learning Style Inventories in the Classroom

LSIs can be administered during orientation, during class time, or independently as an assignment before entering a program or course. A practical application of LSIs is that once an educator knows a student's preferred learning style, that information can be used when tutoring or counseling that student. For example, if a student has difficulty studying or taking tests, the educator could direct the student to use the study methods that would be most helpful for students with his or her preferred learning style.

A variety of teaching strategies can be used to appeal to different learning styles and thus maximize student learning. Different teaching strategies facilitate learning by creating a match between preferred learning style and method of instruction. Students who are exposed to a variety of teaching strategies are also challenged to learn using styles other than their preferred one.

Questions regarding learning style remain: Should students use only their preferred learning style and perhaps risk becoming rigid and unable to learn in different ways? Should educators encourage students to increase their ability to learn in different ways? Students who habitually use only their preferred learning style are disadvantaged when the situation demands that they use a different style.

Heredity, Environment, and Prior Learning

Other factors that influence how students learn are heredity, environment, and prior learning experiences. Genetic makeup does play a part in a person's overall potential for learning. However, this potential is also greatly influenced by what students experience as a children in their homes, schools, and communities. Children who grow up in a stimulating and supportive environment are more likely to feel very positive about learning and be eager to learn. Those children who grow up in an environment that is not stimulating are usually not as eager to learn or as excited about the prospect of learning. In addition, students' prior learning experiences can affect the way they learn new material. To develop the most effective teaching and learning environment, faculty need to assess what skills, attitudes, knowledge, and values the nursing students bring to the learning environment.

Summary

Assessment of students' learning style preferences and prior learning helps faculty to design learning experiences that best meet the diverse learning needs of the students in their program. The use of diverse teaching strategies to meet a variety of learning styles, including culturally influenced styles of learning, can be found in Chapter 10.

ASSESSING CRITICAL THINKING ABILITIES

The National League for Nursing has established criteria for program accreditation that include critical thinking as a major required program outcome. Nursing programs are required to demonstrate that their students are developing the specific critical thinking skills of analysis, reasoning, decision making, and independent judgment (National League for Nursing, 1989).

Critical thinking has been discussed in the nursing literature for the past several years. Experts on critical thinking cannot agree on a definition for it, nor is there one way to measure it or what impact it has on patient care. Critical thinking is not a single way of thinking but rather is a complex process. One reason critical thinking is difficult to define is that nurse researchers lump together problem solving, clinical decision making, and critical thinking (Duchscher, 2003).

Critical Thinking Inventories

Despite the difficulty of defining critical thinking, several critical thinking inventories have been developed. These inventories have been used in nursing and include the Watson-Glaser Critical Thinking Appraisal (WGCTA), the California Critical Thinking Skills Test (CCTST), and the California Critical Thinking Disposition Inventory (CCTDI). A brief description of each follows. The reader should bear in mind that these inventories have been tested with predominantly white middle-class groups and therefore may not work well when used with culturally diverse populations.

Watson-Glaser Critical Thinking Appraisal. One of the earliest definitions of critical thinking was that of Watson and Glaser (1964), who defined critical thinking as a composite of attitudes, knowledge, and skills. This definition was operationalized as a score on the WGCTA. The WGCTA consists of a number of objective items that involve problems encountered in everyday life. The test contains five subtests—deduction, inference, recognition of assumptions, interpretation, and evaluation of arguments—designed to measure different aspects of critical thinking. Each subtest contains 16 questions, and the format is multiple choice. The subtests are weighted evenly to determine the total score, with the maximum score being 80.

Bauwens and Gerhard (1987) found in their study, in which they used the WGCTA to predict the success of baccalaureate nursing students in passing the NCLEX-RN, that there was no significant change in total scores between the first and last semesters. Behrens (1996) found that WGCTA scores did not increase as a result of the nursing school experience. Others (Adams et al., 1999; Frye et al., 1999; Maynard, 1996; Vaughan-Wrobel et al., 1997) also found that critical thinking ability did not change significantly in nursing students from entry to end of the program. In another study Magnussen, Ishida, and Itano (2000) administered the WGCTA to their students in the first and final semesters of their nursing program. Those students who had the lowest critical thinking scores at entry showed significant improvement in the final semester; however, those who received midlevel and high critical thinking scores at entry showed a decline in these scores in the final semester.

California Critical Thinking Skills Test. The CCTST College Level (Facione, 1990) is the first instrument to use the Delphi Report's (American Philosophical Association, 1990) definition of critical thinking. The CCTST has gone through extensive evaluation.

The CCTST is a standardized, 34-item multiple choice test whose purpose is to test core critical thinking skills considered to be essential for college students. There are two statistically equivalent forms: Form A, developed and validated in 1989/1990, and Form B, developed and validated in 1991/1992. The items include analysis of the meaning of sentences and selection of inferences from assumptions provided.

The CCTST reports an overall score for an individual's critical thinking skills plus the scores on five subscales: analysis, evaluation, inference, deductive reasoning, and inductive reasoning. The three subscales of analysis, evaluation, and inference are the major core skills as identified in the Delphi Report for the theory of critical thinking (American Philosophical Association, 1990). There is little in the literature reporting the use of the CCTST with nursing students.

California Critical Thinking Disposition Inventory. The CCTDI uses the Delphi Report's consensus definition of critical thinking (American Philosophical Association, 1990). The Report lists 19 dispositional phases in the description of the ideal critical thinker. Factor analysis and item analysis were used to create seven disposition scales (subscales): open-mindedness, analyticity, cognitive maturity, truth seeking, systematicity, inquisitiveness, and self-confidence (Facione & Facione, 1992).

The CCTDI is a 75-item instrument that measures students' attitudes, beliefs, and opinions relevant to critical thinking. Students respond using a 6-point Likert scale, indicating the extent to which the student strongly agrees (1) to strongly disagrees (6) with the statement. The CCTDI reports eight scores: an overall score plus scores for each of the seven subscales. Cronbach's alpha for the overall instrument is .91, and for the individual subscales alphas ranged from .71 to .80. The scales are scrambled, and the names of the subscales are not on the test instrument. A brief description of each subscale follows:

1. The *open-mindedness subscale* reflects a person's tolerance of opinions different from his or her own and sensitivity to his or her own bias.
2. The *analyticity subscale* measures a person's awareness of potential problems, ability to anticipate consequences, and ability to use reason to solve dilemmas.
3. The *maturity subscale* targets cognitive maturity. The CCTDI score reflects a preference for exercising judiciousness when making decisions. The cognitively mature person approaches problems with the attitude that there may be more than one solution and the realization that some problems are ill structured.
4. The *truth-seeking subscale* reflects a person's eagerness to seek knowledge and ask questions.
5. The *systematicity subscale* reflects how organized, orderly, and focused a person is when approaching problems or specific issues.
6. The *inquisitiveness subscale* measures a person's desire for learning. It also reflects how intellectually curious a person is and how well informed he or she is on a variety of issues.
7. The *self-confidence subscale* reflects the level of trust a person has in his or her own ability to reason.

Summary

Nursing school faculty are expected to evaluate the critical thinking skills of students and to use these data to guide future revision and development of the school's curriculum. Measurement of students' critical thinking skills remains problematic, however, because currently no critical thinking instruments are specific to nursing and none correlate to the clinical decision-making skills required of students.

Adams' (1999) integrative review found no consistent evidence that nursing education contributes to increased critical thinking in nursing students. Myrick (2002) suggested that the use of more qualitative methods to measure the development of critical thinking skills in students is in order. In addition, Sedlak (1997) recommended the design of longitudinal research studies to measure the development of critical thinking skills across the curriculum and further research to identify measures that increase critical thinking ability.

Videbeck (1997) suggested that the incorporation of more active teaching strategies in the classroom is necessary to stimulate critical thinking in students. Gray (2003) introduced a teaching strategy to develop critical thinking skills in senior-level students where they assume the role of leader, participant, or evaluator. Students' evaluations of this teaching strategy indicated that the goal of fostering a deeper discussion of issues and topics was achieved.

Future research efforts will undoubtedly need to be focused on the development of instruments specific to the nursing discipline that measure students' critical thinking and clinical decision-making skills. Identifying teaching and learning strategies and educational environments that foster the development of these skills is also of importance.

ASSESSING COGNITIVE DEVELOPMENT

Cognitive development has been defined as "the way in which individuals reason, view knowledge, manage diversity of opinion and conflicting points of view, and relate to authorities or experts" (McGovern & Valiga, 1997, p. 29). The level of a student's cognitive development can have an impact on his or her ability to think critically and make autonomous clinical decisions.

In his scheme of intellectual and ethical development, Perry (1970) identified four stages of development that students supposedly achieve as they move along the continuum of educational experiences in college: dualism, multiplicity, relativism, and commitment. Research has indicated that many new college freshmen are in the dualistic stage, or lowest level of cognitive development, and many college seniors may have progressed no further than the multiplicity stage by the end of their undergraduate college career (McGovern & Valiga, 1997). It is the responsibility of faculty not only to identify the cognitive skills students have but also to teach students how to further develop and use their cognitive abilities (Doherty et al., 1997).

Determining Cognitive Abilities

Grade point average and standardized test scores, such as Scholastic Aptitude Test (SAT) and American College Test (ACT) scores, have often been used by faculty as a measure of a student's overall cognitive abilities. However, sole reliance on grades and standardized test scores is not enough. These need to be considered in conjunction with other assessments to determine a student's overall potential. A student who scores well on standardized tests or earns high grades might not do well with the psychomotor or psychosocial aspects of nursing. The reverse is also true. A student who does well with the psychomotor and psychosocial aspects of nursing might not be able to analyze and synthesize all of the information needed to make appropriate clinical decisions.

There are several assessment activities that can be used to determine the cognitive abilities of students before they begin a program. These activities can be used to determine students' current level of knowledge and skill development and can occur at the institutional, program, or course level. Data gathered from such activities can be used to recommend and plan a student's program of study and other more specific learning experiences. For example, at the course level, the best way to determine whether a student has a particular psychomotor skill is to have the student demonstrate the skill. Further learning activities can then be planned based on the level of psychomotor skill the student has demonstrated. A written pretest can be effective in determining a student's cognitive knowledge level about a specific concept. If there is not enough time in a course to have each student demonstrate a skill or to conduct a pretest, asking the students as a whole whether they are able to perform certain skills or can demonstrate certain levels of cognitive knowledge may suit the faculty's purposes.

A more inclusive testing process provides a more comprehensive student profile that can be used to design learning experiences. At the institutional and program levels this would include testing of prospective students before acceptance or as part of the acceptance process to the institution, the nursing major, or both. The testing could include assessment of learning style preferences, mathematical abilities, reading and writing abilities, stress and coping strategy preferences, and critical thinking abilities. A program could then be developed to maximize the fit to the student profile.

Several issues are related to the selection and use of assessment/diagnostic instruments. Initially, faculty must consider the time and expense of administering the instrument. Some instruments may require that scoring be performed by the company that sells the tools. This can create a delay in getting the results returned to faculty, which could make it difficult for faculty to make programming decisions in a timely fashion. Other issues include whether all students should take the tests and, if not, which students would benefit the most from the results of the testing information. Once faculty obtain test results, what will they do with that information? Are there enrichment programs available to students? These questions need to be carefully thought through by faculty as they make decisions with regard to the selection of assessment instruments and other measures.

Fostering Development of Cognitive Abilities

McGovern and Valiga (1997) recommended a systematic approach to developing the cognitive abilities of students. If faculty view cognitive development as an ongoing process that occurs throughout the program, it is reasonable to assume that any systematic approach to the cognitive development of students will require frequent assessment of students' abilities, along with appropriate feedback to students.

Within the educational program itself, fostering the development of cognitive abilities in students requires faculty to shift the major focus of concern from *content* to the *student*. This may mean that faculty will need to reexamine the teaching strategies they choose to use in the classroom and their methods of assessment (Doherty et al., 1997; Magnussen, 2001). Learning experiences that require active involvement in the learning process, such as reflective writing, debates, and collaborative group work, are more appropriate for developing cognitive abilities. Qualitative measurements of developing student abilities may yield more meaningful assessment data for faculty and students (McGovern & Valiga, 1997). Such student-centered efforts can help foster the development of self-assessment skills in students, as well as the development of lifelong learning skills.

SUMMARY

This chapter describes the demographic characteristics of today's nursing student and the special needs of culturally diverse students. Information related to assessing the learning styles, critical thinking skills, and cognitive abilities of students has been presented.

Faculty are responsible for creating an environment that is conducive to learning. Likewise, students are responsible for identifying environments that will best help them to learn. The assessment of learning style preferences, critical thinking skills, and cognitive abilities can help faculty and students develop collaborative partnerships that will foster the acquisition of the knowledge and skills necessary to practice professional nursing.

REFERENCES

Adams, B. (1999). Nursing education for critical thinking: An integrative review. *Journal of Nursing Education, 38*(2), 111-119.

Adams, M., Stover, L., Whitlow, J. (1999). A longitudinal evaluation of baccalaureate nursing students' critical thinking abilities. *Journal of Nursing Education, 38*(3), 139-141.

American Association of Colleges of Nursing (1997). Diversity and equality of opportunity. Washington, DC: Author.

American Association of Colleges of Nursing. (2003). *Enrollment and graduations in baccalaureate and graduate programs in nursing.* Washington, DC: Author.

American Philosophical Association. (1990). Critical thinking: A statement of expert consensus for purposes of educational assessment and instrument. *The Delphi Report: Research findings and recommendations prepared for the committee on pre-college philosophy.* (ERIC Document Reproduction Service No. ED 315-423).

Bauwens, E., & Gerhard, G. (1987). The use of the Watson-Glaser critical thinking appraisal to predict success in a baccalaureate nursing program. *Journal of Nursing Education, 26*(7), 278-281.

Behrens, P. (1996). The Watson-Glaser critical thinking appraisal and academic performance of diploma school students. *Journal of Nursing Education, 35*(1), 34-36.

Berlin, L., Stennett, J., Bednash, G. (2003). 2002-2003 Salaries of instructional and administrative nursing faculty in baccalaureate and graduate programs in nursing. Washington, DC: American Association of Colleges of Nursing.

Billings, D. (1991). Assessing learning styles using a computerized learning style inventory. *Computers in Nursing, 9*(3), 121-125.

Billings, D. (1994). Effects of BSN student preferences for studying alone or in groups and attitude when using interactive videodisc instruction. *Journal of Nursing Education, 33*(7), 322-324.

Booth, D. (1989). *Developmental and demographic characteristics of generic and nongeneric students in a baccalaureate nursing program.* Unpublished doctoral dissertation, University of Southern Mississippi, Hattiesburg.

Brown, S., Santiago, D., Lopez, E. (2003). Latinos in higher education. *Change 35*(2), 40-46.

Campbell, A., & Davis, S. (1996). Faculty commitment: Retaining minority nursing students in majority institutions. *Journal of Nursing Education, 35*(7), 298-303.

Carr, S. (2000, February 11). As distance learning comes of age, the challenge is in keeping the students. *Chronicle of Higher Education 16*(23), 15-17. Retrieved June 16, 2003, from www.chronicle.com/free/v46/i23/23a00101.htm

DeCoux, V. (1990). Kolb's learning style inventory: A review of its applications in nursing research. *Journal of Nursing Education, 29*(5), 202-207.

Doherty, A., Chenevert, J., Miller, R. R., Roth, J. L., & Truchan, L. (1997). Developing intellectual skills. In J. G. Gaff, J. L. Ratcliff, & Associates (Eds.), *Handbook of the undergraduate curriculum: A comprehensive guide to purposes, structures, practices, and change* (pp. 170-189). San Francisco: Jossey-Bass.

Dowell, M. A. (1996). Issues in recruitment and retention of minority nursing students. *Journal of Nursing Education, 35*(7), 293-297.

Duchscher, J. (2003). Critical thinking: Perceptions of newly graduated female baccalaureate nurses. *Journal of Nursing Education, 42*(1), 14-27.

Dunn, R., Dunn, K., & Price, G. (1986). *Productivity environmental preference survey*. Lawrence, KS: Price Systems.

Facione, P., & Facione, N. (1992). *The California Critical Thinking Dispositions Inventory*. Millbrae, CA: California Academic Press.

Frye, B., Alfred, N., & Campbell, M. (1999). Watson-Glaser critical thinking appraisal with BSN students. *Nursing and Health Care Perspectives, 20*(5), 253-255.

Gray, M. (2003). Beyond content generating critical thinking in the classroom. *Nurse Educator, 28*(3), 136-140.

Halstead, J. A., & Billings, D. M. (1998). Nursing education. In G. Deloughery (Ed.), *Issues and trends in nursing* (3rd ed.) (pp. 245-269). St. Louis: Mosby-Year Book.

Hesser, A., Pond, E., Lewis, L., & Abbott, B. (1996). Evaluation of a supplementary retention program for African-American baccalaureate nursing students. *Journal of Nursing Education, 35*(7), 304-309.

King, J. (1986). A comparative study of adult development patterns of RN and generic students in a baccalaureate nursing program. *Journal of Nursing Education, 25*(9), 336-371.

Kizilay, P. (1991). *The relationship of learning style preferences and perceptions of college climate and performance on the National Council Licensure Examination for Registered Nurses in associate degree nursing programs*. Unpublished doctoral dissertation, University of Georgia, Athens.

Knowles, M. (1970). *The modern practice of adult education*. New York: Associated Press.

Knowles, M. (1978). *The adult learner: A neglected species* (2nd ed.). Houston: Gulf Publishing.

Kolb, D. (1976). *Learning style inventory: Technical manual*. Boston: McBer.

LaMothe, J., Billings, D., Belcher, A., Cobb, K., Nice, A., & Richardson, V. (1991). Reliability and validity of the productivity environmental preference survey (PEPS). *Nurse Educator, 16*(4), 30-35.

Laschinger, H., & Boss, M. (1989). Learning styles of baccalaureate nursing students and attitudes toward theory-based nursing. *Journal of Professional Nursing, 5*(4), 215-223.

Magnussen, L. (2001). The use of the cognitive behavior survey to assess nursing student learning. *Journal of Nursing Education, 40*(1), 43-46.

Magnussen, L., Ishida, D., & Itano, J. (2000). The impact of the use of inquiry-based learning as a teaching methodology on the development of critical thinking. *Journal of Nursing Education, 39*(8), 360-364.

Mahedy, W., & Bernardi, J. (1994). *A generation alone*. Downers Grove, IL: InterVarsity Press.

Martin-Holland, J., Bello-Jones, T., Shuman, A., Rutledge, D., & Sechrist, K. (2003). Ensuring cultural diversity among California nurses. *Journal of Nursing Education 42*(6), 245-250.

Martinez, T., Martinez, A. (2003). Nursing schools ratchet up recruitment of Hispanics. *Hispanic Outlook, 13*, 10-13.

Maynard, C. (1996). Relationship of critical thinking ability to professional nursing competence. *Journal of Nursing Education, 35*(1), 12-18.

McGovern, M., & Valiga, T. M. (1997). Promoting the cognitive development of freshman nursing students. *Journal of Nursing Education, 36*(1), 29-35.

Morgan, S. (1990). *An investigation of learning styles, effective teaching, and student achievement in the experiential nursing clinical environment*. Unpublished doctoral dissertation, University of Kansas, Lawrence.

Myrick, F. (2002). Preceptorship and critical thinking in nursing education. *Journal of Nursing Education, 41*(4), 154-164.

National League for Nursing. (1989). *Criteria for the evaluation of baccalaureate and higher degree programs in nursing* (6th ed.). New York: Author.

Palloff, R., & Pratt, K. (2003). *The virtual student*. San Francisco: Jossey-Bass.

Perry, W. G. (1970). *Forms of intellectual and ethical development in the college years: A scheme*. New York: Holt, Rinehart and Winston.

Price, G. (1986). *Changes in learning style for a random sample of individuals 18 and older who responded to the PEPS, 1986.* Paper presented at the National Learning Style Leadership Training Conference, New York, July 10, 1986.

Raines, C., & Hunt, J. (2000). *The xers & the boomers.* Menlo Park, CA: Crisp Publications.

Rew, L. (1996). Affirming cultural diversity: A Pathways Model for nursing faculty. *Journal of Nursing Education, 35*(7), 310-314.

Rosenfeld, P. (1994). Profiles of the newly licensed nurse: Historical trends and future implications (2nd ed.). New York: National League for Nursing Press.

Sacks, P. (1996). *Generation x goes to college.* Chicago: Open Court.

Sedlak, C. A. (1997). Critical thinking of beginning baccalaureate nursing students during the first clinical nursing course. *Journal of Nursing Education, 36*(1), 11-17.

Staton-Cross, D. (1988). *Relationship of learning styles, learning preference, and learning autonomy among adult learners in two associate degree nursing programs: Traditional and nontraditional.* Unpublished doctoral dissertation, Boston College.

Stewart, S., Cleveland, R. (2003). A pre-college program for culturally diverse high school students. *Nurse Educator 28*(3), 107-110.

Strauss, W., & Howe, N. (2000). *Millennials rising: The next generation.* New York: Vintage Books.

Swail, W. (2002). Higher education and the new demographics. *Change, 34*(4), 15-23.

Tulgan, B. (2000). *Managing generation x.* New York: W. W. Norton.

U.S. Department of Education. (2001). *Digest of education statistics.* Washington, DC: National Center for Education Statistics.

Vaughan-Wrobel, B., O'Sullivan, P., & Smith, L. (1997). Evaluating critical thinking skills of baccalaureate nursing students. *Journal of Nursing Education, 36*(10), 485-488.

Videbeck, S. L. (1997). Critical thinking: A model. *Journal of Nursing Education, 36*(1), 23-28.

Villarruel, A., Canales, M., & Torres, S. (2001). Bridges and barriers: Educational mobility of Hispanic nurses. *Journal of Nursing Education, 40*(8), 245-251.

Watson, G., & Glaser, E. (1964). *Watson-Glaser critical thinking appraisal manual.* New York: Harcourt Brace & World.

Yoder, M. K. (1996). Instructional responses to ethnically diverse nursing students. *Journal of Nursing Education, 35*(7), 315-321.

3

THE ACADEMIC PERFORMANCE
OF STUDENTS
LEGAL AND ETHICAL ISSUES

Elizabeth G. Johnson, DSN, RN,
Judith A. Halstead, DNS, RN

Nursing faculty have many things to consider as they assist students in the learning process. Developing curriculum content, choosing teaching strategies, and developing student evaluation plans can be major areas of focus. However, in carrying out these functions, faculty must also consider the legal and ethical concepts that influence the process and product of nursing education.

Just as nurses in practice have guidelines, nurse educators are guided by legal and ethical principles and policies. Nursing faculty are responsible for understanding the broad legal and ethical policies and policies that apply in all circumstances, as well as those specific to their own setting. Major problems can occur if faculty lack an understanding of these principles and policies and are unable to apply them appropriately.

Many potential problems can be avoided if faculty take a proactive approach to anticipate student concerns. Faculty members who treat students with respect, provide honest and frequent communication about progress toward course goals and objectives, and are fair and considerate in evaluating performance are less likely to encounter student challenges. A learning environment that supports student growth and questioning is likely to reduce the incidence of problems, especially litigation. Suggestions for avoiding such problems are discussed later in this chapter. The goal of the educational experience remains that students develop knowledge, skills, and values that will enable them to provide safe, effective nursing care. Nursing faculty who are able to apply general legal and ethical principles are much more likely to play their part in effectively meeting that goal.

The purpose of this chapter is to provide an overview of the legal and ethical issues related to student academic performance that nurse educators most commonly face in the classroom and clinical setting. The chapter includes a discussion of the importance of student–faculty interactions and the legal and ethical issues related to academic performance, including the provision of due process, the student appeal process, assisting the failing student, and academic dishonesty.

STUDENT–FACULTY INTERACTIONS

The student–faculty relationship that is developed during the teaching and learning process is a very important one. Students have often identified student–faculty relationships as the relationships that most often affect learning. Emphasizing the importance and centrality of student–faculty relationships to the learning process, Bevis (1989) defined curriculum as "those transactions and interactions that take place between students and teachers and among students with the intent that learning take place" (p. 72).

Research has indicated that the quality of student–faculty interactions has the potential to either positively or negatively affect the outcome of the educational process by affecting student performance in the classroom and clinical settings and student satisfaction with the nursing program (Halstead, 1996). The National League for Nursing (1993) has stated that the nature of student–faculty relationship should be egalitarian and collaborative. Through the development of collaborative student–faculty partnerships in the learning process, an environment is fostered that allows for professional growth and development on the part of both student and faculty.

Supporting the concept of a collaborative partnership between student and faculty, Millar (1996) proposed that the diverse student population on today's college campuses demands a new approach from educators in the classroom. Students' individual learning needs are diverse and are best met by faculty who view teaching as a dialogical process. Millar stated, "Each person comes by knowledge in the course of addressing the other during interactions, not by absorbing transmittable, objective material. Thus, learning is construed as an inherently dialogical process occurring among knowers who depend on their mutual interaction for the development of new knowledge and their own identities" (p. 161). Faculty who interact with students from a dialogical philosophical framework establish an egalitarian relationship with students that allows faculty and students to work together to achieve satisfactory educational outcomes.

The first step in the process of developing a learning environment that encourages collaborative and positive student–faculty interactions requires faculty to carefully examine and develop an awareness of their own beliefs and values about the teaching–learning process. Working collaboratively with students may require faculty to adopt new strategies that involve active student participation and do not place faculty in the role of having sole responsibility for determining learning experiences. Activities such as cooperative group work, debate and discussion, role playing, and problem-solving exercises are examples of interactive teaching strategies that shift the focus from the faculty to the student. Such a pedagogical shift in teaching may also require faculty to leave behind the "safety" and control of the classroom lecture and develop more fully the skills necessary to successfully incorporate interactive teaching strategies into the classroom. Chapter 13 provides further discussion of teaching strategies that promote active learning.

Another important step in the process of developing a positive learning environment is examining attitudes and beliefs that students bring to the learning environment. Upcraft (1996) stated that many college students appear to lack confidence in their ability to learn and need to be empowered by faculty to believe that they can be academically successful. Empowerment occurs in the teaching process when caring, a sense of commitment, mutual respect, and creativity are evidenced in the student–faculty interactions (Chally, 1992). Having a role in developing their own learning experiences can prove to be an empowering experience for students.

How can nursing faculty successfully incorporate this concept of empowerment and equity into student–faculty relationships? Educators can design learning activities and projects that demonstrate collaborative learning and collegial interactions between faculty, students, and nurses in practice settings (Halstead, 1996). For example, the use of computer-mediated communication, such as e-mail and computer conferencing, tends to remove the elements of status and power from communication, thus allowing a freer exchange of information. Integrating content and discussion about empowerment, collaboration, collegiality, and teamwork throughout the curriculum can also help to nurture positive student–faculty interactions. Faculty involvement in orientation programs, mentoring initiatives, academic advising, and student organizations can help to promote positive student–faculty interactions outside the classroom (Halstead, 1996). Ongoing, open dialogue with students that results in a clear communication of mutual expectations and responsibilities is an essential component of all successful student–faculty interactions, as is illustrated in the remaining sections of this chapter.

LEGAL CONSIDERATIONS OF STUDENT PERFORMANCE

An established responsibility of faculty in nursing education programs is the evaluation of student performance in the classroom (didactic) and clinical setting. This responsibility carries with it accountability because the outcomes of such evaluation have a major impact on the student's progress in the course, and even status in the program. The courts have consistently affirmed faculty members' responsibility for evaluation and have for the most part practiced "judicial deference"—meaning that the court has not interfered with the faculty's expertise in evaluation of student academic performance—as long as due process has been provided and evaluation is deemed fair and just (Smith et al., 2001). However, the evaluation process must be based on principles that ensure that students' rights are not violated.

Student Rights

Faculty must be aware that students enter the educational experience with rights, just as faculty have rights. The concept of "student rights" is a relatively new one in the legal system, developing over the last 5 decades (Brent, 2001). However, there is increasing evidence of the judicial system's perception that student rights are important, and cases supporting and detailing this concept are increasing (for information about specific cases, see Brent [2001] and

Guido [1997]). Rights of students that are addressed here are due process, fair treatment, and confidentiality and privacy.

Due Process

Student rights in the broadest sense are protected by the Fourteenth Amendment of the U.S. Constitution, which limits the restrictions that government may impose on an individual. This amendment states that no citizen may be deprived of life, liberty, or property without due process of law and requires that the federal government provide due process for all citizens.

Due process then involves assurances that procedures are "fair under the circumstances" (Brent, 2001, p. 428). Because the Fourteenth Amendment refers to state or government action, a public institution is always accountable for due process. Private institutions may not be held to these same standards because they are not considered a government arm. However, many private institutions have adopted policies ensuring due process for their students even though courts may not always hold them to that standard. Although private institutions may not always be held to the due process standards, to avoid problems and potential litigation, institutions must ensure that faculty actions are not perceived as "arbitrary, capricious, or discriminatory" (Brent, 2001, p. 428).

Student rights have their foundation in two categories of due process: procedural due process and substantive due process. Procedural due process refers to process steps and requires that "individuals whose rights are affected be entitled to appropriate notice and a hearing" (Osinski, 2003, p. 56). These guidelines mandate that individuals be provided with notification of the concerns and provided with an opportunity to be heard—or to present their case to involved parties in the decision-making process. Substantive due process involves the basis for the decision itself (or the substance of the decision) and is based on the principle that a decision should be fair, objective, and nondiscriminatory. Students who might challenge on this principle would seek to prove that a faculty decision was arbitrary or impulsive.

Other legal concepts that influence student rights come from contract law or theory. Students may also use these concepts in seeking action against an institution. Contract law is applied in this circumstance with the understanding that when students enter a university or college, they actually enter into a contract with the school. If students complete the degree requirements and follow the required procedures, then a degree will be awarded. The implied contract between the student and school forms the basis for much student right–oriented precedent law.

Osinski (2003) differentiated between student concerns or grievances based on academic performance and those based on disciplinary circumstances. Academic concerns are based solely on grades or clinical performance, whereas disciplinary misconduct is based on violation of rules or policies within the school or department. Osinski reported that due process for academic challenges requires that students be informed of the problems and the need to improve, be given a time frame for doing so, and have an understanding of the consequences if they do not. When disciplinary action is considered, different rules apply. In this circumstance the individual must receive notice of the specific charge that is being made and the policy and code that has been violated, and the student must have an opportunity to present a defense against the charges, usually at a formal hearing, but at least in writing. Because disciplinary dismissals may have more long-lasting effects on the individual, more complicated due process rules apply.

Fair Treatment

Students have the right to expect that they will be treated fairly, consistently, and objectively. Standards of expectations for the course provide the objective guide for evaluation and must be communicated to students early and often. Course requirements should be consistent for all students, including classroom and clinical assignments. Students should receive equivalent assignments, even if they are not identical, that allow them to demonstrate progress toward meeting course objectives

Confidentiality and Privacy

Legislation that has been passed to protect health information and the privacy of patients should remind faculty of their obligation to protect information from and about students. The need for confidentiality in the faculty role is based in the same code of ethics that guides all nurses. Students have a right to expect that information about their progress in the program, their academic and clinical performance, and their personal concerns will be kept confidential.

In the course of the teaching role, faculty are often privy to information about students that is of a personal and private nature. Students often confide in faculty about events that may influence their performance in the classroom or may simply seek advice from persons they feel they can trust. This information, as in a nurse–patient interaction, must be guarded and held in confidence. Morgan (2001) pointed out the conflicts nursing faculty often feel when deciding whether it is in the student's best interest to divulge information of a personal nature. She suggested that there should be a "compelling professional purpose" (p. 291), such as protection of patients or helping the student achieve the goal of successful completion of the program, for disclosing confidential personal information. Faculty must exercise good judgment in sharing information, making certain that it is in the student's best interest to do so and obtaining permission whenever possible.

In addition to confidentiality, privacy, especially of student records, is essential. The Buckley Amendment provides the basis for protection of student records. Brent (2001) related that this amendment provides for students over the age of 18 years to have access to their own records, to have information about how to obtain that access, and to control to whom those records are released. The amendment also mandates that a procedure to allow students to contest information in their record that they object to must be in place. Schools of nursing generally follow the guidelines of the institution, they but must give particular attention to guarding student health records, which are usually kept in a separate file and should follow Health Information Portability and Accountability Act of 1996 (HIPAA) guidelines. Student records and evaluation notes maintained by faculty during the process of course evaluation must also be guarded to protect privacy.

Guidelines for Providing Due Process to Students
Due Process for Academic Issues

The potential for litigation always exists, even in the best of circumstances; therefore it is prudent to take actions and establish policies that decrease the likelihood that litigation will occur as a result of academic failure or dismissal. These practices help to keep students informed of faculty expectations and their progress in coursework and provide the basis for ensuring that students receive the information they need.

1. *Provide a copy of student and faculty rights and responsibilities in formal documents.* On admission to the program, students should be given a copy of rights, responsibilities, policies, and procedures that apply to students and faculty. Although institutions have the right to establish policies, they also have the responsibility to communicate those policies and guidelines to students and faculty. Policies and procedures that are in effect for all students in the institution, as well as those that are specific to a program, should be available and must be congruent. Policies should address progression, retention, graduation, dismissal, grading, and conduct. Students should also be informed of circumstances that will interfere with progression and those that would result in termination from the program. They should learn the process to follow in filing a grievance. These policies should be readily available and are usually published in faculty and student handbooks. Strategies that ensure that students have read and understand the information contained in these documents should be a part of the orientation process. In every course faculty should plan to reinforce this information, including providing specific expectations for the course. Written specifics of requirements should be contained in the course syllabus and discussed with students on the first day of class.

2. *Review and update policies in the handbook and catalog periodically.* Published materials given to students and faculty should contain current information about academic policies and procedures. This serves to keep students and faculty informed about the policies and procedures they are subject to, and it is a requirement of institutional and program accreditation agencies. Regular review by faculty of policies and procedures ensures that faculty are aware of current policies and increases the likelihood that they will be consistent in following them.

3. *Course requirements and expectations should be clearly established and communicated at the beginning of the course.* The course syllabus should explain course requirements, critical learning experiences, and faculty expectations of student performance to satisfactorily complete the course. Schools commonly establish guidelines for information to be included in all syllabi developed for nursing courses, and faculty should follow these criteria. A course syllabus should include the

following information, at a minimum: description of the course and the course objectives; course credit hours, faculty responsible for the course, class schedule, attendance policies, teaching strategies used in the course, topical outlines, evaluation tools and methods, due dates for assignments, late work policy, and standards that must be met for students to pass the course. Many institutions also require that course syllabi include a statement about the need for students to notify faculty about desired accommodations for a disability. The syllabus for a course should be distributed the first day of class to provide students the opportunity to understand and clarify course requirements.

4. *Retain all tests and written work in a file until the student has successfully completed at least the course requirements, and in some cases the program requirements.* Student assignments, tests, and evaluations are invaluable, especially in cases of academic deficiency that may result in a student challenge. All evidence of a student's performance in a class should be kept at a minimum until that course is completed. Faculty must be aware of institutional policy or standards that govern maintenance of records and should follow that policy. There are no universal rules for how long student files should be maintained, and the policy may vary from institution to institution. Student clinical evaluations often become a part of the student's permanent file, although in some programs these are only retained until the student completes the program.

   The maintenance of files of student work and tests may also serve to decrease the likelihood of plagiarism of other students' work. Knowing that faculty keep a copy of assignments and tests may make students less likely to attempt to claim other students' work as their own. Files of student work may also serve as examples of assignments to share with evaluators during accreditation visits or to assist in outcome assessment efforts. Samples of student work may also be used to provide positive examples to other students. Faculty must obtain a student's permission to share his or her work with others. Some schools choose to have students sign a standard form granting such permission and keep this on permanent file.

5. *Students should have the opportunity to view all evaluation data that are placed in the student file.* Students have the right to see all documentation that has been used to determine an evaluation of their performance. Students also have the right to disagree with the appraisal of their performance and should be provided with an opportunity to respond to the comments of the evaluation with comments of their own. Faculty should ask students to sign and date the evaluation form to indicate that the evaluation has been discussed with them, while providing an opportunity for them to register their own comments on the form.

6. *When students are not making satisfactory progress toward course objectives and the potential for course failure or dismissal exists, students must receive notification of and information about their academic deficiencies.* Students should receive regular feedback about the progress they have made toward meeting class and clinical objectives throughout the course.

If deficiencies occur, students must receive details of what behavior is unsatisfactory, what needs to be done to improve that behavior, and the consequences if improvement does not occur. Faculty should hold formal conferences with students who are in academic jeopardy, identify the deficiencies in writing, and work with the student to determine a plan to address the deficiencies. Both the faculty member and the student should sign the document to indicate mutual involvement in and agreement to the plan. Subsequent follow-up conferences should be held to note progress or lack of progress made toward achieving the agreed upon goals and note revisions or additional strategies employed. All conferences should be documented in writing, and both parties should receive a copy of the documentation.

Faculty who fail to evaluate a student's unsatisfactory performance accurately, through either a reluctance to expose the student to the experience of failure or a fear of potential litigation, are guilty of misleading the student, potentially jeopardizing patient care, and placing faculty peers in a difficult situation. Nursing faculty and even the university are responsible for preparing safe and competent practitioners and can be held accountable if they relinquish their responsibility for doing so (Smith et al., 2001). Student deficiencies will eventually be identified and dealt with by faculty. Students might legitimately ask why they were not notified earlier in the educational experience of these deficiencies and accuse the "failing" faculty of prejudicial behavior. It is much fairer to inform students of their unsatisfactory behaviors when such behaviors are first identified. Informing students of deficiencies in a caring, constructive manner allows students the opportunity to improve performance; to not inform them denies them this opportunity and right.

These procedures help ensure that students receive the due process related to academic failure that is their right by law. Maintaining open lines of communication with a student who is not progressing is a key component in resolving such situations satisfactorily and decreasing faculty liability. Students are much less likely to sue if they perceive that they have been treated in a fair and impartial manner and have been given information throughout the process.

Due Process for Disciplinary Issues

Students who are dismissed because of misconduct or disciplinary reasons should receive additional assurances that due process has been followed. Students must receive in writing a copy of the charges or concerns that are cited (Osinski, 2003). The information should include details about what policy or rule was violated, and enough information must be provided to ensure that the student can develop a defense against the charges. Osinski reports that students are usually granted the opportunity to speak on their own behalf and provided an opportunity to explain their actions. Students often are allowed to hear the evidence against them and to present oral or written testimony, and they may be allowed to call witnesses in their defense (Smith et al., 2001). If the student desires, legal counsel can be present to provide the student with advice but not to question or interview other participants in the proceedings. Legal counsel for the institution is usually available as well. No action should be taken by the faculty or university until a formal hearing has occurred.

Grievances and the Student Appeal Process

Even when a student has been treated in accordance with due process with a clear communication of policies and expected academic standards, it is possible that the student may wish to seek legal recourse in the face of an academic failure or dismissal. In such cases the student may appeal to the court on the basis that faculty has acted in a capricious or arbitrary manner. Courts have traditionally not overturned academic decisions unless the student can prove that faculty did not follow "accepted academic norms so as to demonstrate the person or committee responsible did not actually exercise professional judgment" (*Ewing v. Regents of the University of Michigan*, 1985, p. 225).

There are other reasons that students may choose to bring suit against an institution. Breach of contract, described earlier, may be charged by students, particularly in private institutions, who may not be provided with due process protections. The court has generally followed the "well-steeled rule that relations between a student and a private university are a matter of contract" (*Dixon v. Alabama Board of Education*, 1961, p. 157). However, there is inconsistency in court cases that address grievances of contract issues depending on the substance of the case. Students may also make charges of defamation or violation of civil rights, including discrimination. Courts generally have not hesitated to analyze cases in which discrimination based on any parameter (e.g., race, gender, age, or disability) has been charged. Brent (2001) reported that the best way to avoid such litigation is to maintain policies that clearly state the institution's and program's guidelines, including a statement that they follow all federal and state laws regulating civil rights.

Goudreau and Chasens (2002) pointed out that recent cases in which nursing faculty have been charged with negligence in terms of protecting students from injury have also occurred. Student safety in the classroom, in the clinical area, and on clinical experiences must be a consideration of nursing faculty. Students must receive adequate preparation and instructions to avoid foreseeable risks, and as these authors stated, "Faculty members are obligated to be as concerned about students' personal safety as they are about patient safety" (p. 45).

The Student Appeal Process

Before seeking the assistance of the court system, students must first use all available recourse within the institution. Guido (1997) reported that the courts have generally relied on academic institutions to deal with grade disputes and have intervened only when due process questions come into consideration. Institutions of higher learning have established policies for hearing student grievances and appeals. An example of such a procedure is available on pp. 50-51. The purpose of these guidelines is to establish common procedures to ensure that students are provided due process and that faculty rights are supported.

STUDENT GRIEVANCE AND APPEAL POLICY FOR INDIANA UNIVERSITY SCHOOL OF NURSING

Policy

The purpose of the Subcommittee on Appeals is to review student-identified problems relevant to student academic and professional status as these have emerged within the context of the student's enrollment at IUSON. The student must be able to provide supporting evidence relevant to the identified problem. This Subcommittee hears and makes recommendations on those appeals brought to the committee that are not resolved at the student-faculty level.

The Subcommittee on Appeals deals only with problems related to student academic and professional standards. Academic problems are defined as those problems/ sets of circumstances that threaten the quality of a student's academic standing. Professional problems are defined as those problems that are viewed by a student as threatening the student's professional reputation or status. Problems involving personality conflicts should be handled on the student-faculty level unless directly related to academic or professional standards. The Subcommittee on Student Appeals has the authority from the Student Affairs Committee of the Council of Nursing Faculties to make recommendations concerning cases that come before its members.

General Procedure

1. The Subcommittee reads the initial problem statement and supporting evidence and makes a decision regarding whether the issue is within the scope of the Subcommittee.
2. The Subcommittee recommends a course of action with respect to the original complaint.

Procedure for Resolution of Appeal Involving Committee Action

1. The student shall attempt to reconcile the conflict or question in face-to-face interaction with the involved party within 10 academic days of the incident.
2. If this attempt at resolution is not satisfactory, the student may request mediation from the administrative person immediately responsible for the involved faculty member. This attempt at mediation shall occur within 5 academic days after the initial attempt at resolution.
3. If no resolution is reached, the appeals procedure may be initiated by the student.

Submission of Evidence

1. Written presentation of evidence
   a. Within 3 academic days after attempts at verbal mediation, the student may formally initiate the process for submission of appeal.
      (1) The student obtains the Student Appeals Application (Form A) from the Chairperson of the Committee on Student Affairs.
      (2) Form A should be completed and returned to the Chairperson of the Committee on Student Affairs within 5 academic days of obtaining Form A. (If the Chairperson determines extenuating circumstances have prevailed, requirements for time limitations regarding submission of the appeal may be waived.)
2. After Form A has been submitted, the Subcommittee (comprised of the Chairperson and six additional people from the Student Affairs Committee) determines whether the student appeal will be processed further. This Subcommittee consists of three faculty members and three students and will be convened as soon as possible by the Chairperson.
3. If the Subcommittee determines that the appeal does not warrant further process, the student will be informed and the next step in the School of Nursing appeal process explained. (The student talks to the appropriate Academic Dean, then the School of Nursing Dean, and finally will be referred to a University level Dean.)
4. If the Subcommittee determines that a full hearing should be given the student
   a. The Chairperson of the Committee on Student Affairs provides a copy of the submitted Form A to the faculty member(s) involved in the complaint, within *5 academic days* after the Subcommittee meets.
   b. The faculty member(s) involved in the complaint has 5 academic days after receipt of notification in which to respond (via Form B) to the Chairperson of the Committee on Student Affairs.
   c. Within 5 academic days after receiving Form B, the Chairperson of the Student Affairs Committee forwards copies of Form A and Form B to members of the Subcommittee on Student Appeals and the administrative person immediately responsible for the faculty member. Should there be no response from the faculty member involved in the appeal, the Subcommittee will process the appeal within 10 academic days.

STUDENT GRIEVANCE AND APPEAL POLICY FOR INDIANA UNIVERSITY SCHOOL OF NURSING—cont'd

Submission of Evidence—cont'd

d. All transactions involving exchange of written materials require signatures of all parties on Form C.

e. New evidence may be submitted in writing at any time before action on the appeal by contacting the Chairperson.

f. The Chairperson (or a faculty member designated by the Chairperson) shall be available to both the student and faculty member for technical advice regarding compilation of data and filing of the appeal. Any designated faculty member shall be knowledgeable about the function of the Student Appeals Subcommittee, but not a member thereof.

5. Verbal presentation of evidence

   a. In the event that the Subcommittee needs further information from any of the parties involved in the appeal, the Chairperson may ask those involved to meet with the Subcommittee in person.

   b. Persons or witnesses involved in the appeal, who wish to underscore their position in the appeal verbally, may meet with the Subcommittee by contacting the Chairperson. The Subcommittee determines whether the request is granted and informs all involved parties.

Access to Evidence

1. All parties receive all completed forms at least 5 academic days before the scheduled Appeals Meeting in which the appeal will be processed.

2. All parties involved in the appeal may be present during verbal presentation of evidence in the Appeals Meeting.

Committee Recommendation Regarding the Appeal

1. Merits of the evidence for the appeal presented in written and verbal form will be discussed while the subcommittee is in session. The six members constitute a quorum. The Chairperson of the Student Affairs Committee is an ex-officio member.

2. If new data are obtained as a result of the statements and questioning of the complainant, respondent, or witnesses, any member of the Subcommittee, the student, or the faculty member shall have the right to request a postponement of the vote. A postponement would have to be voted by a majority of the Subcommittee members. If a postponement is voted by the majority, the hearing would reconvene at a date specified by the Subcommittee.

3. Voting regarding the appeal will be done by secret ballot.

4. The final vote on the appeal indicates one of the following

   a. That the appeal has justification (The Subcommittee then recommends any action that is to be taken.)

   b. That the appeal does not have justification.

5. Each Subcommittee member will support his/her vote with an unsigned written statement explaining the rationale for the recommendation. This written rationale will be filed with other appeals documents and kept in the archives for at least 2 years.

Communication of Appeal Process and Decision

1. Audiotapes of any full appeal procedure will be made and will be available to all parties for review on request for a period of 2 calendar years.

2. The Subcommittee recommendation shall be written to include majority and minority opinions, each accompanied by the respective rationales and given to the parties involved, namely, student, faculty member, the administrative person immediately responsible, and the appropriate Associate Dean in the Academic Program office, within 5 academic days.

Appeal of Committee Action

1. Higher appeal of the Subcommittee's recommendation may be made through the Office of the Dean of the School of Nursing.

Prepared by Subcommittee on Student Appeals at Indiana University School of Nursing, Indianapolis, Indiana.

Institutional and program policies related to student appeals and grievance procedures should be made available in writing to students and faculty. Faculty are usually given this information in the faculty handbook on orientation to the institution. Faculty must be familiar with the policies that guide their practice as educators and should refer to them periodically as changes are made.

Likewise, students should be informed that a formal grievance process policy exists and that it is their responsibility to initiate the procedure. It is recommended that programs distribute this information to students when they are first admitted to the institution and document that students have received such notification. Students may choose not to initiate the grievance procedure that is their right, but they should always be aware of the option of doing so. Information about the appeal process should be reviewed with an individual student if the situation warrants.

When a grievance occurs and the appeal process is implemented, there are two possible outcomes. It is possible that the appeals board may review the information provided and find that there are insufficient grounds for the student's charge and that the assigned grade or faculty action should stand. The other option is that a recommendation for corrective action may be made based on a review of evidence that indicates that the student's charges have merit. This may mean a change of grade or an opportunity for further evaluation. Implementation of the recommendations may vary depending on the specific charges and circumstances. If, at the conclusion of the institutional appeal process, the student is not satisfied with the outcome, the student has the right to pursue further recourse in the court system.

Faculty Role in the Appeal Process

Being involved in the appeals process can be a stressful experience for both the faculty member involved and student. When a student indicates dissatisfaction with an assigned grade or evaluation and is considering an appeal, the faculty member should give consideration to reevaluation. If the faculty member finds the student's evidence is legitimate and that the student truly deserves a higher grade, then the grade should be changed. If the faculty member believes no changes are justified after reviewing the situation and finding that all procedures and standards have been applied consistently and justly, then the faculty member should maintain the assigned grade. However, a faculty member should not act in haste or out of fear in reaction to the threat of a grievance procedure. Changing a grade without justification sets a dangerous precedent and should be avoided. Clear, consistent use of standards for grading that are made known to students will help to effectively support grades that are assigned. Planning before the implementation of a course assignment or activity and providing clearly established grading criteria may help to decrease student misunderstanding.

ACADEMIC PERFORMANCE IN THE CLINICAL AND CLASSROOM SETTINGS

One major responsibility of nursing faculty is the evaluation of student academic performance. In many circumstances faculty are charged with evaluating students both in the classroom (didactic) and clinical settings. Student evaluation is an expectation of faculty at all levels, and one that requires careful consideration for many reasons.

The outcome of evaluations has a major impact on students, and faculty must always be aware of this. Boley and Whitney (2003) report that university faculty do take this responsibility seriously, contrary to what students may believe. The outcome of an evaluation usually means that students progress in the program; however, an unsatisfactory evaluation means that students may face repeat of a course, a delay in their education, and/or removal from the program. These outcomes have financial, emotional, and other costs for students. In addition, faculty may also experience negative consequences, such as emotional distress, pressure from administration to maintain numbers, and a sense of personal failure, when it is necessary to assign a failing grade. In the context of this stressful situation for all involved, faculty must be aware of the legal concepts important to the evaluation process.

Academic Failure in the Clinical Setting

Faculty who teach clinical nursing courses are responsible for guiding students in the development of professional nursing skills and values. Faculty must ensure that the learning experiences chosen provide the student with the opportunity to develop those skills that ensure that they will become safe, competent practitioners. Applying a theoretical knowledge base, developing psychomotor skills, using appropriate communication technique with patients and staff, exhibiting decision-making and organizational skills, and behaving in a professional manner are examples of the types of competencies that nursing students are expected to achieve through their clinical experiences. Faculty are also expected to make judgments and decisions about the ability of students to satisfactorily meet the objectives of the clinical experience. When students are unable to meet the objectives of the clinical experience in a satisfactory manner, faculty have the legal and ethical responsibility to deny academic progression.

Legal and ethical grounds exist for dismissal of a student who is clinically deficient. Nurse Practice Acts exist in all states to regulate nursing practice and nursing education within that given state. Successful graduation from a nursing program should indicate that the student has achieved the minimum competencies required for safe practice.

When providing clinical care, nursing students are held to the same standards as the RN; that is, what would the reasonably prudent nurse with like education and experience do (Guido, 1997). Patients should expect that the care provided be safe, quality care at the level that is needed. In addition, students and faculty are expected to follow professional standards of practice and codes of ethics that have been developed to guide the profession, even though the students' educational experiences are not completed. Individual students are also accountable for their actions and may be held liable for their negligence (Guido, 1977). Students do not "practice on the instructor's license" and are accountable for their own actions, assuming that they have received adequate information and orientation to the clinical assignment.

When engaged in clinical learning experiences, the nursing student is under the supervision of the clinical faculty and the RN in the facility. Both the clinical faculty and the RN in the clinical facility are responsible for the quality of care delivered by students under their supervision. The clinical agency contract that allows for nursing students and faculty to use the facility for learning experiences may also contain a clause stipulating that the school of nursing will provide supervision of students. It is also for the agency to retain the right to request removal of students and faculty if the level of performance does not meet the standard of practice acceptable to the institution. This could also result in the loss of the clinical agency as a site for future clinical experiences. Faculty must accept responsibility for ensuring that students practice with an acceptable level of competence. Failure of clinical faculty to intervene when an unsafe situation exists with a student's level of performance could conceivably place the faculty member, the clinical agency, and the educational institution in a legally liable situation (Guido, 1997).

Clinical faculty have several responsibilities related to the instruction of students. First, clinical faculty must set clear expectations for student performance and communicate these expectations to students before the onset of any learning experience. These expectations must be reasonable for students to meet and must be consistently and equitably applied to all of the faculty member's assigned students. Second, faculty must determine the amount of supervision to provide to students. When determining the appropriate level of supervision, faculty should consider the severity and stability of the assigned patient's condition, the types of treatments required by the patient, and the student's competency and ability to adapt to changing situations in the clinical setting. Therefore it is clear that although individual faculty member expectations must remain consistent for all students, the level of supervision that each student receives may vary depending on the student and the assigned learning experience (Orchard, 1994).

Another responsibility of clinical faculty is to judge the ability of the student to transfer classroom knowledge to the clinical setting (Orchard, 1994). Application of theory to nursing care is an important component of safe nursing practice, and faculty must engage in data collection to determine the level of student performance in this area. Faculty may collect these data in multiple ways. For example, before providing care, students may be asked to develop written care plans and provide the rationale for their proposed nursing interventions. Faculty may also verbally ask students to explain the significance of patient assessment data they have gathered, or students may be asked to keep a weekly journal that provides insight into their clinical decision making. Chapters 15 and 23 provide further discussion of clinical teaching and evaluation. Whatever data collection methods are used by faculty to assess student performance must be consistently applied to all students. It is the clinical faculty's responsibility to remove students from the clinical setting if their performance is unsatisfactory and potentially harmful to patients (Boley & Whitney, 2003).

Fearing legal action, faculty may hesitate to fail a student who performs poorly in the clinical setting. However, federal and state courts have frequently upheld the responsibility and right of faculty to evaluate students' clinical performance and dismiss students who have failed to meet the criteria for a satisfactory performance. The courts have indicated that faculty, as experts in their profession, are best qualified to make decisions about the academic performance of students (Brent, 2001; Guido, 1997; Smith et al., 2001). When teaching a clinical course, faculty can implement a number of steps that will decrease the likelihood that legal action would occur as a result of assigning a failing clinical grade to a student. Faculty must clearly establish and communicate the course and clinical objectives; they must document student performance and effectively communicate with students on an ongoing basis about their progress in the clinical area. These measures are discussed in greater depth in Chapter 15. Key to the success of any of these measures is that there has been clear communication of expectations to students.

As part of this communication faculty should clearly identify at the beginning of the course the clinical objectives and the level of clinical competence that students will be expected to achieve. These requirements should be stated in the course syllabus, along with information about how the clinical grade will be determined for the course. It is also important to identify in writing the types of data that will be used to determine the clinical grade, such as preceptor evaluations, written care plans, patient feedback, direct observation, participation in clinical conferences, skills testing, professional behavior and appearance (Smith et al., 2001), and any other data that are to be used in the evaluation process. Chapter 23 provides more information about the process of clinical evaluation. Students must be informed about how these data will be obtained and whether the clinical evaluation of the student will be formative and/or summative. Students must receive continuing input through a formative evaluation process, periodically providing information about progress and suggestions for improvement. Students must have time to demonstrate the course competency requirements during the clinical experiences and cannot be required to master those competencies until the end of the course.

The consequences of not meeting course objectives should also be clearly communicated to students. All identified course requirements should be congruent with any institutional policies that exist regarding grade assignment and student progression.

Written records of all clinical experiences and student–faculty conferences should be kept for each student during the course. Smith, McKoy, and Richardson (2001) noted that anecdotal records make a significant contribution to the process of clinical evaluation. These records should include notes of the student's daily and weekly assignments and "must be factual and nonjudgmental and should identify both strengths and weaknesses" (p. 37). Written records of a student's learning experiences provide documentation that the student has been provided with adequate opportunity to meet the clinical objectives. Students have the right to expect that they will have clinical experiences that will enable them to meet the course objectives. If opportunities to meet clinical objectives have not been provided, students cannot be evaluated or failed on unmet objectives (Orchard, 1994).

Anecdotal records should be objectively written, describe both positive and negative aspects of a student's performance, and address the objectives of the course. Faculty should avoid commenting on the personality of the student but instead should reflect on what the student has or has not accomplished in relation to the course objectives. Dwelling on the negative aspects of the student's performance to the exclusion of any positive aspects could convey the impression that the faculty member is negatively biased toward the student (Smith et al., 2001). Documenting both aspects of performance indicates that the student's total performance was taken into account when the final clinical grade was assigned.

Throughout the clinical experience, faculty should provide consistent, constructive feedback to students. Identifying positive aspects of a student's clinical performance and areas needing improvement will help that student develop self-esteem and confidence as a practitioner. Feedback is best conveyed in privacy, away from peers, staff, and patients, thus maintaining student confidentiality. Persistent clinical deficiencies should be addressed in conferences with the student, ideally away from the clinical setting. Written records of student–faculty conferences are used to document areas of faculty or student concern that have been discussed, along with the measures that are being taken to correct these deficiencies. Information about the progress the student makes toward correcting clinical deficiencies and any lack of progress should be included in follow-up notes. Both the faculty member and student should sign these written records.

Communicating effectively with a student who is not performing satisfactorily can be difficult. When feedback is given to a student about deficiencies in performance, it is essential for the faculty member to convey to the student a sense of genuine concern about helping the student to improve his or her performance, as well as to convey the faculty member's responsibility for ensuring patient safety in the clinical setting. Students should be allowed the opportunity to clarify and respond to the feedback given by the faculty member. Sometimes an objective third party, such as a department chairperson or course coordinator, can assist by providing an objective perspective of the circumstances and serving as an impartial witness to what was said by both the faculty member and the student.

When notifying a student that course requirements are not being met and failure of the course may result, the faculty member must follow the institutional guidelines that have been established for such situations. Informing a student of unsatisfactory clinical performance can produce a stressful situation for the student. However, it also provides the due process that is the student's right in cases of academic deficiency. It enables the student to understand that his or her performance is unsatisfactory and provides the student with the opportunity to correct deficiencies. It is equally important that the faculty member communicate information about the student's performance to other faculty who are administratively responsible for the course.

Assisting the Failing Student in the Clinical Setting

How do clinical faculty determine when a student's clinical performance is unsatisfactory and warrants failure of the course? How many opportunities should the student be given to learn before being evaluated? These are questions that have been debated in nursing education for decades without resolution. Faculty are responsible for evaluating the cognitive, psychomotor, and affective behaviors of students during clinical learning experiences. Even with reliable and valid evaluation tools, it can be difficult to objectively evaluate the behavior of students, especially in the affective domain. Scanlan, Care, and Gessler (2001) reported that nursing faculty have great difficulty defining behaviors that make a student "unsuited" to nursing. However, once having determined that a student's performance is unsatisfactory and that failure of the course is likely to occur, faculty must implement actions to protect the student's right to due process and assist the student through what will undoubtedly be a stressful experience.

Graveley and Stanley (1993) stated that nursing faculty in public institutions have three legal obligations when working with a student who may potentially fail a clinical course. The first obligation is to strictly follow any institutional policies that have been established for students who are in academic difficulty and face dismissal. Second, the faculty must notify the student of the reasons for the academic dismissal. The student should be referred to any academic review procedures that exist within the school. Third, faculty are obligated to maintain student confidentiality and not speculate about the student's intellectual abilities or lack of preparation for course work with individuals external to the immediate academic setting. Adhering to theses obligations helps to protect the student's right to due process.

There are several guidelines for faculty to use when working with students whose clinical performance is unsatisfactory. For example, as previously mentioned, unsatisfactory clinical behaviors should be identified and discussed with the student as early as possible. Documentation of the student's performance and all conferences with the student should be maintained. At this time faculty should cite the positive aspects of the student's performance in addition to the unsatisfactory aspects (Smith et al., 2001).

Working in collaboration with the student, faculty should develop a plan or "learning contract" in which the needed areas of improvement are identified, along with appropriate measures to ensure improvement of performance. The student should be made aware that isolated instances of good or inadequate performance will not lead to a passing or failing grade. Instead, it is essential that the student strive to develop a consistency of behavior that portrays continuing improvement in performance and the delivery of safe patient care. The student should also understand that successful completion of any remedial work identified in the plan may not be sufficient to ensure a passing grade for the course; satisfactory completion of the course objectives will be required. After the plan has been detailed in a document, both the student and faculty should sign and date it. The student should be given a copy of the plan to refer to and keep for the student's own records.

Frequent feedback sessions are essential during this time as the student attempts to make an improvement in performance. The number of sessions depends on the situation, but it is often helpful to agree to meet on a regular basis, for example, weekly. The faculty member should maintain objective and factual records of all sessions held with the student, including a description of strategies for intervention that were developed. Student self-appraisal should be a part of the process.

The student should also understand that during this period of evaluation increased supervision and observation by faculty may be necessary to continue to ensure that patient safety is maintained. The student may report feeling being treated unfairly or harassed and indicate that the increased faculty supervision is creating a stressful situation. It may be helpful at this time to refer the student to a counselor or other qualified individual for assistance with stress management. The clinical faculty member should refrain from assuming the role of counselor to the student because a conflict of interest could develop that would interfere with the objective and unbiased judgment of the instructor. Morgan (2001) cautioned that faculty, like counselors and therapists, have a responsibility to avoid assuming dual roles, such as counselor and faculty supervisor, when establishing relationships with students.

At times a clinical instructor may experience a sense of concern about a student's performance but has difficulty clearly identifying the unsatisfactory behaviors. The instructor may wish to seek input from another faculty member about the student's performance. Faculty have the right, but no legal responsibility, to obtain an objective evaluation by another faculty member. If this is done, the faculty member must make the student aware of the purpose of this observation and that the results of the objective evaluation may have an impact on the grade awarded.

If the student continues to provide unsafe patient care despite the interventions to improve performance, faculty can withdraw the student from the course before the end of the semester. Students who might qualify for removal from the clinical setting are those who demonstrate a consistent lack of understanding of their limitations, those who clearly and repeatedly cannot anticipate the consequences of their actions or lack of action, and those who consistently fail to maintain appropriate communication with faculty and staff about patient care. A student's being dishonest with faculty and staff about the care provided to a patient has potentially serious legal and ethical implications.

In all of these cases patient care may be jeopardized and unsafe situations may be created for patients. Clinical faculty can refuse to allow a student to continue to provide care in the clinical setting; however, if the student's performance is safe, the student must be allowed to complete the clinical requirements of the course, even if the student is not meeting course objectives. Students are not required to achieve course objectives until the end of the course.

Following the mentioned procedures helps to ensure that students' rights to due process have been upheld. Maintaining effective communication with the student throughout the experience is essential to achieving a satisfactory resolution to the situation for both faculty and student. When students perceive that they have been treated fairly and objectively, most will accept that they were unable to satisfactorily meet the objectives required of the course. Faculty should avoid excessive self-blame for the clinical failure of a student. Scanlan, Care, and Gessler (2001) stated, "Failing students can be viewed as an uncaring practice, when, indeed, it may be more caring to fail students than to allow them to continue" (p. 26).

Academic Failure in the Classroom Setting

Nursing program curricula, which typically include a strong liberal arts and science base, in addition to the many hours of required nursing courses, are by necessity academically rigorous. Academic classroom failure, with a subsequent attrition from the nursing program, is not uncommon, and retention of nursing students is a familiar concern of nurse educators.

The reasons for academic failure in the classroom are numerous. First, students may initially underestimate the amount of time that they will need to devote to course study to be successful in the pursuit of a nursing degree. Students may be unprepared and lack the study and time management skills necessary to organize their schedule and study time appropriately. Students can quickly become overwhelmed with the academic demand of a nursing program, and the resulting stress serves to further increase anxiety and the inability to deal with course requirements.

Second, many of today's nursing students are attempting to fulfill numerous roles, simultaneously juggling the responsibilities and demands of work, family, and school. Role overload becomes excessive, and the student's grades are adversely affected.

Third, some students have difficulty with the level of cognitive ability required in nursing courses. Although adept at memorizing facts and information, they are not able to apply the concepts and develop the appropriate decision-making abilities. This is usually demonstrated by their inability to perform well on tests that demand application, analysis, and synthesis levels of cognition. Students who have never before been required to think on these levels may become frustrated when they spend much time memorizing information but still do not perform well on tests.

Some students may have learning disabilities that affect their ability to read with comprehension, successfully take tests, memorize information, or maintain concentration. These are students who often have satisfactory clinical performance but are unable to perform well in the classroom setting. See Chapter 4 for further discussion of students with learning disabilities. Students for whom English is a second language may also experience these difficulties.

Faculty have an ethical responsibility to identify students who are considered to be at high risk for academic failure in the classroom. Examples of high-risk characteristics include low grade point average, low standardized test scores, decreased critical thinking skills, attendance at several universities without attaining a degree (Donovan, 1989), and difficulty achieving satisfactory grades in required science courses. When students who have these characteristics are accepted into a nursing program, academic support services must be provided to increase their chances of success.

Faculty also have the responsibility for developing and providing supports services that increase students' chances for success and thus increase student retention in the nursing program (Donovan, 1989). Examples of services that can assist students academically are tutoring programs, study sessions, faculty–student mentoring programs, test taking support, and time and stress management training. Faculty should be aware of resources within other departments in the institution that can offer valuable assistance to students in need. They should also encourage activities that provide a support system for students, such as participation in student clubs and organizations. Developing and providing support services for students with academic difficulties helps to ensure that students receive the assistance they need at the earliest possible intervention point.

Assisting the Failing Student in the Classroom Setting

When designing intervention programs that will assist students to be academically successful in a nursing program, faculty must consider the academic experience from the perspective of the student because this may have major implications for student retention and success. Faculty should obtain feedback from students in the program about their areas of concern, both academic and nonacademic. For example, if students believe that large class size is interfering with their ability to learn, strategies that provide students with access to faculty in small groups could be implemented. Student focus groups can provide much feedback, and faculty can use this information to develop interventions. Faculty also need input about what programs or interventions are working (e.g., tutoring services, orientation programs, peer-to-peer study assistance groups) so that these can be continued or eliminated according to their success in meeting student need. Faculty need to know what concerns students have that can be addressed with appropriate resources. Using this information, faculty would be able to develop a retention intervention program designed to maximize students' positive experiences and enhance academic success.

More specifically, faculty can implement several proactive strategies that support students' academic efforts in the classroom. First, faculty should remain aware of the changing student population and students' different learning styles. Nurse educators need to develop innovative, flexible programs designed to support the academic needs of the increasing numbers of nontraditional adult learners, graduate students, and culturally diverse students. Flexible class scheduling, the use of technology for convenient learning times for students, campus child care, recognition of students' life experiences, and support for students with English as a second language can all help students achieve their educational goals. The learning expectations and strategies of today's college students are likely to be different than those of students of the past. Much literature has been published that addresses the varying learning styles of the current generation, and information gained from those studies should be used to provide meaningful learning experiences for students.

Courage and Godbey (1992) suggested that interaction with faculty, peers, and staff is important for students' successful integration into the academic environment. Students who are successfully integrated academically and socially into the academic environment will more likely be retained in the system. Institutions must realize that students bring diverse needs to the educational process. The role of the faculty advisor is key in assisting students to successfully adjust to their academic responsibilities. Faculty need to be informed about academic policies that have an impact on student advisement so that they are able to provide accurate, timely information.

Williams (1993) also emphasized the importance of the faculty advisor in aiding student retention in nursing programs. In addition, Williams suggested that improving the cultural competence of faculty and developing orientation programs and support services for new students can assist in decreasing student anxiety and increase the likelihood of success in nursing studies. Nursing associations or organizations can be a source of encouragement for students and can serve as a vehicle for socializing students into the nursing profession.

Fisher and Parkinson (1998) reported success with involving students in the process of determining what strategies support a positive classroom learning environment. They suggested that students are able to identify what kinds of faculty activities significantly contribute to their learning and that students be actively involved in evaluating and establishing the classroom environment.

Individually, faculty members can take several steps to assist students who are doing poorly in the classroom. When a student demonstrates evidence of a lack of understanding of content of the course, such as failing a test or not completing an assignment properly, the faculty member should meet with the student to identify the student's perspective of the problem. Students are often able to recognize the problem themselves, such as not enough time spent in preparation, lack of understanding of the material, or personal problems. Each of these reasons for poor performance requires the use of different intervention strategies, and the student should be involved in determining what actions are to be taken. Tests should be reviewed to assess the areas of difficulty and to determine whether the problem is potentially related to, for example, lack of knowledge about content, reading difficulties, anxiety associated with test taking, poor study skills, or personal difficulties. Once the potential causes have been identified, intervention strategies can be designed and implemented to help correct the situation. Faculty must realize that it is the student's responsibility to learn, as well as the student's responsibility to use the resources available to improve academic performance. Students must take responsibility for carrying out the plan of action developed in conjunction with the faculty member. Faculty cannot assume responsibility for ensuring that all students are successful in the course, but they must make certain that students are active participants in identifying concerns, developing strategies to address deficiencies, and improving performance.

If, despite various efforts, a student cannot satisfactorily meet the course requirements, faculty have no alternative but to assign a failing grade. At this point the student will require guidance and support as the available options are reviewed. If this is the first nursing course that the student has failed, it is commonly program policy to allow one retake of the course. If this is the second nursing course failure for the student, the student may be dismissed from the program. The student should receive appropriate academic advice as he or she plans future educational goals.

ETHICAL ISSUES RELATED TO ACADEMIC PERFORMANCE

The previous discussion related to academic performance and assisting the failing student emphasized the importance of student–faculty interactions that are characterized by mutual respect and open communication. It is apparent, though, that there is the potential for student–faculty conflict to develop in these interactions. Faculty should consider the ethical implications that exist in relationships developed with students. This section addresses ethical issues that can develop in student–faculty relationships, including academic dishonesty and the nature of interactions occurring between students and faculty. Suggestions for avoiding the development of unethical situations are provided.

Academic Dishonesty

A student copies from another student during a test or uses "crib" notes; another student agrees to help an academically weaker student by providing answers to a test. Lacking the time it takes to write term paper, a student turns in a paper written by another student, yet another student plagiarized portions of a term paper, taking the chance that the professor will never detect the omission of appropriate reference citations. During a clinical experience, a student forgets to administer a medication on time. Fearing the consequences of admitting the error, the student instead documents it as "given." After all, the patient experienced no "real" harm, did he? These are all examples of academic dishonesty, or "cheating," representing one of the most difficult situations faculty have to deal with in their interactions with students. Unfortunately, such incidents are not uncommon. Numerous reports detail alarming statistics that demonstrate an increasing occurrence and acceptance of cheating in schools at every level.

What are some of the factors influencing a student's decision to be dishonest? Jeffreys and Stier (1995) divided the possible influencing factors into two categories: student factors and faculty factors. Student factors that influence student dishonesty include (1) psychological factors, such as stress resulting from pressure to perform well, test taking anxiety, and the student's own expectations for success; (2) ethical factors, such as valuing success at any price; (3) social factors, such as competitiveness and the belief that "everyone else cheats"; and (4) environmental factors that encourage cheating, such as a large class size and reuse of test items. Faculty factors that may influence student dishonesty include difficulty confronting students and fear of potential grievance procedure if one accuses a student of dishonesty. In addition, a faculty member's own values and standards will influence perceptions of student actions (Jeffreys & Stier, 1995).

Faculty can take a number of actions to deter cheating in their courses. One of the most common forms of academic dishonesty is cheating on classroom tests. This may be done by copying from another student's test, with or without the cooperation of the other student, concealing and bringing into the classroom potential answers to the test, or obtaining test questions from students who were previously enrolled in the course. Developing alternate test forms that can be used in subsequent semesters can help decrease the likelihood of questions being shared between classes of students. Alternative test forms can also be used among students in the same class, thus decreasing the chance that students can cheat by looking at the test of the student sitting next to them. Requiring students to leave books and other personal items at the front of the classroom or under their desks and rearranging the seating can also make it more difficult for students to cheat. Directing students to look only at their own tests can serve to remind students that their behavior is being observed and that they are responsible for not conveying the appearance of cheating.

Another common method of cheating is plagiarism of written work, either through the use of papers written by other students or the inappropriate citation of references. Students may be unclear about what constitutes plagiarism; therefore faculty might consider clarifying this at the beginning of the course, including how and when citing is to be done and what consequences will take place if plagiarism occurs. This may reduce the number of "I did not know that was wrong" excuses from students. Requesting that copies of the references cited in written work be turned in with the assignment can facilitate faculty review of the materials and reduce the likelihood that the student will deliberately plagiarize. Keeping on file copies of past student papers can also decrease the likelihood that students will be able to represent a previous student's work as their own. Sometimes students are pressured into helping another student cheat on course work, either through a misguided sense of feeling sorry for and wanting to "help" the student or sometimes through fear. It can be helpful to periodically review the institution's policy on academic dishonesty with students in the class, especially if the faculty member suspects there may be a problem. Many students do not realize that institutional policies commonly state explicitly that a student participating in and enabling another student to cheat is also guilty of academic dishonesty and may be disciplined as well. Also, most institutions have policies that provide guidance for students who feel that they are being verbally and otherwise harassed by another student.

Solomon and DeNatale (2000) described the use of a programwide convocation to discuss the issue of academic dishonesty, maintaining that drawing the analogy between academic dishonesty and professional ethics is an important first step in socializing students into the nursing profession. Davis et al. (1996) recommended the development of an academic honor code as a proactive stance to discourage dishonesty and to foster the development of a professional value system. An academic honor code should define what activities constitute academic misconduct, what disciplinary action could result if the student engages in such activity, and the student grievance and appeal procedure. McCabe and Trevino (1996) reported that some evidence exists to suggest that the presence of a campus academic honor code creates an environment where cheating is not a socially acceptable behavior and decreases the number of incidences of student dishonesty. It is also helpful if written statements on course syllabi are used to remind students of the institution's policy on academic dishonesty and the academic code of honor if one exists.

The consequences of cheating and violating the honor code should also be clearly delineated in the course syllabus. If cheating has occurred, does the student get an F for the assignment or an F for the course? Or, are other options a possibility? This information can be included in the evaluation section of the syllabus and lets students know that any incidents of cheating will be taken seriously by the faculty member.

If a faculty member has evidence that a student has engaged in some form of academic dishonesty, it becomes necessary for him or her to confront the student about the incident. Jefferys & Stier (1995) recommended that the following steps be followed when discussing an incident of academic dishonesty. Privacy should first be ensured for the student when initiating discussion of the incident. It is appropriate to include an impartial third party, such as the department chairperson or another faculty member, in the discussion. Faculty must clearly communicate to the student the identified dishonest behavior and the potential consequences resulting from this behavior. It is important that faculty convey this information in an objective manner, avoiding blame or anger. The student should be informed of institutional policies and the importance of adhering to professional standards of conduct. The conference should be documented by the faculty member. As mentioned previously in the section regarding disciplinary action and due process, the student's right to due process should be ensured before any action is taken.

Student–Faculty Relationships

The nature of the relationships that students develop with faculty in the classroom and clinical setting can have a profound influence on the quality of the students' education experiences. Students commonly identify collegial relationships with faculty as those characterized by mutual respect and collaboration. Such relationships promote personal and professional growth opportunities for both students and faculty. Student–faculty interactions can have ethical implications as well, however.

Novice faculty often are uncertain about how to appropriately develop relationships with students. This can have a major impact on the success of faculty in the classroom and their personal satisfaction with their role as an educator. A lack of supportive, collaborative interactions between a faculty member and a student can also affect the student's learning outcome. Faculty may indeed be very knowledgeable about the content they teach, but if they cannot relate in a positive manner to students, the students may not listen to the substance of the information being conveyed. Novice faculty should be encouraged to seek guidance on how to develop an effective interpersonal style with students (Halstead, 1996).

Behaviors that help develop effective relationships with students are those that have been described throughout this chapter. Open, ongoing dialogue with students throughout the educational process is essential. Students have the right to expect from faculty respect for their ideas and opinions (although not necessarily agreement); constructive, helpful feedback on their academic performance; a willingness to answer questions and address concerns the student may have; and a respect for student confidentiality. Displaying an appropriate sense of humor and warmth with students is also important and allows students to see the human side of faculty.

Behaviors that are inappropriate and unethical in the teaching situation include using sarcasm or belittling the student, threatening the student with failure, criticizing the student in front of others, acting superior, discussing confidential student issues with other faculty, and displaying inappropriate sexual behavior. Showing favoritism in the treatment or grading of students, refusing to answer students' questions, behaving rudely, and being an authoritarian are other examples of unethical teaching behaviors. Student–faculty interactions that are based on the inappropriate use of power and control cannot result in caring, collegial relationships.

Faculty can foster the development of positive student–faculty relationships through the design of learning experiences that promote collaborative, collegial learning exchanges between faculty and students. Faculty need to examine their beliefs about the teaching–learning process and student–faculty relationships to gain an understanding of their own attitudes. Conceptualizing the student–faculty relationship as a collaborative partnership, instead of an authoritarian relationship, is a first step in the process of fostering a learning environment that is empowering for both faculty and students (Halstead, 1996).

SUMMARY

This chapter has provided an overview of the legal and ethical issues that are related to the academic performance of students. Academic failure in the classroom and clinical setting was discussed, as were methods of assisting students through this difficult experience, while ensuring their rights to due process. The importance of clear, mutual communication of expectations between students and faculty was emphasized.

Nursing students in today's classroom exhibit different characteristics from those exhibited by students when many current nursing faculty members were students. They bring a richness of life experiences and provide diversity in values, beliefs, and ideals. Each student is an individual possessing a variety of knowledge, skills, values, beliefs, and needs that will help form the nursing professional the nursing student wishes to become. It is important for nurse educators to meet the needs of these students by establishing professional relationships that are positive and empowering in nature, ultimately providing students with a learning environment that supports their personal and professional goals.

REFERENCES

Bevis, E. (1989). Nursing curriculum as professional education: Some underlying theoretical models. In E. Bevis & J. Watson (Eds), *Toward a caring curriculum: A new pedagogy for nursing*. New York: National League for Nursing Press.

Boley, P., & Whitney, K. (2003). Grade disputes: Considerations for nursing faculty, *Journal of Nursing Education, 42*(5), 198-203.

Brent, N. (2001). *Nurses and the law: A guide to principles & applications*. Philadelphia: W. B. Saunders.

Chally, P. (1992). Empowerment through teaching. *Journal of Nursing Education, 31*(3), 117-120.

Courage, M. M., & Godbey, K. L. (1992). Student retention: Policies and services to enhance persistence in graduation. *Nurse Educator, 17*(2), 29-32.

Davis, M., Johnston, S., DiMicco, W., Findlay, M., & Taylor, J. (1996). The case for a student honor code and beyond. *Journal of Professional Nursing, 12*(1), 24-30.

Dixon v. Alabama State Board of Education, 294 F.2d 150. (5th Cir. 1961).

Donovan, M. (1989). The "high-risk" student: An ethical challenge for faculty. *Journal of Professional Nursing, 5*(3), 120.

Ewing v. Regents of University of Michigan, 474U.w. 214, 106 S. Ct 507 (1985).

Fisher, D. L., & Parkinson, C. A. (1998). Improving nursing education classroom environments. *Journal of Nursing Education, 37*(5), 232-236.

Goudreau, K. A., & Chasens, E. R. (2002). Negligence in nursing education. *Nurse Educator, 27*(1), 42-46.

Graveley, E. A., & Stanley, M. (1993). A clinical failure: What the courts tell us. *Journal of Nursing Education, 32*(3), 135-137.

Guido, G. (1997). *Legal issues in nursing.* Stamford, CT: Appleton & Lange.

Halstead, J. (1996). The significance of student-faculty interactions. In K. Stevens (Ed.), *Review of research in nursing education: Vol VII.* New York: National League for Nursing.

Jeffreys, M. R., & Stier, L. A. (1995). Speaking against student academic dishonesty: A communication model for nurse educators. *Journal of Nursing Education, 34*(7), 297-304.

McCabe, D. L., & Trevino, L. K. (1996). What we know about cheating in college: Longitudinal trends and recent developments. *Change, 28*(1), 28-33.

Millar, S. (1996). New roles for teachers in today's classrooms. In R. Menges, M. Weimer (Eds.), *Teaching on solid ground: Using scholarship to improve practice.* San Francisco: Jossey-Bass.

Morgan, J. E. (2001). Confidential student information in nursing education. *Nurse Educator, 26*(6), 289-292.

National League for Nursing. (1993). *A vision for nursing education.* New York: Author.

Orchard, C. (1994). The nurse educator and the nursing student: A review of the issue of clinical evaluation procedures. *Journal of Nursing Education, 33*(6), 245-251.

Osinski, K. (2003). Due process rights of nursing students in cases of misconduct. *Journal of Nursing Education, 42*(2), 55-58.

Scanlan, J., Care, W., & Gessler, S. (2001). Dealing with the unsafe student in clinical practice. *Nurse Educator, 26*(1), 23-27.

Smith, M., McKoy, Y., & Richardson, J. (2001). Legal issues related to dismissing students for clinical deficiencies. *Nurse Educator, 26*(1), 33-38.

Solomon, M., & DeNatale, M. (2000). Academic dishonesty and professional practice: A convocation. *Nurse Educator, 25*(6), 270-271.

Upcraft, M. (1996). Teaching and today's college students. In R. Menges, M. Weimer (Eds.), *Teaching on solid ground: Using scholarship to improve practice.* San Francisco: Jossey-Bass.

Williams, R. P. (1993). The concerns of beginning nursing students. *Nursing and Health Care, 14*(4), 178-184.

4

TEACHING STUDENTS WITH DISABILITIES

Betsy Frank, PhD, RN, Judith A. Halstead, DNS, RN

Nursing students with special needs present a challenge to nursing faculty in both the classroom and clinical settings. Students who have special needs include those who have a physical disability, such as a visual or hearing impairment; a chronic illness; a learning disability; or a chemical dependency problem. Many nursing programs have had some experience in meeting the needs of these students. Magilvy and Mitchell (1995) surveyed 200 undergraduate nursing programs (associate and baccalaureate) to determine how many have had experience with educating students with special needs. The following experiences were reported by 68 of the schools responding to the survey: 57% had experience with learning disabled students, 40% had experience with students who had social or emotional problems, 37% had experience with students with auditory problems, 25% had experience with students who had a chronic illness, 19% had experience with students with a mobility impairment, 12% had experience with visually impaired students, and 7% had experience with students who had mixed disabilities. More recently Colon (1997) surveyed 54 nursing programs. Of the 45 schools that responded, one half admitted students with learning disabilities and one third graduated students with learning disabilities. Persaud and Leedom (2002) surveyed schools in California. Of the 52 schools that responded, the majority had admitted students with a variety of emotional and physical disabilities, including mental illness, impaired vision, back injury, and hearing loss. Most schools (82%) responded that the accommodations that had to be made were reasonable, but 16% thought that the accommodations were not reasonable. Their results show that what are considered reasonable accommodations causes some conflict for nursing faculty. Persaud and Leedom go on to challenge nursing faculty to consider what are essential nursing functions and how can these functions be met in a variety of ways.

This chapter addresses the issues related to the education of students with disabilities. It specifically focuses on students with learning disabilities, physical disabilities, mental health problems, and chemical impairment problems because of the more common occurrence of these problems among college students. The Rehabilitation Act of 1973, the Americans with Disabilities Act of 1990, and the significance of these acts to nursing education are also addressed.

LEGAL ISSUES RELATED TO STUDENTS WITH DISABILITIES

Faculty should be aware of the legal issues that are associated with teaching students with disabilities. In recent years two laws in particular, the Rehabilitation Act of 1973 and the Americans with Disabilities Act of 1990, have greatly influenced the educational environment for students with disabilities on college campuses.

Rehabilitation Act of 1973

The Rehabilitation Act of 1973 states that individuals with disabilities cannot be denied access to, or participation in, any program or activity that receives federal funding. Section 504 of this act specifically addresses higher education and prohibits public postsecondary institutions that receive federal funds from discriminating against individuals with disabilities. As a result of this act, colleges and universities have experienced an increased number of students with disabilities admitted to their programs.

The Americans with Disabilities Act of 1990

The Americans with Disabilities Act (ADA) protects the rights of individuals with disabilities in the arenas of education, employment, and environmental accessibility. In higher education, individuals with disabilities are guaranteed equal access to educational opportunities. Discrimination against individuals with physical and mental disabilities is prohibited by the ADA. However, the ADA does not guarantee that an admitted student will achieve academic success—only that the student has the opportunity to achieve academic success (Gordon & Keiser, 1998).

The full impact of the ADA on professional education has yet to be determined. However, as Magilvy and Mitchell (1995) stated, "It is clear that the criteria for admission to professional educational programs must be stated in terms of the program's academic requirements, not in terms of the student's functional abilities" (p. 31). Failure of an institution to make reasonable accommodations to a student who is disabled is considered discrimination (Helms & Weiler, 1993), and the institution and faculty may be sued for failing to make reasonable accommodations.

Implications for Nursing Education

By law it is considered the student's responsibility to notify the institution that a disability and need for accommodation exist (Helms & Weiler, 1993; Letizia, 1995). Students who have a disability and require accommodation are encouraged to share this information with the institution's office for students with disabilities. See Box 4-1 for an example of a statement of services provided for students with disabilities. Sharing this information is voluntary, however, because students are not legally required to inform the institution that a disability exists. If the student does share this information with the office for students with disabilities, the office may not share this information with faculty unless the student has provided written consent to such notification. When consent is provided, faculty are told that a disability exists and what type of accommodation is required. Even when student consent is given to share information with faculty, the nature of the disability is not disclosed to faculty unless the student decides to disclose it. Faculty are not allowed to inquire about the nature of the disability. In fact, decisions regarding whether accommodation is possible must be made after the student has been admitted, unless essential abilities are published and all students are asked before admission whether they possess the abilities needed for academic success (Christensen, 1998).

When considering the admission of a student who has a disability, admission committees in schools of nursing must consider the following questions:

- Disregarding the disability, is the individual otherwise qualified to be admitted to the program?
- What reasonable accommodations can the school make to enable the student to be successful in the pursuit of becoming a nurse?

Although institutions are not expected to lower or alter academic or technical standards to accommodate a student with a disability, they are expected to determine what accommodations would be reasonable for a student who is disabled. Examples of reasonable accommodations would include altering the length of test taking times or methods, providing proctors to read tests or write test answers, allowing additional time to complete the program of studies, providing supplemental study aids such as audiotapes of texts, providing note takers, or altering the method of course delivery. The same considerations must be given to students who become disabled during their

---

Box 4-1
STATEMENT OF SERVICES PROVIDED FOR STUDENTS WITH DISABILITIES

Services for Persons with Disabilities

Students who need adaptations in their learning environment may obtain help through the services located in the Student Academic Services Center. Services include assistance in accessing recorded textbooks or readers for the blind and learning disabled. This office also arranges for note takers or signers for hearing impaired persons. Alternate testing procedures may be arranged as needed. Services for persons with disabilities are based on individual needs and the University's intent to offer appropriate accommodations according to the student's documentation of need for same. These services are coordinated by the Student Support Services Grant Program. It is recommended that persons with disabilities visit Indiana State University before making a decision to enroll.

Courtesy Indiana State University Undergraduate Catalog, 2003-2004.

enrollment in a nursing program. Questions to be asked would include the following:

- Disregarding the disability, is the student otherwise qualified to continue in the nursing program?
- What reasonable accommodations can be made to allow the student to continue?

Regulations established by the U.S. Department of Education have stated "that only those academic requirements that are essential to the program or the license will not be required to be modified so as to meet the needs of a student with disabilities" (Helms & Weiler, 1993, p. 359). Faculty should consider in their decision making that just because a student has a disability he or she is not necessarily ill, and the type of support needed is not the type needed to cure an illness but to support health (Sowers & Smith, 2002). Marks (2000) suggests that how those with a disability are viewed is a result of social constructs. Whether a person's limitations are viewed as a disability is defined by society rather than through the actual abilities of the person involved. Thus making the decision regarding what is a reasonable accommodation for a person with a disability is a complex process that may be influenced as much by attitude as by actual abilities of the student. Marks goes even further and suggests that by referring to those with disabilities as those with "special needs" invites discrimination against persons with disabilities. As more students with disabilities enter higher education, the advice given by Sowers and Smith and Marks seems worthy of consideration. More recently Sowers and Smith (2002) have challenged nursing faculty to adopt a more open attitude in accommodating those students with disabilities.

As the impact of the ADA on nursing education continues to unfold in the courts, nurse educators must keep current with legal developments that relate to the education of individuals with disabilities pursuing degrees in the health professions. Some suggestions for increasing faculty awareness of the needs of students with disabilities include periodic continuing education sessions related to the legal implications of educating such students and the use of consultants who are experts in working with students with disabilities. Most institutions of higher education have an office dedicated to assisting and supporting students with disabilities who are enrolled on campus. This office can provide resources and expert advice to faculty and students. Another source of information may be individuals with disabilities who have successfully developed a career in nursing. These successful nurses can help nursing faculty understand the issues involved in educating students with disabilities and can also serve as mentors to students with disabilities who are pursuing a nursing education (Magilvy & Mitchell, 1995).

Nursing faculty must begin to separate the truly *essential* components of nursing education from the merely traditional nursing curricula and teaching strategies. Magilvy and Mitchell (1995) and Sowers and Smith (2002) have suggested that nursing faculty need to consider such philosophical issues as whether nursing education might be extended to those individuals who will never practice bedside nursing in the "traditional" manner. Such nursing jobs might include staff development, infection control, and case management. A more recent study of admission and retention practices of California nursing schools (Persaud & Leedom, 2002) shows that despite more than a decade of experience with the ADA, nursing faculty still struggle with what are reasonable accommodations that balance student access with patient safety. In making admission and progression decisions, faculty need to balance student rights, safety, and abilities with issues of patient safety and university responsibility for providing appropriate accommodations according to the ADA (Wadkins & Kurz, 1997). Having an ongoing evaluation plan that shows how making appropriate accommodations affects student outcomes in terms of graduation and subsequent employment is essential (Wadkins & Kurz, 1997). As the role of the nurse continues to evolve in response to societal needs and expectations, this issue deserves the full attention of the nursing profession.

Some schools of nursing, as well as other professional schools, have identified in writing the abilities that students need to possess to be successful in their chosen educational program. The essential abilities that students need to possess for successful progression through the nursing program at one school of nursing are presented in Box 4-2. The skills deal mostly with the cognitive realm of learning.

Many students fear that revealing their disability will jeopardize their student status (Maheady, 1999). Often the barriers for these students are more attitudinal on the part of peers and faculty than physical. However, caring relationships with faculty are the key to successful integration of students with disabilities (Beilke & Yssel, 1998).

THE NURSING STUDENT WITH A LEARNING DISABILITY

Learning disabilities are the most common type of student disability found on college campuses (Eliason, 1992) and in nursing programs (Watson, 1995). Colon (1997) found that more than one third of North Carolina nursing schools had experience with students with learning disabilities. Colon further states that perhaps the other schools had students who had learning disabilities but were unidentified.

Frequently students begin college without their learning disabilities being detected. However, persons with learning disabilities are presumed to have lifelong difficulties with learning, whether the disabilities are diagnosed or not (Selekman, 2002). In nursing education learning disabilities are commonly first detected when faculty notice striking differences between a student's classroom and clinical performance. The student may display an adequate knowledge base and competent skills during clinical experiences but be unable to demonstrate the same degree of knowledge when taking tests in the classroom. Such disparities in performance lead to much frustration and stress for the student and, not uncommonly, academic failure. Faculty should have an understanding of the characteristics of learning disabilities so that they can refer students for the appropriate assistance from counselors.

The National Joint Committee on Learning Disabilities (1997) states the following:

> Learning disabilities is a general term that refers to a heterogeneous group of disorders manifested by significant difficulties in the acquisition and

Box 4-2
ESSENTIAL ABILITIES REQUIREMENTS

The University is committed to helping temporarily and permanently disabled students make t
transition to student life. Students with physical, mental, or learning impairments are enco
aged to consult with counselors from the School of Nursing and Adaptive Educational Services
assistance in meeting degree requirements. Students with disabilities must meet all academic a
technical skill requirements of their program.

The Indiana University School of Nursing faculty have specified essential abilities critical to
success of students enrolled in any Indiana University nursing program. Students must dem
strate the following essential abilities (technical standards) with or without reasonable acco
modations to meet all progression criteria:

- **Essential judgment skills,** including the ability to identify, assess, and comprehend conditi
  surrounding patient situations, for the purpose of problem solving and coming to appropri
  conclusions and/or courses of action.
- **Essential neurological functions,** including the ability to use the senses of sight, heari
  touch, and smell, to make correct judgments regarding patient conditions for the purpose
  demonstrating the competence to safely engage in the practice of nursing. Behaviors t
  demonstrate essential neurological functions include, but are not limited to, observing,
  tening, understanding relationships, writing, and employing psychomotor abilities.
- **Essential communication skills,** including the ability to communicate effectively with fell
  students, faculty, patients, and all members of the health care team. Skills include verbal, w
  ten, and nonverbal abilities consistent with effective communication.
- **Essential emotional coping skills,** including the ability to demonstrate the mental health n
  essary to safely engage in the practice of nursing as determined by professional standards
  practice.
- **Essential intellectual and conceptual skills,** including the ability to measure, calculate, analy
  synthesize, and evaluate, to engage competently in the safe practice of nursing.
- **Other essential behavioral attributes,** including the ability to engage in activities consiste
  with safe nursing practice without demonstrated behaviors of addiction to, abuse of,
  dependence on alcohol or other drugs that may impair behavior or judgment. The stude
  must demonstrate responsibility and accountability for actions as a student in the School
  Nursing and as a developing professional nurse.

Data from Campus Bulletin 2002-2004 IUPUI. Retrieved February 25, 2004, from http://www.bulletin.iupui.e

use of listening, speaking, reading, writing, reasoning, or mathematical
skills.

These disorders are intrinsic to the individual, presumed to be due to central nervous system dysfunction, and may occur across the life span. Problems
in self-regulatory behaviors, social perception, and social interaction may
exist with learning disabilities but do not, by themselves, constitute a learning disability. (¶ 2 & 3)

Characteristics of Learning Disabilities

Learning disabilities may manifest as a number of characteristics, each necessi-
tating a different treatment and accommodation. Some students may have reading or spelling difficulties or difficulty with language, memory, or nonverbal
processing, whereas others have math difficulties. It is estimated that 80% to
90% of students with learning disabilities have difficulty with language, memory, or both. Memory difficulties, such as trouble remembering details and

sequencing, commonly lead to reading and spelling difficulties. Additional characteristics that may indicate the presence of a learning disability include poor handwriting; distractibility with difficulty concentrating; a history of poor academic performance; difficulty meeting deadlines; anxiety and low self-esteem (Shuler, 1990); difficulty following verbal instructions; and difficulty organizing ideas in writing, or the inability to articulate ideas verbally but the ability to articulate them in writing. Students may also have auditory processing deficits that have an impact on their ability to recite from memory (Selekman, 2002).

Nursing faculty must remember that learning disabilities are highly individualized and that each student manifests a different grouping of characteristics (Selekman, 2002). Also, faculty should remember that students with learning disabilities have average or above average intelligence and have often developed significant strengths that offset the identified weaknesses. Having a learning disability does not mean that a student should not be expected to achieve the same learning objectives as other students. It does mean, however, that the student may need accommodations for the learning disability to be academically successful, and educators are required by law to provide the necessary accommodations.

Accommodating Learning Disabilities

When faculty believe that a student, previously undiagnosed, may have a learning disability, the initial action is to refer the student to an expert in learning disabilities for assessment. After the diagnosis is made, a plan for accommodation of the disability can be developed. Often the plan calls for both remediation activities and accommodation. If the student grants written permission, the learning expert and faculty can communicate to assist in the implementation of the plan for accommodation (Shuler, 1990). Faculty members who are made aware of a student's disability are not allowed to discuss that information with additional faculty members unless the student gives permission.

Depending on the type of learning disability, a variety of accommodations may be appropriate for the student. Students who have memory difficulties may have difficulty with remembering details and taking notes but will be able to grasp concepts. These students find learning to be a fatiguing experience and will usually experience greater success when learning activities that incorporate "hands-on" and observation experiences are included in the teaching strategies (Eliason, 1992). Such students may also benefit from the assistance of an in-class note taker. This allows students to concentrate on classroom discussion without the distraction of trying to take notes. Some students have difficulty processing multiple stimuli at once. These students may need specific step-by-step instructions for tasks and help with time management (Selekman, 2002).

Students who have difficulty reading, and as a result read slowly, often find this disability to be the greatest barrier to their academic success. Helping students overcome this difficulty by providing textbooks on tape, providing them with the required reading assignments early in the semester, or helping them to identify the key sections of reading assignments may help these students to be successful. These students may also need accommodations for testing because slow reading skills can affect the student's ability to complete a test within the time allowed. Questions that are grammatically complex or contain double negatives, although difficult for all students, can be particularly challenging for students with learning disabilities and should be avoided. Providing the student with an extended testing time and a quiet room free from distractions may also be necessary (Eliason, 1992; Klisch, 1994). A test proctor who either reads the test to the student or writes and records the student's dictated answers to the test questions may also be helpful.

An additional strategy that faculty can use to assist students with learning disabilities is incorporating a multimedia approach, such as computer-assisted instruction (Eliason, 1992; Selekman, 2002). Other strategies can benefit both students with learning disabilities and students without them. These include providing copies of PowerPoint slides or other notes before class, placing visual cues within class notes, and checking over nursing notes before placing them on the patient charts (Ijiri & Kudzma, 2000; Selekman, 2002). Use of a pocket speller in the clinical area may also be beneficial (Ijiri & Kudzma). Another strategy that benefits all students, but particularly those with learning disabilities, is to meet with students on a regular basis to ensure that learning goals are being set appropriately and are then being achieved and allowing part-time study (Selekman). Accommodation does not mean that academic standards are lowered but that multiple ways to achieve those standards are provided for all students, including those with learning disabilities. Any one classroom contains students with multiple learning styles. By structuring classes to take into account different learning styles and by providing a variety of learning aids, nurse educators will also help to accommodate those with diagnosed learning disabilities (Ijiri & Kudzma, 2000).

Campus Support Services

As previously mentioned, most institutions of higher education have established an office responsible for providing support services to students who identify themselves as learning disabled. Use of these services is voluntary, and they are usually available at little or no cost to the student. Services vary among institutions but typically include assessment and diagnosis of learning disabilities, identification of appropriate accommodations for the student, guidance counseling, and development of study and test taking skills. Faculty education about students with learning disabilities is another service commonly provided by these offices.

Accommodations for the National Council Licensure Examination

Nurse educators need to be familiar with the accommodations provided for students with disabilities in their states when taking the National Council Licensure Examination (NCLEX). Accommodations are offered to individuals with learning disabilities in accordance with the ADA (National Council of State Boards of Nursing, 2004). Each state individually determines the degree of accommodation offered to students on a case-by-case basis. Educators should investigate and verify the accommodations offered to students in their respective state and encourage students with disabilities to seek appropriate accommodations. One of the most common accommodations has to do with time allotted for the examination. Regulations do change, and the student and faculty are encouraged to check with the National Council of State Boards of Nursing website *(http://www.ncsbn.org)* or the individual State Board of Nursing for further information. The student must provide documentation as to what accommodations have been made during his or her course of study.

THE STUDENT WITH PHYSICAL DISABILITIES

Required abilities that schools use to exclude students may include hearing, seeing, and lifting. Although a court ruled more than 20 years ago that a prospective nursing student with a hearing impairment could be denied admission because of the potential for lowering educational standards (McGuire, 1998), since that time there have been published reports of students with hearing impairments who have achieved success in nursing programs and in subsequent employment (Maheady, 2003; Rhodes et al., 1999). Many aids, such as amplified stethoscopes, are now available, and an interpreter could be used for auscultation (American Association of Medical Professionals with Hearing Losses, 2003; Rhodes et al.). Through the use of note takers and tape recorders, many students with hearing impairments have little difficulty participating in the classroom. Pagers that vibrate may also help students keep in contact with others in the clinical setting.

Some students with impaired vision may be accommodated (Murphy & Brennan, 1998). Providing alternative learning environments and enabling students to work with preceptors may be accommodations that can reasonably be made. For example, a student with a visual impairment might need a magnifier to help with reading printed matter.

Lifting restrictions may not be a barrier because many hospitals and nursing homes are striving for an environment that minimizes lifting (Nelson et al., 2003). Employed nurses have successfully functioned in a wheelchair, and with some creativity students could as well (Maheady, 2003; Nettina, 2003; Yox, 2003).

Students may become disabled during their time in school, and thus reasonable accommodations for students with physical disabilities may include time extensions for assignments and the assignment of an "incomplete" grade for courses that may not be completed on time. Maheady (2003) relates a case study of a nursing student who became wheelchair bound as a result of an accident. The student successfully completed her program and went on to obtain a master's degree in nursing and gainful employment.

THE NURSING STUDENT WITH A CHEMICAL AND ALCOHOL IMPAIRMENT

Nursing students are considered to be at risk for developing a chemical dependency problem during their time in school. According to Coleman et al. (1997), risks factors fall into two categories: familial and external, such as illness or school, and job stress. Other external risk factors for nurses, as well as for other health professionals, are easy access to drugs and, perhaps, society's willingness to deny substance abuse in this population (Haack, 1988; O'Quinn-Larson & Pickard, 1989). It has also been stated that the nursing profession may attract individuals who have a problem with dependency (Marion et al., 1996). Additionally, nurses are often uncomfortable dealing with substance abuse in colleagues (Grover, 1998).

Nurses who are substance abusers often cite that they began alcohol or drug abuse while they were a student (Ball, 2000). It is not uncommon for nursing students to be exposed to high levels of stress during their education. The psychological stressors associated with caring for acutely ill clients while still acquiring the clinical knowledge and skills necessary to do so are considerable (O'Quinn, 1996). Students may also feel powerless to relieve the suffering they see their clients experiencing. In Haack's (1988) longitudinal study of the relationship of stress and impairment in nursing students, students reported increased feelings of burnout and an increase in the frequency of alcohol use as they progressed through their education. Haack noted that those students who reported a lack of social support and exhibited an external attribution style reported higher levels of burnout and alcohol use. In addition to clinical stressors, many students face numerous role conflicts in their life, which increases their level of stress. Coleman et al. (1997) showed that nursing students admitted in 1989 had experimented with drugs less frequently than had pharmacy students. In addition, over a 2-year period, pharmacy students, and following enhanced information in the curriculum regarding substance abuse, exhibited a greater change in attitudes, both positive and negative, regarding drug and alcohol abuse. Also, the college environment can provide students with easy access to alcohol and drugs and can expose them to situations in which alcohol and drug use is considered an acceptable activity. A survey of more than 17,000 college students was conducted by the Harvard School of Public Health (Wechsler, 1996). The results of the survey indicated that 84% of the students drank alcohol during the school year. Of this 84%, close to half (44%) could be classified as "binge" drinkers, drinking four, five, or more drinks in a row, 1 or more times in a 2-week period. Most of these students (91% of women; 78% of men) labeled their drinking habits as "light" or "moderate" and considered these behaviors to be acceptable.

It is difficult to determine the number of nursing students who may be impaired by drug or alcohol use. However, it is possible to project the numbers of nursing students who may be abusing drugs or alcohol by examining the statistics that are available regarding chemical dependency in college students and RNs (O'Quinn-Larson & Pickard, 1989). Haack (1988) estimated the number of RNs in the United States who have a chemical dependency problem to be approximately 90,000. How many of these chemically dependent nurses began their misuse of drugs during their nursing education is unknown. Studies have indicated that alcohol use among college students, including nursing students, is approximately 80% (O'Quinn-Larson & Pickard). In one of the studies (Haack, 1988), 13% of the nursing student sample reported that the use of alcohol had at some time interfered with their school or work. In another study of baccalaureate nursing students, the findings indicated that 21% of the students had a serious drinking problem (Marion et al., 1996). Coleman et al. (1997) surveyed nursing, pharmacy, medical, and allied health students. They found that, for example, 20% of entering nursing students used alcohol on a weekly or daily basis, compared with 14% of pharmacy students. Trinkoff and Storr (1998) have reviewed the literature on substance abuse and have determined that practicing nurses' overall rate of substance abuse mirrored the general population.

Characteristics of Students with Chemical and Alcohol Impairments

It is obvious that the potential for substance abuse exists among nursing students. Faculty need to have an understanding of this issue so that they may assist students in receiving the appropriate professional support necessary to treat their problem. Faculty also have a responsibility to protect clients from the actions of a potentially unsafe student whose clinical performance and judgment may be impaired because of substance abuse (Asteriadis et al., 1995). Faculty should be aware of the characteristics of students who may be chemically dependent, knowledgeable about the policies and procedures within their institution that relate to students who are chemically dependent, and familiar with the support services that are available to students who have a chemical dependency problem.

Clark (1999) identified the following behavioral, personality, and physical characteristics that may be present in students who are chemically dependent: frequent mood swings, irritability or hostility, eating alone and social isolationism, forgetfulness, intolerance of others and other inappropriate responses, nervousness, intricate excuses for behavior, disheveled personal appearance, and odor of alcohol or mints detected on breath. Other characteristics include unsteady gait, affected speech, bloodshot sclera and alteration in pupil size, tremors, difficulty following directions or performing calculations, diaphoresis, and nausea and vomiting (Asteriadis et al., 1995). Frequent absences may also indicate a problem with substance abuse (Clark).

Faculty Responsibilities Related to Students with Impairments

What are the responsibilities of faculty if they suspect that a student is displaying characteristics that are indicative of chemical dependency? Faculty have ethical responsibilities toward the student and the student's clients and therefore should not ignore or make excuses for such behavior. O'Quinn-Larson and Pickard (1989) indicated that overprotective behavior toward an impaired student is an enabling behavior that does not help the student deal with the problem. However, any measures that faculty take should be assistive in nature rather than punitive (Asteriadis et al., 1995).

Before taking any measures, faculty need to clearly understand the policies and procedures for assisting chemically dependent students that are in place within their institution. Behavior must be documented, and it is helpful if it is documented by more than one faculty member (Clark, 1999). A faculty member might have to take immediate action if, for example, a student appears impaired in the clinical area. In cases where the student does not impose an immediate danger to clients but is suspected of substance abuse, an appointment might be made with the student for the purpose of making the student aware of institutional policies regarding substance abuse. Clark suggests that in addition to the faculty member who has identified the problem, someone else, such as a department chair and/or the Director of Student Affairs, should be present.

Written policies about chemical impairment that include the institution's definition of chemical dependency, the nursing faculty's philosophy on chemical dependency, and student and faculty responsibilities related to suspected chemical dependency should be clearly stated in the student handbook. Without such policies faculty may not be legally supported if they implement actions against a student for chemical impairment (Clark, 1999; Polk et al., 1993). Furthermore, adhering to the institution's established policies helps to ensure that the student's right to due process is not denied.

The American Association of Colleges of Nursing (1996) provides guidelines for policy development for the management of substance abuse. These guidelines include recommendations for education, identification of students with substance abuse problems, intervention, treatment, and reentry into the program if the student must enter into treatment and take a break from the educational course of study. The guidelines emphasize the use of professional resources for students instead of the use of faculty as counselors. Many colleges and universities offer treatment programs and support groups for students who are chemically impaired. It is highly recommended that faculty maintain a listing of effective counselors and programs located within the campus vicinity that can be used for student referrals. Another resource for faculties may be their respective State Board of Nursing Peer Assistance of Impaired Professionals program. Students should also be made aware that clinical agency policies may require blood or urine testing of individuals, including students, suspected of chemical dependency.

Some schools of nursing have developed their own intervention program for nursing students who are impaired. The following are key considerations: (1) ensuring the confidentiality of students who access the program; (2) clarifying the responsibilities of individuals associated with the program (i.e., faculty, students, administrators, alumni, counselors, and substance abuse professionals); and (3) orienting the student population to the purpose, activities, and responsibilities of the program (Greenhill & Skinner, 1991).

As the Harvard study on alcohol (Wechsler, 1996) indicates, substance abuse among students remains a common problem on many college campuses. Many colleges and universities are attempting to deal with this problem by increasing student awareness of the effects of substance abuse through campus educational programming. Incorporating information about substance abuse among health care professionals into the nursing curriculum may raise nursing students' awareness of the significance of the problem (Coleman et al, 1997). Helping students to identify appropriate coping strategies to use when they are feeling stressed and promoting an environment within the school that fosters supportive student–faculty interactions and student–peer relationships may also affect the potential development of substance abuse among students (Haack, 1988; O'Quinn-Larson & Pickard, 1989).

NURSING STUDENTS WITH MENTAL HEALTH PROBLEMS

Despite the fact that it has been suggested that nursing students may be at a high risk for developing mental health problems because of the high levels of stress that are generally reported among nursing students (Mental health risk is highest for students, 1999), little has been written on how to deal with nursing students with a specific mental illness diagnosis. What has been written focuses on behaviors, such as signs of anxiety, stress, and anger. One study by Patton and Goldenberg (1999) suggested that those nursing students with higher degrees of hardiness can handle personal stress better than students with lower degrees of hardiness. Their research is particularly timely because, overall, college students of today have more mental health problems before enrollment than did college students of the past (Levine & Cureton, 1998). Some nursing students may also have mental health problems before enrolling in nursing school, which lead them to be attracted to a "helping" profession. Students who experience mental health problems may need assistance in identifying and addressing these problems.

Because of their close interaction with students, nursing faculty are often the first to note the signs of mental health problems in nursing students. Some behavioral indicators, either in the classroom or in the clinical setting, may include frequent absenteeism, disruption of logical thought patterns, and a decrease in the quality of work (Lambert & Nugent, 1994).

FACULTY RESPONSIBILITIES RELATED TO STUDENTS WITH MENTAL HEALTH PROBLEMS

The process used to assist students with suspected mental health problems is similar to the approach used with any student whose academic progress is jeopardized by unsatisfactory performance. First, the ADA prohibits discrimination against individuals who are mentally impaired. Second, all actions taken by faculty must be congruent with existing institutional policies and afford students the due process that is their right. Keeping detailed anecdotal notes that describe the events of concern, sharing these notes and concerns with the individual student, and informing administrators of these concerns are all appropriate steps to be taken by the faculty members involved (Lambert & Nugent, 1994). Those with specific diagnoses may need some accommodation, such as permission to take tests in an alternate setting, more time to complete assignments, and written contracts for completing assignments (Job Accommodation Network, Office of Disability Employment Policy of the United States Department of Labor, 2003)

Students should be made clearly aware of the behavior that is adversely affecting their academic performance and what they need to do to correct this behavior. A learning contract may be used in this instance to indicate what the student needs to do to improve the behavior and the time frame in which this must be accomplished. It is appropriate for faculty to recommend professional counseling with a mental health professional. Many university campuses offer this service to students free or for a reduced fee. Nursing faculty may be tempted to counsel students on their own, but separating the student–faculty relationship from the student–counselor relationship is more effective and indeed safer (Brooke, 1999). If, despite these interventions, the behavior does not improve and the student is unable to perform effectively or client safety is compromised, administrative withdrawal or dismissal from the program may be necessary. As always, the student who is administratively withdrawn or dismissed has the right to pursue the grievance and appeal process in place within the institution (Lambert & Nugent, 1994).

Mental health issues may manifest themselves in a variety of ways. One common way is in the form of test anxiety. Test anxiety in and of itself is not considered to be a disability, but a student's preexisting anxiety may be if it is judged to be greater than that of the average person (Wylonis & Schweizer, 1998). Although nursing students' level of anxiety may be no different than that of their university peers, their level of test anxiety has been found to be significantly higher (Brewer, 2002). For nursing students, passing tests is crucial to program success and ultimately licensure success. Although test anxiety may not always affect a student's level of success in the program, faculty need to help students cope with their anxiety. Brewer has noted that often faculty are very abstract and conceptual in their thinking, whereas students are more concrete and pragmatic. Matching teaching styles with student learning styles and helping students work with their learning styles may help students deal with their anxieties (see Chapters 2 and 12) (Lenehan et al., 1994).

Mental health issues may also manifest themselves in the form of student incivility in the classroom and ultimately in anger in the student–faculty relationship. Lashley and de Meneses (2001) reported on a national survey of nursing programs. Of the 408 schools that responded, 100% reported instances of incivility. In addition to students' tardiness and repeated absences, 24.8% reported that there was objectionable physical contact from students and 42.8% reported that students verbally abused or yelled at instructors in the clinical area (Lashely & de Meneses, 2001). Sadly, anger can be taken to the extreme, which occurred at the University of Arizona when a nursing student shot and killed three nursing faculty members (Rooney, 2002).

Thomas (2003) provides guidelines on how to deal with angry students. First, recognizing signs and risk factors for potential violence may help to avert tragedy. Second, violent students tend to be males in their 30s and 40s who may have had a previous history of violence. Third, depression is often a precursor to violence, and anger and violence are more likely to occur in times of high stress, such as at examination time or program dismissal (Thomas, 2003). Fourth, having policies and procedures in place for dealing with potential violence is important. Threats should be promptly reported to campus security. All schools should have a procedure for dealing with student complaints, and that procedure should be publicized to all students and faculty. Finally, if a faculty member is in a situation in which a student is extremely angry, the student should be asked to make an appointment and discuss the issue when tempers are less heated. If the faculty member thinks that the student may get violent, security should be notified. Having a third party to mediate disputes is sometimes helpful. In addition, a respectful proactive strategy faculty can use is to put classroom behavioral expectations in the course syllabus (Carbone, 1998).

SUMMARY

This chapter has provided information about the legal issues related to teaching students with disabilities and other special needs. The needs of students with learning disabilities, chemical dependency, and mental health problems were presented, along with faculty responsibilities associated with teaching these students. Interventions were identified for assisting students to cope with a disability or impairment and to ultimately be successful in obtaining a nursing degree.

Nursing faculty are responsible for creating a learning environment that supports the teaching–learning process for all students. Working with students who have disabilities or impairments brings special challenges to the faculty–student relationship. No specific rules say what level of disability or impairment rules out admission to a nursing program. However, faculty who are knowledgeable about the legal issues related to students with disabilities or impairments, their institution's and school's policies and procedures related to students with these special needs, and the interventions designed to help students maintain their self-esteem and be successful will find themselves capable of meeting these challenges in a caring, facilitative manner. Viewing persons with disabilities through a nonmedical paradigm paves the way for lessening the discrimination that those persons often face in the educational environment and in the workplace (Marks, 2000). Further, if faculty are open to working with students who have disabilities, students might be more apt to disclose, without fear of adverse consequences, that they have a need for accommodations (Maheady, 1999). Developing strong partnerships with clinical agencies may also be a key to successfully integrating those students with disabilities into the nursing program (Murphy & Brennan, 1998). Educating nursing students about various disabilities will also help future generations of nurses and nursing faculty to view disabilities as differences rather than deficiencies.

As more persons with disabilities seek enrollment in nursing programs, faculty may need to consult resources that give guidance on how to accommodate those with disabilities. In addition to the resources available on individual campuses, the following websites contain much information regarding how to accommodate students with disabilities:

http://www.exceptionalnurse.com: This website contains many resources for those with disabilities and links for faculty that teach students with disabilities.

http://www.amphl.org: This website for the Association of Medical Personnel with Hearing Losses contains case studies and other resources to aid faculty who have students who are hearing impaired.

http://cdrc.ohsu.edu/selfdetermination/education/postsecondary/resources.html: This website for the Center for Self Determination at Oregon Health Sciences University contains a bibliography of the latest research, in addition to other links.

http://www.healthsciencefaculty.org/resource_center/nursing.html: This website for the Health Sciences Faculty Education Project contains links to many resources for professionals and professional students who are disabled.

CASE STUDIES FOR FUTURE DISCUSSION

Case Study 1

Charlie was a 49-year-old construction worker who fell while building an addition to a hospital. He sustained a severe head injury and was in a coma and suffered hemiplegia. With aggressive rehabilitation, Charlie regained full movement of all extremities and was able to pursue a new career. He enrolled in an associate degree nursing program because he felt he needed to redirect his work life. He was able to successfully complete the program in 4 years and to pass the NCLEX. Accommodations made during his program of study that contributed to his achievement included allowing his testing to take place in isolation from other students, having tests read to him if needed to promote understanding of what was asked, and permitting added time to complete tests. In addition, he was permitted, as were all students, to pursue part-time study. Support from faculty was crucial to his success. One faculty member in particular had experienced a head injury and was able to help Charlie improve his reading comprehension skills by teaching him to place transparent colored film over and a line above the text he was reading.

Case Study 2

Paula was a nursing student who had a hearing impairment before enrollment. Only one instructor knew of her hearing impairment, and Paula was able to self-accommodate by sitting in the front in class and walking up and down hospital hallways to detect which direction alarms came from because her hearing loss was on one side. In her junior year she injured her back and had to drop out for a year. When she returned to the program, she had a lifting restriction, which she did not share with the faculty. She again self-accommodated by asking for lifting help or ignoring the restriction. She was able to successfully complete her program and gain employment that did not require lifting. During her program, however, she thought that other students and some faculty resented her disabilities.

From Donna Maheady (personal communication, August 23, 2003).

REFERENCES

American Association of Colleges of Nursing (1996). Policy and guidelines for prevention and management of substance abuse in the nursing education community. *Journal of Professional Nursing, 12*(4), 253-257.

American Association of Medical Professionals with Hearing Losses (2003). *Clinical rotation years.* Retrieved February 24, 2004, from http://www.amphl.org/index.html

Asteriadis, M., Davis, V., Masoodi, J., & Miller, M. (1995). Chemical impairment of nursing students: A comprehensive policy and procedure. *Nurse Educator, 20*(2), 19-22.

Ball, K. (2000). Drinks tonight at 7 PM: Students and alcohol use. *Nursing New Zealand, 6*(4), 18-19.

Beilke, J. R., & Yssel, N. (1998). Personalizing disability: Faculty-student relationships and the importance of story. *Journal for a Just and Caring Education, 4*(2), 212-223.

Brewer, T. (2002). Test-taking anxiety among nursing and general college students. *Journal of Psychosocial Nursing, 40*(11), 23-29.

Brooke, C. P. (1999). Feelings from the back row: Negotiating sensitive issues in large classes. In S. M. Richardson (Ed.), *Promoting civility: A teaching challenge* (pp. 23-33). San Francisco: Jossey-Bass.

Carbone, E. (1998). Students behaving badly in large classes. In S. M. Richardson (Ed.), *Promoting civility: A teaching challenge* (pp. 35-43). San Francisco: Jossey-Bass.

Christensen, R. M. (1998). Nurse educators' attitudes toward and decision-making related to applicants with physical disabilities. *Journal of Nursing Education, 37*(7), 311-314.

Clark, C. M. (1999). Substance abuse among nursing students: Establishing a comprehensive policy and procedure for faculty intervention. *Nurse Educator, 24*(2), 16-19.

Coleman, E. A., Honeycutt, G., Ogden, B., McMillan, D. E., O'Sullivan, P. S., Light, K., & Wingfield, W. (1997). Assessing substance abuse among health care students and the efficacy of educational interventions. *Journal of Professional Nursing, 13*(1), 28-37.

Colon, E. J. (1997). Identification, accommodation, and success of students with learning disabilities in nursing education programs. *Journal of Nursing Education, 36*(8), 372-377.

Eliason, M. J. (1992). Nursing students with learning disabilities: Appropriate accommodations. *Journal of Nursing Education, 31*(8), 375-376.

Gordon, M., & Keiser, S. (1998). Underpinnings. In M. Gordon & S. Keiser (Eds.), *Accommodations in higher education under the American with Disabilities Act (ADA)* (pp. 3-19). Dewitt, NY: GSI Publications

Greenhill, E. D., & Skinner, K. (1991). Impaired nursing students: An intervention program. *Journal of Nursing Education, 30*(8), 379-381.

Grover, S. M. (1998). Nurses' attitudes towards impaired practice. *Journal of Addictions Nursing, 10*(2), 70-76.

Haack, M. R. (1988). Stress and impairment among nursing students. *Research in Nursing & Health, 11*(2), 125-134.

Helms, L. B., & Weiler, K. (1993). Disability discrimination in nursing education: An evaluation of legislation and litigation. *Journal of Professional Nursing, 9*(6), 358-366.

Ijiri, L., & Kudzma, E. C. (2000). Supporting nursing students with learning disabilities: A metacognitive approach. *Journal of Professional Nursing, 16*(3), 149-157.

Job Accommodation Network, Office of Disability of Employment Policy of the United States Department of Labor. *Work-site accommodation ideas for persons with psychiatric disabilities.* Retrieved August 23, 2003, from http://www.jan.wvu.edu/media/Psychiatric.html

Klisch, M. L. (1994). Guidelines for reducing bias in nursing examinations. *Nurse Educator, 19*(2), 35-39.

Lambert, V. A., & Nugent, K. E. (1994). Addressing the academic progression of students encountering mental health problems. *Nurse Educator, 19*(5), 33-39.

Lashley, F. R., & de Meneses, M. (2001). Student civility in nursing programs: A national survey. *Journal of Professional Nursing, 17*(2), 81-86.

Lenehan, M. C., Dunn, R., Ingham, J., Signer, B., & Murray, J. B. (1994). Effects of learning-style intervention on college students' achievement, anxiety, anger, and curiosity. *Journal of College Student Development, 35*, 461-466.

Letizia, M. (1995). Issues in the postsecondary education of learning-disabled nursing students. *Nurse Educator, 20*(5), 18-22.

Levine, A., & Cureton, J. S. (1998). Collegiate life: An obituary. *Change, 30*(3), 14-17, 51.

Magilvy, J. K., & Mitchell, A. C. (1995). Education of nursing students with special needs. *Journal of Nursing Education, 34*(1), 31-36.

Maheady, D. C. (1999). Jumping through hoops, walking on egg shells: The experiences of nursing students with disabilities. *Journal of Nursing Education, 38*(4), 162-170.

Maheady, D. C. (2003). *Nursing students with disabilities change the course.* River Edge, NJ: Exceptional Parent Press.

Marion, L. N., Fuller, S. G., Johnson, N. P., Michels, P. J., & Diniz, C. (1996). Drinking problems of nursing students. *Journal of Nursing Education, 35*(5), 196-203.

Marks, B. A. (2000). Commentary: Jumping through hoops and walking on egg shells or discrimination, hazing, and abuse of students with disabilities. *Journal of Nursing Education, 39*(5), 205-210.

McGuire, J. M. (1998). Educational accommodations: A university administrator's view. In M. Gordon & S. Keiser (Eds.), *Accommodations in higher education under the Americans with Disabilities Act (ADA)* (pp. 20-45). Dewitt, NY: GSI Publications. *Australian Nursing Journal, 6*(8), 13.

Mental health risk is highest for students [Electronic version]. *Australian Nursing Journal, 6*(8), 13.

Murphy, G. T., & Brennan, M. (1998). Nursing students with disabilities. *Canadian Nurse, 94*(10), 31-34.

National Council of State Boards of Nursing (2004). *Candidate examination bulletin.* Retrieved February 25, 2004, from http://www.ncsbn.org/pdfs/NCLEXCandidateBulletin_NCSPearson.pdf

National Joint Committee on Learning Disabilities. (1997, February 1). *Operationalizing the NJCLD definition of learning disabilities for ongoing assessment in schools.* Retrieved August 22, 2003, from http://www.ldonline.org/njcld/operationalizing.html

Nelson, A., Owen, B., Lloyd, J. D., Fragala, G., Matz, M. W., Amato, M., et al. (2003). Safe patient handling and movement. *American Journal of Nursing, 103*(3), 32-44.

Nettina, S. (2003). The untapped nursing workpool: Nurses with disabilities. *Medscape,* Article 452605. Retrieved July 1, 2003, from http://www.medscape.com/viewarticle/452605

O'Quinn, J. L. (1996). Chemical abuse in nursing students: A retrospective view. *Journal of Addictions Nursing, 8*(3), 94-98.

O'Quinn-Larson, J., & Pickard, M. (1989). The impaired nursing student. *Nurse Educator, 14*(2), 36-39.

Patton, T. J., & Goldenberg, D. (1999). Hardiness and anxiety as predictors of academic success in first-year, full-time and part-time RN students. *Journal of Continuing Education in Nursing, 30*(4), 158-167.

Persaud, D., & Leedom, C. L. (2002). The Americans with Disabilities Act: Effect on student admission and retention. *Journal of Nursing Education, 41*(8), 349-352.

Polk, D., Glendon, K., & DeVore, C. (1993). The chemically dependent student nurse: Guidelines for policy development. *Nursing Outlook, 41*(4), 166-170.

Rhodes, R. S., Davis, D. C., & Odom, B. C. (1999). Challenges and rewards of educating a profoundly deaf student. *Nurse Educator, 24*(3), 48-51.

Rooney, M. (2002). Student kills 3 U. of Arizona professors. *Chronicle of Higher Education.* Retrieved July 12, 2003, from http://www.chronicle.com

Selekman, J. (2002). Nursing students with learning disabilities. *Journal of Nursing Education, 41*(8), 334-339.

Shuler, S. (1990). Nursing students with learning disabilities: Guidelines for fostering success. *Nursing Forum, 25*(2), 15-18.

Sowers, J., & Smith, M. (2002). Disability as difference. *Journal of Nursing Education, 41*(8), 331-332.

Thomas, S. P. (2003). Handling anger in the teacher-student relationship. *Nursing Education Perspectives, 24*(1), 17-24.

Trinkoff, A. M., & Storr, C. L. (1998). Substance abuse among nurses: Differences between specialties. *American Journal of Public Health, 88*(4), 581-585.

Watkins, M. P., & Kurz, J. M. (1997). Managing clinical experiences for minority students with physical disabilities and impairments. *The ABNF Journal, 8*(4), 82-86.

Watson, P. G. (1995). Nursing students with disabilities: A survey of baccalaureate nursing programs. *Journal of Professional Nursing, 11*(3), 147-153.

Wechsler, H. (1996). Alcohol and the American college campus. *Change, 28*(4), 20-25, 60.

Wylonis, L., & Schweizer, E. (1998). Mood and anxiety disorders. In M. Gordon & S. Keiser (Eds.), *Accommodations in higher education under the Americans with Disabilities Act (ADA)* (pp. 154-169). Dewitt, NY: GSI Publications

Yox, S. B. (2003). From the editor—February 2003: Do we support nurse colleagues who have disabilities? *Medscape,* Article 449392. Retrieved July 1, 2003, from http://www.medscape.com/viewarticle/449392

CURRICULUM

5

CURRICULUM DEVELOPMENT

AN OVERVIEW

Nancy Dillard, DNS, RN, CS, ANP, *Linda Siktberg,* PhD, RN,
Juanita Laidig, EdD, RN,

In today's world of rapidly shifting resources, institutions of higher education are facing the need to make numerous changes to successfully meet the challenges of the future. Creative, innovative methods of curriculum delivery are being explored in an effort to provide cost-effective, quality programming to an increasingly diverse population of students. Flexible curricula are being developed that allow universities to provide programs that can quickly respond to the needs of the local, regional, and national constituencies to which they are accountable. Some authors have asserted that the quickest way to contain university costs and alleviate financial strain is to maintain quality courses, yet limit the number of electives offered or eliminate selected programs of study (Breneman, 1993; Breneman & Taylor, 1996; Pew Health Professions Commission, 1995). As institutions of higher education reevaluate how to best achieve their stated mission and position themselves for the future, it is apparent that sweeping changes in higher education are affecting the development and delivery of curricula.

Traditionally, faculty autonomy has been closely tied to curriculum. In this era of fewer economic resources and rapidly changing societal forces, faculty will undoubtedly continue to play an important role in the decision-making and evaluation processes concerning curriculum development, and, in addition to financial resources, they must consider the following issues as curricula are redesigned (Breneman, 1993; Denning, 1996; Erickson, 1995):

- Is the curriculum meeting students' needs and the needs of the community?
- Is the curriculum design one that will be appropriate for the future?
- Does the university provide programs that are of higher quality, are more accessible, and are more economically sound than those of other schools?

Students are seeking faster and more economical means of earning a degree in higher education. Universities and nursing programs that expect to survive must respond to the needs of consumers and communities. Curricula must be flexible to accommodate work schedules; offer diversity in courses and programs; teach management of culturally diverse peoples, as well as delegation and negotiation skills; enhance verbal, written, and speaking communication skills; and enhance the decision-making skills needed for this increasingly complex world (Doll, 1996; Erickson, 1995; Lempert, 1996; Pew Health Professions Commission, 1995; Pew Higher Education Roundtable, 1994). Distance education through the Internet has gained popularity as students across the country share ideas in virtual chat rooms, complete discussion board assignments, send electronic papers, and complete quizzes and examinations in online courses without ever seeing the faces of their professor and their colleagues. Educators focus on opening new courses to students; responding to students' learning needs; providing student support resources; and providing well-developed, cost-effective learning materials to distance education students. Potential students compare programs offered through the Internet to determine which will be the best, shortest, and most cost-effective (Hodson Carlton et al., 2003; Melton, 2002).

As the future looms ahead, faculty must consider the following questions:

- Are students really being prepared for a complex and changing world?
- Are students prepared as professionals (socialized to professionalism), or are they prepared to be technicians with high-tech skills?
- Are students prepared to face the increasing complexity of ethical decisions?
- Are students learning essential multicultural and global concepts?
- Are graduates leaving school with the necessary knowledge and skills for their job?
- Are faculty working effectively, efficiently, and productively in designing curricula that will help prepare students for the workforce?
- Are curricula meeting the needs of women, minorities, and vulnerable populations?
- Are curricula being delivered with outdated methods, such as traditional lecture and discussion, or with current methods of instruction, including interactive, computer-mediated technology?

These and other questions should challenge faculty to review curricula and methods of instruction with the goal of preparing graduates for the future (Breneman & Taylor, 1996; Brown & Kysilka, 2002; Erickson, 1995; Fuhrmann, 1997; Garcia & Ratcliff, 1997; Myers et al., 1991; Pew Health Professions Commission, 1995; Rambur, 1991; Ratcliff, 1997a, 1997b; Smith et al., 1993).

The rapid development of technology has also affected curriculum development, and faculty must be cognizant of the implications of technology in education. How is the development of curricula being affected by the technology explosion? How many programs are offered through the Internet? Which programs can be, and should be, offered through electronic means? The Internet will play an increasingly larger role in higher education, and students will expect to be able take more online courses that fit their work schedule. Electronic communication will enhance professional education because certification programs offering advanced knowledge and skills will soon replace traditional degree programs. [Faculty will have to develop new technology skills to be used for course delivery, testing, curriculum design, and networking among professionals] (Brown & Duguid, 1996; Denning, 1996; Halstead et al., 1996; Hodson Carlton et al., 2003; Lindeman, 2000; Pew Health Professions Commission, 1995; Pew Higher Education Roundtable, 1994).

How are professional curricula, such as nursing and health care, being affected, and what are the implications for nursing faculty? Restructure and reforms in the health care system are rapidly changing the focus of nursing education as graduates must learn to survive within a managed care environment that includes hospitals downsizing professional nursing staff, increased numbers of unlicensed personnel providing client care, advancing technology, shortened hospital stays, and increased home care. Nursing education must continue to maintain standards and meet the requirements of state boards of nursing and national accrediting agencies while responding to health care and institutional changes. Nursing practice must be safe and cost-effective across client settings. Competency-based programs have been designed to prepare students for transition into a variety of agencies (Redman et al., 1999)."The Pew Health Professions Commission was created in 1989 to focus on the healthcare workforce. . . . The mission of the Commission . . . was to help policy makers and educators produce health care professionals who meet the changing needs of the American health care system" (Center for the Health Professions, 2003, ¶ 1). Recommendations from the Pew report were to downsize nursing education programs by 10% to 20% (associate and diploma programs), recognize the value of and distinguish between practice responsibilities of the different levels of nursing, strengthen career ladders to enhance mobility through the various nursing levels, and increase the number of master's level nurse practitioner programs by increasing federal funding for students. Additional recommendations were as follows: increasing the knowledge and skills of practicing acute care nurses to enable them to practice in community-based agencies; increasing the knowledge and skills of associate degree and diploma nurses to better prepare them for more complex client care; incorporating a clinical management role for baccalaureate students that includes direct patient care; increasing the scientific base of nursing education; providing cultural experiences to increase cultural sensitivity; and increasing interdisciplinary training (Dochterman & Grace, 2001; Fagin, 1997; Tagliareni & Mengel, 2001).

Lenburg (2002) challenged nurses and nurse educators to consider the following changes that affect the profession and curriculum:

> (1) Rapid knowledge expansion and use of changing information technology; (2) necessity for documented practice-based competencies; evidence-base practice; (3) sociodemographic, cultural, economics, political influences on healthcare, education, community; (4) community-based, collaborative, interdisciplinary healthcare and education; (5) consumer-oriented society and impact on healthcare and education; (6) ethics and bioethical issues, dilemmas; biotechnology, biogenetic advances; (7) shortage of qualified nurses, teachers, and other healthcare personnel; aging; (8) increasing professional and personal responsibility and accountability; required continuing competency; (9) diversity, flexibility, mobility, and delivery of education; changing methods for learning and assessment of competence for practice; and (10) increasing reality of terrorism in various forms; fear, preparedness, consequences. (pp. 6-7)

Thus nursing education faces a great transformation as faculty adapt curricula to prepare graduates for the workforce (Gaff, 1997b; Halstead et al., 1996; Manuel & Sorensen, 1995; Pew Health Professions Commission, 1995; Rentschler & Spegman, 1996).

This chapter provides an introduction to curriculum and the curriculum development process in a rapidly changing world. Several issues affecting curriculum are addressed, including social, economic, and technological forces. Traditions in higher education and nursing are changing as faculty progress to more interactive curriculum models with students and faculty actively collaborating in the learning process.

DEFINITION OF CURRICULUM

The term *curriculum* was first used in Scotland as early as 1820 and became a part of the education vernacular in the United States nearly a century later. Curriculum, derived from the Latin word *currere*, which means "to run," over time has been translated to mean "course of study" (Wiles & Bondi, 1989). Ronald C. Doll (1996) defined curriculum as the "formal and informal content and process by which learners gain knowledge and understanding, develop skills, and alter attitudes, appreciations, and values under the auspices of that school" (p. 15). William E. Doll, Jr. (2002), described curriculum in relation to a shifting paradigm, moving from a formal definition to a focus on one's multiple interactions with others and one's surroundings. He defined curriculum using the following five concepts:

1. *Currere:* "To run a course" . . . "a process or method of 'negotiating passages'—between ourselves and the text, between ourselves and the students, and among all three" (pp. 45-46)
2. *Complexity:* "Looking at curriculum : . . . as a complex and dynamic web of interactions evolving naturally into more varied interconnected forms is a formidable task that will require vision and perseverance" (p. 46)
3. *Cosmology:* Viewing the curriculum as alive, combining "the rigorousness of science . . . the imagination of story . . . the vitality and creativity of spirit" (p. 48)
4. *Conversation:* "Teachers and students respect, honor, and understand their own humanness . . . the 'otherness' of each other . . . [and] the texts studied and the ways of thinking inscribed in them" (pp. 49-50)
5. *Community:* "An extension of community beyond self," which will include "ecological, global, and cosmological issues within which all humans are enmeshed" (pp. 51-52)

Because of the amorphous nature of the term *curriculum*, it has a variety of definitions. Educators prefer particular definitions based on individual philosophical beliefs and the emphasis placed on specific aspects of education. A review of literature revealed that common components in the definition of curriculum include the following (Beauchamp, 1968; Doll,

1996; Longstreet & Shane, 1993; Ornstein & Hunkins, 1993; Wiles & Bondi, 1989):

- Preselected goals/outcomes to be achieved
- Selected content with specific sequencing in a program of study
- Processes and experiences to facilitate learning
- Resources used
- The extent of responsibility for learning assumed by the teacher and learner
- How and where learning takes place

Curriculum is viewed from a variety of perspectives, ranging from narrow and circumscribed to broad and encompassing. Oliva (1992) and others offered additional varied interpretations as follows (Doll, 1996; Erickson, 1995; Klein, 1995):

- Knowledge organized and presented in a set of subjects/courses
- Modes of thought
- Cognitive/affective content and process
- Instructional set of outcomes/performance objectives
- Everything planned by faculty in a planned learning environment
- Interschool activities, including extracurricular activities, guidance, and interpersonal relationships
- Individual learner's experience as a result of schooling

Curriculum Development in Nursing

Curriculum in nursing has also been viewed from a number of perspectives. Heidgerken, a respected nurse educator in the 1940s and 1950s, believed that curriculum entailed all planned and day-to-day learning experiences of the students and faculty, including both organized instruction and clinical experiences (Diekelmann, 1993). Taba (1962), a curriculum expert whose work influenced nursing education, defined curriculum as the following:

> All curricula, no matter what their particular design, are composed of certain elements. A curriculum usually contains a statement of aims and of specific objectives; it indicates some selection and organization of content; it either implies or manifests certain patterns of learning and teaching, whether because the objectives demand them or because the content organization requires them. Finally, it includes a program of evaluation of the out-comes. (p. 11)

Building on curriculum as a plan, Beauchamp (1968), another expert in curriculum development, viewed curriculum as a written document depicting the scope and arrangement of a projected educational program for a school.

For the past 25 years nurse educators have been greatly influenced by the work of Bevis. The definition of curriculum used in her earlier writings reflected her allegiance to the Tyler behaviorist, technical model of curriculum development, an orientation supported by most nurse educators. In 2000 Bevis defined curriculum as "those transactions and interactions that take place between students and teachers and among students with the intent that learning takes place" (p. 72).

Bevis has challenged nurse educators to move from what she termed the *Tylerian/behaviorist curriculum development paradigm* to one that focuses on human interaction and active learning. Relative to this new paradigm, Bevis proposed that the definition of curriculum be changed to incorporate students' and teachers' interactions and the transactions that occur (Bevis, 1989, 2000). Other nurse educators have attempted to broaden Bevis' definition of curriculum. To capture the personal meaningfulness of curriculum, Nelms (1991) defined the term as an intensely personal learning within a transpersonal interaction, stating that curriculum is "the educational journey, in an educational environment in which the biography of the person (the student) interacts with the history of the culture of nursing through the biography of another person (the faculty) to create meaning and release potential in the lives of all participants" (p. 6).

In recent dialogues among nursing educators about the conceptualization of curriculum, there has been a stimulus to reconsider the meaning of the term. "It is the responsibility of nursing education in collaboration with practices settings to shape practice, not merely respond to changes in the practice environment" (American Association of Colleges of Nursing, 1999, p. 60). New opportunities are offered to debate a number of issues, including the following:

- Enhance students' delegation, supervision, and leadership skills to effect change
- Focus on health promotion and disease prevention
- Enhance student–faculty interaction in the learning process
- Use "anticipatory–innovative learning" rather than "maintenance learning" (Watson, 2000, pp. 40–41)
- Use research-based nursing practice
- Focus on quality, cost-effective nursing care
- Expand culturally sensitive nursing practice in community-based agencies

Although various curriculum models are found in the literature, most authors in nursing education agree that for learning to be successful and satisfying, an ongoing, responsive relationship between curriculum and instruction is essential (Baldwin & Nelms, 1993; Manuel & Sorensen, 1995; Morse & Corcoran-Perry, 1996; Rentschler & Spegman, 1996; Wink, 2003).

Types of Curricula

Regardless of the interpretation of curriculum, several curricula may occur concurrently. The *official curriculum* includes the stated curriculum framework with philosophy and mission; recognized lists of outcomes, competencies, and objectives for the program and individual courses; course outlines; and syllabi. Bevis (2000) stated that the "legitimate curriculum . . . [is] the one agreed on by the faculty either implicitly or explicitly" (p. 74). These written documents are distributed to other faculty members, students, curriculum committee members, and accrediting agencies to document what is taught.

The *operational curriculum* consists of "what is actually taught by the teacher and how its importance is communicated to the student" (Posner,

1992, p. 10). This curriculum includes knowledge, skills, and attitudes emphasized by faculty in the classroom and clinical settings.

The *illegitimate curriculum*, according to Bevis (2000), is one known and actively taught by faculty yet not evaluated because descriptors of the behaviors are lacking. Such behaviors include "caring, compassion, power, and its use" (p. 75).

The *hidden curriculum* consists of values and beliefs taught through verbal and nonverbal communication by the faculty. Faculty may be unaware of what is taught through their expressions, priorities, and interactions with students, but students are very aware of the "hidden agendas" (curriculum), which may have a more lasting impact than the written curriculum. The hidden curriculum includes the way faculty interact with students, the teaching methods used, and the priorities set (Bevis, 2000; Posner, 1992; Schubert, 1986).

The *null curriculum* (Bevis, 2000; Eisner, 1985; Schubert, 1986) represents content and behaviors that are not taught. Faculty need to recognize what is not being taught and focus on the reasons for ignoring those content and behavior areas. Examples include content or skills faculty think they are teaching but are not, such as critical thinking. As faculty review curricula, all components and relationships need to be evaluated.

The idea of an interrelationship between curriculum and instruction is also supported by other educators. According to Lempert (1996), a new approach to education and curriculum must be developed: one in which faculty are active participants and guides in learning, not lecturers. Lempert urges an increased involvement in the community, with the university becoming responsible and accountable to the needs of the community. He also favors a curriculum that recognizes and accepts individual differences to enhance multiculturalism. He believes that curriculum and learning should be focused on acquiring skills, not just factual knowledge. After all, knowledge should be measured by the ability of the students and graduates to perform tasks, not recite facts. Therefore it follows that the most effective learning occurs by experience, not just by passively learning facts (Erickson, 1995; Lempert, 1996; Pew Health Professions Commission, 1995; Pew Higher Education Roundtable, 1994).

General education and nursing curricula are becoming more interactive, with classroom and workplace joining to meet learning goals set by diverse groups of students. Students must develop the ability to communicate across cultures; understand and respect others' views and lives; and learn teamwork skills, including management, delegation, and negotiation. The curriculum should offer activities to enable students to gain actual experiences and learn to work collaboratively with other disciplines in seeking solutions to problems (Erickson, 1995; Lempert, 1996; Pew Health Professions Commission, 1995). The concept of service learning, which embodies these principles, is further discussed in Chapter 11.

CURRICULUM COMPONENTS

Components of the curriculum that are used by faculty in the review, restructuring, and development of contemporary curricula include foundations;

philosophy and mission; designs; organizing frameworks; outcomes, competencies, and objectives; educational activities; and evaluation (Doll, 1996; Erickson, 1995; Halstead et al., 1996). These curriculum components are briefly discussed in this overview with further elaboration in following chapters.

Foundations

The foundations of curriculum set the external boundaries for a given field of study, whereas historical perspectives provide a view of the evolving content and roots of the discipline. In nursing, historical perspectives enable students to learn of the development of nursing as a profession, nursing education, and nursing research. Review of sociological and political forces also provides a historical perspective of the effects of various legal actions; economics; and events, such as wars, on the nursing profession. Psychological foundations of curriculum have formulated teaching and learning aspects of nursing education, including evaluation and curriculum revisions (Bevis, 2000; Doll, 1996; Longstreet & Shane, 1993; Ornstein & Hunkins, 1993). Forces and issues that are currently influencing the development of nursing curricula are discussed in Chapter 6.

Philosophy and Mission

The program must integrate the philosophy and mission of the university or college within the curriculum. The mission of the university or college varies with the social forces that affect faculty, students, and curricula. Institutional missions must address the knowledge and technology explosion, critical thinking, problem solving, multiculturalism, and communication in response to the multiple changes occurring in today's workplace. Students learn what to value as they receive a foundation for specialized content and skills.

The philosophy provides the framework for curriculum choices that are made. Most curricula are formulated and based on several philosophies, not just a single one (Ratcliff, 1997b). The values and beliefs on which curricula are founded provide coherence, shape, and consistency for a program. The beliefs set the criteria from which to develop, teach, and evaluate the learning of concepts, such as the concepts of nursing (Bevis, 2000).

Educational philosophies include perennialism, essentialism, progressivism, reconstructionism, and existentialism (Bevis, 2000; Ornstein & Hunkins, 1993; Wiles & Bondi, 1989). In *perennialism* (grounded in realism), the curriculum is based on knowledge and conservative, inflexible, traditional content, including mathematics, grammar, languages, sciences, and strong moral and spiritual teachings. Goals of the curriculum include character training and development of reasoning abilities, and faculty are considered the authorities and experts at developing the content, which is taught primarily by lecture. Students' opinions are not useful in curriculum development because students, as passive recipients, are not able to adequately judge what must be learned. Further studies in realism would include Aristotle and the writings of Thomas Aquinas, Harry Broudy, and John Wild (Ornstein & Hunkins, 1993; Schubert, 1986; Wiles & Bondi, 1989).

Essentialism is another conservative philosophy grounded in idealism and realism, with traditional content and teachings. Students are viewed as having "spongelike" minds that absorb new content provided. The curriculum should be the same across student populations; however, students should be allowed to learn at an individual pace based on ability. Such a philosophical base would be viewed as costly in the contemporary environment if the curriculum were offered on campus and the teacher, a model of ideal behavior, continued to be viewed as the authority (Ornstein & Hunkins, 1993; Wiles & Bondi, 1989). Essentialism can be studied further in works on idealism (e.g., by Plato, Hegel, Fredrich Froebel, J. Donald Butler) and realism.

Both perennialism and essentialism could be considered outdated in a rapidly changing world in which the teacher and student learn from each other. The application of just one of these philosophies implies a lack of flexibility in the curriculum, which is a necessity in today's dynamic and complex U.S. health care system.

Progressivism, rooted in pragmatism, views problem-solving skills, scientific inquiry, and critical thinking as essential to the curriculum. The teacher's role is more participative, and the emphasis is on teaching students how to learn and how to problem solve rather than on the content of a specific subject. Traditional course content is replaced by a set of activities and experiences that encourage group participation and teamwork. Further study on the history of pragmatism is offered in the writings of John Dewey and William James (Bevis, 2000; Ornstein & Hunkins, 1993).

The philosophy of *reconstructionism*, also grounded in pragmatism, focuses education on the needs of society rather than the individual. Social and cultural issues are primary areas of the curriculum, which is viewed as constantly changing. A major goal is that teachers and students will become change agents in a world of crises and controversy. The works of Alvin Toffler and Theodore Brameld can be studied to enhance the understanding of reconstructionism (Ornstein & Hunkins, 1993).

Existentialism focuses on individualism and self-fulfillment, teaching about choices one has to make, freedom of choice, the meaning of choice, and the responsibility one has for choice. There is no established curriculum other than the focus on choices and the human condition. Established standards, authority, and group norms are rejected and replaced by self-expressive activities, experiments, emotions, feelings, and insights. Teachers and students learn by dialogue and discussion in the development of choices. The origin of existentialism can be further studied with a review of the works of Søren Kierkegaard and other existentialist philosophers (Ornstein & Hunkins, 1993; Sartre, 1974; Schubert, 1986; Wiles & Bondi, 1989).

As discussed, various complex philosophical beliefs exist within curricula. Philosophies are being reevaluated by educators as curriculum restructuring occurs. Further discussion of philosophy and mission statements can be found in Chapter 7.

Designs

Curricula today need to incorporate opportunities for students to problem solve, think critically about issues of the day, and communicate in the real world. Ratcliff (1997a) stated that curricula must be coherent to stimulate creativity among students as they prepare for the workplace. He believed curricula must be designed to encourage students to consider divergent ideas and differences among people. Learning about different cultures and considering a variety of beliefs and ideas fosters questioning and intellectual development. In a prescribed curriculum, such as nursing, graduates will be better prepared and equipped to work within a changing society if both the general studies core courses and the clinical courses require students to learn about multicultural peoples and issues. The prescribed goals, objectives, and outcomes of a professional program such as nursing will prepare graduates for oppotunities for divergent thinking.

Curricula today are changing rapidly because of the technology explosion and the "crumbling of the four walls." Software companies are preparing to market high-quality education at costs lower than those charged by universities, thus increasing the demand for curricula offered via distance education. Williamson (1996) described the effects technological changes have on universities and faculty as both struggle to compete in the technological race. Less time is needed to complete course-related paperwork and thus faculty now have more time to spend with students. Computer modules provide more cost-effective use of time in that the modules can be viewed over and over by students to enhance learning, and they are less expensive than faculty time. However, Williamson (1996) identified that faculty must be familiar with current technology. More and more students are entering higher education with greater technological literacy than the faculty. Faculty must have training and equipment, including various types of digital media, that enable them to increase their computer literacy to meet students' needs and adequately address students' different learning styles.

The costs of higher education by means of computer-mediated instruction will need to be evaluated to determine whether electronic education is truly more cost-effective and less expensive than traditional classroom education. The cost savings of the computerized curriculum, although controversial, are anticipated to come primarily through the reduction of faculty positions. Electronic education is projected to be more consumer oriented with regard to the timing of course offerings and the decreased time and costs for students who otherwise would have to drive to and from school. Electronic resources are available for both faculty and students around the clock. Students can now access libraries and other resources electronically, thus decreasing the time required for searches and for extracting journals from a variety of settings (Denning, 1996).

Because of these and other influences, curricula of the future will by necessity be flexible. Chapter 8 provides further discussion of undergraduate and graduate curriculum designs used in nursing education.

Organizing Frameworks

An organizing framework provides faculty with a means of delivering a cohesive curriculum that provides students with the learning experiences necessary to achieve the desired educational outcomes. There are a number of ways to design an organizing framework for a curriculum, and faculty must carefully consider the implications of the framework they have implemented. For example, Ratcliff (1997a) opposed general education programs in which students are permitted simply to choose among arts, humanities, social sciences, life and physical sciences, and mathematics courses. He believed such an approach to general education does not build on the students' abilities, reasoning skills, and intellectual development and leads to failure of students with lesser abilities and lack of stimulation of intellectual development of successful students.

Ratcliff (1997a) also suggested the use of a variety of coursework sequences, rather than a single set curriculum pattern, with assessment measures to evaluate progress and performance as students progress toward meeting degree requirements. Multiple core curricula for general education could be tailored to students' abilities and content majors as the overall organizing frameworks are redesigned.

Whatever organizing framework is used, assessment of outcomes is an essential component of curriculum development. Assessment data must be used to determine whether students have learned and to evaluate the effects of curriculum changes. Assessment findings should be given to students in a timely manner to enable them to evaluate their own learning. The development and assessment of organizing frameworks for nursing education are further discussed in Chapter 9.

Outcomes, Competencies, and Objectives

Outcomes, competencies, and objectives are derived from the philosophical beliefs that create the framework of the curriculum. Learning outcomes became prevalent in the mid 1980s in higher education as accrediting agencies focused on measuring student and graduate performance, holding faculty and institutions of higher learning accountable for student learning (Diamond, 1998; Erickson, 1995; Keith, 1991; Pew Health Professions Commission, 1995).

Lempert (1996) stated that outcomes of curriculum and learning would be stretched beyond the walls of the traditional classroom and focus on building skills for the real world through connecting various disciplines. He stated that the outcome of curricula should be to build better citizens who are productive in the workforce and in the community. As competition for education dollars increases, legislators and other external forces have a greater influence over curriculum development by mandating review of outcomes. The focus on preparation of graduates for the workforce has increased in importance as societal changes have occurred. If educational systems are to continue to maintain accreditation, questions that must be answered include not only how many graduated, but also how many graduates were employed on graduation and are employers satisfied with the graduates' readiness for the workforce.

Traditional outcomes and competencies in nursing and other areas of health care are being challenged and pressured to change. In 1995 the Pew Health Professions Commission projected an evolving health care system that focuses on better management of diminishing resources, promotes wellness education and interventions for the prevention of illness, and emphasizes improving the health of populations. Nurse educators are challenged to recognize and further define the various levels of nursing and to promote educational mobility between the levels. Nurses at each level will have specific responsibilities in the health care system, and the curriculum for each level must be adapted accordingly (Pew Health Professions Commission, 1995).

Halstead et al. (1996) described the development of program outcomes around the essential qualities and competencies as identified by faculty for new nursing graduates. The process of curriculum review as related to real and potential health care reform was discussed, and a list of program outcomes and competencies was created that includes critical thinking, cultural competence, managed care, political awareness, ethical and legal concerns, effective communication, and community aspects. Critical challenges for nurse educators facing an uncertain future were incorporated in the development of outcomes.

Lenburg (1991) and Bevil (1991) discussed assessment outcomes and program evaluation, posing the following several questions for faculty to consider in the process of nursing program evaluation:

- Who will develop the assessment outcomes?
- Who will develop instruments to measure the outcomes?
- Who will maintain records?
- Who will interpret assessment findings, and how will the findings be used?
- What effect will findings have on faculty jobs and salaries?
- Is the success of the program supported by administration? By faculty?
- Are graduates prepared to meet the demands of nursing practice?

Outcomes must incorporate the increasing diversity and technological explosion in the sequence of learning experiences that will prepare the graduate to survive within the workforce (Erickson, 1995; Pew Health Professions Commission, 1995; Ratcliff, 1997b). Institutions will be held accountable for students' performance and will be assessed by how well students meet course outcomes and competencies. Performance indicators will likely be used to fund public institutions (Denning, 1996; Schmidt, 1997). Faculty need to evaluate the learning that occurs in classroom and clinical settings to verify that outcomes are being met. The use of classroom assessment and research techniques (CATs) provides faculty and students with information about strengths and weaknesses in the students' learning. Faculty and students can adapt techniques mid course to increase students' learning in the semester (Angelo & Cross, 1993; Cross & Steadman, 1996). A further discussion of selecting outcomes and competencies is provided in Chapter 9.

Educational Activities

Learning activities provided to enhance students' knowledge and inquisitiveness must also prepare the graduate for real world experiences. Creativity, oral and written communication, problem solving, managing diverse groups of people, and negotiation are among the outcomes necessary for undergraduate curricula (Ratcliff, 1997a). Collaborative learning experiences can be created to enable students to learn from their peers and professionals (Dochterman & Grace, 2001). Activities should be planned to enhance progressive learning, starting with less difficult activities and progressing to activities that require students to synthesize complex concepts. Learning should be assessed and feedback given to students in a timely manner, enabling them to see their progress and make decisions about their learning. Presentations and student projects will become more automated as electronic delivery enhances communication to consumers (Denning, 1996). Clinical experiences, while including traditional acute care, must move into community-based agencies in which students are required to possess and use more critical thinking skills and flexibility to problem solve issues concerning clients' care with interdisciplinary health care teams (Freeman et al., 2002; Kotecki, 2002; Massey, 2001; Matteson, 2000; Wink, 2003).

Poirrier (2001) and others stressed the importance of service-based learning using community-based partnerships to focus on health promotion and prevention in communities. The nursing curriculum emphasis of service learning would broaden students' view of nursing to address human needs in addition to individual patient needs. The curriculum focus would be on the promotion of a healthy lifestyle; the care of underserved, vulnerable populations; environmental concerns; and cultural diversity. Service learning enhances the student's role as a citizen with health care, social justice, and policy responsibilities. Environmental, global health, and bioterrorism issues would be addressed (Bailey et al., 2002; Hamner & Wilder, 2001; Leonard, 2001; Redman & Clark, 2002; Reece et al., 2003; Seifer & Vaughn, 2002; Veenema, 2001, 2002; Wink, 2003; Wright, 2003).

Problem-based learning enables students to engage in complex situations to determine what they need to learn and what skills are needed to arrive at solutions. The teamwork associated with problem-based learning strengthens students' communication, negotiation, and social skills; creative and critical thinking skills; and clinical reasoning abilities (Savin-Baden, 2000).

Finally, as part of curriculum restructuring, increasing the involvement of alumni and other professionals in curriculum design, for example, by integrating their ideas for useful educational activities, should increase curriculum relevance to the workplace. The selection and design of learning activities and service learning are discussed in Chapters 10 and 11.

Evaluation

As stated previously, with the new, consumer-driven curricula, universities and faculty will be evaluated on the basis of how well students and graduates perform (Denning, 1996; Pew Health Professions Commission, 1995; Schmidt, 1997). Breneman (1993) recognized that the challenge to higher education, as related to curriculum, is to mobilize faculty members, who differ in educational beliefs and perceptions about the university, into a team that will work together so that real change can occur. He agreed that universities and faculty would be held accountable for the curriculum by funding sources. Instruments must be found or developed to assess outcomes according to specific procedures (Diamond, 1998). Outcomes would include entry and graduation rates, licensure or certification of graduates, and employment rates. In nursing, the outcome criteria of state boards and national accrediting agencies include pass rates on the National Council Licensure Examination for Registered Nurses (NCLEX-RN) and postgraduation employment rates for basic undergraduate programs (National League for Nursing, 1996). Evaluation of the curriculum is discussed in detail in Unit V.

CURRICULUM DEVELOPMENT AS A PROCESS

Many global changes are rapidly occurring, and these changes will affect curriculum development in higher education. Faculty must remain responsive to the needs of society and students and design curricula that reflect these changes. Faculty in higher education across the nation are engaging in curriculum revision and development in an effort to provide curricula that will produce graduates who possess the skills necessary for success in the workplaces of the twenty-first century.

Curriculum development is a deliberative process that takes concentrated time, effort, and faculty commitment, not just an event (Bevis & Murray, 1990; Civian et al., 1997; Diamond, 1998; Hord et al., 1987; Lindquist, 1997; Oliva, 1992). According to Oliva (1992) and others, curriculum change begins at the level of its current state and continues as a process of making choices from a number of alternatives. If curricula continue to exist, change is inevitable because of the effects of external change agents, such as community pressure, policy changes, and funding sources (Doll, 1996; Fullan, 1991; Gaff, 1997b; Wiles & Bondi, 1989).

Curriculum development, which may consist of changes ranging from simple substitutions or alterations of content from course to course to a complete restructuring of the entire curriculum, should be a cooperative group activity. However, change results only as people alter their thoughts and patterns of behavior. Significant curriculum change is associated with ambiguity, ambivalence, and uncertainty; therefore smooth implementation is often a sign that little change has occurred. Relearning is at the heart of change and may be a powerful inhibitor of change (Oliva, 1992). Faculty engaging in curriculum development would benefit from examining their environment for facilitators and barriers to curriculum development, working collaboratively to maximize the facilitative aspects and minimize the barriers. According to Diamond (1998), "An effective curriculum provides multiple opportunities to apply and practice what is learned" (p. 85).

Facilitators of Curriculum Development

Ritchie (1986) and McNeil (1990) offered suggestions to promote an effective curriculum change process, including faculty development workshops and focus groups. The group of faculty involved initially in the change must be key faculty members who understand the problem and can effectively evaluate strategies for problem solving. Faculty on a curriculum committee need to perceive that their contributions will be heard and have an impact on the outcome of decisions. Faculty also need to believe that their contributions will be recognized and rewarded and be assured that their contributions will promote a greater good for the organization. Mutual respect must be present among participants of the committee, fostered by trust, honesty, and confidence between the committee leader and faculty. Recognition of the components of effective change can help ensure that the change process will produce the desired outcomes (Carmon et al., 1992; Doll, 1996; Fullan, 1991; Lindquist, 1997; Oliva, 1992). However, curriculum change takes time. In today's uncertain world curriculum changes must occur carefully but quickly for nursing schools to survive. Several examples of the process of curriculum change are found in nursing literature (Hamner & Wilder, 2001; Mawn & Reece, 2000; Redman et al., 1999; Webber, 2002).

Barriers to Curriculum Development

Real change causes conflict, and the idea of conflict leads to fear in many faculty members (Erickson, 1995; Mawn & Reece, 2000; McNeil, 1990). In many institutions of higher education real changes need to be made so that the necessary contemporary curricula can be developed. For example, faculty need to be flexible, adaptable, and open to experiential learning if the curriculum is to change to meet workforce and community needs. In the past, any experiential learning was typically viewed as an "add-on" to the curriculum, not an integration of learning that would increase creativity and individual initiative. This viewpoint is no longer compatible with society's needs. Students should actively be involved in real world activities throughout the curriculum, not just during an internship at the end of the program (Lempert, 1996). Working with community leaders and cultural groups enables students to learn to work within the real world and enhances communication and decision-making skills beyond those learned from the textbook and in the classroom (Erickson, 1995). Hamner and Wilder (2001) identified the need to determine possible obstacles to curriculum implementation early so that faculty could address the issues.

To make the changes necessary to integrate experiential learning throughout the curriculum, faculty are required to conceptualize curriculum development differently than they have in the past. Faculty may be uncertain about how to effectively incorporate such changes into the curriculum, with this uncertainty manifesting itself in a reluctance or a refusal to change.

Thus, as this example illustrates, one of the major barriers to curriculum development is the fear of change itself. Faculty who resist change often lack the flexibility, adaptability, and vision to combine theory and workplace skills. Ritchie (1986) described these barriers and others and identified the following 13 reasons that curriculum change is resisted by faculty.

1. Fear of losing control of the curriculum
2. Misunderstanding due to lack of information or confusion about new vocabulary and jargon
3. Perception of lack of ability to progress because of new time and energy demands
4. Different views about what needs to be done

5. Lack of motivation to study the change
6. Lack of perception of a need for change ("If it ain't broke, don't fix it.")
7. Too many changes and too many demands related to the change process
8. Desire to be vindictive and make the leader look bad
9. Idea that "no one can tell me what to do"
10. Threat to current social support systems
11. Lack of resources
12. View that formal methods used to facilitate change are a barrier rather than a help
13. Lack of rewards

Because of these potential barriers, the leader and organizational culture are key players in successful curriculum change (Fullan, 1991; Middlewood, 2001; Ritchie, 1986; Wiles & Bondi, 1989). For example, the future of nursing is faced with many uncertainties as technology and the health care system undergo rapid and dramatic changes. Traditional nursing curricula are threatened as needed skills and program outcomes are changed with little input from nursing education (Pew Higher Education Roundtable, 1994). As external changes such as these occur, leadership characteristics become extremely important. Faculty observe the manner in which the leader (1) responds to critical incidents and crises; (2) supervises, evaluates, praises, handles conflict resolution, directs changes, and represents the organization; and (3) executes rewards and assigns, promotes, and terminates employees.

The leader must acknowledge potential barriers to change and understand that faculty have differing beliefs and opinions about change. When a change is proposed faculty members may each react differently because the change will affect them individually. For example, teaching styles may need to be altered for some faculty members, whereas others already use the needed strategies. Also, courses may be removed from the curriculum or moved to a different location within the curriculum pattern. Faculty would then experience a need to teach new courses, face employment changes, or deal with the problems associated with teaching a different level of students. Effective leadership is important in the change process; if the leader's vision and goals differ greatly from those of the faculty, desired outcomes will likely not occur (Fullan, 1991; Middlewood, 2001).

Curriculum Development as Planned Change

A plan should be developed for a regular review of the curriculum. Diamond (1998) states that curriculum change must be planned. "The needs for . . . improvement are too great and resources too limited to allow us to be inefficient or ineffective in the way we address our curricular problems. We cannot afford to leave things to chance" (p. 15). It is expected that faculty will routinely update individual courses with the latest developments in the given field. The overall curriculum, however, may change without faculty awareness as individual courses change, leading to gaps in content or skills. Faculty must plan to evaluate the curriculum on a regular basis to avoid this pitfall.

The organizational culture must facilitate the innovative ideas of faculty in curriculum change. Administrative support of faculty innovations is important. Creativity may lead to a better product, or graduate, than originally planned. As faculty model development of new ideas, critical thinking skills in students can be fostered.

Also, faculty must view the curriculum committee as a means for program improvement and innovation rather than as a hindrance. By fostering an environment that supports the review of the curriculum on a regular basis, continuous open dialogue about needed changes, and the incorporation of planned changes, leaders can help faculty become more comfortable with the change process. The results will be a curriculum that remains on the cutting edge, meeting the needs of the students, community, and society.

SUMMARY

Rapid changes in today's world mandate review and restructuring of the curricula across the university setting, including health care. Faculty must cope with transition from tradition to an era of information explosion led by massive changes in technology, economics, and the development of multiculturalism. In the past, curricula in higher education were designed to teach students how to inquire, how to perform in a specialty field, and how to do research, with the professor being the central figure (Gaff, 1997a). Faculty felt comfortable with this authority, this belief, and this practice.

In today's world, and in the future, significant change is necessary to lower the cost of education and increase productivity while maintaining high-quality curricula based on sound educational principles. According to Gaff (1997a) and others, faculty and administrators who are restructuring curriculum must do the following:

- Use technology in the classroom and beyond the four walls
- Design interdisciplinary studies
- Develop more holistic, experimental, and integrative models of learning
- Incorporate cultural diversity
- Develop academic majors that will cultivate writing and critical thinking skills and integrate theoretical and practical knowledge
- Internationalize the curriculum
- Assess student learning, provide feedback, and provide supplemental instruction to help at-risk students achieve high academic standards
- Use group work to enhance the learning of students and faculty together.

Administrative personnel need to be visionary in providing leadership and coordination of activities across departments as the restructuring process occurs. Curriculum change must be paralleled with faculty change as students and learning outcomes become the focus of contemporary higher education (Curry & Wergin, 1997; Doll, 1996; Gaff, 1997a, 1997b; Levine & Nidiffer, 1997; Lindquist, 1997; McNeil, 1990; Ratcliff, 1997b; Taba, 1962).

This chapter provided an introduction to curriculum, including a brief comparison of traditional versus interactive and innovative types of curricula. Curriculum was defined according to several authors, and curriculum components were reviewed. The discussion of curriculum changes briefly described the process, barriers, and facilitators of change in curriculum development. The impact of social, economic, and technological forces was also described.

REFERENCES

American Association of Colleges of Nursing. (1999). A vision of baccalaureate and graduate nursing education: The next decade. *Journal of Professional Nursing, 15*(1), 59-65.

Angelo, T. A., & Cross, P. K. (1993). *Classroom assessment techniques* (2nd ed.). San Francisco: Jossey-Bass.

Bailey, P. A., Carpenter, D. R., & Harrington, P. (2002). Theoretical foundations of service-learning in nursing education. *Journal of Nursing Education, 41*(10), 433-436.

Baldwin, D., & Nelms, T. (1993). Difficult dialogues: Impact on nursing education curricula. *Journal of Professional Nursing, 9*(6), 343-346.

Beauchamp, G. A. (1968). *Curriculum theory* (2nd ed.). Wilmette, IL: The Kagg Press.

Bevil, C. A. (1991). Program evaluation in nursing education: Creating a meaningful plan. In M. Garbin, *Assessing educational outcomes* (pp. 53-67). New York: National League for Nursing Press.

Bevis, E. O. (1989). *Curriculum building in nursing.* New York: National League for Nursing Press.

Bevis, E. O. (2000). Nursing curriculum as professional education. In E. O. Bevis & J. Watson, *Toward a caring curriculum: A new pedagogy for nursing* (pp. 74-77). New York: National League for Nursing.

Bevis, E. O., & Murray, J. P. (1990). The essence of curriculum revolution: Emancipatory teaching. *Journal of Nursing Education, 29*(7), 326-331.

Breneman, D. W. (1993). *Higher education: On a collision course with new realities.* Boston: American Student Assistance.

Breneman, D. W., & Taylor, A. L. (Eds.). (1996). *Strategies for promoting excellence in a time of scarce resources.* San Francisco: Jossey-Bass.

Brown, J. S., & Duguid, P. (1996). Universities in the digital age. *Change, 28*(4), 11-19.

Brown, S. C., & Kysilka, M. L. (2002). *Applying multicultural and global concepts in the classroom and beyond.* Boston: Allyn & Bacon.

Carmon, M., Hauber, R. P., & Chase, L. (1992). From anxiety to action. *Nursing & Health Care, 13*(7), 364-368.

Center for the Health Professions. (2003.). *Pew Health Professions Commission 1989-1999.* Retrieved September 1, 2003, from http://www.futurehealth.ucsf.edu/pewcomm/factsht3.html

Civian, J. T., Arnold, G., Gamson, G. F., Kanter, S., & London, H. B. (1997). In J. G. Gaff & J. L. Ratcliff & Associates, *Handbook of the undergraduate curriculum* (pp. 647-660). San Francisco: Jossey-Bass.

Cross, P. K., & Steadman, M. H. (1996). *Classroom research: Implementing the scholarship of teaching.* San Francisco: Jossey-Bass.

Curry, L., & Wergin, J. F. (1997). Professional education. In J. G. Gaff & J. L. Ratcliff & Associates, *Handbook of the undergraduate curriculum* (pp. 341-358). San Francisco: Jossey-Bass.

Denning, P. J. (1996). Business designs for the new university. *Educom Review, 31*(6), 21-41.

Diamond, R. M. (1998). *Designing and assessing courses and curricula: A practical guide.* San Francisco: Jossey-Bass.

Diekelmann, N. L. (1993). Behavioral pedagogy: A Heideggerian hermeneutical analysis of the lived experiences of students and teachers in baccalaureate nursing education. *Journal of Nursing Education, 32*(6), 245-250.

Dochterman, J. M., & Grace, H. K. (2001). Nursing education in transition. In J. M. Dochterman & H. K. Grace, *Current issues in nursing.* (6th ed.). St. Louis: Mosby.

Doll, R. C. (1996). *Curriculum improvement: Decision making and process* (9th ed.). Boston: Allyn & Bacon.

Doll, Jr., W. E. (2002). Ghosts and the curriculum. In W. E. Doll, Jr., & N. Gough, *Curriculum visions* (pp. 23-70). New York: Peter Lang

Eisner, E. W. (1985). *The educational imagination* (2nd ed.). New York: Macmillan.

Erickson, H. L. (1995). *Stirring the head, heart and soul: Redefining curriculum and instruction.* Thousand Oaks, CA: Corwin.

Fagin, C. (1997). How nursing should respond to the third report of the Pew Health Professions Commission. *Online Journal of Issues in Nursing,* December 30. Retrieved December 3, 2003, from http://www.nursingworld.org/ojin/tpc5/tpc5_2.htm

Freeman, L. H., Voignier, R. R., & Scott, D. L. (2002). New curriculum for a new century: Beyond repackaging. *Journal of Nursing Education, 41*(1), 38-40.

Fuhrmann, B. (1997). Philosophies and aims. In J. G. Gaff & J. L. Ratcliff & Associates, *Handbook of the undergraduate curriculum* (pp. 86-99). San Francisco: Jossey-Bass.

Fullan, M. G. (1991). *The new meaning of educational change* (2nd ed.). New York: Teachers College Press.

Gaff, J. G. (1997a). *New life for the college curriculum: Assessing achievements and furthering progress in the reform of general education.* San Francisco: Jossey-Bass.

Gaff, J. G. (1997b). Tensions between tradition and innovation. In J. G. Gaff & J. L. Ratcliff & Associates, *Handbook of the undergraduate curriculum* (pp. 684-706). San Francisco: Jossey-Bass.

Garcia, M., & Ratcliff, J. L. (1997). Social forces shaping the curriculum. In J. G. Gaff & J. L. Ratcliff & Associates, *Handbook of the undergraduate curriculum* (pp. 118-136). San Francisco: Jossey-Bass.

Halstead, J. A., Rains, J. W., Boland, D. L., & May, F. E. (1996). Reconceptualizing baccalaureate nursing education: Outcomes and competencies for practice in the 21st century. *Journal of Nursing Education, 35*(9), 413-416.

Hamner, J., & Wilder, B. (2001). A new curriculum for a new millennium. *Nursing Outlook, 49*(3), 127-131.

Hodson Carlton, K. E., Siktberg, L. L., Flowers, J., & Scheibel, P. (2003). Overview of distance education in nursing: Where are we now and where are we going? In M. H. Oermann and K. T. Heinrich, *Annual review of nursing education.* New York: Springer.

Hord, S. M., Rutherford, W. L., Huling-Austin, L., & Hall, G. E. (1987). *Taking charge of change.* Austin, TX: Southwest Educational Development Laboratory.

Keith, N. Z. (1991). Assessing educational goals: The national movement to outcomes evaluation. In M. Garbin, *Assessing educational outcomes* (pp. 1-23). New York: National League for Nursing Press.

Klein, M. F. (1995). Alternative curriculum conceptions and designs. In A. C. Ornstein & L. S. Behar, *Contemporary issues in curriculum* (pp. 28-33). Boston: Allyn & Bacon.

Kotecki, C. N. (2002). Community-based strategies: Incorporating faith-based partnerships into the curriculum. *Nurse Educator, 27*(1), 13-15.

Lempert, D. H. (1996). *Escape from the ivory tower.* San Francisco: Jossey-Bass.

Lenburg, C. B. (1991). Assessing the goals of nursing education: Issues and approaches to evaluation outcomes. In M. Garbin, *Assessing educational outcomes* (pp. 25-52). New York: National League for Nursing Press.

Lenburg, C. B. (2002). Changes that challenge nursing education. *Alabama Nurse, 29*(4): 6-7.

Leonard, B. J. (2001). Quality nursing care celebrates diversity. *Online Journal of Issues in Nursing, 6*(2). Retrieved December 3, 2003, from http://www.nursingworld.org/ojin/topic15/tpc15_3.htm

Levine, A., & Nidiffer, J. (1997). Key turning points in the evolving curriculum. In J. G. Gaff & J. L. Ratcliff & Associates, *Handbook of the undergraduate curriculum* (pp. 53-85). San Francisco: Jossey-Bass.

Lindeman, C. A. (2000). The future of nursing education. *Journal of Nursing Education, 39*(1), 5-12.

Lindquist, J. (1997). Strategies for change. In J. G. Gaff & J. L. Ratcliff & Associates, *Handbook of the undergraduate curriculum* (pp. 633-646). San Francisco: Jossey-Bass.

Longstreet, W. S., & Shane, H. G. (1993). *Curriculum for a new millennium.* Boston: Allyn & Bacon.

Manuel, P., & Sorensen, L. (1995). Changing trends in healthcare: Implications for baccalaureate education, practice and employment. *Journal of Nursing Education, 34*(6), 248-253.

Massey, C. M. (2001). A transdisciplinary model for curricular revision. *Nursing and Health Care Perspectives, 22*(2), 85-88.

Matteson, P. S. (2000). Preparing nurses for the future. In P. Matteson, *Community-based nursing education* (pp. 1-7). New York: Springer.

Mawn, B., & Reece, S. M. (2000). Reconfiguring a curriculum for the new millennium: The process of change. *Journal of Nursing Education, 39*(3), 101-108.

McNeil, J. D. (1990). *Curriculum: A comprehensive introduction* (4th ed.). Glenview, IL: Scott, Foresman.

Melton, R. (2002). *Planning and developing open and distance learning.* New York: Routledge Falmer.

Middlewood, D. (2001). Leadership of the curriculum: Setting the vision. In D. Middlewood & N. Burton, *Managing the curriculum.* Thousand Oaks, CA: Sage.

Morse, W. A., & Corcoran-Perry, S. (1996). A process model to guide selection of essential curriculum content. *Journal of Nursing Education, 35*(8), 341-347.

Myers, S. T., Stolte, K. M., Baker, C., Nishikawa, H., & Sohier, R. (1991). A process-driven curriculum in nursing education. *Nursing & Health Care, 12*(9), 460-463.

National League for Nursing. (1996). *1996 Criteria for accreditation of baccalaureate and higher degree programs.* New York: Author.

Nelms, T. (1991). Has the curriculum revolution revolutionized the definition of curriculum? *Journal of Nursing Education, 30*(1), 5-8.

Oliva, P. J. (1992). *Developing the curriculum* (3rd ed.). New York: Harper Collins.

Ornstein, A. C., & Hunkins, F. P. (1993). *Curriculum: Foundations, principles and issues* (2nd ed.). Boston: Allyn & Bacon.

Pew Health Professions Commission. (1995). *Critical challenges: Revitalizing the health professions for the twenty-first century.* San Francisco: Author.

Pew Higher Education Roundtable. (1994, April). To dance with change. *Policy Perspectives, 5*(3), 1A-12A.

Poirrier, G. P. (2001). *Service-learning: Curricular applications in nursing.* Sudbury, MA: Jones & Bartlett.

Posner, G. J. (1992). *Analyzing the curriculum.* New York: McGraw Hill.

Rambur, B. (1991). Human environments, phenomena, crises, and lifestyles. *Nursing & Health Care, 12*(9), 464-468.

Ratcliff, J. L. (1997a). Quality and coherence in general education. In J. G. Gaff & J. L. Ratcliff & Associates, *Handbook of the undergraduate curriculum.* San Francisco: Jossey-Bass.

Ratcliff, J. L. (1997b). What is a curriculum and what should it be? In J. G. Gaff & J. L. Ratcliff & Associates, *Handbook of the undergraduate curriculum* (pp. 5-29). San Francisco: Jossey-Bass.

Redman, R. W., & Clark, L. (2002). Service-learning as a model for integrating social justice in the nursing curriculum. *Journal of Nursing Education, 41*(10), 446-449.

Redman, R. W., Lenburg, C. B., & Walker, P. H. (1999). Competency assessment: Methods for development and implementation in nursing education. *Online Journal of Issues in Nursing,* September 30. Retrieved December 3, 2003, from http://www.nursingworld.org/ojin/topic10/tpc10_3.htm

Reece, S. M., Mawn, B., & Scollin, P. (2003). Evaluation of faculty transition into a community-based curriculum. *Journal of Nursing Education, 42*(1), 43-47.

Rentschler, D. D., & Spegman, A. M. (1996). Curriculum revolution: Realities of change. *Journal of Nursing Education, 35*(9), 389-393.

Ritchie, J. B. (1986). Management strategies for curriculum change. *Journal of Dental Education, 50*(3), 97-101.

Satre, J. P. (1974). *Between existentialism and Marxism.* New York: Pantheon Books.

Savin-Baden, M. (2000). *Problem-based learning in higher education: Untold stories.* UK: SRHE and Open University Press.

Schmidt, P. (1997, April 4). Rancor and confusion greet a change in South Carolina's budgeting system. *The Chronicle of Higher Education,* pp. A26-A27.

Schubert, W. H. (1986). *Curriculum: Perspective, paradigm, and possibility.* New York: Macmillan.

Seifer, S. D., & Vaughn, R. L. (2002). Partners in caring and community: Service learning in nursing education. *Journal of Nursing Education, 41*(10), 437-439.

Smith, B. E., Colling, K., Elander, E., & Latham, C. (1993). A model for multicultural curriculum development in baccalaureate nursing education. *Journal of Nursing Education, 32*(5), 205-208.

Taba, H. (1962). *Curriculum development: Theory and practice.* New York: Harcourt, Brace & World.

Tagliareni, M. E., & Mengel, A. (2001). Broadening clinical education in basic nursing programs. In J. M. Dochterman & H. K. Grace, *Current issues in nursing.* (6th ed.). St. Louis: Mosby.

Veenema, T. G. (2001). An evidence-based curriculum to prepare students for global nursing practice. *Nursing and Health Care Perspectives, 22*(6), 292-298.

Veenema, T. G. (2002). Chemical and biological terrorism: Current updates for nurse educators. *Nursing Education Perspectives, 23*(2), 62-71.

Watson, J. (2000). A new paradigm. In E. O. Bevis & J. Watson, *Toward a caring curriculum: A new pedagogy for nursing.* New York: National League for Nursing.

Webber, P. B. (2002). A curriculum framework for nursing. *Journal of Nursing Education, 41*(1), 15-23.

Wiles, J., & Bondi, J. (1989). *Curriculum development: A guide to practice* (3rd ed.). Columbus, OH: Merrill.

Williamson, S. R. (1996). When change is the only constant: Liberal education in the age of technology. *Educom Review, 31*(6), 39-41.

Wink, D. M. (2003). Community-based curricula at BSN and graduate levels. In M. H. Oermann & K. T. Heinrich, *Annual review of nursing education.* New York: Springer.

Wright, D. J. (2003). Collaborative learning experiences for nursing students in environmental health. *Nursing Education Perspectives, 24*(4), 189-191.

6

Forces and Issues Influencing Curriculum Development

Joanne Rains Warner, DNS, RN

The magnitude, pace, and intensity of change within the health care arena have astonished providers, consumers, and financers of health care. Sweeping health care reforms affect everyone, including the nursing profession. Nurse educators are challenged to develop relevant curriculum to prepare practitioners equipped for new roles and responsibilities. Curriculum does not occur in a vacuum but is instead a contextual representation of global trends, national circumstances, professional priorities, and faculty values. Curriculum must be congruent with this social context, the interrelated conditions, and factors in the setting. Without a fit between the curriculum and the broad practice environment, nurses would not have the relevant skills and attitudes necessary to effectively intervene in contemporary health care challenges or have adequate knowledge of the populations needing care.

The context of interrelated forces and issues that influence the development and direction of curriculum is complex and ever changing. Some of these forces and issues are external to the nursing profession, including societal patterns, demographic trends, and economic characteristics that shape the general environment. Some are current forces within higher education, including issues of affordability, access, and accountability. Some forces and issues are specific to the nursing profession, including workforce trends and practice competencies. Other forces, such as health policy trends or work redesign, are both internal and external to the nursing profession.

This influential social context is dynamic and involves interrelating factors that are regularly prompting change. To remain relevant, curriculum must be responsive to these changes. Garcia and Ratcliff (1997) described curriculum as a "social construct undergoing continuous revision and modification" (p. 118). To plan and develop meaningful curricula, faculty must closely examine and analyze the various forces that provide direction for curriculum change (Lenburg, 2002). Faculty need assessment strategies and tools to monitor the pulse of the curriculum context. These tools should monitor the strength and regularity of the signs coming from the practice environment and suggest times and ways for curriculum adaptation.

This chapter describes the current social context for curriculum development, including issues and forces in the environment external to the nursing profession, the higher education environment, and the profession's internal environment. This chapter also describes four strategies to identify the forces and issues that significantly influence nursing practice and education. Faculty can use these tools to develop curricula that match the populations needing care, the leading health challenges, and the skills and abilities needed to promote health and prevent illness.

FORCES AND ISSUES IN THE CURRENT CURRICULUM CONTEXT

The issues that are currently influencing curriculum development can be explicated. In attempting to describe a time so proximate, faculty run the risk of either overlooking what will become an enduring feature of the time or underestimating the difficulty in winnowing the significant issues from the irrelevant ones. However, faculty do not have the luxury of waiting until history tells the story of our times. They must be proactive developers of a dynamic curriculum, one that will provide students with the skills and competencies necessary to successfully practice in today's global society.

In an effort to describe the current setting and environment for curriculum development, the following issues are discussed: issues external to the nursing profession, issues of higher education, and issues specific to the nursing profession. Each section is by no means an exhaustive discussion of the topic but an identification of major current and projected themes.

Issues External to the Nursing Profession

Increasingly, health issues are related to the sociopolitical and economic characteristics of the communities where people live, work, and play. Curriculum must acknowledge the broad determinants of health to prepare practicing nurses to effectively intervene in complex problems such as bioterrorism, homelessness, global and domestic violence, teen pregnancy, and emerging infectious diseases.

The issues external to nursing relate to curriculum in several ways. First, they provide the setting for the world in which nurses practice and learn. Collectively, they describe the current states of humanity and health. Second, they comprise the risk factors for health and disease and contribute to the complex web of causation. Nurses need to have a working knowledge of these issues as they strive to prevent health problems and promote wellness. From both of these perspectives, issues external to nursing provide a crucial foundation for nursing's understanding of societal needs and characteristics and therefore form an essential piece of the foundation necessary for contemporary curriculum development.

Five trends capture significant developments and concerns for society and are presented as the broad sociopolitical and economic context of nursing practice and education. These trends are global violence and the threat of violence, demographic revolutions, the technological explosion, globalization and the rise of global economy, and environmental challenges.

Although these trends are discussed separately, their interconnectedness is undeniable.

Global Violence and the Threat of Violence

On September 11, 2001, hijacked airplanes hit the World Trade Center towers in New York City and the Pentagon near Washington, DC. A fourth plane crashed in rural Pennsylvania. These events and their aftermath play significantly into the sociopolitical, economic, and cultural landscape of our nation. The attacks are understood by many as acts of terrorism and as part of an international series of retaliations against perceived wrongs. They marked an end to a sense of national invulnerability, and a "watershed in human expectations" about the world and life (Lewis, 2003, p. 291). *Terrorism* became part of our nation's daily lexicon.

The societal reverberations of the attacks have been many, including two economic consequences: The events aggravated the economic downturn of 2001, and they shifted national spending toward security and antiterrorism strategies and away from social programs and human needs (Wiener & Tilly, 2002). The health implications from both consequences are tremendous. The health care system has focused resources on disaster and mass trauma preparedness, bioterrorism responses, and a multitude of strategies to prepare for unpredictable and diverse catastrophic events. Nurses need the skills and knowledge to help create emergency response systems and work within the public health infrastructures characterized by community-wide collaboration, communication, and appropriate public policy. Nurses need clinical knowledge related to biological agents, as well as skills to address the emotional stresses in the face of war and perceived vulnerability.

The Demographic Revolutions

The United States is aging. The U.S. Census Bureau (2000) projects that between the years 2000 and 2050, the number of people aged 65 years and older will increase by 135% and those aged 85 years and older will increase by 350%. When the baby boomer cohort enters long-term care, they will be "disproportionately widowed women with high rates of disability and poverty; many will be members of racial and ethnic minorities" (Wallace et al., 2001, p. 217).

Issues surrounding geriatric health have obvious curricular implications because educators have the responsibility to prepare nurses to promote health and prevent disease and disability in the large aging population. Not only will nursing care's emphasis be shifted from acute to chronic illnesses, but it will increase in complexity for the ongoing management of multiple disabilities and diseases. Initiatives such as those of the John A. Hartford Foundation Institute for Geriatric Nursing are excellent examples of bringing best practices and resources to improve the health care of older adults.

The disproportionate growth of the aged population is juxtaposed a slower growth in the working population age cohort. The number of people aged 16 to 64 years is projected to grow 33% between the years 2000 and 2050. Not only does this project a workforce shortage of health care providers, particularly nurses, to care for elderly patients, but also relatively fewer individuals contributing to the tax resources required to support needed social programs (Wiener & Tilly, 2002). Family and community resources to assume the burdens of care are stressed, with difficult policy discussions required relative to resource allocation (Gorman, 2002). Curricula should include opportunities to develop the political advocacy skills needed to influence public policy decisions relative to the allocation of resources toward health and human needs.

Another demographic phenomenon in the United States is the growth of Hispanic and Asian American populations. Klineberg (1997) notes that the immigration patterns are changing the composition of the country, where the Anglo/European majority is a historic trend, into a microcosm of the world's peoples. The conflict and controversy that accompany that significant of a demographic shift are exacerbated by the economic insecurity and volatility of our times. Multicultural diversity and ethnic understanding have major curriculum implications. Also, recruitment and retention of faculty and students who reflect the diversity of the population being served are significant issues for schools of nursing.

Whether the demographic shifts include age, diversity, or other population features, there are implications for health and the resources needed to promote health. Preparing tomorrow's nursing practitioners requires attention to all demographic revolutions of both developed and developing areas of the globe, including patterns of growth, migration, and ethnic/racial composition.

Technological Explosion

America's transition from a resource-based, industrial economy characterized by semiskilled factory workers and raw materials to a knowledge-based, Information Age economy has been reshaping society for decades, and new technological possibilities continue to revolutionize life. Information and digital technologies have changed the pace and possibilities in communication, data management, and information access (Heller et al., 2000).

Access to education and knowledge is access to wealth, which can widen the gap between the rich and the poor. Issues in biotechnology, genetic engineering, information management ethics, and robotics accompany the technological progress, each with multiple implications for nursing practice and education. Billings et al. (2001) suggest that technology's influence on educational practice should be driven by pedagogical goals rather than the lure of technology itself, or as "a learning vision pull rather than as a technology push" (p. 42).

Globalization and the Rise of the Global Economy

National boundaries are becoming less relevant in an era of instantaneous telecommunications, free trade, and multinational corporations. The globe operates as a single worldwide production system, and the important skills are investing, strategic planning, and securing a market presence. The consequences of globalization are staggering and depend, in part, on a country's state of development.

The health implications of globalization are both negative and positive. According to Heller et al. (2000), globalization marks the "'death of distance' in the spread of disease and the delivery of health care" (p. 10), meaning that disease may be transmitted rapidly beyond borders and continents and that health knowledge regarding treatment and causes of disease can also spread between countries and health systems.

Nursing curriculum should acknowledge the realities of a market-driven or demand-driven health care system based increasingly on a global economy. Curriculum should also acknowledge that health care is a significant industry whose profit margins, stock prices, and bottom lines influence salaries and employment opportunities. Curriculum should help nurses understand the influence of globalization on the transmission and treatment of disease. Nurses best prepared for changes due to economic forces understand the significance of globalization and the global economy.

Environmental Challenges

Just as currency more readily crosses borders, so can environmental and epidemiological hazards. Besides health issues across the globe, there are concerns of sustainable development, energy availability, pollution-free water, and global warming, to name a few. Environmental health involves understanding and intervening to improve the impact people have on the environment and the impact the environment has on the health of the people (Allender & Spradley, 2001).

Increasingly, Americans are becoming aware that the threats to public health and life are found in "the fragility of the web of life, in the limits to the earth's waste-absorptive and cleansing capacities, in the delicate interdependence that support the process of life itself on this planet" (Klineberg, 1994, p. 236). Nursing curricula should address the content and competencies related to environmental health, preparing nurses to factor environmental issues into the web of disease causation and to intervene to improve environmental health.

Summary

These recurring issues from the broad sociopolitical and economic setting have current and future influence on the practice of nursing. Curriculum needs to acknowledge the possibilities and implications of global violence; demographic revolutions in number, age, and ethnic composition of populations; the technological explosion; the globalization of the economy and health; and the increasing awareness of environmental fragility.

Issues in Higher Education

Institutions of higher education sit at an interesting juncture of at least two global themes: the technological explosion and the globalization of the economy. As learning, knowledge, and skills become the primary resources of a country, the public and private financing of quality higher education becomes more challenging. Therefore "affordability, access, and accountability are the three key issues facing public higher education at the start of the new millennium" (Heller, 2001, p. 1). Each issue affects the other, for affordability determines access, and as public concerns related to these issues mount, there are increasing calls for accountability.

Affordability

Heller (2001) defines college affordability as a combination of the price of tuition, fees, and other costs, as well as the student's ability to pay for college. The concern for affordability was noted as early as 1947 yet persists today as economic and societal factors promote an increased value of a college degree in labor markets; higher education is considered an avenue to a livable wage, or a salary to support a middle-class lifestyle.

Because of societal concern for a living wage, the financing of higher education becomes a crucial public policy debate. Within that debate, the academy should prepare persuasive arguments for the merits of education beyond salary, for societal obligation to invest in human infrastructure, and for the importance of public commitment to higher education. The specific charge for schools of nursing is to articulate the cost-effective contribution nursing makes to the improvement of the health of the nation.

Access

Another historic issue that persists today is access to higher education. Callan (2001) highlights the importance of access by noting that society's transformation from an industrial economy to an information-based, global economy makes education beyond high school a necessity for a middle-class lifestyle. "If opportunity is broadly defined as the chance to participate fully in society, higher education has become the only road to opportunity for most Americans" (p. 85).

Opportunity, therefore, requires public policies and political will that support access, as well as higher education institutions that make real the opportunities. As administrators of nursing schools pursue robust enrollments of diverse and talented students, affordability and access are crucial considerations for the profession.

Accountability

Worldwide, governments and taxpaying publics are questioning the allocation of scarce public resources. The concept of high-quality, affordable public education is threatened by the competition for funding of other public needs. Before World War II the U.S. public regarded higher education with trust and respect, granting substantial autonomy; today taxpaying publics are demanding accountability in the form of data, outcomes achieved, and a variety of performance goals (Zumeta, 2001).

Several forces prompt this increased accountability for higher education. In times of cost cutting and corporate downsizing, business and private sector management looks to education, and its products, for competitive strategies. Also, drastic state budget cuts have caused policymakers and taxpayers to require justification for higher education funding. Legislatures have tended to disallow tuition hikes and request internal moves toward efficiency. These economic forces are fueled by a values clash, termed *cultural critiques of higher education*, that accuse the academy of setting weak standards, overresponding to multiculturalism and affirmative action, giving disproportionate emphasis to PhD preparation and esoteric research, light faculty workloads, and administrative bloat (Zumeta, 2001). Each of these forces promotes increased public scrutiny and higher expectations.

Accountability, therefore, becomes a multidirectional force. Institutions of higher education depend on the government for funding and therefore are highly accountable to the pubic for academic productivity and fiscal prudence. Schools of nursing are accountable to state legislatures, Congress, and the public regarding the preparation of adequate numbers of competent nurses. Governments, in response to their perceived accountability to the public, act to regulate and reform higher education. Accountability will continue as a significant theme in higher education.

Summary

Institutions of higher education are affected by major trends in the environment and very specifically by the need to create an educated and skilled workforce and by the financial challenges of doing so. The financial challenges include both private costs from individuals and families and public expenditures from state tax budgets. There is a potential for dissonance because the public both desires education and scrutinizes public expenditures in light of other societal needs. Increased accountability will be required of higher education in terms of measurable outcomes for quality education.

Issues Specific to the Nursing Profession

This chapter began by looking through the lens of the broad socioeconomic and sociopolitical issues that shape our world and influence contemporary life. Within that context, forces in higher education influence the education of the present and future nursing workforce. This section focuses the lens more specifically on the profession, highlighting issues of particular consideration within the profession. It is a false dichotomy to separate issues as internal and external to the profession, for it denies an interactive exchange between issues. Included are the context of nursing care, the nursing shortage, and competencies for the twenty-first century.

Context of Nursing Care Delivery

The nursing profession influences and is influenced by the health care delivery system, which provides a context for nursing services. Coile (2001) summarizes six trends, acquired through a health care environmental assessment, that have implications for nursing practice and education: informed consumers, technology, rising costs, managed care, health policy, and human capital.

First, Internet-savvy health care consumers often approach providers with extensive information, requesting treatments or drugs and expecting quality ratings on provider and institution report cards. "The central idea behind the consumer-driven quality revolution is to repair the buy–sell dynamic of the market by collecting and disseminating to consumers information about provider performance" while rewarding providers who practice exemplary health care (Billett, 2002, p. 9). Nursing needs to appreciate these empowered consumers, create satisfying patient–provider relationships, and demonstrate skills in helping families optimize and manage their own health needs (Heller et al., 2000).

Second, technology continues to revolutionize the health care possibilities. For example, the Human Genome Project presents a multitude of individualized genetic therapies, as well as ethical quandaries. Electronic health records and telehealth technologies require nurses to acquire significant technological proficiencies, and schools are challenged to use sophisticated simulations for skill acquisition and critical thinking development. Informatics education within schools of nursing assists students to understand data, combine data and knowledge, and make decisions, often through the use of technology (Carty, 2000). "Students immersed in high-technology education settings will be better prepared to practice in tomorrow's health care environment" (Simpson, 2002, p. 15).

The third trend involves the continued surge of health costs and the need for hospitals and providers to manage care more efficiently within finite budgets. Hospital budgets will be challenged by labor shortages and increased pharmaceutical and supply costs. Research that documents nursing's contribution to efficient, quality care is needed to advocate in budget negotiations and hospital changes.

Coile's (2001) fourth trend envisions managed care's waning market power, declining enrollment in health maintenance organization (HMO) membership, and the switch by employers from offering defined health benefits to offering defined contributions. One consequence could be that employees forego health benefits or choose the lowest-cost plans. These changing market forces may not result in a healthier population with access to health care, a goal that the nursing profession monitors and cares about.

Health policy, the fifth trend, becomes an increasingly significant strategy to shape, finance, and regulate the health care system. With costs of health care approaching 15% of the total gross national product, state and federal policies seek to regulate costs, shift care to less expensive settings, and use market forces to control costs when possible (Heller et al., 2000).

According to French (2002), policy analysts also ask two other questions: Does greater use of care produce greater health? and How does the nation meet the needs of the 45 million uninsured Americans? Nurses need political advocacy skills to campaign for reforms at both the state and national levels to bring nursing's voice to the policy debates and to play a meaningful role in policy development.

Finally, human capital becomes a significant trend, with nursing and physician shortages and the potential unionization of health care providers. Retention of satisfied employees will be the goal of viable organizations, which is related to the creation and maintenance of healthy and safe work environments. In part, respecting human capital means attention to work relationships and sanctions against verbal abuse by physicians, patients, and nurse colleagues; sexual harassment; and workplace violence, including horizontal violence or hostile behaviors within a group of nurse colleagues (Robinson, 2001).

These trends inform educators as they determine what and how to teach the next generation of nurses. Future practitioners will need knowledge and abilities to assist informed health care consumers, use technology, stem rising costs, work within managed care, advocate for effective health policy, and work to create a health care system with competent human capital.

Nursing Shortage

The current paucity of nurses, the aging of the practitioners and educators, and the prediction of worsening shortages threaten patient safety and the quality of health care delivery. Cycles of excesses and shortages are not new to nursing, but this shortage is more complex and threatens to be more severe. The shortage presents significant challenges to the profession, practice settings, and nursing programs.

Heinrich (2001) summarized the multiple factors contributing to these complex phenomena, including a decreased number of younger nurses entering the profession, more career options for bright men and women that compete with the choice of nursing, and job dissatisfaction that hinders retention and recruitment. Factors contributing to job dissatisfaction include inadequate staffing, inadequate support staff, heavy workload, employer expectation to work overtime, inadequate wages, and the rigors of treating increasingly ill patients, as well as issues mentioned previously related to verbal abuse and workplace violence. These factors are known by most within the profession and must be articulated to policymakers, physicians, hospital administrators, and society at large.

Long-term strategies will be needed to address the contributing factors, rather than short-term "bandages" that avoid root causes and undermine the autonomy, identity, and professionalism of nursing. The Tri-Council (2001), which includes the American Association of Colleges of Nursing (AACN), the American Nurses Association (ANA), the American Organization of Nurse Executives, and the National League for Nursing, proposed a comprehensive framework of strategies. Recommendations related to education include career progression initiatives; staff development programs that assist nurses to stay current, to switch specialties, or with reentry employment; and early recruitment into the profession. Strategies of workplace redesign include creating a partnership environment in which nurses can contribute fully and equally and making concerted retention efforts. Legislation and regulation would be written and passed to fund education and support equitable reimbursement systems, and technology, research, and data collection would be needed to justify and support these initiatives.

In September 2001 the ANA convened a strategic planning process, the Call to the Nursing Profession summit. The process resulted in a document entitled *Nursing's Agenda for the Future;* the summit and the ongoing implementation work demonstrate nursing proactively responding to the professional challenges contributing to the shortage and envisioning their own future. The desired future involves 10 areas of focus, itemized in Box 6-1, and a time line extending to 2010. The chief objective of the education domain is to increase the congruence between education and societal health needs (ANA, 2002).

In addition to there being a shortage of practicing nurses, too few educationally prepared nursing faculty present a "continuing and expanding problem" (American Association of Colleges of Nursing [AACN], 2003). The faculty shortage begins with a deficit; Hinshaw (2001) notes that as few as half

> **Box 6-1**
> **NURSING'S AGENDA FOR THE FUTURE: TEN DOMAINS FOR ACTION**
>
> 1. Delivery systems
> 2. Diversity
> 3. Economic value
> 4. Education
> 5. Leadership and planning
> 6. Legislation/regulation/policy
> 7. Professional/nursing culture
> 8. Public relations/communication
> 9. Recruitment/retention
> 10. Work environment

of nursing faculty in programs across the nation have met the academic norm of holding an earned doctoral degree. Add to the equation the "graying professoriate," the narrowing pipeline of baccalaureate and master's prepared nurses, and the older age of nurses completing their doctorate, and the severity of the shortage expands. At risk is not only a restriction in nursing school enrollments during a time of increased need, but also reduction in scientific knowledge generation from nurse scholars and fewer professional leaders shaping policy and bringing a nursing voice to interdisciplinary discussions.

The nurse educator shortage is an invitation for creative solutions: rethinking faculty roles, academic resources, and teaching methods; using retired yet vibrant faculty in creative "intellectual homes"; supporting senior faculty with resources and rewards to prolong productivity; and recruiting individuals into doctoral programs at a younger age. As with the shortage of practicing nurses, strategies that present a positive message of the discipline and the opportunities within a career of scholarship and teaching can address the shortage (AACN, 2003; Goodin, 2003; Hinshaw, 2001).

These shortages therefore present opportunity and challenge. Nursing professionals are taking steps to seize the opportunity to create nursing programs that will adequately prepare future practitioners for societal health needs and care settings that optimize the contribution nursing makes to the health of the nation. The challenges are undertaken in partnership with nursing colleagues within service and education, policymakers and business leaders, the media, and society in general.

Competencies for the Twenty-first Century

Not only does the profession need robust workforce numbers, but it also needs practitioners with requisite knowledge, abilities, and work behaviors to meet the health demands of the population. Educators are challenged to prepare individuals who, upon graduation, deliver competent and compassionate care and have the ability to navigate future changes in the system and acquire future abilities associated with evolving roles. O'Neil and the Pew Health Professions Commission (1998) proposed competencies needed for contemporary and future practice and suggest that they serve as evaluation criteria as

Box 6-2
TWENTY-ONE COMPETENCIES FOR THE TWENTY-FIRST CENTURY

1. Embrace a personal ethic of social responsibility and service
2. Exhibit ethical behavior in all professional activities
3. Provide evidence-based, clinically competent care
4. Incorporate the multiple determinants of health in clinical care
5. Apply knowledge of the new sciences
6. Demonstrate critical thinking, reflection, and problem-solving skills
7. Understand the role of primary care
8. Rigorously practice preventive health care
9. Integrate population-based care and services into practice
10. Improve access to health care for those with unmet health needs
11. Practice relationship-centered care with individuals and families
12. Provide culturally sensitive care to a diverse society
13. Partner with communities in health care decisions
14. Use communication and information technology effectively and appropriately
15. Work in interdisciplinary teams
16. Ensure care that balances individual, professional, system, and societal needs
17. Practice leadership
18. Take responsibility for the quality of care and health outcomes at all levels
19. Contribute to continuous improvement of the health care system
20. Advocate for public policy that promotes and protects the health of the public
21. Continue to learn and help others to learn

From Bellack, J. P., & O'Neil, E. H. (2000). Recreating nursing practice for a new century: Recommendations and implications of the Pew Health Professions Commission's final report. *Nursing & Health Care Perspectives, 21*(1), 14-21.

educators review curricula for currency and relevance. These competencies, presented in Box 6-2, represent an expansion and update of the list proposed in 1991 as requirements for health practitioners in 2005.

Bellack and O'Neil (2000) discuss the recommendations from the Pew Health Commission's fourth and final report, a continuing effort to support the health profession's education reform and align educational programs more fully with the health needs of the population. They present five recommendations for all health professions schools and eight specific to nursing. These recommendations provide excellent guideposts for nurse educators as they pursue the preferred future via the current reality. The first general recommendation prompts educators to recognize the characteristics of the new health care system and cease preparation for "yesterday's health care system" (p. 15). Included is the advice to form creative and reciprocal relationships with clinical partners and to be an active agent in the creation of "tomorrow's" system.

The second recommendation is an imperative for a diverse workforce, noting that the configuration of diversity varies by region. A diverse workforce allows consumers of health care to see practitioners who share their diversity and presupposes greater resources in addressing the challenges of our most vulnerable populations.

Interdisciplinary competence, recommendation three, requires that professions dismantle the "silos" that isolate practitioners and inhibit the sharing of perspectives and potential solutions. Interdisciplinary competence does not diminish individual professions but strengthens the processes and outcomes of health care. The fourth recommendation, an emphasis on ambulatory practice, is compatible with interdisciplinary competence. Community-based care experiences benefit from creative partnerships between the community, agencies, and educational programs.

The fifth recommendation emphasizes the value of community service and suggests it as an integral component of the educational process. Service-learning experiences benefit the learner and the community partner. As faculty model service through their community engagement, they enrich themselves, the community, and student learning.

Consideration of each recommendation can bring a curriculum and an educational experience closer to the envisioned future for the health system and competent workforce. The eight specific suggestions for nursing, summarized in Box 6-3, further refine the possibilities for curricular revision.

Summary

Through intentional efforts and collaboration with other stakeholders, nursing has worked within the societal and higher education contexts to advance health and continually refine the process that produces tomorrow's workforce.

Box 6-3

EIGHT RECOMMENDATIONS FOR RECREATING NURSING FOR A NEW CENTURY

---

1. Adjust educational programs to meet local or regional demand for numbers and types of nurses
2. Delineate the knowledge and outcome competencies for each level of nursing
3. Radically revamp the curriculum to produce graduates prepared for differentiated practice
4. Integrate research, teaching, and practice to further nursing's professional and practice goals
5. Reorient AP educational programs to meet changing practice situations and settings
6. Request that federal funding be made available to support AP education
7. Develop standard guidelines for AP and reinforce them in curriculum, examination, and accreditation regulations.
8. Emphasize AP styles that include preventive, health-promoting interventions and attention to psychosocial, environmental, and resource factors.

Modified from Bellack, J. P., & O'Neil, E. H. (2000). Recreating nursing practice for a new century: Recommendations and implications of the Pew Health Professions Commission's final report. *Nursing & Health Care Perspectives, 21*(1), 14-21.
AP, Advanced practice.

Nursing has shaped and is shaped by the context of care and by the challenges of the nursing shortage; nursing remains mindful of the competencies needed for the twenty-first-century practice.

STRATEGIES TO IDENTIFY INFLUENTIAL FORCES AND ISSUES

To develop a curriculum that is relevant and current, faculty must continually monitor the environments internal and external to the institution and the profession. This section presents four strategies that faculty can use separately or in combination to identify influential forces and issues: environmental scanning, forecasting, epidemiology, and survey research and consensus building.

Environmental Scanning

Environmental scanning involves various activities that monitor and evaluate information from the external environment. The goal is to become aware of general trends and events affecting health care and higher education generally and nursing specifically. Information can be acquired in various ways, including careful review of scientific and professional journals, as well as lay literature and newspapers, and attendance and networking at professional meetings.

Environmental scanning has been successfully used by colleges and universities to determine the context of the forces that have an impact on curriculum development (Garcia & Ratcliff, 1997). An example of environmental scanning at one university was a blue-ribbon commission composed of and chaired by nursing faculty. The Commission included a diverse cross section of faculty of different rank, research interests, and specialty areas. The purpose was to review recent literature to identify key professional and societal issues and trends related to nursing and health care. The resulting document, including a 100-item reference list, became the springboard for discussion and curriculum revisions in both undergraduate and graduate programs. Cognizant of the timely issues and trends, faculty were better equipped to shape a relevant curriculum.

In curriculum development, environmental scanning allows faculty to be simultaneously reactive and proactive. Through awareness and acknowledgment of significant trends (reactive), faculty can more actively choose a future direction for nursing education and curriculum (proactive). The use of environmental scanning as a strategy to obtain a broad scope of information and evaluate its relevance to nursing is the foundation of the other strategies that follow.

Forecasting

Forecasting is a process of producing likely futures on the basis of factual information about the present. Dunn (1981) described three forms of forecasting: projection, prediction, and conjecture. The forms can be differentiated by the basis of their forecast. Projection is based on current and previous trends taken into the future. Using projection and inductive reasoning, nursing faculty can extrapolate from present data (e.g., morbidity rates or census data) what a future rate will be. Prediction is based on explicit theoretical assumptions. Using prediction and deductive reasoning, nursing faculty can forecast the future using laws, propositions, or theories. Conjecture is based on subjective judgments about the future and applies retroductive reasoning. In this form of reasoning nursing faculty rely on insights, creativity, and tacit knowledge to present a claim about the future. The claim is related back to, and supported by, information and assumptions. These three forms of forecasting show that descriptions of a future can be created using current or previous data, theory, or subjective judgments and that the reasoning can be inductive, deductive, or retroductive.

Forecasting is not an exact science but is an art that includes judgments and assumptions. Errors can occur with incomplete data, superficial analysis, and flawed communication about the data. Even with the limitations inherent in the art and science of forecasting, it is a tool for nursing faculty to develop a curriculum that prepares students for the future.

Epidemiology

Epidemiology is the study of the distribution and determinants of states of health and illness in human populations. Epidemiology provides nursing faculty with systematic ways to understand patterns of disease, characteristics of people at high risk for disease, environmental factors, and shifts in demographic characteristics of the population. Valanis (1999) described the application of epidemiology in health care, including the activities of health planning and health policy development. Using epidemiological data with groups or populations, nurses understand and document the need for programs and policies to reduce risk and promote health. Epidemiology can, therefore, be seen as a method for planned change.

In the same way, nursing faculty responsible for the development of curriculum can use epidemiological data and methods to understand factors affecting the health of populations and trends occurring in health and illness states. Epidemiology provides faculty with methods for understanding that part of the context that involves the broad determinants of health and patterns of disease and disability in the population.

Survey Research and Consensus Building

Another tool at the disposal of faculty is survey research. Surveys involve systematically collecting information from individuals and deriving statistical statements, such as some measure of central tendency, or consensus statements from groups of experts or involved individuals. If the design is iterative and involves a series of surveys, feedback, and more surveys, it is considered a form of Delphi technique.

Surveys and consensus-building processes provide an opportunity to sample the perspective of various stakeholders and knowledgeable persons, for example, employers or consumers. They facilitate tapping the rich diversity of group wisdom related to complex issues.

The strategies of environmental scanning, forecasting, epidemiology, and survey research and consensus building have utility in preparing for curriculum development or revision. Using some combination of the four strategies presented here, faculty can be equipped to develop curriculum compatible with the current and projected issues influencing nursing and health care.

SUMMARY

The forces and issues that influence and are influenced by nursing curriculum originate in the external, higher education, and internal environments. Educators sensitive to major sociopolitical and economic trends can develop curriculum that matches global characteristics. Educators aware of prevailing higher education issues can assist schools of nursing to be leaders in the academy. Educators attuned to prevailing and visionary thinking within the profession can shape the future through progressive curriculum and pedagogy. Nursing deserves curriculum that is both compatible with the contemporary health care context and flexible enough to be relevant for emerging circumstances and needs.

REFERENCES

Allender, J. A., & Spradley, B. W. (2001). *Community health nursing: Concepts and practice.* Philadelphia: Lippincott Williams & Wilkins.

American Association of Colleges of Nursing. (2003). *Faculty shortages in baccalaureate and graduate nursing programs: Scope of the problem and strategies for expanding the supply.* Retrieved August 29, 2003, from http://www.aacn.nche.edu/Publications/WhitePapers/FacultyShortages.htm/

American Nurses Association. (2002). *Nursing's agenda for the future.* Retrieved July 10, 2003, from http://nursingworld.org/naf/

Bellack, J. P., & O'Neil, E. H. (2000). Recreating nursing practice for a new century: recommendations and implications of the Pew Health Professions Commission's final report. *Nursing & Health Care Perspectives, 21*(1), 14-21.

Billett, T. C. (2002). Driving toward a revolution in health care quality. *Employee Benefit News, 16*(1), 4, 9.

Billings, D. M., Connors, H. R., & Skiba, D. J. (2001). Benchmarking best practices in web-based nursing courses. *Advances in Nursing Science, 23*(3), 41-52.

Callan, P. M. (2001). Reframing access and opportunity: Problematic state and federal higher education policy in the 1990s. In D. E. Heller (Ed.), *The states and public higher education policy: Affordability, access and accountability* (pp. 83–99). Baltimore: Johns Hopkins University Press.

Carty, B. (2000). *Nursing informatics: Education for practice.* New York: Springer.

Coile, R. C. (2001). *Futurescan 2001: A millennium forecast of health care trends 2001-2005.* Chicago: Health Administration Press.

Dunn, W. N. (1981). *Public policy analysis: An introduction.* Englewood Cliffs, NJ: Prentice-Hall.

French, H. E. (2002, summer). The competitive revolution. *Regulation, 25*(2), 52-57.

Garcia, M., & Ratcliff, J. (1997). Social forces shaping the curriculum. In J. G. Gaff & J. L. Ratcliff & Associates (Eds.), *Handbook of the undergraduate curriculum: A comprehensive guide to purposes, structures, practices, and change* (pp. 118-133). San Francisco: Jossey-Bass.

Goodlin, H. J. (2003). The nursing shortage in the United States of America: An integrative review of the literature. *Journal of Advanced Nursing, 43*(4), 335-343.

Gorman, M. (2002). Global ageing: The non-governmental organization role in the developing world. *International Journal of Epidemiology, 31*, 782-785.

Heinrich, J. (2001, July 10). Emerging nurse shortages due to multiple factors. *FDCH Government Account Reports.* Washington, DC: Federal Document Clearing House.

Heller, B. R., Oros, M. T., & Durney-Crowley, J. (2000). The future of nursing education: 10 trends to watch. *Nursing and Health Care Perspectives, 21*(1), 9-13.

Heller, D. E. (Ed.). (2001). *The states and public higher education policy: Affordability, access and accountability.* Baltimore: Johns Hopkins University Press.

Hinshaw, A. S. (2001). A continuing challenge: The shortage of educationally prepared nursing faculty. *Online Journal of Issues in Nursing, 6,*(1). Retrieved August 29, 2003, from http://www.nursingworld.org/ojin/topic14/tpc14_3htm

Klineberg, S. L. (1994). Envisioning the next fifty years: Six revolutionary trends. In T. Mullen (Ed.), *Witness in Washington: Fifty years of friendly persuasion* (pp. 222-236). Richmond, IN: Friends United Press.

Klineberg, S. L. (1997) *Is science the salvation to society?* Retrieved June 20, 2003, from the Phi Beta Kappa Society website: http://www.pbk.org/news/views/klineberg.htm

Lenburg, C. B. (2002). The influence of contemporary trends and issues on nursing education. In B. Cherry & S. R. Jacob (Eds.), *Contemporary nursing: Issues, trends & management* (pp. 65-94). St. Louis: Mosby.

Lewis, R. D. (2003). *The cultural imperative: Global trends in 21st century.* Yarmouth, MA: Intercultural Press.

O'Neil, E. H., & The Pew Health Professions Commission. (1998). *Recreating health professional practice for a new century.* Retrieved July 10, 2003, from http://futurehealth.ucsf.edu/pdf_files/recreate.pdf

Robinson, C. (2001). Magnet nursing services recognition: Transforming the critical care environment. *AACN Clinical Issues: Advanced Practice in Acute and Critical Care, 12*(3), 411-423.

Simpson, R. L. (2002). The virtual reality revolution: technology changes nursing education. *Nursing Management, 9,* 14-15.

Tri-Council Members. (2001). *Strategies to reverse the new nursing shortage.* Retrieved June 6, 2003, from http://www.nursingworld.org/pressrel/2001/sta0205.htm

U.S. Census Bureau. (2000). *Projections of the total resident population.* Retrieved July 8, 2003, from http://www.census.gov/population/projections/nation/summary/np-t4-f.pdf

Valanis, B. (1999). *Epidemiology in health care.* Stamford, CT: Appleton & Lange.

Wallace, S. P., Abel, E. K., Stefanowicz, P., & Pourat, N. (2001). Long-term care and the elderly population. In R. M. Andersen, T. H. Rice, & G. F. Kominski (Eds.), *Changing the U.S. health care system: Key issues in health services, policy, and management* (pp. 205-223). San Francisco: Jossey-Bass.

Wiener, J. M., & Tilly, J. (2001). Population ageing in the United States of America: Implications for public programmes. *International Journal of Epidemiology, 31*(4), 776-781.

Zumeta, W. (2001). Public policy and accountability in higher education: Lessons from the past and present for the new millennium. In D. E. Heller, (Ed.), *The states and public higher education policy: Affordability, access and accountability* (pp. 155-197). Baltimore: Johns Hopkins University.

7

Philosophical Foundations of the Curriculum

Judie Csokasy, PhD, RN

Philosophical beliefs of the university in tandem with the nursing faculty provide a framework to guide all curricular activities. Educational philosophy provides a framework for developing the mission, philosophy, goals and objectives, curricular framework, evaluation methods, and the environment in which the educative process takes place. It is essential that the philosophical beliefs developed in the written documents be lived out in the learning activities designed for students.

Presented in this chapter is a basic framework from which to make decisions about the development of mission and philosophy statements as a foundation for curriculum planning. A mission statement describes the unique purpose and reason for the existence of the institution. The statement of philosophy raises questions, describes beliefs, and explores basic issues faced by nurse educators as they explore the relationship of human beings to their world. Faculty who interact with students in their learning experiences model their philosophical beliefs about how people learn. Through planned discourse faculty have the opportunity to develop an educative experience that is empowering and student focused, away from historical pedagogy in which the teacher holds the power and the student spends his or her learning time figuring out "what the teacher really wants." Nurse educators are charged with preparing professionals to deal with the political and social challenges of a diverse and global society; engage in collaborative, community nursing practice; and respond to the future advances of health care (Ironside, 2001; Kritek, 2001).

This chapter focuses on the importance of mission and philosophy statements in guiding decisions about teaching, learning, measurement, and evaluation strategies. An introductory discussion about the philosophical frameworks of idealism, realism, pragmatism, and existentialism demonstrates that there is a relationship between philosophy and educational theoretical frameworks and describes how these beliefs guide faculty activities, curriculum development, and student activities. Strategies for developing mission and philosophy statements are presented to stimulate activities in developing a shared vision that can be operationalized in the collective undertaking of curriculum development.

HISTORICAL ROLE OF EDUCATIONAL PHILOSOPHY

There have always been philosophers who were well-grounded in education. Although the ancient Greek philosophies ruled the social, cultural, political, and educational process, philosophers such as Aquinas, Locke, Plato, and Dewey wrote eloquently about the necessity of philosophical foundations for education. It was not until the nineteenth century that philosophy of education, with its own literature and tradition, began to have an influence in the United States (Blake et al., 2003). The establishment of the American Philosophical Society in 1941 and the publication in the 1960s of various journals, including the *Journal of Philosophy of Education* and *Studies in Philosophy and Education*, influenced universities to expand their teaching about philosophies of education.

There is no longer "a one size fits all" belief about philosophy, and although many educators believe that philosophy can be useful for identifying problems and as a source for solving problems, the way in which philosophy influences theory and praxis is constantly changing. When reviewing philosophical curricular frameworks in nursing education, one notices that there is a marked absence of the vast body of nursing research and theories (Ironside, 2001; Kirkham & Anderson, 2002; Romyn, 2001). It is possible that nurse educators are more focused on their clinical knowledge and scholarship than on the educational foundations of their teaching scholarship and are more comfortable with the conventional and traditional theories of education than with the emerging body of nursing knowledge and theories applicable to nursing education.

As more educators enter the discussion about philosophy, nursing professors teaching in this exciting time can design new and innovative ways of implementing curricula for nursing students. The effects of the new-market economy, globalization, and emerging ideas about teaching and learning can provide educators with valuable tools and insights to change the way nursing is taught and practiced throughout the twenty-first century.

The history of formulating a philosophy for nursing education begins with Nightingale's writings and continues to the present. Nursing leaders now and in the past have struggled with the definition and content of a philosophy statement. Stewart (1943) described philosophy in nursing education as a blend of personal beliefs and values—authoritarian and autocratic—whereas others are liberal and democratic. Stewart credits Florence Nightingale with developing the first well-rounded philosophy on nursing education and supported Nightingale's clear and practical application of ancient and contemporary philosophers. Early nursing educators tended to focus on curriculum development through design of didactic and experiential strategies to "professionalize" the work done by nurses. The philosophical foundations initially advocated by Stewart took years to develop because of the need to recruit an educated faculty capable of curriculum design, implementation, and evaluation.

In the 1960s the National League for Nursing (NLN) promoted discussion about curriculum design and provided education for nurse educators on how to develop curricula. Philosophy was described as the foundation to "make value judgments relative to the curriculum, and to provide justification of a way of life through a background knowledge of theory, knowledge and beliefs" (Skipper, 1962, p. 40). Schindel (1962) also wrote about curriculum development in the NLN publications and advocated that philosophy should "(a) serve as a touchstone or primary criterion, for judging the soundness, goodness, or the validity of its formulated objectives, its selected content, and organization and sequence learning experiences; (b) and, serve as a means of evaluating the methodology, policies, learning outcomes, and the total curriculum" (p. 60).

Recent nurse educators see philosophy as one part of curriculum foundation but caution against great reliance on philosophy as a framework. Bevis (1983) stated that philosophy provides a "value system for ordering priorities and selecting from various data; that philosophy alone is a weak cornerstone for curriculum development, but in conjunction with other components of the curriculum framework it strengthens the curriculum design" (p. 35). As Bevis has continued her call for curricular change, she calls for a curriculum design that is "more responsive to societal needs, more successful in humanizing the highly technical milieus of health, more caring and compassionate, and more capable of critical thinking" (Bevis & Watson, 2000).

When faculty begin to develop a philosophy statement, they must be aware that in addition to institutional values and the individual faculty member's belief, many societal and political influences must be considered when developing and implementing a curriculum. The divergent forces influencing curriculum and the components of philosophy can be seen in Figure 7-1. A more thorough discussion of these and other forces influencing curriculum are included in Chapter 6. In a pluralistic society, the expectations of patients, students, and the community, along with the goals of the institution, may change. Placing the process of education and the nuances of curriculum development into a philosophical framework and seeking to come to agreement about personal beliefs can help to clarify what is happening in an institution.

As the body of nursing knowledge has evolved, there is a clarion call from nurse researchers and educators for faculty to integrate the unique body of knowledge that is nursing into philosophical frameworks for curricula that empower and transform (Newman, 2002), reflect epistemic diversity (Georges, 2003) and emancipatory paradigms (Romyn, 2001), focus on interpretive experiences (Diekelmann, 2001), and consider an emancipatory and activist stance in a praxis-oriented curriculum (Kirkham & Anderson, 2002). How then should nursing faculty proceed to arrive at some agreement about the basic philosophical foundations of curriculum? In light of the number of increasingly meaningful nursing theories, perhaps beginning with a study of the historical context of philosophy and then moving to the personal belief system one has developed through education and professional practice will assist nursing faculty to define and develop their collective belief systems.

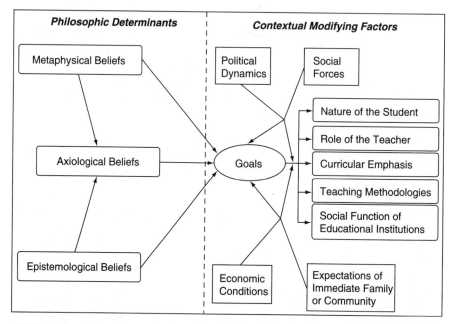

FIGURE 7-1   The relationship of philosophy to educational practice. (From Knight, G. R. [1982]. *Issues and alternatives in educational philosophy*. Berrien Springs, MI: Andrews University Press.)

COMPONENTS OF PHILOSOPHY

Historically, the body of knowledge called *educational philosophy* has been based on an understanding of the components of philosophy as described by the Greeks: metaphysics, epistemology, and axiology. Metaphysics seeks to answer the basic question of what is real; epistemology involves the study of the nature, sources, and validity of knowledge; and axiology includes exploring the nature of values, ethics, and logic.

Metaphysics

The study of what is reality versus what is fantasy or illusion is the primary concern of metaphysics. What is real for one person may be different for another. Educators' application of metaphysical principles includes theology, the reality of God, and anthropology, the study of human beings. Each person carries beliefs about the nature and function of human beings that have their origins in the cultural and societal group.

Two well-known nursing theorists, Madeline Leininger (1978) and Jean Watson (1979), have their theoretical beliefs rooted in metaphysics. Leininger, an anthropologist, writes of the need for nurses to understand culture to plan their patient's holistic care. Watson's work on caring theory has a base in her metaphysical belief about persons. Watson has taken this philosophy and combined it with existentialist/humanistic philosophy to lead the discussion about the role of caring as a theoretical nursing framework.

Epistemology

The focus of epistemology is the question, What is truth? (how one arrives at truth and how truth differs from opinion). The issue of truth and one's perception of truth presents a challenge for the nursing educator. Tradition, instinct, and feelings are not considered to be valid sources of knowledge. Instead, knowledge is subjected to rigor and investigation about what it means.

The nursing theorist Martha Rogers (1961) was a proponent of a metaphysical/epistemological foundation of moving nursing education toward a professional model. As outlined in her development of nursing theory she stated, "the development of a substantial organized body of theoretical knowledge fundamental to nursing is imperative" (Rogers, 1961, p. 23). To develop this theoretical framework, nurses must possess a philosophical perspective of persons that includes a definition of the person; his or her role in the universe; and the knowledge, skills, and abilities necessary to develop rational thinking models. Most philosophers, except those of the analytic school, have interpreted the question of knowledge in similar ways.

A different interpretation of epistemology is seen in analytical philosophy, a type of logical and linguistic analysis that is described as linguistic analysis, logical empiricism, and Cambridge analysis, among other terms. The analytical philosophers believe that the basic question of epistemology is not truth but meaning. Their concern is for the meaning of language or words that human beings use within the context of the culture in which they live. Members of the analytical movement believe that reality consists of what is knowable or that which can be verified by experience. The discussion about words and meaning has gained importance in theoretical frameworks of feminist theory, in environmental and ecological theories, and in the broadening understanding of diversity and cultural similarities and differences and their influence on the worldview of learning.

Kritek (2001) describes how "30 years of the cognitive and linguistic sciences have fostered a new respect for the power of meaning" (p. 907). She supports the epistemology of healing practices in nursing and gives importance to "what we know and how we know it" (p. 910). She speaks eloquently of the need for a philosophy that reflects what is uniquely nursing and owned by members of the profession to deal with emerging definitions of health and nursing.

Axiology

The third question of philosophy, What is good? is generally interpreted by society as what is good or bad for the group. The study of this philosophical question is approached through the study of axiology, or value. Human beings are capable not only of knowing and understanding but also of placing a value on certain thoughts and behaviors. The values we hold are better indicators of our humanness than how much knowledge we have accumulated. Proponents of this view propose that presenting information and developing the intellect is not the only task of the educator. They advocate that a teacher should be encouraged to serve as a role model of those behaviors that the school values. In other words, to teach a philosophy is not enough. One must also live it as an example to students.

EDUCATIONAL PHILOSOPHIES

The advent of educational philosophy as a field of study is a recent phenomenon when compared with the classical philosophies dating back 2500 years to early Greece. John Dewey (1916) wrote of his belief that philosophy is useful for identifying problems and as a source for solving the problems. Dewey advocated a strong philosophical foundation when implementing curricular reform because the primary purpose of philosophy could serve to prevent the pitfalls of responding to the latest educational fads. He supported curriculum revision as a deliberative process and cautioned teachers "to avoid yielding to precipitately short term contemporary currents, abandoning in panic, things of enduring and priceless value" (Dewey, 1916, p. 3). Dewey emphasized the value of experiential, problem-based learning and of students' active involvement in learning (Fuhrmann, 1997). Dewey's writings are timeless and can be useful to nursing educators today as health care reform causes many faculty to rethink the role of philosophy in developing contemporary curricula.

When studying philosophical frameworks, faculty often perceive them to be obtuse and abstract. However, unless one becomes familiar with one's personal philosophy and is able to develop curriculum and learning activities within a sound framework, students are subjected to faculty who are erratic, inconsistent, and may lurch from one end of the philosophical spectrum to the other—from strict behaviorism to unbridled humanism—leading to confusion on the part of both teachers and students. Educational theories have evolved from the attempt of educators through the years to place teaching and learning activities within a framework of beliefs. Figure 7-2 illustrates the relationship between the traditional philosophies of idealism and realism, the modern philosophies of pragmatism and existentialism, and the educational theories that have evolved as educators have attempted to operationalize their philosophical belief systems.

Every time a teacher makes a decision about curriculum, he or she is confronted with options. Decisions about content, course sequence, and evaluation strategies will reflect a teacher's belief system. Table 7-1 presents an overview of philosophical beliefs related to the role of student, teacher, and curriculum goals, and the beliefs' relation to nursing education.

School of Traditional Philosophers

The traditional schools of philosophy date back to the early Greek philosophers. The classical philosophers influenced educational philosophy, especially in the area of liberal arts and the role of the humanities in higher education. Currently, nursing educators are dealing with the issues of the humanities as faculty in higher education are strengthening the requirements for the core curriculum of undergraduate education and the incorporation of

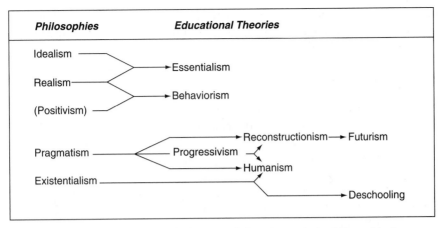

FIGURE 7-2 The relationship of educational theories to their philosophical sources. (From Knight, G. R. [1982]. *Issues and alternatives in educational philosophy.* Berrien Springs, MI: Andrews University Press.)

capstone experiences to document outcomes. The way in which faculty view the role of society and education is reflected in the differences between the two main schools of traditional philosophy: idealism and realism.

Idealism and Realism

Idealism states that the individual is wanting to live in a perfect world of high ideals, beauty, and art. Idealism focuses on truth as universal. In the Western world, Augustine, who combined Christianity and idealism, said that the "ultimate aim of education was to prepare man for life after death through an understanding and practice of the Christian virtues of faith, hope, charity, and humility" (Elias & Merriam, 1995, p. 15). Mission statements from religious institutions often reflect the idealistic school of philosophy when they speak of assisting students in their search for ultimate truth through an emphasis on humanities and liberal arts.

Realism, on the other hand, proposes that the world is composed of natural laws that regulate all of nature. For Aristotle, true happiness came from wisdom and the contemplation of truth. The origin of a liberal arts education is in the writings and culture of realism. Realists believe that the student should be rewarded for learning and responding to new experiences with scientific objectivity and analysis. The teacher is one who presents learning material in a highly efficient, orderly, and sequential process.

Educational Theory: Essentialism

Essentialism encompasses both idealism and realism. The essentialists view knowledge as key and an effective teacher as one who is responsible and who possesses and passes on this truth to the student. In turn the student will acquire this knowledge and store it for future use. They believe that the goal of education is to transmit and uphold the cultural heritage of the past. The emphasis on a liberal arts curriculum and upholding the Great Book Series as a foundation for all learning is a strongly held belief of the essentialists.

TABLE 7-1   Application of Philosophical Beliefs to Educational Practice

PHILOSOPHY	EDUCATIONAL THEORY	ROLE OF STUDENT	ROLE OF TEACHER	CURRICULUM DESIGN	APPLICATION TO NURSING EDUCATION
Idealism					
Truth is universal; values are unchanging	Essentialism	Expected to expand his or her mind by inquiry, discovery, aesthetics, synthesis, and application of knowledge to life; reality is unchanging	Functions as a model of what the student may become, both intellectually and morally; focus is not just on how and what to think	Foundation in the humanities to foster intellectual growth; education is truth accumulated through the history of civilization	Belief in strong liberal arts foundation on which to build the role of professional nursing is the basis of several nursing theorists
Realism					
Reality is found in physical world; truth is an observable fact (positivism)	Behaviorism	Subject to natural law; motivated to learn through positive reinforcement; rewarded for scientific objectivity and objective analysis	Provides information in an efficient, disciplined manner; facts must be mastered in a sequential process; emphasis is on critical analysis, not normative criteria	Purpose is intellectual development of physical world (life and natural sciences); emphasis is on science and math; organized by subject matter content	Has been the driving model of most schools of nursing, state boards of nursing, and accrediting bodies 1950-present
Pragmatism					
Sought to combine the dualism of idealism and realism through the testing of ideas and scientific methods; "truth" is what works	Reconstructionism	Experience inquiry through active learning and exploration; must have involvement in social and community activities	Facilitates learning to a group or individual; disdain for assignments, tests, and lecture fosters an environment in which student gains control of his or her life	Develop experimental learning in many environments; exploration is encouraged	Early nursing educators were social and community activists and used learning to develop social and community health services

Progressivism	Process by which individuals gain entrance to a democratic society; belief in an organic holism	Supports social adaptation and change through the education process; assumes the role of guide/facilitator	Assisted to develop the self through field trips, labs, and simulation; apply learning to daily life and society	Goal-oriented inquiry to move toward unity of thought unity of thought and action; experiential learning leads to problem solving
Existentialism Reality is in the individual; freedom to choose is of the essence				
Humanism	Experience available to student to develop self-knowledge and assist in maximizing his or her potential	Collaborates and facilitates as a nondirective resource for student to meet individual needs and goals	Encouraged to freely choose own path to learning; assume responsibility for life	Movement from a teaching model to emphasis on the student as collaborator to identify and meet his or her personal learning needs
Postmodernism	A process of encouraging student input and control over his or her own learning while creating a process of learning	Downplays the role of the expert and fosters inclusiveness and cultural–political foundations of learning	Formulates his or her own reality from interests, personal needs, and traditional culture; believes in no single theoretical framework of study	Heideggerian phenomenology; transformative learning; emancipatory curricula

From Bevis, M. (1989). *Toward a caring curriculum.* New York: National League for Nursing; Scales, F. (1985). *Nursing curriculum: Development, structure and function.* Norwalk, CT: Appleton-Century-Crofts.

Educational Theory: Behaviorism

The behaviorist movement served a useful purpose in early nursing education. The publication by Tyler (1949) on goals, objectives, and curriculum has provided a framework for nursing education up to and including the present. The goal of behaviorism has been to develop mental discipline through an efficient educational process, such as memorization, drill, and recitation. Holmquist (1960) and other nursing leaders saw behaviorism as providing the structure and step-by-step process from statement of philosophy through evaluation necessary to move nursing education toward a professional model. As humanistic theories and postmodern philosophies gain prominence, the behaviorist framework is seen less often but continues to work well in community and technical colleges where the goal is to prepare the student for employment after 2 years of education. A philosophy statement based on behaviorism often includes behaviorist strategies about teaching and learning. Learning is described as systematic and sequentially building on previous learning, and the faculty member is the primary decision maker about the educational experience.

School of Modern and Postmodern Philosophers

The modern philosophers moved the discussion of philosophy away from the metaphysical or relativist point of view to a focus on epistemology and axiology as having more relevance for society. The modern schools of philosophy either have embraced the scientific method or, as in the case of existentialism, have sought to move education away from the scientific method and into the human potential movement.

Pragmatism

Pragmatism has been considered a uniquely American philosophy that arose in response to the rapid scientific and technological changes of the late nineteenth and early twentieth centuries. The pragmatists attempted to combine the dualism of idealism and realism through the testing of ideas through science to declare their usefulness and validity. The changing demographics and influx of immigrants influenced the American public to question a belief system based on an absolute reality and instead see truth as relative to man's experience. John Dewey (1916) propelled pragmatism into the arena of educational philosophy. Dewey's original work was directed toward the nation's secondary schools, but his writings have become an integral part of the evolution of broadening the role of education to include social reform and support of democracy through the individual growth of each citizen.

Educational Theory: Reconstructionism

The reconstructionist viewed the role of the school as the major vehicle for social change. The reconstructing of society began as individual students were given a sense of social direction and responsibility. Reconstructionism embraced the social ideal of a democratic life, the Utopian view of the political as a means to provide the learner with everything necessary for life. The social reforms supported by the reconstructionist did not occur, and a new movement called *progressivism* began to spread across the country.

Educational Theory: Progressivism

Progressivism carried Dewey's work further into relative truth and away from the absolutism of the early Greek philosophers. The progressivists saw the student as able to make choices about what is important and further relegated the teacher to the role of facilitator of learning. The progressive movement was heavily influenced by the settlement movement of the late nineteenth century and is responsible for incorporating the pragmatic framework into the public schools. For the immigrant population the goal of a democratic life was operationalized through the educational experience. As the immigrants became acculturated into society and subscribed to democratic ideals, they moved away from the mechanistic idea of personhood. Along with the unrest during the two world wars, an influx of immigrants, and a changing workforce—into an industrial society—the groundwork was being laid for existentialism and the view that individual values should not be subverted for the group or society.

Educational Theory: Existentialism

Existentialists seek to find personal meaning in a world of impersonal rational thought and believe the function of education is to help the individual explore the reason for existence. In the late nineteenth century Friedrich Nietzsche in Germany and Søren Kierkegaard in Denmark began the early existential movement through their writings on alienation in a technical society (Tanner & Tanner, 1990). Kierkegaard hoped to reformulate Christianity by uplifting the place of the individual's role of personal choice and commitment. Nietzsche fought to declare the death of God, and by denouncing Christianity he was one of the first to advocate the image of a superhuman race capable of finding personal meaning for their existence.

In the era between World War I and World War II, the political and social climate provided fertile ground for the writings of the existentialist. Schools were no longer viewed as just preparation for college but became places where the social ideals and democratic ideas were institutionalized. Education was viewed as a process to personal growth and achievement, and curriculum was becoming more controversial as behaviorism clashed with existential ideas. Nursing educators are concerned about the role of behaviorism versus existential/humanistic frameworks, and much of the dialogue about the curriculum revolution is about which philosophical framework will guide curriculum development and implementation in the future.

Benner and Wrubel (1989) used Martin Heidegger's phenomenological approach as a foundation for their framework of caring. Heidegger, a deconstructionist of the existentialist school, believed that a person has understanding in an effortless and nonreflective manner, that meaning and interpretation offer fresh insight. Human beings have this understanding because they are always placed within a context that has meaning.

According to Benner and Wrubel (1989), Heidegger's hermeneutical analysis has implications for nursing theory and practice through the application of his phenomena to individual interpretation. They write of the need to see the person as a self-interpreting human being, uniquely defined by his personal beliefs, concerns, and experiences of life. Their application of Heidegger's work has influenced nursing care to patients as nurses move away from the Cartesian belief of mind–body dualism and toward a more holistic, empowering view of the patient as one capable of interpreting his or her own lived experience. Diekelmann (1993, 2001) and Rather (1994) supported this theoretical framework in their use of hermeneutic interpretation as an empowering and liberating framework for the returning nursing student.

Educational Theory: Humanism

Humanism as an educational theory is a natural outgrowth of the existentialist view of the rights of an individual. The primary concern of humanism as an educational theory is the autonomy and dignity of human beings. Humanism has continued in a modified movement to promote many of the progressive principles of student-centered education and the role of the teacher as guide. The existentialist thought in educational humanism has led to an emphasis on a search for personal meaning in human existence. The writings of Carl Rogers (1969) and Abraham Maslow (1954) have emphasized the importance of helping individuals become "humanized or self-actualized," thereby assisting the individual to develop his or her real self and full potential.

The humanist movement dates back to fifteenth century Italy and members of the Italian renaissance. As a revolt against the church-dominated focus on glorifying a rigid educational system through a study of the classics, humanism spread rapidly throughout Europe. The modern humanists rebelled against the industrial–military complex, the mechanistic philosophy of the scientific world, and the spread of communism that promoted a godless society (Elias & Merriam, 1995). Existentialists and humanists have shared a common value in the role of education as vital to assist the individual toward human happiness through becoming all he or she can be. Bevis and Watson (2000) encouraged faculty to study and implement curriculum that is "existential/humanistic, holistic, subjective, intuitive, phenomenological, and human experience oriented" (p. 5). See Box 7-1 for an example of one school of nursing's philosophy statement that uses many concepts from the existential/humanistic paradigm.

Postmodernist Theories

The last decade has seen an explosion of postmodernist thought, research, and theory building. Definitions are as varied as the theories. Jencks (1996) has recorded 70 related words and definitions from 1870 to 1996 that define postmodernism. In general terms, postmodernism refers to that period after the modern philosophies and is now viewed as a complex amalgam of many different philosophies and theories. The postmodernists do not view the schools of idealism and realism with their conservative frameworks and explanation of the world to be an adequate way to deal with the diversities of people and problems in today's world. They do not view religion and science as being the only two alternatives for framing the world of philosophical thought. Their

Box 7-1
PHILOSOPHY STATEMENT

- **We believe that professional caring is a function of the whole person, in which concern for the growth and well-being of another is expressed through application of nursing knowledge.** Integrating the art, science, theory, and practice of nursing requires a synthesis of the nurse's professional knowledge and humanity.

- **We believe that caring involves learning about and understanding human needs and human responses in varying states of health.** It involves understanding universal human patterns in constructing lives and restructuring meaning. It involves understanding and valuing human individuality and diversity. By extending a human presence, nurses reinforce self-esteem, enhance spirituality, nurture strengths, and facilitate healing.

- **We believe that nurses should actively seek self-knowledge and engage in self-care to maintain personal wellness, balancing responsibilities to themselves, others, and their profession.** This requires personal attributes of stamina, responsibility, flexibility, adaptability, creativity, curiosity, compassion, constructive skepticism, assertiveness, courage, and humor. Nurses should examine personal experiences, attributes, values, and lifestyle for their impact upon the professional role.

- **We believe it is important for nurses to engage in critical thinking and decision making and that critical thinking skills enhance both interpersonal and cognitive functioning.** Nurses who can analyze, synthesize, examine, compare and contrast, question, anticipate, investigate, inquire, reflect, recognize insights, intuit, and find patterns and meanings in situations will be effective nurses. Nurses who value these intellectual modes will use higher-level thinking in making judgments and decisions and will be better able to set goals, engage in dialogue, and engage in self-evaluation.

- **We believe it is important for nurses to know how to seek, find, and use health information and resources.** There are many complex, multifaceted sources of information, help, and support available within the health care environment. Using written, technological, and human sources is necessary because nursing's knowledge base is rapidly changing, ever expanding, and increasingly specialized.

- **We believe it is important for nurses to acquire clinical competency through experience in various health care settings so that professional standards of care are met.** Each clinical milieu is unique, requiring the integration of role, technical, and interpersonal skills. Although it is not possible to experience the entire breadth and depth of nursing, nurses can use principles and concepts to deliver care in a safe, skilled, quality-focused manner across health care settings.

- **We believe it is important for nurses to communicate effectively with clients, health care professionals, and other members of the community concerning health-related issues.** Nurses continuously use nonverbal, verbal, and technological communication skills as an integral part of positive and effective interpersonal relationships.

Continued

> **Box 7-1**
> **PHILOSOPHY STATEMENT—cont'd**
>
> - **We believe that nurses cultivate a spirit of community, teamwork, and partnership by collaborating with and empowering others.** Nurses are part of a larger health care community that includes both professional and nonprofessional caregivers. Nurses provide the leadership, management, delegation, consultation, and supervision required in today's health care milieu.
> - **We believe it is important for nurses to commit to professional values, professional development, and lifelong learning.** Such values are incorporated into an ethical framework that includes respect for diversity, individual worth and dignity, autonomy, truth, and justice. Professional development includes engaging in activities to evaluate the quality and effectiveness of nursing practice; keeping current in skills and knowledge; contributing to the professional development of peers, colleagues, and others; and becoming a consumer of, and contributor to, nursing research.

theories can be seen in feminism, ecology, culturally diverse ideas, and multitudes of other theoretical frameworks now under discussion.

Postmodernism influence is not just found in the study of philosophy but is also found in the arts (e.g., dance and music, architecture, and literature) and in other fields of study. As a cultural phenomenon, postmodernism challenges convention, has a high tolerance for ambiguity, emphasizes diversity of culture and thought, and encourages innovation and change (Beck, 1993). The discourse between postmodernists and other philosophers continues to evolve as the attempts to define certainty, power, identity, and the belief about truth and knowledge as being absolute continues throughout the academy.

DEVELOPING MISSION AND PHILOSOPHY STATEMENTS

Mission Statements

Curriculum development must be guided by and reflective of the mission and philosophy of the institution (Reardon & Ramaley, 1997). As faculty begin the process of curriculum development, they must first engage in collegial dialogue about the mission of the institution and the nursing school's contributions to all institutional initiatives. In a pluralistic society, the expectations of patients, students, and the community, along with the goals of the institution, may change (Fuhrmann, 1997).

A mission statement is a "declaration of the special purposes of an institution and whom it intends to serve." The mission statement is the public statement about what the institution is and why it exists, whereas the vision statement is what the institution wishes to become, and philosophy provides the framework or context in which all educational activities take place. The mission statement provides direction for the planning of educational activities and commonly includes the following: (1) the target patients or constituencies, (2) the geographic area (this is usually seen in public universities), (3) the goal of the institution (teaching, service, research), (4) the quality indicators (often the word *excellence* is used to describe the standard to which the school aspires).

A mission (purpose) statement is a brief statement that answers the questions of why and for what purpose the organization exists. To maintain congruence between the mission statement and curriculum implementation, faculty should decide the curriculum within the context of the mission of the university. Along with the mission statement, many faculty groups choose to develop a vision statement (the future the institution seeks to create, core values), a description about the preferred behavior of the institution, and goals (what the institution is committed to do). The mission statement should be derived from the characteristics of the institution (Reardon & Ramaley, 1997).

Development of a program's mission statement can take place after the institution's statement is completed. There will be more buy-in for the mission statement when all stakeholders, faculty, staff, and administration have an opportunity for input into the decision-making process. When the mission statement is being developed, the context within which the institution and program are placed must be carefully considered (Reardon & Ramaley, 1997). Is the program situated in a private or public institution? What is the program's relationship to the community it serves? What are the characteristics of the student body served? What is the scope of educational offerings provided within the program and institution? Developing an understanding of the answers to questions such as the ones listed here will help faculty design a mission statement that clearly reflects the uniqueness of the institution and program and provides direction to curriculum development. Many of the strategies identified later in this chapter for developing a philosophy statement can be applied to mission statement development.

Philosophy Statements

As the philosophical discussion begins, institutional values and the faculty member's beliefs, along with many societal and political influences, must be considered. Watson (1995) speaks of this when she describes how nursing's "caring–healing and health model have been largely ignored, dismissed, or controlled by medicalizing of the health care philosophy and educational practices" (p. 81). A more thorough discussion of these and other forces influencing curriculum are included in Chapter 6.

In reviewing philosophy statements developed for nursing education, certain commonalities may be found that reflect nurses' belief systems about human beings and their place in the world. The school of nursing philosophy statement in Box 7-1 demonstrates how the components of philosophy combine to make an articulate, easy-to-understand document that is useful to students and faculty. The following common elements of the nursing metaparadigm appear in most philosophy statements: nurse, patient, environment, and health. Many schools also include beliefs about nursing, teaching, learning, and nursing education.

The development of a philosophy of education is a thoughtful, introspective process and commonly includes a basic understanding of the traditional, modern, and postmodern philosophers and their subsequent educational theories. Conflicting interpretations of philosophy can occur as faculty attempt to resolve the dualism seen in many educational issues. These different interpretations of philosophical concerns are reflective of the pluralistic society that is the United States.

Philosophical questions about teaching and learning have continued through the ages. For example, is curriculum product or praxis? Grundy (1989) writes of product as behaviorist and more technical, whereas praxis is rooted in collaborative understanding and shared activity. Other questions arise about what should be the goal of education: Is it to meet the individual needs of the learner or to benefit society? Should student interest guide the curriculum or should all subjects be sequential and progress from simple to complex? Are students capable of designing and selecting their educational experiences, or must faculty retain these rights in order to ensure passage of National Council Licensure Examination (NCLEX) examinations? Faculties make decisions about these issues every day, often not in a conscious manner. Some faculties make decisions from an informed and broad base of understanding, others using a more casual and intuitive process.

Ideally the philosophy statement will proceed from the philosophical beliefs and educational practices of all members of the faculty. An experienced faculty is aware that the view of a university as a community of professionals who come to agreement and then proceed with one voice is not reality. Faculty pride themselves on their academic freedom, and this brings a rich diversity to the educational experience. However, if an institution has a clear mission to guide institutional advancement, faculty must grow in the process of shared vision and goals, while maintaining their own integrity and unique experiences as educators. A work environment that supports collegial dialogue in a nonthreatening environment through seminars, discussion groups, or "brown bag" lunches can be valuable in building communication about how to develop mission and philosophy statements.

Strategies to Develop the Mission and Philosophy Statements

Nursing faculty are a diverse group. There may be many faculty members who have never taken a philosophy course and are unfamiliar with the importance of the philosophical foundations of education. Offering opportunities for faculty to attend seminars to prepare them for curricular development activities, along with mentoring by senior faculty, can do much to encourage new faculty members to study and apply readings in philosophy. Otherwise, faculty will continue to "teach as they were taught," thus perpetuating the same educational process devoid of the growing body of nursing theories and research that can provide frameworks for new curricular frameworks. Stimulating and informative discussions can take place when time is set aside to dialogue in a collegial manner about philosophy. To focus only on the outcome of completing the philosophy statement for accrediting bodies eliminates the role of inquiry and discovery and turns the process into just another task to complete for the self-study report.

The use of computer technology can facilitate communication and is especially useful in multicampus systems. Computer interaction using groupware technology, also known as *workforce productivity software* (Webopedia, 2003a), allows the interconnected parties to view and edit documents in real time from a variety of locations. A subset of groupware is instant messaging, which allows a document to be prepared in real time when participants are separated by distance. Webinars, an Internet-based seminar tool, allows the giving and receiving of contributions to the discussion during the time the meeting is held (Webopedia, 2003b). Webinars, when combined with groupware, can accommodate large groups, thus encouraging a synergy that will facilitate faculty commitment and accountability to the newly developed curriculum.

Various strategies can facilitate the process of enlightened discourse, such as small group activities, critical incident/role play, Delphi process, and storyboarding. Ground rules are useful to generate positive group outcomes. The goal of consensus versus consent needs to be clarified. Is the group working toward consensus, where all members agree to support and implement but some may not be satisfied with the decision, or is unanimous consent the goal, where everyone agrees with the decision? Other considerations include using a neutral facilitator to uphold a community of trust and support with equal airing of ideas; ground rules for civility; time limits for meetings and for when a final decision is due; agreement about how voting will occur; and the role of faculty, staff, and administration in decision making.

Critical Incident/Role Play

Because philosophy is sometimes difficult to implement, faculty may benefit from the use of examples of case studies and role play that illustrate specific philosophical frameworks. A group could develop a critical incident around a student–faculty encounter in a classroom involving some specific learning situation and portray the interaction in behaviorist and humanistic frameworks, thus comparing and contrasting the two frameworks. This is an excellent opportunity for faculty to observe, question, and apply to what they observe to their own educational practice.

Delphi Process

The Delphi process is a useful strategy for gaining input about the development of the philosophy from all faculty. The strength of the Delphi process is that it allows a person time for reflection and personal inquiry to clarify personal meanings and values about curriculum. Faculty can write their thoughts on index cards and submit the cards to a task force of faculty, who then assemble the thoughts for the next round of feedback. By the second round of Delphi, comments can begin to be categorized according to the components of a philosophy statement—human beings, health, nursing, environments, and so forth—with attention to unexpected headings that may reflect group thinking. The method for using a Delphi survey to write a curriculum philosophy using a feminist, humanistic/existential, and phenomenological orientation with input from both practice and education was described by Beddome et al. (1995).

Storyboarding

Another strategy to be used for large groups of faculty is storyboarding. Faculty brainstorm ideas and then write on small pieces of adhesive paper as many ideas as they may have about a philosophical concept. If desired, each philosophical concept has a heading. For example, faculty could use storyboarding to identify all of their beliefs about patients, nursing, and health. These ideas are then categorized on large pieces of easel paper under broad headings. After everyone has written as much as they wish about each concept, the statements are compiled and listed. The next step is organizing and ranking the concepts. The third step is to select the top belief statements and begin the process of statement development. Although this process takes place over time, it is an excellent way to ensure that everyone has input into the process.

SUMMARY

As nurse educators participate in the dialogue about the role of nursing in the nation's health care system, faculty are designing innovative and cutting-edge curricula to prepare graduates capable of assuming responsibility for nursing in the twenty-first century. The development of a mission statement and a philosophy statement forms the basis for sound curriculum design. Philosophy may serve as both the source of and influence for curriculum development. The ability to articulate and apply one's philosophical beliefs to the educational process is the mark of a professional educator. If no guiding philosophy exists, tradition and past practice continue to be the prevailing forces driving the educational process.

Faculty often perceive philosophical frameworks to be obtuse and abstract. However, when faculty develop curriculum and learning activities within a sound framework, the quest for new philosophical foundations and subsequent curriculum initiatives can be a rewarding and satisfying experience for the nurse educators and learners alike.

REFERENCES

Beck, C. (1993). *Postmodernism, pedagogy, and philosophy of education!* From the University of Illinois at Urbana-Champaign website: http://www.ed.uiuc.edu/EPS/ PES-Yearbook/93_docs/BECK.HTM

Beddome, G., Budgen, C., Hills, M., Lindsey, E., Duval, P., & Szalay, L. (1995). Education and practice collaboration: A strategy for curriculum development. *Journal of Nursing Education, 34*(1), 11-15.

Benner, P., & Wrubel, J. (1989). *The primacy of caring.* Menlo Park, CA: Addison-Wesley.

Bevis, E. O. (1983). *Curriculum building in nursing: A process.* New York: National League for Nursing.

Bevis, E. O., & Watson, J. (2000). *Toward a caring curriculum: A new pedagogy for nursing.* (1st ed.). Boston: Jones and Bartlett and the National League for Nursing.

Blake, N., Smeyers, P., Smith, R., & Standish, P. (2003). *The Blackwell guide to the philosophy of education.* Malden, MA: Blackwell.

Dewey, J. (1916). *Democracy and education.* New York: Macmillan.

Diekelmann, N. (1993). Learning as testing: A Heideggerian hermeneutical analysis of the lived experiences of students and teachers in nursing. *Advanced Nursing Science, 14*(3), 72-83.

Diekelmann, N. (2001). Narrative pedagogy: Heideggerian hermeneutical analyses of lived experiences of students, teachers, and clinicians. *Advanced Nursing Science, 23*(3), 53-71.

Elias, J., & Merriam, S. (1995). *Philosophical foundations of adult education*. Malabar, FL: Krieger Publishing.

Fuhrmann, B. S. (1997). Philosophies and aims. In J. G. Gaff & J. L. Ratcliff & Associates (Eds.), *Handbook of the undergraduate curriculum* (pp. 86-99). San Francisco: Jossey-Bass.

Georges, J. (2003). An emerging discourse: Toward epistemic diversity in nursing. *Advances in Nursing Science, 26*(1), 44-52.

Grundy, S. (1989). *Curriculum: Product or praxis*. Philadelphia: Falmer Press.

Holmquist, E. (1960). *Steps in curriculum planning* (pp. 360–364). New York: National League for Nursing.

Ironside, P. (2001). Creating a research base of nursing education: An interpretive review of conventional, critical, feminist, postmodern, and phenomenologic pedagogies. *Advanced Nursing Science, 23*(3), 72-87.

Jencks, C. (1996). *What is post-modernism?* (4th ed.). London: Academy Editions.

Kirkham, S., & Anderson, J. (2002). Postcolonial nursing scholarship: From epistemology to method. *Advances in Nursing Science, 25*(1), 1-17.

Kritek, P. (2001). Toward a philosophy of healing practices in nursing. In N. Chaska (Ed.), *The nursing profession tomorrow and beyond* (pp. 907-918). Thousand Oaks, CA: Sage.

Leininger, M. (Ed.). (1978). *Transcultural nursing: Concepts, theories and practices*. New York: Wiley.

Maslow, A. (1954). *Motivation and personality*. New York: Harper & Row.

Newman, M. (2002). The patterns that connects. *Advanced Nursing Science, 24*(3), 1-7.

Rather, M. (1994). Schooling for oppression: A critical hermeneutical analysis of the lived experience of the returning RN student. *Journal of Nursing Education, 33*(6), 263-271.

Reardon, M. F., & Ramaley, J. (1997). Building academic community while containing costs. In J. G. Gaff & J. L. Ratcliff & Associates (Eds.), *Handbook of the undergraduate curriculum* (pp. 513–532). San Francisco: Jossey-Bass.

Rogers, C. (1969). *Freedom to learn*. Columbus, OH: Merrill.

Rogers, M. (1961). *Educational revolution in nursing*. New York: Macmillan.

Romyn, D. (2001). Disavowal of the behaviorist paradigm in nursing education: What makes it so difficult to unseat? *Advanced Nursing Science, 23*(3), 1-10.

Schindel, A. (1962). The application of criteria and principles to curriculum development in the diploma school. In *Aspects of curriculum development* (pp. 59-61). New York: National League for Nursing.

Skipper, D. (1962). Principles of curriculum development. In *Aspects of curriculum development* (pp. 38-50). New York: National League for Nursing.

Stewart, I. (1943). *The education of nurses*. New York: Macmillan.

Tanner, D., & Tanner, L. (1990). *History of the school curriculum*. New York: Macmillan.

Tyler, R. (1949). *Basic principles of curriculum and instruction*. Chicago: University of Chicago Press.

Watson, J. (1979). *Nursing: The philosophy and science of caring*. Boston: Little, Brown.

Watson, J. (1995). Advanced nursing practice and what might be. *Nursing and Health Care, 16*(2), 78-80.

Webopedia.com. (2003a). *Groupware*. Retrieved April 3, 2003, from http://www.pcwebopedia.com/TERM/g/groupware.html

Webopedia.com. (2003b). *Webinar*. Retrieved April 3, 2003, from http://www.pcwebopedia.com/TERM/W/Webinar.html

Further Reading

Brosio, R. (2000). *Philosophical scaffolding for the construction of critical democratic education*. New York: Peter Lang.

Philosophy of Education Society. Journals, online publications, and valuable links and information. Website: http://www.philosophyofeducation.org/

Philosophy of Education Society of Great Britain (PESGB). Website: http://www.philosophy-of-education.org

Studies in Philosophy and Education. An international journal with editors and contributors from around the world. Website: http://www.kluweronline.com/issn/0039-3746

8

CURRICULUM DESIGNS

Donna L. Boland, PhD, RN, Linda M. Finke, PhD, RN

Curriculum, by its very nature, holds a different element of promise for different groups of faculty. For some faculty, curriculum is a product to be delivered. For those who focus on consumerism, curriculum is a program that can and should be available for purchase at a fair market value. For external and internal constituencies whose intent is to evaluate, curriculum is conceived as a well-articulated statement about intended learning outcomes. There are also those with a gestalt view who believe that curriculum is to be experienced and that what is learned can only be interpreted from the perspective of the learner (Beane et al., 1986).

However one views curriculum, there is no argument that a well-designed curriculum is critical to the preparation of practicing nurses at all levels. Curricula in general, and undergraduate curricula specifically, have been under scrutiny for the last decade. Stark and Lattuca's (1997) summarization of reports critical of higher education suggested that "the reports urged colleges and universities to place more emphasis on common learning for all students. The curriculum, variously viewed as skills to be learned, courses to be pursued, and subject matter to be transmitted, was the central concern of all three reports [noted]" (pp. 81-82).

Regardless of the view of general education or professional education, the underlying theme is that curriculum designs must be responsive to the needs of society. Within the nursing profession, curriculum designs must reflect the current health care system and be fluid and flexible. These curriculum changes follow Bevis' (1988) original call for a

> [R]evolution that attacks the basic tenets of nursing curriculum development; that deinstitutionalizes the Tyler curriculum model and its mandated products; that makes nursing philosophy, research, and education congruent; that distinguishes between learning that is training and learning that is education; that alters our perception of teaching and the role of teacher; that abandons the industrial metaphor; that restructures the relative roles of classroom and clinical practice; that de-emphasizes curriculum development and concentrates on faculty development; that develops a national strategy for change; and, above all, that provides new guideposts for a new age. (pp. 27-28)

Using this formula, nursing faculty have been busily at work creating curriculum models that reflect contemporary needs.

This chapter discusses the issues of undergraduate and graduate education that have had an impact on program and curriculum designs, as well as current designs for all levels of nursing programs. It is important to have a sense of the issues that have shaped, and continue to shape, nursing curricula as faculty make decisions about the design of curriculum in their programs.

UNDERGRADUATE EDUCATION IN NURSING

Constituencies Invested in Undergraduate Curriculum Design

Undergraduate nursing curricula are assumed to set the stage for entry into nursing practice and to provide a foundation essential to graduate education and advanced nursing practice. Given the importance of these expectations, many different constituencies are invested in specific perceptions of undergraduate nursing programs. These constituencies have placed a number of often competing controls on the development, implementation, and evaluation of undergraduate curricula. As a professional education program, nursing is seemingly one of the most regulated educational enterprises on campuses of higher education today. One advantage enfolded into the desire to regulate is the consistency by which the quality of educational processes and resulting outcomes are scrutinized. A disadvantage to the control is the perceived decrease in latitude to be unique and creative in the design and delivery of the curriculum.

State Boards of Nursing

The first constituents interested in nursing education programs and curricula are the individual state boards of nursing. Early in the history of state boards of nursing, rules and regulations were set for programs that often specified content areas that must be covered, minimum hours that must be spent by all students in specified health care areas, and competencies or skills that all students must possess at the completion of a nursing program leading to licensure. Although these rules and regulations have tended to become less prescriptive, they are still state specific and varied. Their purpose is still to guide the development and implementation of undergraduate nursing curricula. The establishment of state regulations stems from the need to hold licensed health care personnel to standards of social responsibility and public accountability for actions taken on behalf of others. It can be argued that the education of nurses is and should be independent of regulatory licensure agencies, whose sole interest should be the protection of the consumer of nursing services. It is apparent that regulatory controls do have an impact on creativity and flexibility within nursing programs, especially undergraduate curricula.

Accrediting Bodies

Other constituents interested in nursing education programs are accrediting bodies. The National League for Nursing (NLN) historically served the role of the professional accrediting body for the evaluation of undergraduate nursing programs. Through the establishment and refinement of program assessment criteria, the NLN also affected the development, implementation, and evaluation of undergraduate nursing curricula across the country. These criteria, which address the mission and governance of the institution, faculty, students, curriculum, resources, and program effectiveness, had to be met by all programs seeking or renewing accreditation. The curriculum was developed by the nursing faculty and provided learning experiences consistent with the nursing unit's mission and stated outcomes of the program.

The National League for Nursing Accrediting Commission (NLNAC) was established in 1996 to act as an independent body that would carry out the accreditation activities that were once controlled through the NLN. The NLNAC continues to accredit all levels of nursing curricula. In the late 1990s there were five required NLNAC program outcome criteria: (1) critical thinking skills, (2) communication skills, (3) therapeutic nursing intervention skills, (4) graduate performance on licensing or certifying examinations, and (5) employment rates. Programs were also to evaluate any two of the five optional outcome criteria: (1) graduate satisfaction with the program, (2) employer satisfaction with the abilities of the program graduates, (3) graduation rates, (4) scholarship, and (5) public service (NLNAC, 1999). Today, student achievement is measured against graduation rates, performance on licensure examinations, job placement rates, and program satisfaction (NLNAC, 2003).

The Commission on Collegiate Nursing Education (CCNE) is a fairly new entity in the arena for the professional accreditation of nursing programs. CCNE began accrediting baccalaureate and graduate nursing programs in 1997. Unlike the NLNAC, with its broad accreditation scope, CCNE focuses its accrediting efforts on baccalaureate and higher degree programs exclusively. This commission has also identified standards for judging the degree to which nursing programs meet these published expectations. Although these evaluation criteria are not meant to be prescriptive, nursing faculty have used these accreditation standards in designing curricula. This effect can be seen in the balance between nursing and general education distribution credits, the sense of a need for theoretical frameworks on which to design curricula, the need for rationale for course sequencing, and credit hour limits.

Accrediting bodies will continue to influence program development and curricula design because these constituencies hold public accountability as their primary focus of interest. See Chapter 24 for additional information about curriculum evaluation.

Institutions of Higher Education

Historically, nursing has been viewed as having or needing regulatory oversight from those outside its discipline. Institutions of higher education that house nursing programs often actively influence the development and implementation of nursing curricula. This involvement takes many forms, including the development of general education requirements, procurement of clinical sites, hiring of teaching faculty, defraying the cost of undergraduate nursing education, supporting faculty practice, and equipping learning resource centers to keep pace with the advances in technological support for teaching and learning.

Market Forces

The marketplace also has had a strong voice in the design and implementation of nursing curricula throughout modern day nursing. The first schools of nursing were hospital based and generally administered by the director of the hospital, with the direct supervision of the students being delegated to the nursing staff affiliated with the institution. Class content was identified and taught by medical staff members, who had a large investment in what these young women were being prepared to do. This strong voice has changed both in tone and expression over the last 100 years. Today, nursing educators collaborate with their nursing practice counterparts in the design, implementation, and evaluation of nursing curricula. The challenge before nursing educators and practicing nurses is to design and deliver curricula that meet expectations for those entering today's practice arena, while equipping graduates with the skills and competencies necessary to adapt to tomorrow's demands. The concept of lifelong learning is the most powerful tool nursing professionals possess in meeting tomorrow's challenges.

Summary

The list of constituents interested in the education of nurses is varied. Although these constituents can complicate the creation process of undergraduate nursing curricula, they also bring heightened awareness of and enthusiasm for nursing programs and their faculty. The benefit is usually large amounts of goodwill. The cost is most often a higher level of accountability and scrutiny.

Historical Implications for Understanding Undergraduate Curricula

Florence Nightingale has been credited as the founder of modern nursing. As a prolific writer who spoke in eloquent tones about the education and practice of nurses, Nightingale envisioned nursing as more than the understanding of disease. She is quoted as having said, "pathology teaches the harm that disease has done. But it teaches nothing more" (Nightingale, 1969, p. 133). Her nursing orientation focused on health as a broad and encompassing concept that requires an understanding of human nature and the ability of that nature to affect individual health. Nightingale's thinking that nurses need to acquire an understanding of the science and art of human existence has continued to permeate undergraduate education from its original, hospital-based training programs to its current degree-granting educational programs.

Most nurse theorists have continued to define or subscribe to the characteristics of art and science as integral to understanding the profession of nursing. Nursing philosophy and theory are crucial to nursing curricula because philosophy and theory state what nursing is and what it should be. Salsberry (1994) stated that "philosophy of nursing identifies what is believed to be the basic or central phenomena of the discipline, relates nursing to a particular world view, and provides some information on how one may come to learn about the world" (p. 13). These often divergent thinkers, starting with Nightingale, have provided nursing with the theoretical foundation for educational philosophies, mission statements, curriculum models, and delivery of curriculum content. Despite the disagreement among recognized nursing theorists, they, like the curriculum models that have been predicated on their thinking, have focused on the nature of humans, society, and nursing practice.

The focus on human beings and their society complements the aims of general education that date back to Hellenic times, when education examined both "human nature and the nature of society" (Brubacher & Rudy, 1976, p. 287). The desire to understand human nature and society is still a prevailing factor in shaping undergraduate curricula, especially nursing curricula.

Undergraduate Program Designs

The design and development of undergraduate nursing programs that reflect the mission of the university or college, the philosophy of the faculty, current and projected nursing practice trends, changes in the health care system (real and theorized), changes in the demographics of the potential learner pool, and stakeholders' expectations require creativity, political savvy, negotiation skills, analytical rigor, psychic energy, and a modest amount of altruism. Faculty involved in designing programs and building curricula must possess a clear sense of purpose, a commitment to procuring resources, an understanding of market forces, the ability to predict the future, and the ability to know when goals have been accomplished. Once programs are designed, curriculum building becomes a never-ending task that is indispensable to, but separate from, the acts of teaching and learning. Curriculum is a dynamic, evolving entity shaped by learner needs and faculty's beliefs about the science and art of nursing.

Factors Affecting Program Design

Certain factors need to be considered in the development of nursing programs. Stark and Lattuca (1997) identified the following five dimensions or characteristics that are unique to the discipline of nursing, social work, and pharmacy:

- Service/technical role as it relates to conceptual and technical competency
- Connections related to the application of theory to practice
- Discourse communities that are interpreted as interpersonal skills in nursing
- Methods of inquiry related to the questions asked and answered in nursing practice, education, and research
- A value component that nursing teaches as professional identity and ethics

Also essential to program design are the following premises (Bevis, 1989b):

- Students have responsibility for their learning, and faculty have responsibility for structuring the learning setting to facilitate this learning
- The curriculum is designed to provide more structure to the beginning student and less to the more advanced student
- The curriculum is structured to focus on student–faculty interactions that facilitate learning
- Caring is a moral imperative and is therefore fundamental to all configurations of interactions within the learning environment

Nursing faculty must keep these dimensions of a practice profession in mind as they make decisions about program curriculum design.

The choice of approach to curriculum development depends on the beliefs and values that faculty hold about teaching and learning. According to Bevis (1989a) critical points that need to be identified and decided on in curriculum building include the following:

- A determination of the desired characteristics of the graduates of the program
- The identification and structure of knowledge that is critical to nursing practice
- The understanding of the culture of nursing as it relates to roles, ethics, and acceptable practice parameters
- An articulation of nursing's role in society in general and health care in particular
- An identification of curriculum content that will foster and further nursing's contribution to society
- The identification and organization of health care problems that graduates will be dealing with, both in today's reality and tomorrow's possibilities
- Identification of teaching and learning strategies that will foster critical thinking, inquiry, and the ability to meet one's learning needs
- The ability to assist students in developing the context (both within and outside of nursing) in which to understand the discipline of nursing

Various types of undergraduate nursing programs have been developed to allow multiple entry points into the profession. Generally there are many similarities among program designs, with variations occurring within the internal configuration of courses and course content. The three most common program designs are the 2-year associate degree, the 4-year baccalaureate degree, and the 3-year diploma program. In addition to these three educational avenues, there are accelerated baccalaureate program configurations for those with a recognized nonnursing degree, including an accelerated master's degree program for those with a nonnursing degree, a generic master's degree, and the nursing doctorate (ND) program. Diploma, associate, and baccalaureate degree program designs are discussed in further detail in this section.

Diploma Programs

Diploma programs represent the first curriculum model developed for training nurses in the late nineteenth and early to mid-twentieth centuries. Initially affiliated with hospitals, many of today's diploma schools of nursing are also affiliated with institutions of higher education. Diploma programs prepare technical nurses, who provide direct patient care in a variety of health care settings. Typically the curriculum is designed to be completed in 3 years and provides an emphasis on clinical practice. General education courses in the biological and social sciences are provided through affiliation with a local college or university. These college course credits can commonly be applied toward a baccalaureate degree in nursing if the student chooses to continue his or her education. With the shift of nursing education into colleges and universities, diploma schools gradually have been closing over the last 20 years or have been reconfiguring themselves as single-purpose institutions or merging with existing colleges or universities. Currently there are 68 diploma programs accredited with the NLNAC.

Associate Degree Programs

Associate degree nursing programs (ASN, ADN) were first developed in 1952 by Mildred Montag in response to a critical nursing shortage. The intent of the associate degree programs, as originally envisioned by Montag, was to prepare in 2 academic years a technical nurse who would provide direct patient care in acute care settings under the supervision of a professional nurse (Dillon, 1997). Despite the call for increasing the level of preparation of the RN, associate degree programs continue to be very popular. The graduates of associate degree programs taking the RN-CLEX have been steadily decreasing since 1995. However, in 2000, graduates of associate degree programs still comprised approximately 40% of the first time test takers (American Nurses Association [ANA], 2003). Although the emphases within associate degree curricula have usually been placed on subacute and long-term care in the educational preparation of students, many associate degree nurses can be found practicing in health care settings outside the structured hospital environment, even in community-based home health care settings (Neighbors & Monahan, 1997). The apparent overproduction and widespread use of associate degree–prepared nurses with little role differentiation from the baccalaureate graduate is an issue nursing faculty must consider as they design programs and develop and revise curricula to meet the challenges of nursing practice today and tomorrow.

Associate degree programs are commonly located in community or vocational colleges but may also be located in 4-year colleges and universities. The typical curriculum requires 2 academic years to complete and consists of approximately 30 credit hours of general education courses in the biological and social sciences and approximately 38 credit hours of nursing courses. The nursing courses include concepts and content related to the practice of medical–surgical, pediatric, maternity, and psychiatric/mental health nursing care. Some programs may also include management, community health, and gerontological concepts (Dillon, 1997). On completion of the program, graduates are prepared to practice in acute and long-term health care settings.

Baccalaureate Degree Programs

Baccalaureate degree programs (BSN, BS, BA) are offered by 4-year colleges and universities; some may also be independent, freestanding programs affiliated with a health care institution and university (Halstead & Billings, 1995). The graduate of a baccalaureate nursing program is prepared to deliver care to individuals, families, groups, and communities in institutional, home, and community settings. In addition to content related to specific nursing areas, baccalaureate curricula also include concepts related to management, community health, nursing theory and research, group dynamics, and professional issues. Health promotion, illness prevention, and patient education may also be emphasized.

The baccalaureate curriculum offers a strong foundation of liberal arts and sciences in addition to nursing courses. The program may be designed to require students to take prerequisite courses in the sciences, arts, and humanities before admission to the nursing major, or students may be directly admitted to the nursing program and take these courses concurrently with nursing courses. Faculty must consider the issues related to each program design, their philosophical beliefs about education, the characteristics of the program's student population, and the institution's mission as decisions are made about the design of the curriculum.

Educational Mobility Options

Many undergraduate nursing program options have been developed to allow learners educational mobility within the profession. These programs are called *mobility* or *bridging* programs. Program designs vary and depend on the philosophy of the nursing faculty and the expectations of the parent institution. The most popular of these are the LPN to ASN (1-2 + 2) programs and the ASN to BSN (2 + 2) programs. Additionally, programs exist for diploma to BSN students and LPN to BSN students. Some accelerated nursing programs also exist for holders of nonnursing baccalaureate degrees to facilitate their acquiring a BSN or MN. In light of the nursing shortage that is projected to worsen over the next decade (U.S. Department of Health and Human Services, Bureau of Health Professions, 2002), it is conceivable that nursing educators will continue to design educational options that facilitate educational transitioning for individuals coming from a nontraditional background. As a result, individuals wishing to pursue a nursing career will have a richness of opportunities and choices among educational program offerings.

This richness has created challenges for nursing faculty and for the public, who deal with the products of these educational programs. As noted previously, the factors that affect a program choice are related to the type of degree being granted. This decision then dictates credit hours, program length, required courses, and types of learning experiences that are consistent with the degree being awarded. With educational mobility options, faculty must make decisions about how to recognize and credit previous learning experiences. This may be accomplished through articulation agreements, advanced placement opportunities, credit transfers, and validation of previous learning through testing and portfolios.

As the nursing profession seeks to increase the number of nurses prepared at the baccalaureate and advanced practice levels, mobility programs will continue to be a quality, cost-effective means of supporting career mobility and accomplishing this goal. There are no set patterns to this process; what faculty will need to possess as they design future programs is a willingness to engage in flexible, creative curriculum development. Driving the call for creativity is the need to design structured learning experiences that draw on the prior knowledge and experiences of this nontraditional student population. Nursing faculty will be challenged to design curricula and learning experiences that facilitate the building of knowledge and skills on a foundation of what is known or has been experienced in a way that creates a meaningful context for additional knowledge (Marienau & Fiddler, 2002).

Designing the Curriculum

Choosing a specific program design, such as an associate or a baccalaureate degree program, does not automatically dictate the design of the program's curriculum. Faculty should develop a curriculum structure that will support the type of program desired and the outcomes that are envisioned. Chapter 9 provides a discussion on developing program outcomes and competencies. After deciding on desired program outcomes and competencies, faculty are ready to provide additional structure to the curriculum.

There are a number of different ways to think about the construction of a curriculum design. The more traditional approach to designing curricula offers structured courses in a specific sequence. This approach identifies what the student is to learn, when the learning is to occur, and what the outcome of the learning should be. The delineation of nursing and support content, nursing skills, critical learning experiences, and evaluation methods for assessing learning outcomes are emphasized. These pieces are structured into any one of a number of curriculum patterns. Two common curriculum patterns, that of "blocking" course content and that of integrating or "threading" course content, are described.

Blocking Course Content

Patterns can be built on the premise of sequencing specific courses and corresponding clinical learning experiences. The courses usually consist of blocks of content that are structured around particular clinical specialty areas, by patient population, or by body systems. Although each course or group of courses provides the foundation for the courses that follow, the content and focus of each course tends to be unique to that course.

A number of approaches can be used to organize the curriculum when blocking content. Content can relate to specific practice settings and content areas (e.g., medical–surgical nursing, mental health nursing, critical care nursing, pediatric nursing, maternity nursing, gerontological nursing, and community nursing). Faculty may also want to define, or block, content around developmental stages (e.g., birth, infancy, childhood, adolescence, adult, and older adult). Another potential conceptual blocking scheme is to construct courses around body systems (e.g., respiratory system, circulatory system, lymphatic system, regulatory system, digestive and elimination system, neurological system, and skeletal system).

The idea of blocking brings order or organization to both teaching and learning. It facilitates faculty course assignments and complements faculty expertise because this approach to curriculum building allows faculty to teach in areas in which they are most knowledgeable. It is also relatively easy for faculty to trace placement of content within the curriculum; faculty can be reasonably assured that students have been presented the content at a particular point in the curriculum. However, the segregation or blocking of content into specific courses can often cause content to become isolated from previous or following courses and can impede the learner's ability to integrate knowledge and transfer concepts, information, and experiences from one course to another. By and large, this approach produces a curriculum that is highly structured, with little latitude for deviation from specified teaching and learn-ing objectives and meeting individual learning needs.

Integrating Course Content

In a more conceptual approach to curriculum design, selected nursing phe-nomena may be integrated throughout the curriculum. In this approach fac-ulty identify concepts considered core to nursing practice and then integrate, or thread, these concepts throughout the curriculum. For example, some undergraduate program curricula have been developed based on a particular nursing theory. In this approach faculty use a specific nursing theory to help define concepts core to the understanding of nursing practice. Faculty then develop learning experiences that illustrate how the theoretical concepts are expressed in various patient populations in a variety of settings and how they are used to guide nursing practice.

Another example of content integration may be seen in the following description. The concept of pain is one of many concepts that are commonly integrated, or threaded, into a curriculum design. In coursework early in the curriculum, students would first learn about the pathophysiology of pain, the causes of pain, the cardinal characteristics of pain, factors that shape or affect pain, and how to assess and evaluate the characteristics of pain. As students moved through the curriculum, they would increase their understanding about the manifestation and treatment of pain, review research related to the concept of pain, and identify appropriate therapeutic nursing interventions related to the care of the patient with pain, thus progressing from a global understanding of pain to a more specific, in-depth understanding of the con-cept. Eventually, students would learn about pain as it relates to acute and chronic pain, to physical or non-disease-based causes, or specific situations such as surgery and childbirth in various clinical populations.

Other concepts that are commonly integrated through a curriculum include life span development, nutrition, and pharmacology. In a more con-ceptual or integrated approach to curriculum design, there are no boundaries to knowledge development and skill acquisition as noted in the blocking approach. Students use clinical experiences to learn the essence of those concepts identified and are encouraged to transfer their knowledge of these concepts to different settings and experiences. Disadvantages to a more conceptual approach to curriculum design include difficulty in maintaining the integrity of the curriculum because of the lack of discrete boundaries for content and the potential for inadvertently eliminating from the curriculum key aspects of the concept. Another potential disadvantage is that student learning styles may favor a less conceptual approach to learning.

Summary

The more traditional approach to curriculum where structure is critical to suc-cess of program outcomes supports knowledge as being absolute. In this situ-ation faculty have the responsibility to identify what knowledge students need to know and the resources that are most appropriate for obtaining the knowl-edge and the responsibility for imparting or verifying that knowledge in the classroom and clinical practice settings (Welte, 1997). In the conceptual approach to curriculum design, students' learning is reflective of partially known knowledge or truth. The remaining knowledge is gained from experience, inquiry, and application as students actively pursue learning experiences that foster knowledge acquisition.

Curriculum design requires an approach to curriculum development that is "based upon a belief in human freedom" and "calls for encouragement of self-reflection wherein the educators can come in touch with their own humanity and encourage the release of the human spirit in teaching–learning processes" (Watson, 1989, p. 37). This call for change is consistent with knowing as being an integral part of each individual's beliefs (Welte, 1997). Students bring to the learning situations their beliefs and values and learn through discourse and dialogue with self and others. Knowledge can also evolve through this exchange as knowledge is discussed and evaluated on its merit. In this context, knowledge is integrated and applied based on its merits. Welte (1997) referred to this knowledge as contextual, where learning occurs in an environment of critique between and among students and instructors. Problem-based learning ascribes to this tenet.

There is no one template to use in designing or changing undergraduate nursing curricula. However, the curriculum must be dynamic and capable of quickly changing as needed or desired. Nursing faculty can no longer afford to adopt curricula that are rigid and inflexible for learners and teachers alike, or overwhelmingly time consuming to construct. Nursing education's traditional approach to curriculum development as a "series of objectives with the content outlines that are expected to achieve those objectives" (Bevis, 1989a, p. 120) is now believed by some neither to meet the learning needs of students nor to satisfactorily prepare graduates to meet the changing needs of tomorrow's health care system.

Most faculty agree that today's undergraduate nursing students need to have a sense of the "bigger picture" of health care. In this picture, the broader concepts of patient care needs and learning outcomes help frame the learning and practice context, not the context of patient populations or care settings. This vision is a reflection of real and perceived changes in the health care industry. Nursing faculty must respond to these changes by creating a diversity of educational opportunities for an increasingly diverse population of students.

GRADUATE EDUCATION IN NURSING

Historical Development of Graduate Nursing Education

Graduate nursing education initially was developed in the early 1900s when nursing faculty, needing to be prepared at the graduate level, earned a graduate degree in a related field. The first doctoral program in nursing, an EdD, was offered at Teachers College, Columbia University, New York, in 1924 for the purpose of preparing educators and administrators of nursing schools (Peplau, 1966). Doctor of nursing science (DNS) programs were later developed as the need for doctorally prepared nursing faculty grew. The DNS programs were seen as professional clinical degrees and as symbols of nursing's autonomy and control over the programs. Although the DNS programs had a strong research base, they grew primarily from the clinical base of nursing.

As the need for additional, qualified nursing faculty continued to grow with the development of nursing's knowledge base, more educational programs that emphasized the strong clinical base of nursing were needed. Graduate nursing programs were developed to prepare nurses to meet the crucial shortage of nursing faculty and to promote the continued growth of the science of nursing. As the graduate programs in nursing multiplied, an increased need for researchers and not just educators became evident (Stevenson, 1988), thus leading to an increased number of PhD nursing programs across the country to prepare nurse researchers.

The rapid growth in the scientific knowledge base of nursing witnessed a corresponding increase in the number of doctoral programs. Although there was only an increase from 4 to 21 nursing doctoral programs in the United States from 1960 to 1980, there were 34 programs by 1985, and 64 programs by 1995 (American Association of Colleges of Nursing [AACN], 1995; Marriner-Tomey, 1990). There are currently 83 doctoral programs in nursing (AACN, 2002). Most of these programs are PhD programs. In recent years the trend has been toward the establishment of academic research doctoral programs (PhD) that prepare researchers; however, the new degree of Doctor of Nursing Practice (DNP) has been established. The DNP was developed to prepare an expert in professional clinical nursing practice leadership.

The need for an advanced level of nursing practice, beyond baccalaureate preparation, to meet the health care needs of individuals and families was recognized in the 1960s and led to the development of master's degree programs. Rutgers University began a master's degree program to educate clinical specialists in psychiatric nursing. A nurse practitioner program that prepared pediatric nurse practitioners was founded at the University of Colorado in 1965 (Watson, 1995). In the 1990s there was an explosion of master's degree nursing programs, which continues today.

In an effort to meet the needs of working nurses and those in underserved areas, graduate education has moved to the incorporation of distant education learning strategies. There are a number of master's degree programs and a few doctoral programs that are totally accessible through the Internet. Even more graduate degree programs combine distant education strategies with brief face-to-face courses and experiences.

Program Designs for Master's Education

The purpose of education at the master's level is to prepare advanced practice nurses. The role of a master's prepared nurse has evolved from being solely that of an educator, administrator, or researcher to being that of a practitioner or clinician. The role continues to be based on a theory and research foundation that applies knowledge to the care of individuals, families, groups, and communities. The roles of the advanced practice nurse include practitioner, clinical specialist, administrator, nurse midwife, and nurse anesthetist (ANA, 1993).

A master's degree education was not always a requirement for the preparation of advanced practice nurses. At the 1993 national convention of the NLN a resolution was passed that the graduate degree be the minimal educational preparation for advanced practice in nursing (NLN, 1993). Although the clinical specialist had always been prepared at the master's level, the other roles were often prepared at the certificate level. At about the same time the agencies that certify nurse practitioners and nurse anesthetists also adopted the requirement that nurses wishing to be certified in these roles complete a master's program in the appropriate specialty.

Program Characteristics

Master's level programs in nursing vary in length and focus. Most programs are 2 years in length, but some programs are 12 to 18 months in length. The length of the program is determined by a variety of factors, including the entry level of the student, curriculum design, credit hours per semester or quarter, and clinical hours required. Many students also enroll in part-time study, thus lengthening the program.

Most programs require an earned baccalaureate in nursing for entry. However, some programs have been developed for nonnurses with an undergraduate degree in another field. Mobility options are also available (e.g., RN to MSN programs) for nurses without a baccalaureate degree in nursing. Options also have been developed to meet the needs of nurses who already hold a master's degree in nursing but wish to pursue a different specialty.

With health care reform, the need for advanced practice nurses has been recognized by the public and health care agencies, and the establishment of master's level nursing programs has boomed. The programs that have enjoyed the greatest growth are those established to prepare nurse practitioners (AACN, 1995). Nurse practitioner programs prepare advanced practice nurses to meet frontline primary care health care needs.

Faculty and Student Qualifications

The quality of graduate nursing education programs is maintained through the appointment and selection of well-qualified faculty and students. Fifty percent of the faculty teaching in a master's program in nursing must hold the doctorate. This is one of the criteria for program accreditation by NLNAC (NLN, 1996) and CCNE (AACN, 1996a). Most faculty should be certified in the nursing specialty in which they teach. They should be active in advanced nursing practice or in nursing research.

Students admitted to a master's program should have the potential for academic success as indicated by past academic success, standardized tests such as the Graduate Record Examination (GRE), and references. Other common requirements for admission to a master's program are graduation from an NLN-accredited baccalaureate program, current licensure as an RN, a specified amount of work experience, completion of health assessment and statistics courses, and participation in an admission interview (Stokes et al., 1997). Potential students should also have the skills needed to provide leadership and practice in autonomous nursing roles.

Curriculum

From 1993 to 1995 the AACN worked with nursing faculty across the country to develop *The Essentials of Master's Education for Advanced Practice Nursing* (AACN, 1996b). The model identified three types of master's programs: administration; community health; and advanced practice, which includes nurse practitioners, clinical nurse specialists, certified nurse midwives, and certified RN anesthetists. Content that was identified as core for all master's programs includes research; policy, organization, and financing of health care; ethics; professional role development; theoretical foundations of nursing; and human diversity and social issues. Core content for advanced practice was also identified and includes advanced health assessment, advanced physiology and pathology, and advanced pharmacology (AACN, 1996b). In addition to the requirements set forth by the AACN, some master's programs provide students with the opportunity to complete elective or cognate coursework in a specialty area of their choice.

Accrediting Bodies

Master's degree programs in nursing have the choice of seeking accreditation through NLNAC or CCNE. The established accreditation criteria are those cited earlier. A paradigm shift away from prescribed curricula to outcome-based assessment in the early 1990s opened the door for diversity and creativity in curriculum design. Master's level education in nursing is goal oriented and is guided today in a significant way by the requirements of the certifying agencies of advanced practice nurses. Accrediting agencies particularly focus on the number of clinical hours included in an educational program. Most certifying agencies establish minimums for clinical hours that must be met by nurses before taking the certification examination.

Program Designs for Doctoral Education

As stated earlier, during the 1990s the number of doctoral programs in nursing grew rapidly, and according to the AACN (2002), 83 schools of nursing now have doctoral programs. Several suggestions have been made on how to categorize nursing doctoral programs (Forni & Welch, 1987; Gortner, 1990; Grace, 1989; Peplau, 1966). Forni and Welch (1987) suggested that doctoral programs in nursing could be placed in one of three categories: first professional degree, terminal degree, or academic degree.

First Professional Degree

The first professional degree is the ND, which prepares graduates for clinical practice (Fitzpatrick et al., 1986). The ND curriculum assumes the need for nursing education to be at the postbaccalaureate level. The focus of the first 2 years of the program is on the acquisition of clinical knowledge and skills. Advanced clinical practice is the emphasis of the third year. Graduates are qualified to take the NCLEX-RN for RNs. This curriculum model, which was proposed by Schlotfeldt (1978), has not been widely adopted.

Terminal and Academic Degrees

The terminal degrees in nursing include the DNS, the doctor of science in nursing (DSN or DNSc), and the DNP. The terminal degree fulfills the mission of practice or clinical practice (Forni & Welch, 1987). The academic degree is the PhD in nursing science degree. The academic degree fulfills the mission of research. In reality there is little difference in the two types of degrees (Gortner, 1990; Grace, 1989; Meleis, 1988). Both prepare nursing researchers and both are grounded in nursing theory and practice. It is argued that many of the first terminal degree programs were established in the 1960s before nursing science was acknowledged in academe and were therefore offered by the school of nursing instead of the institution's graduate school. Most of these programs have evolved into PhD programs. Educators such as Meleis (1988) have encouraged nursing faculty to either make distinct the differences between the terminal and academic doctoral programs in nursing or phase out the terminal degree programs.

The terminal and the academic degree programs follow the traditional model of graduate education. Doctoral curricula are unique to each institution but commonly include content related to theory construction; philosophy; development of research skills; nursing knowledge; and important social, political, and ethical issues affecting the profession (Ziemer et al., 1991). Although most doctoral programs require a master's degree in nursing for admittance, some will admit students with a baccalaureate degree in nursing (BSN to doctorate programs). Students who enter a doctoral program after earning the baccalaureate in nursing usually study full time for 5 years and complete a dissertation. Students who enter after they have a master's degree in nursing study full time for approximately 3 years and must also complete a dissertation. Many curricula are designed to allow part-time study. Traditional experiences such as a 1-year residency requirement and qualifying examinations (oral, written, or both) following coursework are often part of the program; however, such practices vary among institutions.

There must be a critical mass of nursing faculty who are active researchers to support either the terminal degree or academic degree program. Faculty must be not only excellent teachers but also scholars to guide and advise students in their development as researchers. As members of the scientific community, faculty disseminate their research findings through publication in peer-reviewed journals and presentations at scientific meetings. Students learn by participating with faculty in their research and dissemination of the findings.

Accrediting Bodies

Doctoral programs in nursing are not accredited by a separate nursing body. However, the AACN published *Essentials for Doctoral Programs in Nursing*, which was revised in 1994. Evaluation is always an important aspect of curriculum development. Feedback from the evaluation of program outcomes should lead to curriculum revision, implementation, and further evaluation of the doctoral curriculum.

Summary

Health care reform, with the increasing emphasis on advanced practice nurses as primary care providers who can provide quality, cost-effective, community-based health care, has led to increasing numbers of graduate nursing programs, especially nurse practitioner programs. Nursing education has historically responded to the health care needs of our nation's citizens. Master's level education responded to the demand for advanced practice nurses; doctoral education responded to the need for qualified nursing faculty and then the need for nursing researchers. The continuing faculty shortage has a dramatic effect on the further development of graduate education in nursing. Creative strategies are needed to prepare nursing faculty for the future.

Major issues related to the program design of graduate nursing programs will continue to revolve around maintaining quality standards for educational programs; recruiting and maintaining a culturally diverse student population reflective of our society's increasing multiculturalism; resolving certification and accreditation issues, especially in the area of advanced practice nursing; and developing flexible curriculum models that will facilitate the preparation of the large numbers of advanced practice nurses necessary to meet primary health care needs. Doctoral programs will need to continue to develop curriculum models that foster the development of nursing knowledge in the areas of clinical practice, research, and education. By vigorously addressing issues such as these, graduate education in nursing will continue to produce practitioners capable of meeting the demands of today's health care system.

FUTURE TRENDS IN NURSING EDUCATION

With health care reform, new constituents are now playing more dominant roles in shaping nursing education. Although health care financing, technology development, and modes of delivering health care services have always had an impact on nursing education, competition among health care providers, the increased knowledge of the consumer, and the shift to community-based health care will increasingly shape nursing education in the future. The changes occurring with health care reform have mandated that the nursing profession, both practice and education, work together to address the issue of the appropriate mix of nursing personnel to provide quality health care. Differentiation of roles and responsibilities, based on the educational preparation of the nurse, is becoming increasingly necessary to effectively meet the health care needs of society and must be addressed by the profession (AACN, 1993; Boland, 2000; deTornyay, 1993; Fagin & Lynaugh, 1992; Greiner & Knebel, 2003).

The world of higher education is in the midst of accelerating change. This change will extend beyond the learning environment to the organization and finances of higher education (American Association of University Professors, 2003). To this end, future trends in nursing education will include an increase in the number of collaborative partnerships between nursing practice and education. Such efforts will focus on maintaining congruence between nursing curricula and contemporary nursing practice, developing initiatives that will help new graduates with the transition into nursing practice, and establishing mechanisms to reward and retain the experienced nurse in the workforce (Greiner & Knebel, 2003; Malloch & Laeger, 1997). There also will be an increased emphasis placed on collaboration between disciplines. There is support in the literature that teamwork increases quality and safety in care (Dichter, 2003). Students will be encouraged to participate on interdisciplinary practice and research teams that include a wide spectrum of disciplines.

According to a just released statement from the Health Professions Education Summit committee, "all health professionals should be educated to deliver patient-centered care as members of an interdisciplinary team, emphasizing evidence-based practice, quality improvement approaches, and informatics" (Greiner & Knebel, 2003, p. 3). The members of this committee identified five competencies they believe should drive undergraduate curricula. These five competencies are not new to most faculty, but faculty must continue to create curriculum models that will optimally prepare graduates with knowledge and skills to provide patient-centered care within a disciplinary team based on up-to-date science. The committee identified a number of skills that nurses will need to possess on entry into the profession of nursing. These skills include but are not limited to critical thinking as a process that supports diagnostic reasoning, problem identification, problem resolution, and the optimization of individualized care. Nurses now more than ever must be effective "knowledge workers" who have the ability to effectively communicate within interdisciplinary teams and to collect, organize, retrieve, and apply diverse sources of information that supports care that leads to high quality care outcomes.

The change in academia will include the increased development of educational products by nonacademic and for-profit organizations. Tools and content that can be incorporated by faculty into their teaching will be available. Creative use of this content can assist with the faculty shortage that will continue. Students will also have increased resources at their fingertips to reach new levels of understanding.

Barriers to career mobility and articulation will continue to be removed. Past barriers have included the use of expensive, time-consuming validation examinations; duplication of learning; lack of flexibility; student-perceived attitudinal problems toward the RN student on the part of faculty; and difficulty with transferring credits (Kish et al., 1997). Articulation models that remove these barriers and support career mobility with flexibility and minimal duplication of previous learning are increasingly being proposed and developed (Fagin & Lynaugh, 1992; Kish et al., 1997; Redmond, 1997). Distance learning will continue to play a prominent role in successfully delivering education to geographically dispersed students. Faculty will seek new teaching strategies that will support distance learning using evolving technologies. These new strategies will play an important role in facilitating the learning of nontraditional learners through curricula that will be taught more from an integrated conceptual orientation especially designed for the distant learner.

New educational models are being designed based on the premise that nurse educators must seek new ways of preparing the next generation of nurses. Nurse educators cannot hold onto the traditional models given the rapidly changing nature of health care and education. Educators must design new or modify traditional curriculum models if graduates are to have the relevant skills to practice nursing as it is today, as well as the abilities to shape nursing practice for the future. The ways and means of educating the next generation of nurses must clearly be on the agenda at all nursing schools. Nurse educators must be able to step away from "what has been" to envision "what can be" (Boland, 2000). The AACN is presently proposing a new type of nursing graduate. The projected curriculum for this new nurse provider has been shaped by the recommendations of the Health Professions Education Summit committee. However, it is not clear that suggesting the creation of yet another nurse care provider will result in curriculum clarity for today's nurse educators. This new curriculum model tends to blur the distinctions between undergraduate and graduate education. As new articulation and educational mobility models continue to emerge these lines will become more obliterated, with continued drift to graduate preparation for entering professional nurses. Faculty will also be looking at the addition of some type of intensive practicum experience before graduation or in partnership with health care partners as part of an orientation program that bridges the gap between graduation and full nurse practice privileges.

The nature of undergraduate nursing education will be particularly scrutinized. Oesterle and O'Callaghan (1996) posed several questions about undergraduate curricular issues that warrant discussion in the profession:

- With the increasing use of assistive personnel in the health care setting, what basic skills are essential to include in baccalaureate curricula?
- If increasing numbers of nursing graduates are not likely to find positions in acute care practice settings, why are faculty continuing to prepare most students to work there?
- Is nursing education currently producing graduates that meet the needs of the changing health care environment?
- With knowledge advancing so rapidly, can faculty continue to develop curricula that are structured around specific content?

These are difficult questions to respond to, yet nursing faculty have no choice but to address these and similar questions.

Responding to a health care environment that focuses more on community-based health care between individuals who are well and those who have chronic illnesses, Wilkerson (1996) proposed the consideration of a curriculum that allows for differentiation and specialization of practice at the undergraduate level. Such role specialization has historically been reserved for graduate education, but with the increasing knowledge and technology explosion and the different skills and competencies required for caring for patients with acute illnesses, as opposed to the skills and competencies necessary for teaching health promotion, illness prevention, and caring for patients with chronic illnesses, this approach to undergraduate education warrants consideration. Faculty and students can no longer attempt to "do it all" in a 2- to 4-year span; the careful balance that must be achieved between theory and practice will continue to be an issue, with faculty making difficult decisions about which learning experiences are most essential to developing a competent practitioner.

Professional education, by its very nature, faces several critical issues that faculty must continue to address at the undergraduate and graduate levels. These issues are of importance to all involved in professional education today, not just the discipline of nursing. First, professional schools, such as professional schools of nursing, must continue to abide by the social contract that exists between them and society by producing competent practitioners. Increased consumerism has lead to greater scrutiny and questioning of the cost–benefit value of professions to society (Curry & Wergin, 1997). Historically, nursing has proved its worth to society. Faculty must continue to design nursing programs that produce graduates with the knowledge, skills, and attitude necessary to function effectively and competently in a changing profession. Schools of nursing must also accept responsibility for providing continued professional development to help practitioners maintain competence. Among the number of reforms identified by the Health Professions Education Summit committee were the need for the use of a common language among health care workers and the need for more consistency of learning outcomes across programs and disciplines (Greiner & Knebel, 2003). These two recommendations will have a significant impact on current nursing programs, which enjoy the latitude to create innovative curricula that reflect the values and beliefs of their stakeholders.

Faculty must also continue to be involved in discussions related to defining, measuring, evaluating, and certifying competence in the profession (Curry & Wergin, 1997). Ongoing evaluation and assessment will be one of the most important tools faculty will use in developing future nursing curriculum models and in determining what knowledge and skill sets today's and tomorrow's nurses must have (Boland & Laidig, 2001). Faculty will address the issue of practice relevancy by adding an intensive practice capstone to the curriculum. Capstone experiences will allow faculty the opportunity to evaluate the ability of their students to meet the program competencies and to determine the effectiveness of their students to deliver patient-centered care in an interdisciplinary model. This is especially important as the traditional configuration of clinical practice learning becomes significantly altered because of cost, environmental factors, best learning practices, and alteration of educational competencies.

A major force in nursing education will be the need to teach evidence-based practice. Nursing curriculum must not perpetuate knowledge built on tradition but must build a foundation on evidence that supports the nursing interventions. This will mean a retraining of some faculty and a retooling of much of the curriculum that has been taught over time. Nursing students must learn practice based on evidence and also how to continue the process of evidence seeking and application. Nursing curriculum will be dynamic, with a focus on finding evidence to determine best practices.

In the world of higher education, the nursing profession has long been the source of much educational innovation. The issues identified here are critical to the future of nursing education, but by no means are they an exhaustive listing of the issues nursing faculty must consider as they design future nursing programs and curricula. The innovation and creativity that nursing faculty have demonstrated in the past will no doubt continue to identify them as leaders in professional and higher education into the future. If nurse educators are to become more collaborative in designing curricula at both the undergraduate and graduate levels, then nurse faculty and administrators will need to take the lead in creating educational models that their academic colleagues will embrace.

SUMMARY

Nursing leaders such as Jean Watson (1995) have envisioned a future in which nurses play a predominant role in leading the delivery of health care instead of responding to the demands by others. As nurses take an active role in developing health care delivery, nursing education will need to prepare graduates at all levels with appropriate leadership skills and an understanding of change. Nursing curricula will need to move away from rigid requirements to flexible learning opportunities to prepare nurses for the ever changing future.

Designing curriculum provides an opportunity for faculty to use their scientific knowledge base, clinical competence, and creativity. Curriculum development at all levels is guided by the need to consistently include in the students' educational experiences opportunities to acquire the knowledge, skills, and competencies that are needed by graduates. Careful attention must be paid to accreditation requirements and preparation for licensure and certification examinations. Perhaps most important, students must be encouraged not only to learn new knowledge but also to enhance the critical thinking and lifelong learning skills that will be needed as they meet the challenges of the changing health care environment.

REFERENCES

American Association of Colleges of Nursing. (1993). *Nursing education's agenda for the 21st century.* Washington, DC: Author.

American Association of Colleges of Nursing. (1995). *1994-95 Special report on masters and post-masters nurse practitioner programs.* Washington, DC: Author.

American Association of Colleges of Nursing. (1996a). *Standards for accreditation of baccalaureate and graduate nursing education.* Washington, DC: Author.

American Association of Colleges of Nursing. (1996b). *The essentials of master's education for advanced practice nursing.* Washington, DC: Author.

American Association of Colleges of Nursing. (2002). *List of doctoral programs.* Washington, DC: Author.

American Association of University Professors. (2003). *Distance education and intellectual property issues.* Washington, DC: Author.

American Nurses Association. (1993). Council of nurses in advanced practice. *Advanced Nursing Practice Conference. Council perspectives, 2*(2).

American Nurses Association. (2003). *Nursing facts: Today's registered nurse—Numbers and demographics.* Retrieved July 14, 2003, from http://nursingworld.org/readroom/fsdemogrpt.htm

Beane, J. A., Toepfer, C. F., & Alessi, S. J., Jr. (1986). *Curriculum planning and development.* Boston: Allyn & Bacon.

Bevis, E. O. (1988). New directions for a new age. In *NLN curriculum revolution: Mandate for change.* New York: National League for Nursing.

Bevis, E. O. (1989a). Clusters of influence for practical decision making about curriculum. In E. O. Bevis & J. Watson (Eds.), *Toward a caring curriculum: A new pedagogy for nursing* (pp. 107-152). New York: National League for Nursing.

Bevis, E. O. (1989b). Nursing curriculum as professional education: Some underlying theoretical models. In E. O. Bevis & J. Watson (Eds.), *Toward a caring curriculum: A new pedagogy for nursing* (pp. 67-106). New York: National League for Nursing.

Boland, D. L. (2000). The future of nursing education: Helping to determine if nursing is to be or not to be. In N. Chaska (Ed.), *The nursing profession: Tomorrow and beyond* (pp. 867-880). Thousand Oaks, CA: Sage.

Boland, D. L., & Laidig, J. (2001). Assessment of student learning in the discipline of nursing. In C. Palomba & T. Banta (Eds.), *Assessing student competence in accredited disciplines* (pp. 71-95). Sterling, VA: Stylus.

Brubacher, J. S., & Rudy, W. (1976). *Higher education in transition: A history of American colleges and universities, 1636-1976.* New York: Harper & Row.

Curry, L., & Wergin, J. F. (1997). Professional education. In J. G. Gaff & J. L. Ratcliff & Associates (Eds.), *Handbook of the undergraduate curriculum: A comprehensive guide to purposes, structures, practices, and change* (pp. 341-358). San Francisco: Jossey-Bass.

deTornyay, R. (1993). Nursing education: Staying on track. *Nursing & Health Care, 14*(6), 302-306.

Dichter, J. (2003). Teamwork and hospital medicine: a vision for the future. *Critical Care Nurse, 43*(3), 8-11.

Dillon, P. (1997). The future of associate degree nursing. *N&HC: Perspectives on Community, 18*(1), 20-24.

Fagin, C. M., & Lynaugh, J. E. (1992). Reaping the rewards of radical change: A new agenda for nursing education. *Nursing Outlook, 40*(5), 213-220.

Fitzpatrick, J., Boyle, K., & Anderson, R. (1986). Evaluation of the doctor of nursing (ND) program: Preliminary findings. *Journal of Professional Nursing, 2*(6), 365-372.

Forni, P. R., & Welch, M. J. (1987). The professional versus the academic model: A dilemma for nursing education. *Journal of Professional Nursing, 3*(5), 291-297.

Gortner, S. R. (1990). Nursing values and science: Toward a science philosophy. *IMAGE: Journal of Nursing Scholarship, 22*(2), 101-105.

Grace, H. K. (1989). Issues in doctoral education in nursing. *Journal of Professional Nursing, 5*(5), 266-271.

Greiner, A. C., & Knebel, E. (2003). Executive summary. In A. C. Greiner & E. Knebel (Eds.), *Health professions education—A bridge to quality.* Washington, DC: National Academies Press.

Halstead, J. A., & Billings, D. M. (1995). Nursing education. In G. Deloughery (Ed.), *Issues and trends in nursing* (pp. 249-275). St. Louis: Mosby.

Kish, C., Newsome, G., Dattilo, J., & Roberts, L. (1997). Georgia's RN-BSN articulation model. *N&HC: Perspectives on Community, 18*(1), 26-30.

Malloch, K., & Laeger, E. (1997). Nursing partnerships: Education and practice (NPEP). *N&HC: Perspectives on Community, 18*(1), 32-35.

Marienau, C., & Fiddler, M. (2002). Reflection across the curriculum: Bringing students' experience to the learning process. *About Campus, 7*(5), 12-19.

Marriner-Tomey, A. (1990). Historical development of doctoral programs from the middle ages to nursing education today. *Nursing and Health Care, 11*(3), 133-137.

Meleis, A. I. (1988). Doctoral education in nursing: Its present and its future. *Journal of Professional Nursing, 4*(6), 436-446.

National League for Nursing. (1993, June). *Resolution of advanced nursing practice.* Paper presented at the twenty-first biennial convention of the National League for Nursing Convention, New York, NY.

National League for Nursing. (1996). *Criteria and guidelines for the evaluation of baccalaureate and higher degree nursing programs.* Council of Baccalaureate and Higher Degree Programs, Pub. No. 15-6916. New York: National League for Nursing Accrediting Commission.

National League for Nursing Accrediting Commission. (1999). *1999 Interpretive guidelines.* Retrieved June 30, 2002, from http://www.nlnac.org

Neighbors, M., & Monahan, F. D. (1997). Are ADNs prepared to be home health nurses? *N&HC: Perspectives on Community, 18*(1), 15-18.

Nightingale, F. (1969). *Notes on nursing.* New York: Dover Publications.

Oesterle, M., & O'Callaghan, D. (1996). The changing health care environment: Impact on curriculum and faculty. *N&HC: Perspectives on Community, 17*(2), 78-81.

Peplau, H. (1966). Nursing: Two routes to doctoral degrees. *Nursing Forum, 5*(2), 57-67.

Redmond, G. M. (1997). LPN-BSN: Education for a reformed health care system. *Journal of Nursing Education, 36*(3), 121-127.

Salsberry, P. J. (1994). A philosophy of nursing: What is it? What is it not? In J. F. Kikuchi & H. Simmons (Eds.), *Developing a philosophy of nursing.* Thousand Oaks, CA: Sage.

Schlotfeldt, R. (1978). The professional doctorate: Rationale and characteristics. *Nursing Outlook, 26*(5), 302-311.

Stark, J. S., & Lattuca, L. R. (1997). *Shaping the college curriculum: Academic plans in action.* Needham Heights, MA: Allyn & Bacon.

Stevenson, J. S. (1988). Nursing knowledge development: Into era II. *Journal of Professional Nursing, 4*(3), 152-162.

Stokes, E., Whitis, G., & Moore-Thrasher, L. (1997). Characteristics of graduate adult health nursing programs. *Journal of Nursing Education, 36*(2), 54-59.

U.S. Department of Health and Human Services, Bureau of Health Professions. (2002). *Projected supply, demand and shortage of registered nurses: 2000-2020.* Retrieved June 30, 2002, from http://bhpr.hrsa.gov/healthworkforce/reports/rnproject/

Watson, J. (1989). A new paradigm of curriculum development. In E. O. Bevis & J. Watson (Eds.), *Toward a caring curriculum: A new pedagogy for nursing* (pp. 37-60). New York: National League for Nursing.

Watson, J. (1995). Advanced nursing practice and what might be. *Nursing and Health Care, 16*(2), 78-83.

Welte, S. L. (1997). Transforming educational practice: Addressing underlying epistemological assumptions. *Review of Higher Education, 20*(2), 199-213.

Wilkerson, J. M. (1996). The C word: A curriculum for the future. *N&HC: Perspectives on Community, 17*(2), 72-77.

Ziemer, M. M., Brown, J., Fitzpatrick, M. L., Manfredi, C., O'Leary, J., & Valiga, T. M. (1992). Doctoral programs in nursing: Philosophy, curricula, and program requirements. *Journal of Professional Nursing, 8*(1), 56-62.

Ziemer, M. M., Fitzpatrick, M. L., Valiga, T., Manfredi, C., & Brown, J. (1991). Curricula of doctoral programs in nursing. In M. Garbin (Ed.), *Assessing educational outcomes* (pp. 123-131). New York: National League for Nursing.

9

DEVELOPING CURRICULUM
FRAMEWORKS, OUTCOMES, AND COMPETENCIES

Donna L. Boland, PhD, RN

This chapter describes the use of curriculum frameworks for the purpose of conceptualizing and organizing the delivery of the knowledge, values, beliefs, and skills necessary for professional nursing practice. Various factors that shape the process of curriculum development are discussed. Because curriculum development begins with the need to conceptualize the discipline of nursing, a discussion of organizing frameworks is presented. This chapter also focuses on historical factors that have affected the design of nursing curricula and ends with a discussion of outcomes and competencies and how they are related to faculty's conceptualization of the discipline. Examples of outcomes and competencies are presented to illustrate their link between curricula, faculty expectations, and student learning.

CURRICULUM FRAMEWORKS

A curriculum is designed to provide a sequence of learning experiences that will enable students to achieve desired educational outcomes (Ratcliff, 1997). To determine the desired educational outcomes of a curriculum, faculty must first ask themselves what students should know and be able to do on completion of their educational experience. What competencies, in terms of knowledge, skills, and attitudes, must students possess to successfully demonstrate the desired outcomes? In addition, faculty must also decide what learning experiences will facilitate students' attainment of these competencies and how the attainment of these competencies and the resulting outcomes will be evaluated (Banta, 1996). Curriculum frameworks provide faculty with a means of conceptualizing and organizing the knowledge, skills, values, and beliefs critical to the delivery of a coherent curriculum that facilitates the achievement of the desired curriculum outcomes.

For a determination of what it is that needs to be taught and learned, the phenomenon of focus, which in this case is nursing, must first be identified. The faculty's philosophical beliefs about how teaching, learning, and the discipline of nursing should be viewed, described, and evaluated guide the development of the curriculum framework (see Chapter 7). Organizing frameworks for the curriculum offer a further delineation of the constructs that are discussed in the philosophy statement. Organizing frameworks are still conceptual and reflect a systematic array of ideas and symbols. However, they do provide faculty with a tool that turns mental images of nursing phenomena into visual structures that represent the phenomena and their relationships.

The faculty's philosophical beliefs and values provide the basis for the selection of a particular organizing framework. Fawcett's (1989) work on conceptual models and frameworks can provide readers with a classical discussion of theories, models, and concepts that are beyond the scope of this chapter. Apple (1979) connects the ideas of curriculum with organizing frameworks by suggesting that curriculum exists as a means for creating access to knowledge about the phenomena of interest or the importance to the discipline. Organizing frameworks provide the logical structure for cataloging and retrieving knowledge, which are essential to the processes of teaching and learning. Additionally, organizing frameworks provide the models to assist the learner in building the context for knowledge and helping to promote an understanding and application of nursing knowledge.

Purposes of Organizing Frameworks for Curriculum

Organizing frameworks, or conceptual models, for curriculum serve several purposes. The purpose in constructing frameworks is to systematically design a mental picture that is meaningful to the faculty and students when determining what knowledge is important to nursing and how that knowledge should be defined, categorized, and linked with other knowledge. Therefore organizing curriculum frameworks provide a blueprint for determining the scope of knowledge (i.e., which concepts are important to include in the teachers' and learners' mental picture) and a means of structuring that knowledge in a distinctive and meaningful way for faculty and students.

Organizing frameworks also facilitate the sequencing and prioritizing of knowledge in a way that is logical and internally consistent with theoretical explanations about the concepts included in the curriculum and help to explain how these ideas or concepts apply to nursing practice. Organizing frameworks act as a guide for faculty and students alike in considering the research and practice questions appropriate to ask as they strive to better understand the discipline of nursing and share this understanding with colleagues (Fawcett, 1989). Essentially, organizing frameworks for curriculum "highlight the purposes they serve, their goals and objectives, content, and the methods of instruction and evaluation they promote" (Langenbach, 1988, p. 8).

A number of approaches are used in defining and shaping frameworks. However, an organizing framework must reflect the domain of nursing practice, the phenomena of concern to nurses, and how nurses relate to others who are dealing with health concerns (Bevis & Watson, 1989; Hills et al., 1994). Organizing curriculum frameworks are the educational road maps to teaching and learning. As with any road map, multiple route options are available for arriving at a given destination or outcome.

As faculty move toward the adoption of an outcome orientation in curriculum building, organizing frameworks or models will continue to serve the same purposes noted earlier but will be driven by philosophical views and futuristic mental pictures regarding the practice of nursing. An example of this approach can be seen in the curriculum model designed through the work of the South Carolina Colleagues in Caring project. This model was based on concepts imbedded in the participants' view of differentiated practice for entry level nursing (Loquist & Bellack, 1999).

Developing an Organizing Framework for Curriculum

It is not easy to decide on a specific organizing framework that will best serve a program. Faculty can use two traditional approaches in determining the kind of organizing framework they wish to construct. The first approach is to select a single, specific nursing theory or model on which to build the framework. The second approach is more eclectic: to select concepts from multiple theories or models. Both approaches are discussed further.

Developing a Single Theory Framework

One traditional approach to constructing an organizing framework is to use a particular nursing theory or model to help shape the visual image that is consistent with the philosophy of the faculty. For example, if faculty believe that "health encompasses conditions known as disease and that it is an expansion of a person's consciousness" (Newman, 1997, p. 22), faculty will probably adopt Newman's theory of health as the vehicle for organizing knowledge for that particular nursing program. However, if faculty believe that caring is at the core of nursing, Watson's theory of caring might better serve when explaining the discipline to students and cataloging knowledge about the discipline of nursing.

The advantage to building an organizing framework on a single theory or model is the ability to use a single image with a defined vocabulary that is shared by both the learner and the teacher. Drawing further on Watson's theory, as an example, she says that "the transpersonal caring relationship and authentic presencing translate into *ontological caring competencies* of the nurse, which intersect with *technological medical competencies*" (Watson, 1997, p. 50). The image put forth in this description is "transpersonal caring relationship," which is at the core of Watson's theory. "Ontological caring competencies" and "technological medical competencies" evolve from this caring relationship. It is the development of these competencies that students would be expected to demonstrate in a program in which Watson's theory guided the knowledge to be learned and determined the expected performances of the program's graduates.

Using a single theory or existing conceptual model has limitations and poses challenges. One theory or model may not reflect everybody's visual image or view of nursing and nursing practice. This becomes problematic when faculty have developed or been educated in curricula that have used a different theory or orientation to the discipline.

One of the more common challenges in using a theory is being able to take an ethereal explanation of reality and make it understandable for students being newly introduced to the discipline. The language of a theory also can pose challenges for faculty and students. Especially for beginning nursing students, the language of the theory and the definitions of the critical concepts may be too abstract to be helpful in promoting shared understanding and a common vision for learners and teachers. A good theory must also stand the test of time. Theories must continually be tested to determine relevance with current reality. As the practice of nursing is being transformed by a dynamic evolving health care system, it is imperative to determine the degree to which any single theory is useful or practical. It is clear that nursing educators and/or practitioners of nursing will not, at least in the foreseeable future, agree on a single theory. Students educated in a curriculum driven by a single theory are likely to experience frustration and confusion when they find themselves in clinical practice settings that do not ascribe to the same theory, or any theory for that matter.

Developing an Eclectic Framework

Given the challenges and limitations of using a single theory as an organizing framework, faculty choice does not have to be constrained by a single theory or model. Those believing that a combination of many theories or concepts is more reflective of their beliefs about nursing may use an eclectic approach to developing a curricular framework. For example, an eclectic framework might include the concept of nursing as defined by Florence Nightingale, the concept of needs as defined by Maslow, the concept of self-care as defined by Orem, and the concept of a caring relationship as defined by Watson. All are critical concepts, but each concept comes from a different theory or theoretical orientation.

The use of a more eclectic approach when designing an organizational framework is not without its pitfalls. Some view this approach as an impediment to the development of a comprehensive nursing theory and the development of a body of knowledge that is uniquely nursing. The advantage to an eclectic approach is the ability to "borrow" concepts and definitions that best fit the faculty's beliefs and values from nursing and nonnursing theories. However, if faculty develop an eclectic framework, where concepts and their definitions are "borrowed" from a number of theories, they need to ensure that in the act of borrowing they have not changed conceptual meaning. It is important to retain the original definitions and the characteristics or attributes used to explain or validate the existence of borrowed concepts in altered contexts.

For example, the concept of *hope* may be perceived as critical to the understanding of how individuals make decisions about self-care. If a person has hope that a certain self-care action will have positive results, he or she is more likely to perform that self-care behavior. A person without hope is less likely to initiate that self-care behavior. If a market analyst were to use the concept of hope in a model to predict sales trends, that analyst must determine whether hope has meaning that is altered by, or separate from, the current context in which it will be used. Borrowing concepts from other disciplines is acceptable as long as those doing the borrowing are cognizant of how, in the act of borrowing, the concept may have changed some of its characteristics. Therefore it is important to clarify the meaning of concepts that will be used in an organizing framework so that faculty and students are clear about the phenomena being studied.

Examples of Nontraditional Curricular Frameworks

Accreditation standards and performance expectations have had a significant impact on many organizing frameworks as faculty have moved to incorporate or add into their organizing frameworks and curriculum models such concepts as critical thinking, problem solving, communication, caring, diversity, and therapeutic nursing interventions (McEwen & Brown, 2002). Although these concepts can be compatible with the essence of nursing, they are often not well enough defined to be consistently used by the teacher or applied by the learner. Faculty adopting an outcome orientation to curriculum must be able to construct the context and meaning that these outcomes will have in the curriculum structure. Critical thinking is one outcome that most undergraduate programs have adopted. A number of nationally normative tools have been created to measure critical thinking both on entry into and exit from a program. However, critical thinking as a cornerstone of an organizing curriculum framework is often not well defined, nor are its attributes identified for systematic and purposeful incorporation into nursing curriculum or assessment activities.

As faculty move away from the more traditional use of theory or theories in designing curriculum frameworks, a number of rather unique designs have been identified. One interesting approach to an eclectic curriculum design is the "MSVME framework" (Webber, 2002). This framework is constructed around five "conceptual cornerstones[:] nursing knowledge, nursing skills, nursing values, nursing meanings, and nursing experience" (Webber, 2002, p. 17) and incorporate many of the recognized concepts present in today's nursing curricula.

The Healing Web is another example of a collaborative effort to design an organizing framework whose conceptual orientation is woven into a "collaborative clinical practice in a differentiated practice model" (Nelson et al., 2001, p. 404). The Health Web draws components from Newman's health theory and Watson's caring theory to construct the essential building blocks of this "transformative model" (Nelson et al., 2001).

The emancipatory curriculum, designed to focus less on structure and content and more on the dynamic of learning through discovery, dialogue, and critical reflection, is yet another approach to creating a more meaningful educational experience (Schreiber & Banister, 2002). Although this curriculum design was conceived as the antithesis of the traditional structured curriculum designs, it is still anchored in philosophical conceptualizations from phenomenology, feminist theory, and critical social theory (Schreiber & Banister, 2002, p. 41).

These nontraditional approaches to thinking about curriculum frameworks appear to be driven by the need to make the education of nursing students relevant to tomorrow's practice of nursing. Relevancy is being defined around such concepts as differentiated practice, evidence-based practice, and care outcomes. As faculty and practitioners of nursing struggle to reinvision nursing practice for the next century, these concepts will assume center stage in the various curriculum dialogues. It is crucial that practice and education recognize and assume active roles in all future curriculum development activities because without shared understanding and common goals there is little to ensure the relevancy of graduates.

Designing a Graphic of the Framework

Although it is unnecessary to accompany the description of the organizing framework with a graphic or model, it can be helpful for those trying to grasp concepts or ideas enfolded within the framework. A graphic can provide clarification, especially when the framework is complex or abstract. When developing organizing frameworks, faculty should be guided by a "less is better" approach. Faculty should remember that curriculum-organizing frameworks are roads to a specified destination, not the trip itself. If the framework is too complex, students and faculty spend more time trying to interpret and understand the framework than they do actually implementing and evaluating it. This tradeoff is devastating because time is often perceived as the rarest of commodities in today's undergraduate and graduate nursing programs.

   An example of a simplistic curriculum structure might include the concepts of health, person, and environment. In this example, if health has been defined with a continuum, with wellness at one end and illness at the other, the graphic or model may look something like this:

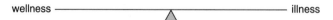

Adding the concept of person to this model requires that person first be defined. If a person is believed to have the ability to balance wellness and illness to achieve a high level of wellness, additional symbols could be added to the model so that it now looks like this:

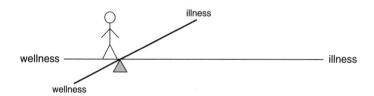

The concept of environment is incorporated into the image by adding a symbol that represents a chosen definition of environment, which suggests that it is an external force that affects a person's ability to balance along the health continuum. As the model now shows, person and health occur within the context of the environment, and the environment affects the person's ability to balance along the wellness–illness continuum.

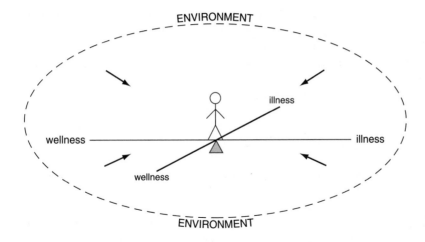

This example demonstrates how busy a framework can get when concepts are added.

Summary

However faculty decide to approach the work of developing a framework for the curriculum, the framework eventually constructed must be consistent with the school's mission and philosophy statements, faculty values and beliefs, and current and future nursing practice trends. Faculty should have broad-based agreement on the curriculum framework because such agreement is fundamental to the consistent interpretation, implementation, and evaluation of the curriculum. This aspect of curriculum development can be very time-consuming and is currently under some scrutiny within the profession.

Additionally today's higher education environment is reemphasizing a strong general education foundation for all undergraduate students. An example of standards that can be expected to inform college and university general education approaches are the "standards for success," which were born out of a collaborative effort of the Association of American Universities and The Pew Charitable Trusts (2003). These standards tend to reflect lifelong learning skills that will continue to serve the learner. Because nursing programs have long built their nursing curricula on strong general education foundations, standards such as these will need to be addressed as part of any framework faculty identify or refine in the future.

Guiding Principles for Developing a Curriculum Framework

Although there are no specific steps or "how to's" for developing organizing frameworks for curriculum, there are some guiding principles to follow. The first principle is to choose those concepts that most accurately reflect the faculty's beliefs about the practice and discipline of nursing. The concepts identified should also reflect or complement the philosophy, mission, and goals of the college or university in which the program is embedded. By creating an organizing framework that reflects concepts valued by both the discipline of nursing and the parent institution, faculty have begun to articulate the contributions their nursing program makes to both stakeholding entities. Mission statements, goals, or expected outcomes are the starting point for choosing concepts for inclusion in the curriculum framework.

Most traditional undergraduate curriculum frameworks minimally contain the concepts of health, person, environment, and nursing. These four concepts were first collectively discussed by Florence Nightingale (Nightingale, 1969) and are still considered cornerstones of many nursing theoretical models despite the fact that they are defined differently by different theorists. Many philosophy and mission statements of schools of nursing still speak to these concepts from their own unique perspective. Faculty often expand their mission and philosophy statements to include such additional concepts as caring, self-care, growth and development, nursing process, and adaptation. However, there is no edict that faculty must follow when determining the concepts or configuration of concepts that will form the framework for the curriculum. As noted earlier, some of the newer curriculum models have focused on nursing practice–related concepts and less on nursing discipline–related concepts. Requisite knowledge and competencies are categorized around what nurses do rather than on what nursing is. This refocusing will continue to be prevalent in both practice and nursing arenas because both practitioners and educators of nursing are being asked to articulate their unique contributions to the health care and education systems.

The second principle is to clearly define these concepts. Consensus should be established in this process because it will fall to the faculty to articulate these concepts to the students. Concepts that are too obtusely, concretely, or narrowly defined are problematic, especially for undergraduate curricula that typically have espoused a "generalist" conception of nursing practice. If faculty wish to adopt a specific theory or theoretical orientation that they find congruent with their mission and philosophy, the concepts and definitions are derived directly from the theory or theoretical model. If faculty select a more open or eclectic approach, the definition of these concepts should reflect back to the philosophy, mission statement, or discipline in which the concepts were originally conceived.

The third principle to attend to in this development process is to explain the linkages between and among the concepts identified. This is critical because the linkages are the basis for how students comprehend, apply, analyze, synthesize, and evaluate knowledge learned throughout the educational process. These principles are analogous to putting together a jigsaw puzzle in which the concepts are the puzzle pieces. Puzzles come in various numbers of pieces. Usually the greater the number of pieces a puzzle has, the greater the challenge in its construction. The outline and coloring of the pieces are the definitions of the concepts. The more clearly the puzzle pieces are defined and the sharper the color delineations, the easier it is to fit the puzzle together. The linkages between the concepts can be related to the coupling of the puzzle pieces themselves into a picture that reflects a mental image that will be easily recognized. Recognition is the outcome that one hopes to achieve in the development of curriculum frameworks. The resulting framework or model must present a "gestalt" of the nursing theory or models from which the concepts were taken. It is critical that faculty and students grasp an understanding of the framework without an intensive investment of time and energy. "To maintain curriculum integrity, it is critical that faculty design all curricular activities to reflect the selected philosophical framework" (Csokasy, 2002, p. 33). The cornerstones of all frameworks must be reviewed on a regular basis to ensure continued relevance to the education and practice of nurses. Lindeman (2000) suggests that "nurse educators must prepare nurses for the emerging health care system and not the system of the past or one that they wish were in place" (p. 7).

THE ROLE OF OUTCOMES AND COMPETENCIES IN CURRICULUM FRAMEWORKS

If curriculum frameworks are the road maps to understanding the discipline of nursing, outcomes can be equated with the trip's destination and competencies with the mileage markers seen along the way. Outcomes, in the simplest of terms, are those characteristics students should display at a designated time. Competencies are the behaviors needing to be acquired to develop those characteristics. Competencies are written to specify the levels of achievement the learner must demonstrate (Stark & Lattuca, 1997).

For higher education, outcomes have become the published measuring stick for public and professional accountability. This need for public accountability has grown out of a perception that the American educational system should be superior in educating students for the challenges of world leadership. The public has increasingly demanded that higher education be held accountable for the product produced and demonstrate that the cost of production is consistent with the quality of the product. Some think that the current emphasis on outcomes will improve both teaching and learning, keeping American education in a place of global prominence (Boland & Laidig, 2001; Lindeman, 2000; Reyonds, 1986).

Identifying Curriculum Outcomes

When identifying curriculum outcomes, faculty must have an understanding of the qualities and characteristics they want graduates of their nursing program to possess on graduation. In nursing there has been an acknowledged need to move from a curriculum that is "politically correct to one that is theoretically pluralistic; to incorporate caring and humanitarianism as core values rather than the dominations of technology; and the centrality of the student–teacher relationship over esoteric scholarship" (National League for Nursing [NLN], 1993, p. 11). As part of this curriculum reform, educators have discussed the need to emphasize "critical thinking, skills in collaboration, shared decision making, social epidemiological viewpoint, and analyses and interventions at the systems and aggregate levels" (NLN, 1993, p. 13). These skills are becoming the basis for outcome development in both undergraduate and graduate curricula.

Rentschler and Spegman (1996) shared the experiences of one school's faculty, who attempted to move away from a more behavioralistic view of curriculum to one that is more humanistic. In discussing the changes experienced by faculty, they suggested that this shift to a humanistic–educative model from a behavioralistic approach to learning had a profound effect on "faculty's beliefs about nursing education, professional practice roles, and the manifestations of these beliefs in the undergraduate curriculum" (p. 390). The premises for moving to a more humanistic–educative model suggest that our traditional model of curriculum development is too narrow in interpretation and too mechanistic to foster creativity among learners (Walton, 1996).

Changes in the health care system are also having a significant impact on how program outcomes are shaped and what those outcomes are designed to achieve, especially in relation to the competence of graduates. Health care trends that have a direct impact on curriculum development and program outcomes include the increasing severity of patients' illnesses in acute care settings, shifting emphasis from acute care settings to community-based settings, increasing consumer knowledge and interest in and control over health care, and increasing demands from the public for high-quality health care at an affordable price. In addition, the competencies nurses need to develop for professional practice are being influenced by shifting demographics in the population; growing competition among traditional and new health care providers; increasing sensitivity to cultural differences and the impact of these differences on lifestyle and health care practices; spending limitations in the face of increasing health care costs; and continuing growth of health-related technology, accompanied by a decrease in affordability of this technology for everyone (NLN, 1993; Pew Health Professions Commission, 1995). See Chapter 6 for further discussion of these trends.

With the need for nursing educators to ensure that the curricula they design keep pace with the ongoing changes in health care and higher education, more emphasis will continue to be placed on the school's ability to demonstrate success. Outcome assessment has been seen as the key by which school programs can document strengths and weaknesses (Study Group on the Conditions of Excellence in American Higher Education, 1984). A comprehensive assessment program can help faculty determine what works and what does not in achieving academic quality and producing the desired program outcomes (Banta, 2001; Keith, 1991). This logic is a significant departure from the predominantly process-oriented Tylerian approach to curriculum and evaluation, in which the emphasis was placed on detailed course objectives, the identification of content needed to meet course objectives, and the appropriate pedagogical approaches to complement the type of content needing to be taught.

The idea that course and terminal objectives have been retitled *outcomes* and changed in name only ignores the differences between the traditional approach to designing curricula that are objective driven and the humanistic–educative approach that is more learner and practice oriented (Bevis & Watson, 1989; Rentschler & Spegman, 1996). In outcome assessment the emphasis is placed on what students have actually learned in their educational experiences, not merely on the knowledge and experiences that were designed with the intent of achieving these results (Boland, 2003; Keith, 1991). These differences, which may seem like nuances to many, are at the core of the "curriculum revolution" in higher education and nursing education.

As discussed earlier in this chapter, the traditional approach to curriculum design has been to conceptualize the curriculum as a process that is constructed from a mission or philosophy statement; a conceptual model that reflects the mission and philosophy; a curriculum design woven by interlinking the concepts together, often in intricate "grids" and knowledge maps; and a complex network of objectives leveled by course, semester, year, and end of program. These interlinks are further developed in this approach by determining the content to be taught in each course, the required learning experiences, and the evaluation methods used. This beginning-to-end curriculum design approach dictates a systematic, logical, mechanistic sequencing of activities, each critical to the next activity and has served nurse educators well for many years, ensuring program integrity. However, it requires full commitment of the faculty, takes a good deal of time and energy to develop and maintain, and requires even more energy to change. It also assumes that learning is a logical, sequential, orderly process in which faculty are able to exert control over the knowledge links identified, specified, and recreated in the learning environment.

Today this assumption is being challenged. Instead, it is believed that learning is more chaotic in nature, although not without specific patterns for individual learners, and that what and how students hear and retain is shaped by their background and experiences. The focus is now on the learner, and as a result faculty need to develop curricula that focus on outcomes, acknowledging that individuals take different paths to reach these outcomes, which suggests that a generic, well-scripted road map may not meet every student's patterns of learning (i.e., gaining, retaining, retrieving, and using knowledge). These curricula need to reflect the essential nursing and general education knowledge, concepts, theories, and skills, which should be organized in such a way that students can connect them together and demonstrate these connections in a nursing practice context (Feiman-Nemser, 2001). Students must be actively engaged in identifying what they already know and how they best learn given what they need to learn. It is critical that students develop lifelong learning skills, as well as the knowledge and competencies needed for the immediacy.

When moving to a curriculum that is more centered on the development of outcomes relevant to nursing practice, it is often easier to think about curriculum development as starting at a program's end rather than its beginning. This method of curriculum development places a different emphasis on the need for organizing frameworks. Approaching curriculum development from the outcome, or end stage, first, then working toward the beginning of the curriculum, provides faculty with an opportunity to identify those essential outcomes and competencies that they wish to see their students demonstrate. The organizing framework is then shaped by the theories and concepts embedded in the outcomes and competencies. For example, if faculty believe that students need to possess critical thinking, communication, or management skills, these concepts will shape the organizing framework. In an outcome-focused curriculum the driver of faculty conversations is not what content must be taught but what students must be able to demonstrate to be relevant to current and future nursing practice.

Before they can think about curriculum from the outcome, or end stage, faculty first must identify the desired program outcomes. They will need to discuss the societal trends that have or will have an impact on health care and nursing practice, identify assumptions about the future of nursing practice, and examine both the institution's and the school's educational mission (Halstead et al., 1996). In addition, faculty will need to call on various interest groups to help them identify outcomes that are relevant to today's practice of nursing and to speculate on requisite knowledge and skills for tomorrow's nursing practice (Boland, 2000).

Outcomes should initially be viewed as core characteristics, or those qualities faculty want graduates to display. For example, one school of nursing's faculty, after reflecting on the driving forces in today's health care delivery system and the skills needed to practice in a contemporary health care environment, decided that graduates from their baccalaureate program should possess the following essential qualities (Halstead et al., 1996, p. 414):

1. Critical thinker
2. Culturally competent
3. Knowledgeable coordinator of community resources
4. Politically aware
5. Ethically and legally grounded
6. Effective communicator
7. Competent provider of health care
8. Modeler of the professional role
9. Responsible manager of human, fiscal, and material resources

These essential qualities were then used to guide the development of related outcomes and competencies.

Once faculty have identified the core characteristics, or attributes, it is time for them to describe the context in which the characteristics are to be expressed. The process of concept clarification or analysis can be used by faculty with some modification to define the core characteristics believed to be critical to the professional nurse graduate of their program. In the process of concept clarification, as described in the classic work of Walker and Avant (1988), the first step is to describe the qualities that most clearly express the phenomenon of professional nurse. The next step is to describe the context of the qualities identified by linking the attributes together in a meaningful way. For example, if faculty decide that one quality of a professional nurse is that he or she is a critical thinker, and faculty define critical thinking as thinking that occurs within the context of intellectual curiosity, rational inquiry, problem solving, and creativity in problem framing, the program outcome may read as "a critical thinker who is able to demonstrate intellectual curiosity, rational inquiry, problem-solving skills, and creativity in framing problems" (Halstead et al., 1996, p. 414). Faculty must link these behaviors to nursing practice outcomes. Specifically, by being a critical thinker a nurse can better frame care problems and seek care initiatives that decrease the length of hospital stays or decrease the number of complications.

Identifying Competencies

After the desired program outcomes have been established, the next step in the curriculum development process is to identify the competencies that students need to possess to attain the outcomes. Competency statements identify the knowledge, skills, and attitudes students need to develop if they are to achieve the program outcomes. They are behaviorally anchored and student focused.

Competency statements are important in assessing student learning because they become the foundation that drives evaluation. When identifying competencies, faculty should give attention to determining the right student, the right level of behavior, and the right context of the behavior. Here, *student* refers to the type of student from whom faculty are expecting these behaviors (e.g., prenursing, nursing sophomore, nursing senior); *level of behavior* refers to the level of learning or performance at which the behavior is to be demonstrated; context of the behavior refers to the environment in which the behavior should occur. For example, if faculty believe that it is essential for students to exhibit a particular skill, knowledge, or attitude across a continuum of health care settings or with a select population of patients, the competency statement should indicate the parameters in which the behavior should be expressed. It is equally important for faculty to remember not to be so specific as to "paint themselves into a corner" from which there is no escape (e.g., if faculty specify that a certain behavior will be demonstrated with postoperative patients in an outpatient surgical setting, all students must be guaranteed this type of experience for faculty to make an accurate and consistent assessment).

The baccalaureate program outcomes and competency statements developed by Indiana University School of Nursing (IUSON, 1995) can be used to illustrate this process:

Program outcome: A critical thinker who demonstrates intellectual curiosity, rational inquiry, problem-solving skills, and creativity in framing problems

Senior-level competency: Evaluates decisions through logical organization, validation of information, and critical examination of assumptions underlying the processing of information and analyzes the conclusions drawn from the information (Halstead et al., 1996, p. 414)

Junior-level competency: Validates care decisions with appropriate persons to determine the degree to which decisions are consistent with client–system information and environmental clues (IUSON, 1995)

Sophomore-level competency: Participates in selected problem-solving exercises that promote critical examination of the professional care role (IUSON, 1995)

In the above example, the identified competency related to critical thinking skills requires students to develop the ability to make reasoned decisions when providing patient care. Sophomore students, who are relative novices at providing client care, could reasonably be expected to participate with other health care professionals in the decision-making process in selected care situations. This competency could also be developed in classroom discussions with peers. A junior-level student would be expected to have developed some independence in gathering assessment data, using these data to make competent patient care decisions, and assuming responsibility to validate those decisions with appropriate individuals. By the end of the senior year, nearing graduation, students who are about to enter the workforce would be expected not only to exhibit problem-solving skills that result in appropriate patient care decisions but also to demonstrate the ability to evaluate the quality of the decisions they have made. Faculty expect students to exhibit these identified competencies regardless of the health care setting; thus the "right" environment has not been explicitly identified in these examples. Faculty and students would use these competency statements to guide the development and implementation of appropriate learning experiences across the curriculum. The process by which students would achieve this competency has not been specified, allowing for flexible learning experiences to be developed according to students' individualized learning needs.

Once outcomes and competencies have been identified, faculty must consider the antecedents, or factors, that need to be in place for the outcomes and competencies to be achieved. Antecedents are defined as the prerequisite knowledge needed to develop or foster the identified attributes or characteristics. If faculty believe that one of the desired program outcomes for graduates should be critical thinking, faculty need to identify the knowledge and skills necessary for students to develop and refine their critical thinking abilities (Table 9-1).

For faculty to develop an outcome-focused, competency-based curriculum, they must emphasize the development of the knowledge and skills required to achieve a specified outcome. Key to students' achieving an educational outcome is faculty's creation of an environment in which students can direct their learning toward achieving the outcome. It is the expression of this product, or outcome, that then drives the assessment of learning. Again, the outcomes that nursing faculty identify should be clearly relevant to health care outcomes such as cost of care, length of stay, effectiveness of patient education, and number of complications.

Developing Outcomes and Competency Statements

Nursing faculty must approach curriculum development from the premise that nursing knowledge and skills are built on or interwoven with general education

TABLE 9-1 Attributes and Antecedent Factors Related to Critical Thinking

CHARACTERISTIC VALUED	ATTRIBUTES OF THE CHARACTERISTIC	ANTECEDENT/KNOWLEDGE AND SKILLS
Critical thinking	• Creativity • Intellectual curiosity • Problem solving • Rational inquiry	• Ability to ask probing questions • Intellectual ability • Understanding of problem solving

knowledge and skills. Outcomes and related competencies should reflect the "essential knowledge, skills, and attitudes students need to acquire" for their lifetime (Association of American Colleges and Universities, 1994, p. ii). Outcomes should include those skills that are specific to the nursing discipline, as well as those skills that establish a foundation for lifelong learning (Boland, 2003; Lindeman, 2000). Outcomes for undergraduate education that have emerged from the work of the Strong Foundation (Association of American Colleges and Universities, 1994, pp. iii-iv) suggest that students should do the following:

- Receive a generous orientation to the intellectual expectations, curriculum rationale, and learning resources of the institution
- Acquire specific skills of thought and expression, such as critical thinking and writing, that should be learned "across the curriculum" and imbedded within several courses
- Learn about another culture and the diversity that exists within our own culture in terms of gender, race, ethnic background, class, age, and religion
- Integrate ideas from across disciplines to illuminate interdisciplinary themes, issues, or social problems
- Study some subjects—beyond their major—at an advanced, not just an introductory, levels
- Have an opportunity near the end of their course of study to pull together their learning in a senior seminar or project
- Experience a coherent course of study, one that is more than the sum of its parts

Although these suggestions are not necessarily new to nursing education, faculty need to become clearer about how they are integrated into meaningful program outcomes and how the faculty will ensure that students are held to these outcomes throughout their educational experience. The latter takes both coordination and cooperation. This coordination effort is especially important for nursing programs that are housed in liberal arts schools, in schools where general education is the main mission or receives a strong emphasis, or in those institutions that have established an undergraduate general education core curriculum.

Within this coordinated effort nursing faculty should determine the role nursing education plays in the general education enrichment efforts of the college or university. The issue that faculty need to address is the added value that the nursing program contributes to the growth or development of students (Boland, 2001; Pascarella, 1986). Nursing faculty are usually well prepared to meet this challenge because they tend to come from different disciplines and have been shaped by these interdisciplinary experiences. In addition, nursing faculty have commonly led the way in higher education in defining outcomes and determining how to articulate them in ways that are meaningful to the broader university or college mission and the nursing discipline (Boland, 2003; Lindeman, 2000).

Guidelines for Writing Outcomes and Competency Statements

When writing outcome statements, nursing faculty need to have one foot firmly anchored in today's practice reality while the other foot seeks the future for nursing graduates. The focus of faculty writing must be on how to express outcomes and competency that clearly focus on the transformation of nursing practice. Nursing faculty need to have the input of the practice sector when putting outcomes and competencies into words to ensure that what is being expressed relates to today's and tomorrow's reality as viewed by the practice experts.

Outcomes are general statements that refer to characteristics graduates must acquire by the end of the program. When writing outcome statements, faculty should determine the readiness of the learners to meet the outcomes identified and the length of time it will take the learners to demonstrate the characteristics. As faculty put outcomes and related competencies in writing, they should ask themselves the "why" question. The "why" or "what good is it" question helps faculty to explain the importance of these outcomes and competencies as stated to various stakeholders (e.g., Why is it important that nursing students and graduates be able to think critically? It appears to be a value that is strongly held by nursing faculty, but to what end?).

Outcome statements should be written to emphasize what is to be accomplished. For example, an outcome statement might read, "A competent care provider who individualizes nursing care to maximize client care outcomes." In this case the outcome is a *competent care provider* who can demonstrate the competency of *individualizing nursing care* to meet a valued expectation: *maximization of patient care*. What is emphasized in this statement is the competency of the care provider, not a particular skill. Also emphasized is that the ability to demonstrate this characteristic has a direct bearing on patient care outcomes.

What faculty must determine next are the competencies that students must develop to be able to express this characteristic. Once the competencies have been defined, faculty will identify what skills and knowledge are consistent with the development of these competencies.

Outcomes, like behavioral objectives, address accountability issues. Students need to demonstrate their ability to meet outcome expectations to ensure a level of acceptable nursing practice for graduates. Outcomes, like objectives, are designed to communicate expectations and suggest appropriate means of measurement for judging student performance. However, in today's environment of public accountability, it is critical that faculty are able to collect data on actual outcomes achieved. Therefore faculty must not only identify curriculum outcomes but also clearly establish internal standards for outcomes identified. Graduate performance is not only compared with these internal standards but is often also compared with state, regional, or national benchmarks. For example, the national pass rate on the National Council Licensure Examination for Registered Nurses (NCLEX-RN) is one benchmark graduate performance is measured against on an annual basis. However, in an outcome orientation, performance on the NCLEX-RN needs to be linked to a specific outcome.

Precision is needed when writing outcome statements. The language of the competencies must reflect a continued sense of development. Development may take the form of increasing complexity, differentiation, delineation, or sophistication. Again, using the example of a "competent care provider" as an outcome, building this idea of development into course competencies might include the following:

- **Carries out procedures ordered for assigned patient.** This might be a realistic expectation for a beginning student. To develop this competency the student will need to be able to read a care plan to determine the interventions that are to be performed for the assigned client.
- **Modifies a standard plan of care consistent with desired patient care outcomes.** To achieve this competency the student is expected to do more than carry out procedures ordered for the patient. The student is now in control of modifying the care plan based on the assessment information collected. The student will have to demonstrate good decision-making skills in knowing how to use evaluation data to make corrections to obtain the desired outcomes.
- **Develops care plans that reflect the individual goals of the patient and desired medical treatment goals.** This competency requires a higher level of functioning than the previous competency statements because the student must again add to his or her skill mix. Individualizing care plans presumes that the student knows the most acceptable medical and nursing interventions for a specific patient and is able to use this information in conjunction with what is known about the patient to develop a plan of care that is consistent with both client desires and medical outcomes.

Note how each competency or skill identified leads to the eventual development of a competent care provider.

Leveling Competencies

In leveling, or specifying, competencies, faculty must recognize the level at which the knowledge and skills need to be demonstrated to obtain the outcome desired. The learning environment will need to be configured to enable the students to acquire knowledge at the level identified. Evaluation measures also need to be consistent with the level of learning identified to ensure consistency in evaluation from the time of input of information through the time of output of the behavior or skill required. Learning occurs at various levels, and the level of learning needs to be explicitly stated in the competencies faculty generate.

Once competencies have been leveled to a year or semester or academic level, faculty will need to carefully examine these competencies and determine how their particular courses can add to the ongoing development of these competencies. The behaviors imbedded in each competency become the focus for writing course-level competencies. Not all competencies will or should be included in all courses that make up the curriculum. Competencies at the course level are more concrete and detail how the chosen competencies explicitly relate to the course. If, for example, faculty believe that the individualization of a standard care map is critical to student learning, then the course competency will reflect this behavior. The faculty will then need to identify what prerequisite and requisite knowledge and skills the students will need to possess to demonstrate this behavior. Faculty must also determine where, when, and how this knowledge and skill set will be developed. As part of course development faculty must also identify how this competency will be assessed and what standard or benchmark will be established to note acceptable performance of this competency.

Benchmarking competencies is important because the use of this process generates information as to what skills and knowledge students are able to demonstrate from the beginning to the end of the program. These data are also valuable when trying to determine the impact the program had on the students' ability to develop all critical competencies chosen. Such data can also provide insight into resources needed for students to achieve an acceptable level of performance both within a course and across the curriculum.

SUMMARY

Organizing frameworks and outcomes should reflect the concepts most valued among the faculty, the professional community, and other identified stakeholders. Organizing frameworks are designed to provide faculty and students with a tool to define, interpret, and communicate the essence of nursing. For some, organizing frameworks reflect a particular theoretical orientation. For others, organizing frameworks present a more eclectic theoretical view of nursing. However organizing frameworks are viewed, faculty should carefully consider the usefulness of the chosen framework in the face of a rapidly changing health care industry. Faculty must also give thought to the outcomes and competencies that they believe graduates must possess on graduation for competent nursing practice. The hallmark of today's curricula must be a flexibility that allows for change to accommodate the health care environment. Faculty will therefore be called on to find ways of building dynamic, fluid curricula that reflect the values of education and nursing.

REFERENCES

Apple, M. (1979). *Ideology and curriculum*. London: Routledge and Kegan Paul.

Association of American Colleges and Universities. (1994). *Strong foundations: Twelve principles for effective general education programs*. Washington, DC: Author.

Association of American Universities and The Pew Charitable Trusts (2003). *Standards for success*. Eugene, OR: Center for Educational Policy Research.

Banta, T. (1996). Using assessment to improve instruction. In R. J. Menges & M. Weimer & Associates (Eds.), *Teaching on solid ground: Using scholarship to improve practice* (pp. 363-384). San Francisco: Jossey-Bass.

Banta, T. (2001). Assessing competence in higher education. In C. A. Palomba & T. W. Banta (Eds.), *Assessing student competence in accredited disciplines* (pp. 1-12). Sterling, VA: Stylus.

Bevis, E. O., & Watson, J. (1989). *Toward a caring curriculum: A new pedagogy for nursing*. New York: National League for Nursing.

Boland, D. L. (2000). The future of nursing education: Helping to determine if nursing is to be or not to be. In N. Chaska (Ed.), *The nursing profession: Tomorrow and beyond* (pp. 867-880). Thousand Oaks, CA: Sage.

Boland, D. L. (2004). Program evaluation and public accountability. In M. Oermann & K. Heinrich (Eds.), *Annual review of nursing education, vol. 2*. New York: Springer.

Boland, D. L., & Laidig, J. (2001). Assessment of student learning in the discipline of nursing. In C. Palomba & T. Banta (Eds.), *Assessing student competence in accredited disciplines* (pp. 71-95). Sterling, VA: Stylus.

Csokasy, J. (2002). A congruent curriculum philosophical integrity from philosophy to outcomes. *Journal of Nursing Education, 41*(1), 32-33.

Fawcett, J. (1989). *Conceptual models of nursing*. Philadelphia: F. A. Davis.

Feiman-Nemser, S. (2001). From preparation to practice: Designing a continuum to strengthen and sustain teaching. *Teachers College Record, 103*(6), 1013-1055.

Halstead, J. A., Rains, J., Boland, D. L., & May, F. E. (1996). Reconceptualizing baccalaureate nursing education: Outcomes and competencies for practice in the 21st century. *Journal of Nursing Education, 35*(9), 413-416.

Hills, M. D., Lindsey, A. E., Chisamore, M., Bassett-Smith, J., Abbott, K., & Fournier-Chalmers, J. (1994). University-college collaboration: Rethinking curriculum development in nursing education. *Journal of Nursing Education, 33*(5), 220-225.

Indiana University School of Nursing. (1995). *Baccalaureate program outcome statements*. Indianapolis: Author.

Keith, N. Z. (1991). Assessing educational goals: The national movement to outcome evaluation. In M. Garbin (Ed.), *Assessing educational outcomes* (pp. 1-23). New York: National League for Nursing.

Langenbach, M. (1988). *Curriculum models in adult education*. Malabar, FL: Robert E. Krieger.

Lindeman, C. A. (2000). The future of nursing education. *Journal of Nursing Education, 39*(1), 5-12.

Loquist, R. S., & Bellack, J. P. (1999). A model for differentiated entry-level nursing practice by educational program type. *Journal of Nursing Education, 38*(7), 301-305.

McEwen, M., & Brown, S. C. (2002). Conceptual frameworks in undergraduate nursing curricula: Report of a national survey. *Journal of Nursing Education, 41*(1), 5-14.

National League for Nursing. (1993). *A vision for nursing education*. New York: Author.

Nelson, M. L., Howell, J. K., Larson, J. C., & Karpiuk, K. L. (2001). Student outcomes of the healing web: Evaluation of a transformative model for nursing education. *Journal of Nursing Education, 40*(9), 404-413.

Newman, M. (1997). Evolution of the theory of health as expanding consciousness. *Nursing Science Quarterly, 10*(1), 22-25.

Nightingale, F. (1969). *Notes on nursing*. New York: Dover Publications.

Pascarella, E. T. (1986). Are value-added analyses valuable? In *Assessing the outcomes of higher education*. Proceedings of the 1986 ETS Invitational Conference. Princeton, NJ: Educational Testing Services.

Pew Health Professions Commission. (1995). Clinical challenges: Revitalizing the health professions for the twenty-first century. San Francisco: UCSF Center for the Health Professions.

Ratcliff, J. L. (1997). What is a curriculum and what should it be? In J. G. Gaff & J. L. Ratcliff & Associates (Eds.), *Handbook of the undergraduate curriculum* (pp. 5-29). San Francisco: Jossey-Bass.

Rentschler, D. D., & Spegman, A. M. (1996). Curriculum revolution: Realities of change. *Journal of Nursing Education, 35*(9), 389-393.

Reyonds, W. A. (1986). Higher learning in America: Aims and realities. In *Assessing the outcomes of higher education*. Proceedings of the 1986 ETS Invitational Conference. Princeton, NJ: Educational Testing Services.

Schreiber, R., & Banister, E. (2002). Challenges of teaching in an emancipating curriculum. *Journal of Nursing Education, 41*(1), 41-45.

Stark, J. S., & Lattuca, L. R. (1997). *Shaping the college curriculum: Academic plans in action*. Needham Heights, MA: Allyn & Bacon.

Study Group on the Conditions of Excellence in American Higher Education. (1984). *Involvement in learning: Realizing the potential of American higher education* (ed246 833.127, p. 55). Washington, DC: National Institute of Education.

Walker, L. O., & Avant, K. C. (1988). *Strategies for theory construction in nursing*. Norwalk, CT: Appleton & Lange.

Walton, J. (1996). The changing environment: New challenges for nursing education. *Journal of Nursing Education, 35*(9), 400-405.

Watson, J. (1997). The theory of human caring: Retrospective and prospective. *Nursing Science Quarterly, 10*(1), 49-52.

Webber, P. B. (2002). A curriculum framework for nursing. *Journal of Nursing Education, 41*(1), 15-24.

10

Selecting Learning Experiences to Achieve Curriculum Outcomes

Pamela R. Jeffries, DNS, RN, Barbara Norton, RN, MPH

The purpose of the curriculum is to present students with a cohesive body of knowledge, attitudes, and skills that are necessary for professional nursing practice. A curriculum provides the means of delivering a course of study designed to support the achievement of intended outcomes (Sell & Lounsberry, 1997). The curriculum is activated for both faculty and students through teaching strategies and learning activities. This chapter focuses on designing and selecting appropriate learning activities that are essential for effective implementation of the teaching–learning process. The rationale that guides the design and selection of appropriate learning activities is reflected in the belief that students should be educated for self-development and the various roles in nursing that serve society. The selecting of experiences that enable curriculum outcomes to be met cannot be accomplished through a casual, hit-or-miss approach; learning activities must be thoughtfully designed to offer students the opportunities necessary to achieve the intended curriculum outcomes.

DEFINING TEACHING STRATEGIES AND LEARNING ACTIVITIES

Terms commonly used in teaching literature include instructional strategies, teaching strategies, teaching methods, and teaching techniques. These are *faculty-centered* strategies that are used to describe the kinds of activities faculty engage in when teaching. Faculty need to select instructional strategies that match the objectives, competencies, and outcomes of the curriculum so that students have the opportunity for maximum learning.

When faculty design an instructional strategy to provide specific kinds of student learning experiences, the instructional strategy is then referred to as a *learning activity* or a *learning experience*. Learning activities are *student-centered* activities that serve as a vehicle to facilitate the students' acquisition of the desired knowledge, competencies, behaviors, and values specified by the curriculum.

STUDENT LEARNING ACTIVITIES

Faculty are responsible for arranging the learning activities and conditions necessary to ensure that learning occurs. It is essential that faculty understand that learning activities are an integral part of the curriculum and courses, and as such they must be purposeful, planned, and organized. Learning activities are designed to engage students in listening to and interacting with others, observing, thinking, and doing in a manner that highlights the knowledge, attitudes, competencies, and skills to be acquired. For example, problem-focused learning activities allow students an opportunity to experience relating content and processes. Active student participation in the learning activities, accompanied by faculty feedback, comprises one of the most powerful experiences in the learning process (Dick & Carey, 1985).

Examples of learning activities include attending lectures; reading assigned materials; viewing media; writing assignments such as journaling, developing care plans and pathways, and term papers; engaging in discussions or debates; participating in role play or games/simulations; using case studies; and using computer-mediated activities and resources such as computer-assisted instruction and the World Wide Web. Learning activities can be designed for use by individual students, pairs of students, or small groups of three to five.

Designing Learning Activities

Learning activities should be designed to incrementally contribute to the achievement of the major objectives or competencies of a course and the curriculum. Any learning activity should articulate with previous and subsequent activities, providing continuity in such a way that students are able to see the connections and relationships between facts, concepts, and principles. Learning activities that require students to create concrete examples from abstract content stimulate learning. Activities should provide students with opportunities not only to acquire knowledge and skills but also to apply specific areas of content and processes. Faculty need to plan and organize class time so that students become actively involved in the learning process because active involvement can result in increased retention and a deeper understanding of the concepts.

PASSIVE AND ACTIVE LEARNING

Bevis (1973) described the learning process as consisting of three phases: input, operations, and feedback. During the input phase, the learner acquires and mentally organizes information; during the operation phase, the learner is actively responding to the information in some manner that may or may not be observable to faculty; and during the feedback phase, the learner is testing or assessing and then validating, modifying, or changing the information obtained during the first phase. These three phases of learning may not occur in sequence within the same period; however, when they occur close together in time, learning is more meaningful. Learning may be a passive or an active process. Students typically experience both types of learning throughout their educational career.

Passive Learning

Passive learning, a mode of learning commonly present in many classrooms, occurs when students use their senses to take in information from a lecture, reading assignments, or some form of audiovisual media. Passive learning is commonly used to acquire ideas and information that are subsequently available through recall (Bevis, 1989b).

Advantages

Passive learning provides faculty the opportunity to present a great deal of information within a short period, and lecture notes, handouts, and audiovisual media can be selected and prepared in advance. Faculty usually feel comfortable with these teaching methods because they can present the information that students need to learn in a controlled environment. For a faculty member who is new or one who is teaching new content for the first time, the instructional strategies used in passive learning may enable him or her to feel more comfortable in the teaching situation when presenting the content.

Because many students have been socialized to passive learning, they often prefer this approach to learning. Important concepts and content are identified for students in a concrete manner that helps them to organize the material in a meaningful way. With passive learning, students tend to have lower anxiety levels and feel secure in their belief that listening to a lecture, reading the assignments and handouts, taking notes, and copying information from visual media will provide them with all or most of the information they need to be successful in the course.

Disadvantages

Passive learning activities may leave faculty with little opportunity to understand how well students are learning the content. Unless designed otherwise, the time used for presentation of the content may leave little time for questions, clarification, or discussion. Students may not feel comfortable letting faculty know that they do not understand key points or relationships; furthermore, they may be reluctant to ask questions in class or they may not ask enough questions to clarify their misunderstandings. In addition, students may be unable to articulate what it is they do not know or understand.

Listening to a presentation, taking notes, and copying from printed media require little cognitive effort from students and no consistent use of higher-level cognitive skills. Even reading activities, although important, do not provide students with opportunities to apply the concepts about which they are reading. Although many students may prefer passive learning, over time passive learning experiences tend to become tedious.

Active Learning

Active learning involves the student through participation and an investment of energy in all phases of the learning process (Bevis, 1973). Active learning is more apt to stimulate higher cognitive processes such as those associated with critical thinking (Bevis, 1989b).

Advantages

Learning experiences that actively engage students in their learning can have positive benefits for both the faculty and students. Active learning strategies may increase critical thinking skills in students. Evidence also suggests that faculty who are rated more highly by students are faculty who (Phoenix, 1986):

- Accept student feelings
- Are accepting of different points of view
- Are attentive to student comments
- Ask for student contributions
- Enable students to show more initiative
- Give explanations of why praise or criticism is given
- Give students alternative courses from which to choose
- Have less sustained lecture time
- Involve students by stimulating them to talk more
- Provide more praise
- Use more student ideas

It is not always possible to determine whether students are actively involved in learning because their responses during a learning activity may be either overt or covert. Although covert participation may provide a meaningful learning experience, using learning activities that require some overt participation makes it easier for faculty to assess student learning. Activities that require overt active participation cause students to use their mental processes and sensory modalities and require some degree of physical activity. They also enable faculty to meet the needs of students with varying learning styles (Van Hoozer et al., 1987). (See Chapter 4 for more information on learning styles.) Fostering active learning in the classroom is a faculty goal, and some evidence exists to support the view that active learning is preferred by some students (Phoenix, 1986).

Disadvantages

Faculty need to be expert in the content and aware of those content elements and relationships among concepts that usually pose difficulty for students. Organizing learning experiences so that students are engaged in active learning requires faculty to learn about and design teaching strategies that shift the focus from faculty activities in the classroom to student activities and feedback. Examples of such strategies include increased opportunities for student involvement in discussion, increased use of student ideas and comments, and more opportunities to explore the appropriateness of various responses to a given situation. This shift in behavior may be stressful for faculty. Furthermore, faculty may have legitimate concerns about receiving less favorable evaluations of instruction. Continuing awareness of and sensitivity to the behavioral and attitudinal changes required of students to adapt to the pedagogical strategies used for active learning are essential.

Students are often resistant to changes in the way in which they receive instruction because adapting to new ways of learning is stressful. They may be impatient with the process and unwilling to put forth the effort needed to alter their learning style. Student concerns about the way in which learning experiences are organized may be overtly or covertly expressed. Support from faculty, administration, and peers is important to faculty who choose to incorporate more interactive learning activities into their teaching.

MATCHING LEARNING ACTIVITIES TO DESIRED OUTCOMES

To determine the match of learning activities with the desired course outcomes, faculty can create a matrix to examine the relationships between the means (learning activities) and the ends (outcomes). Advance planning for how the learning activities relate to the course objectives facilitates the selection of a variety of activities for the course. Faculty and students enjoy and benefit from a variety of learning experiences. Variety helps to prevent students from becoming bored and makes it more likely that different learning style preferences will be accommodated. Faculty may find it helpful to use a systematic approach in designing and selecting the learning activities for a course before actually teaching the course. The learning activity plan shown in Box 10-1 provides a useful approach for planning and evaluating learning activities for each of the course's class sessions.

Box 10-1
LEARNING ACTIVITY PLAN

Date:_____

Class content focus: _____

Learning objective/competency: _____

Domain/domain level: _____

Type of activity: _____

Brief description of activity: _____

Key concepts to be learned: _____

Number of students in class: _____

Types of resources needed: _____

Time allowed for activity: _____

Time allowed for debriefing/discussion: _____

Issues/problems encountered: _____

    Students: _____

    Faculty: _____

Future revisions: _____

PRINCIPLES FOR SELECTING LEARNING EXPERIENCES

Several principles can guide faculty in the planning of learning activities (Davis, 1993; Heidgerken, 1953; Muse, 1950). Learning activities should do the following:

1. Clearly relate to the desired objectives/competencies, learning domain, and domain level
2. Be geared to and appropriate for the cognitive, affective, or psychomotor development of the students
3. Be challenging so that they move students to higher levels of cognitive and affective development
4. Be emotionally satisfying for students
5. Stimulate the development of alternative perspectives of the problem or issue
6. Be clearly obvious that they are
   a. a means for acquiring the expected professional development
   b. an essential component for enabling students to progress
   c. representative of the type of activity in which professional nurses engage
7. Be sufficiently varied to
   a. prevent boredom
   b. allow for and exploit the potential for individual student differences
   c. enable participation in some transcultural experiences
8. Articulate with and allow application of some previous learning experiences within the same course and experiences from previous and concurrent courses
9. Provide a foundation for subsequent learning
10. Permit faculty to guide and monitor the students' practice when appropriate

Structuring Course Materials

The structure of a course can be presented in the course materials provided to students (Weimer, 1993). It is advantageous to include the learning activities in the materials students receive at the beginning of the course. Placing learning activities in the same logical order as the content, in the sequence in which they will be used, and in proximity to the appropriate objectives or competencies enables students to have a holistic sense of how the learning activities relate to the course objectives and content. Students should be able to determine from the course materials the sequence and patterns of the course. Informing students of the learning activities at the beginning of a course also allows students to have some idea of the amount of preparation the course will entail and allows them to plan their time (Davis, 1993).

Structured and Unstructured Learning Activities

Learning activities may be structured or unstructured. Structured learning activities are most commonly used because they are prescriptive with a highly specific focus that guides students' learning (Bevis, 1989a). Although unstructured learning activities may be used at the undergraduate level, they are more apt to be used in honors or honors option courses, independent study courses, and capstone courses. Faculty may also choose to allow students to use unstructured learning activities for extra work for bonus credit.

Structured Learning Activities

In structured learning activities the stimuli for learning are specifically selected. A structured activity consists of a clear, concise description of the purposes, objectives, and competencies related to the activity; the content and processes to be used while engaged in the activity; specific directions presented in a logical sequence indicating each of the steps to be followed; the time for the activity; and the method to be used to report its completion.

A well-structured activity allows students to function with a great deal of independence while working to achieve the desired outcomes. For example, when assigning students a text, article, or other form of media to study, providing specific questions directly related to the desired objectives and competencies directs students' focus to the essential concepts. Faculty may choose any one of several methods for students to share the results of their learning experiences. For example, students may be required to do the following:

1. Complete an answer sheet that will be evaluated by peers, faculty, or both
2. Write a general or specific summary report that addresses the content or processes and submit it to faculty
3. Present a report to the class
4. Discuss the experience with another student or small group of students
5. Initiate a small group or class discussion of the major points, issues, or problems that came up during their work

These methods can be used separately or in combination with each other. Faculty may also choose to allow the student to select the preferred method of sharing.

Unstructured Learning Activities

Unstructured learning activities are designed to allow students to acquire knowledge and skill with much less specific direction from faculty. This form of activity is derived from Bruner's discovery learning (Bruner, 1977). Faculty provide guidance by posing open-ended or directed questions and hints; however, the answers or responses students are to elicit from the activity are not given in the resource materials or by faculty (DeYoung, 1990). Discovery learning is believed to do the following:

1. Promote a disposition toward inquiry
2. Promote independent thinking and enhanced problem solving
3. Stimulate student motivation and interest
4. Improve knowledge retention
5. Facilitate transfer of learning by stimulating the student to seek and find relationships between information and the situation at hand

A major limitation associated with discovery learning is the increased time students require to attain a desired learning outcome from the activity (DeYoung, 1990).

In an unstructured learning activity, students may be given an assignment in which they are asked to apply their previous and current knowledge, skills, and experiences either to a specific faculty-designated situation or a situation of their choice that fits a general profile described by faculty. The situation may be an actual event in the practice setting or an event that is depicted through a simulation, case study, or a form of media. For example, in a community health nursing course a learning outcome for students may be for them to become familiar with the kinds of activities and interactions that occur during a community meeting. Students would be directed to act as a participant–observer at a community-based meeting of their choosing. The meeting could be a support group for a particular health problem, a meeting of constituents with their legislator, a town board meeting, or a neighborhood association meeting. Students could be given the option of describing their experience verbally in class or at a clinical conference or by writing in a journal.

Unstructured learning activities also allow students to individualize the learning experience according to their own interests. This approach is particularly useful for RN to BSN students and for graduate students.

CRITICAL LEARNING EXPERIENCES

Critical learning experiences are those that are considered to be essential to the curriculum. They are specific types of experiences that faculty have agreed that all students must achieve before successfully completing the course or program. Critical learning experiences are clearly and directly tied to one or more course objectives or program outcomes. These experiences are carefully selected so that each student engages in an activity that enables him or her to attain the specific essential competencies by the completion of the course or program.

When faculty decide to designate certain learning experiences as "critical" to the curriculum, it becomes necessary for faculty to make sure that all students will have the opportunity to participate in the experience. This does not mean, however, that all students must have exactly the same experience under the same or similar conditions. For example, when teaching about the care of patients with musculoskeletal disorders, faculty may decide that a critical learning experience for all students is to provide care to patients in skin and skeletal traction. The age of the patient, the setting in which the care is provided, and the specific type of skin or skeletal traction would not necessarily be specified in the learning objective. The identification of the concept of care of patients with skin and skeletal traction as a critical learning experience, however, would provide students the opportunity to develop the necessary competencies in caring for a patient in traction but still allow some flexibility and individualization regarding how that experience is designed.

Faculty and students in collaboration with faculty may also elect to create different types of experiences that are expected to yield similar results consistent with the course objectives. For example, if a course learning objective states that all students are to develop a family nursing care plan, faculty may decide that this is such an essential part of the course that it will be identified as a critical learning experience. The objective for the critical learning experience would simply state, "Students will develop a family nursing care plan." Faculty may agree on more than one appropriate way in which students may complete this critical learning experience. The following two examples demonstrate how this may be done:

Example 1. Students are required to make a series of visits over a period of weeks to a family in any community setting, such as their home, a daycare center, a senior center, an extended care facility, a homeless shelter, or a church function. Over the course of the visits, students use the nursing process to develop a plan of care with the family and provide verbal or written reports to faculty, peers, and agency staff on the visits and the progress they are making. On completion of the visits, students will have completed a family nursing care plan. Faculty may choose to have students share their care plan with others in any one of a variety of ways. For example, students may present their completed care plan either verbally or in writing, either in clinical conference or as a case study, to faculty, peers, and agency staff. When a student develops a case study, faculty may want to obtain the student's permission to use it as a teaching tool with future students.

Example 2. In the event that not enough families are available for students to visit, faculty may choose to have students use case studies or simulations presented in a videotape or computer-assisted instruction that present a scenario representative of the type of experience in which the students would engage in actual practice. These alternative activities could be used by a small group of clinical students, and care plans could be shared in the manner described in Example 1.

Both of these examples provide students with the opportunity to complete the desired critical learning experience of developing a family care plan, although different learning strategies are used in each example.

Learning Experiences with Simulation

A simulation is an event or situation made to resemble clinical practice as closely as possible to teach theory, assessment, technology, pharmacology, and skills (Rauen, 2001). The emphasis is often on the application and integration of knowledge, skills, and critical thinking. Unlike the traditional classroom setting, a simulation allows the learner to function in an environment that is as close as possible to a real-life situation and provides the opportunity for the learner to think spontaneously and actively rather than passively. Simulations should present realistic situations, require active involvement in problem solving, provide feedback on the process, and require the learner to act on the effects of the harmful actions.

When faculty decide to use simulation in the classroom or clinical teaching, simulations should be developed at an appropriate level for the beginner or advanced beginner. Simulations should provide opportunities for students to select relevant assessment data, infer patient problems, and take appropriate actions (Rauen, 2001; Johnson et al., 1999; Weis & Guyton-Simmons, 1998). Ideally simulations present clinical situations that vary in complexity depending on the number of decisions that must be made, the clarity or ambiguity of the possible choices, and the urgency of the underlying problem. The complexity of each case has to be appropriate for the targeted learners.

When using a simulation, faculty should guide the students' understanding of why the data are relevant, what the critical issues are, and how the actions relate to the data and the issues. Assistance is also needed in viewing the clinical situation as a whole rather than as isolated segments of information.

AcheyCutts (2002) discusses the challenge in education is to create an enriched classroom environment. Simulations can help to enrich an environment by promoting interaction with students' minds, the content, and the equipment. Good educators attempt to make learning meaningful so that students can make connections, problem solve, and think critically, and simulations are one way of doing that. When faculty are deciding whether to develop and incorporate simulation in the learning environment, they should consider both the advantages and challenges/barriers to its use (Table 10-1) (Rauen, 2001).

TABLE 10-1   **Advantages and Challenges/Barriers in Using Simulation within the Curriculum**

ADVANTAGES	CHALLENGES/BARRIERS
Mistakes can be made without patient harm	More faculty preparation time to set up and conduct simulations
Clinical situation can be manipulated	Performance anxiety for student and faculty
Planned learning time can be designated	Only a small number of students per session
Controlled learning environment	Expense (resources; equipment; assistance with set up, evaluation, tear down)
Multiple users for the same simulation	Needed physical space for simulation and equipment
Psychomotor skills can be enhanced	All events in simulation cannot necessarily be replicated
Can present complex clinical situations for the learner	Resource availability (equipment, use of manikins, lab facility, faculty time, etc.)
Active learning	Technical support and computer literacy may be needed if simulation is computer based
Opportunity for immediate feedback	Inclusion of all realistic variables within an actual clinical setting
Can promote activities for problem solving and critical thinking	Clear communication of expected outcomes and skills from the simulation experience

Modified from Rauen, C. A. (2001). Using simulation to teach critical thinking skills: You can't just throw the book at them. *Critical Care Nursing Clinics of North America, 13*(1), 93-103.

Online Learning Experiences

"E-learning is use of the Internet learning tools such as discussion forums, chats, testing, and e-mail to support teaching and learning in an online community" (Billings, 2002, p. 3). Educators, professional experts, and students are the members of the community where the teaching is done and the learning takes place. Because e-learning involves separation of the educator and the learner in time and space, it is considered "distance learning."

Learning experiences in online courses must be selected with the same amount of attention to activating identified competencies or learning outcomes as they are in face-to-face courses. In online courses the educator has an opportunity to select experiences that take advantage of the learning environment offered, using the tools of the learning management system such as threaded discussion, chat, e-mail, and testing to promote active learning and interaction among students and with the course faculty (see Chapter 19).

The role of the educator changes when he or she is teaching on the Web. There is limited to no face-to-face contact with the students. Electronic interaction occurs either synchronously or asynchronously. When teaching on the Web, the educator becomes a "facilitator of learning" and not necessarily the primary source of information as in a traditional classroom. Learning experiences are designed to encourage active learning among the students. The instructor facilitates the students to meet the learning goals and achieve expected outcomes. The teacher guides the students to assume responsibility for identifying their own needs and to be self-directed in the process of achieving expected outcomes. Many educators who have experience teaching on the Web state that the timeliness of communication with students is important to the success of the teaching. Halstead (2002) describes two essential teaching behaviors for online education: (1) to communicate established evaluation criteria to the learner and (2) to provide prompt feedback to the learner on the performance. Table 10-2 lists differences between online and traditional teaching in the curriculum. Faculty must evaluate the content of their courses and decide whether any of the material or instruction should be Web based. Web-based instruction can provide opportunities for the learner to access rich resources and explore Web links that enhance the content delivered. According to Chastain (2002), technology is imperative in nursing education and practice. Information technology must be a fixture in today's nursing curriculum; therefore nurse educators and nurses must accept the challenge of incorporating information technology into nursing programs and not run the risk of becoming obsolete.

DOMAINS OF LEARNING AND LEARNING ACTIVITIES

Cognitive, psychomotor, and affective domains of learning provide a systematic framework for designing a series of appropriate learning activities that will facilitate students' achievement of course objectives and desired competencies and outcomes (Davies, 1976). Although the domains address the three aspects of learning (knowledge, skills, and attitudes) separately, they are actually interdependent (Bloom, 1956; Krathwohl et al., 1964; Reilly & Oermann, 1990).

TABLE 10-2   Traditional Teaching versus Online Teaching

TRADITIONAL TEACHING	ONLINE TEACHING
Learning is teacher centered	Learning is student centered
Classroom environment with a set time for class	Learning can take place anytime, anywhere
Instructor can read verbal and nonverbal cues	Instructor can interact in discussion forums, e-mails, chats, and other online activities
Face-to-face interaction with students	Electronic interactions and communication with students
Typically a fixed academic schedule (e.g., a semester or quarter)	Students may have more freedom in their course start dates and completion times
Student interaction in the classroom	Student interaction in a Web format via discussion forums, e-mails, chats, and other forums
Teaching occurs at a set time (e.g., Tuesdays 9-12)	Teaching is flexible: synchronous or asynchronous

After the desired outcomes related to each domain have been clearly delineated, faculty can then think creatively about the types of learning activities that will actively engage students in the process of learning. Learning activities need to be appropriate for the domain and domain level. One learning activity can be designed to meet several objectives; those with a broad focus are especially helpful.

A sequence of learning activities is designed to provide continuity with previous learning and experiences. Although the same concepts may be used repeatedly, they should be applied to increasingly complex situations. Learning activities are designed to enable students to integrate concepts and recognize relationships. Combining and unifying concepts from the cognitive, psychomotor, and affective domains facilitates integration. For example, an activity focused on a specific skill such as taking a blood pressure requires knowledge, technical skill, communication skills, and valuing the importance of an accurate measurement.

Because nursing is a practice discipline that ultimately requires the application and synthesis of acquired knowledge, skills, and attitudes, faculty must keep in mind that the levels of the domains are sequenced in a hierarchical order progressing from the simple to the complex, thus enabling the learner to move toward these higher levels of learning. The underlying assumption is that each subsequent level builds on and integrates the prior set of knowledge, skills, and attitudes (Bloom, 1956).

For example, the hierarchical order presented by Bloom's (1956) taxonomy for the cognitive (knowledge) domain consists of six categories: knowledge, comprehension, application, analysis, synthesis, and evaluation. The following objectives reveal progression from the simple to the most complex cognitive processes:

1. Identifies steps in the epidemiological process (knowledge)
2. Differentiates among the steps in the epidemiological process (comprehension)
3. Applies the epidemiological process to common health conditions (application)
4. Relates the epidemiological process to patients' health conditions (analysis)
5. Proposes interventions based on the epidemiological process for patients' health conditions (synthesis)
6. Determines priorities for patients' health conditions based on the epidemiological process (evaluation)

Krathwohl et al.'s (1964) taxonomy for the affective (attitude) domain consists of five categories: attending, responding, valuing, organization, and characterization by value set. The following objectives reveal progression from the simple to the most complex affective processes:

1. Listens for patients' concerns about health conditions (attending)
2. Accepts patients' concerns about health conditions (responding)
3. Assumes responsibility for involving patients in decisions about self-care practices (valuing)
4. Develops nursing care plans incorporating patients' belief systems (organization)
5. Revises nursing care plans in accord with patients' preferences (characterizes values)

The separation of the cognitive, psychomotor, and affective domains is intended for classification purposes only because they are closely interrelated. Behaviors in each domain have dimensions in the others, and one domain may be used as a vehicle to attain the others (Krathwohl et al., 1964). Knowledge must be possessed if it is to be applied, professional nursing values must be internalized if they are to be implemented in practice, and skills must be well practiced if they are to be safely executed in a variety of circumstances. Faculty need to guard against selecting domain levels that are too low on the hierarchy for the outcomes they want students to achieve.

Matching the Learning Activity with the Learning Domain

When choosing instructional materials, faculty need to consider the match between the learning materials, the desired outcomes, the learning domain and domain level, and student attributes. All instructional materials used during the course, such as textbooks, course handouts, articles, and media, including computer-assisted instruction programs, should be selected in accord with their appropriateness for the learning objective, learning domain, and domain level. Faculty must also take into account the students' academic level, cognitive maturity, learning readiness, motivation, and interests, as well as the complexity of the course content, processes, and skills (Reilly & Oermann, 1990).

Faculty can expect the time required for students to attain the desired learning outcome in each domain to increase according to the complexity of the domain level. A reasonable amount of time for the teaching–learning process to occur needs to be allocated. The learning activity should facilitate learning and also be cost-effective in terms of the use of time, effort, and resources for both faculty and students.

The Cognitive Domain

The categories in this domain include knowledge, comprehension, application, analysis, synthesis, and evaluation. Knowledge represents the lowest, or simplest, level of learning in the cognitive domain. At this level the learner focuses primarily on the acquisition and recall of specific facts, concepts, and principles. Ideally learners progress to a higher order of intellectual ability and through the more complex stages of cognitive learning. Higher levels of learning are the ability to understand the meaning of new information (comprehension), the ability to apply this information to a new situation (application), the ability to break down the information into its component parts (analysis), the ability to put together elements to form a new whole (synthesis), and the ability to make judgments about information and ideas (evaluation) (Reilly, 1980).

The lecture is perhaps the most commonly used teaching method to instruct learners in the cognitive domain. When using this method, faculty are primarily responsible for presenting the content to the students. Research on this method has focused on teacher characteristics or behaviors in the classroom. Menges (1994) notes that student performance in relation to the use of lecture is dependent on two variables: presentation characteristics of the lecturer and student characteristics. One of the more important lecturer characteristics associated with greater student learning is teacher organization and clarity in presenting the content. Studies have shown that highlighting the structure for the content and emphasizing the relationships among concepts throughout the lecture enhances student achievement (Menges & Austin, 2001). Lecture can be effective if cognitive involvement is fostered by using reflection during the presentation, illustrating points with relevant examples, and providing a framework for organizing information (Garrison & Archey, 2000).

The challenge in this domain is to select an appropriate action verb that clearly describes the desired level of student performance. When designing and selecting learning activities to fit the appropriate domain level, faculty need to consider all aspects of the activities and determine whether they provide students with the opportunities necessary to learn and practice the desired competencies. The following example written for a community health nursing course illustrates how an objective at the application level and learning activity can be matched:

Learning objective: Students will apply the epidemiological process to common disease conditions.

Learning activity: The following directions are provided to students for the learning activity: *Before class read the assigned text section describing the steps of the epidemiological process. At the beginning of class form into groups of four to discuss your understanding of the reading, then select one disease condition to which you will apply all of the steps in the process. Write a brief summary of your* *work on a transparency and be prepared to report your work to the class. You have 25 minutes to complete your group work and 10 minutes for your presentation. Faculty will be available for consultation.*

This activity requires that the group members agree on a single disease condition, share and clarify their knowledge of the content and understanding of the task, and actually apply the epidemiological process as it would be done in actual community health nursing practice. Although designed primarily for the cognitive domain, this activity also focuses students on the affective domain by raising their consciousness (level one) with regard to the importance of and opportunities for disease prevention, which is the primary focus of public health practice.

The Affective Domain

The affective domain of learning encompasses attitudes, beliefs and values, and feelings and emotions. Classification of affective behaviors, like that of the cognitive domain, is hierarchical. The categories are organized along a continuum of stages of internalization that reflect changes in personal growth, moving from an external to an internal locus of control (Krathwohl et al., 1964).

Storytelling, with the use of vivid images, has been recommended as a way of enhancing the development of the affective domain. The story could be an experience, a fantasy, or a combination of both. Learning activities that involve case studies, clinical decision making, group work, practice experiences, and writing also enhance the development of the affective domain.

Competency statements must be clearly written so that faculty can design learning experiences that help students develop the desired competencies and outcomes. It is also important for faculty to develop a systematic manner for assessing and evaluating students' progress (Krathwohl et al., 1964). The following example written for a community health nursing course illustrates how an objective at the valuing level of the affective domain and a learning activity can be matched:

Learning objective: Students will assume responsibility for involving their patients and families in decisions about disease prevention self-care practices.

Learning activity: The following directions are provided to students for this learning activity: *You are to be prepared to discuss in clinical conference your plan to engage your patient or family in preventive health care decisions. Present your analysis of the patient and family assessment data that led you to identify the existence of an actual or potential problem that could be averted through the use of preventive self-care practices. Describe the approaches you will use to stimulate involvement of your patients in appropriate self-care practices. Be prepared to give a report on your progress in a future clinical conference.*

Although this activity is designed to focus primarily on the affective domain, it is clear that students need to possess some in-depth knowledge of the epidemiology of specific health problems and be able to use data collection and communication skills. This activity directs students to integrate disease prevention strategies in the context of promoting self-care practices within the family.

The Psychomotor Domain

For the psychomotor domain, Reilly and Oermann (1990) described three types of skills: fine motor, manual, and gross motor. These are the skills most commonly used in the clinical techniques of nursing practice. Fine motor skills are those needed to implement tasks requiring exactness. Nursing skills such as preparing and administering parenteral medications, manipulating instruments to prepare and apply dressings, and manually adjusting intravenous fluid drip rates are examples of skills that fall into this category. Manual skills are those involving some common coordinated movements of the hand, arm, and eye. Nursing skills involving different types of touch, such as personal hygiene, suctioning, and the physical assessment skills of palpation and percussion, are examples of skills included in this group. Gross motor skills are those that use large muscle masses in body movements. Some nursing skills that require the use of gross motor skills are bed making, transferring and positioning, exercising, and cardiopulmonary resuscitation.

The psychomotor taxonomy suggested by Reilly and Oermann (1990) as the most useful for nursing was the one published in *Psychomotor Levels in Developing and Writing Objectives* (Dave, 1970). Dave's taxonomy is based on neuromuscular movement and coordination; the five levels in the taxonomy are imitation, manipulation, precision, articulation, and naturalization. Reilly and Oermann (1990) created criteria for the levels that they believe are consistent with the developmental stages of competency; the criteria may be used to write learner objectives/competencies. The criteria for each level are as follows:

1. *Imitation level:* The necessary actions are taken with some errors, there are some weaknesses in the smoothness of the gross motor actions, and the time used to complete the actions depends on the learner's needs
2. *Manipulation level:* Written directives are followed with some degree of accuracy, and variations occur during the coordination of movements and the time taken to execute the actions
3. *Precision level:* Actions are carried out in a logical sequence with few errors occurring only during some noncritical actions, movements are well coordinated, the time needed to execute the actions continues to be variable
4. *Articulation level:* Coordinated actions are carried out in a logical sequence with limited errors, and the time used to execute the actions is reasonable
5. *Naturalization level:* The skill performance demonstrates professional competence in that it is automatic with good coordination (p. 84)

Within the nursing curriculum students can learn psychomotor skills in various traditional and nontraditional settings. Different teaching strategies requiring considerable instruction, explanation, support, and facilitation about the process are needed by the educators teaching psychomotor skills. Faculty must orient students to the mechanism of the skill and encourage students to learn and practice the skills in the environment provided. Faculty can use a variety of instructional methods to provide learning, including "hands-on" instruction, even though the content may originally not be delivered in a traditional mode.

The teacher role of the educator in teaching psychomotor skills is evolving. Several studies (Darr, 2000; Jeffries et al., 2002) describe the teacher's role when teaching psychomotor skills as a facilitator or guide for the student learner. One resource discussed the talents needed by educators who teach psychomotor skills as described in Box 10-2. With the use of simulations, simulators, computer-based training, and other innovative teaching strategies, traditional faculty activities are still required to validate learning, stimulate problem solving and critical thinking questions, and validate the correct procedures to be used when performing a skill. Overall the educator is still needed when new, innovative methods are used to teach psychomotor skills, but the educator role may need to be modified to ensure that learning outcomes are positive and competencies are being met.

The following example created for a physical assessment course in the first semester of a baccalaureate nursing program illustrates how an objective at the articulation level in the psychomotor taxonomy and learning activity can be matched.

Learning objective: Students will be skillful in using auscultation, palpation, and percussion to assess a person's pulmonary status.

Learning activity: Students are given the following directions: *Read the assigned text and view the assigned videotapes in preparation for your rehearsal and practice session in assessing pulmonary status. Sign up on the schedule posted for the examining room to rehearse and practice these skills in triads. As a group, first discuss the equipment and manual technique you will use to implement the skills. Describe the sequence, positions, and patterns you will use on the chest during each skill. When you have finished this part of the activity, decide who will be the exam-*

Box 10-2
TEACHER ABILITIES NEEDED TO TEACH PSYCHOMOTOR SKILLS

- Knowledge of instruction in all three domains of learning: cognitive, affective, and psychomotor
- Clinical competence
- Facilitation skills to progress students from a beginning level
- Awareness of students' unique learning styles
- Knowledge about general principles in nursing in addition to specific procedures
- Facilitation skills to promote critical thinking and adaptability in the clinical area
- Empowerment skills to promote students to provide safe, competent nursing care

From Minnesota Baccalaureate Psychomotor Skills Faculty Group. (1998). Conversations: An experience of psychomotor skills faculty. *Journal of Nursing Education, 37*(7), 324-325.

iner, the examinee, and the participant–observer for the first round of practice. Begin your examination by describing to the examinee what you will be doing and then perform a complete assessment of your peer's chest in a systematic manner. At the completion of each separate assessment make a written record of all of your findings. The participant-observer is to provide feedback on the skill and systematic approach used by the examiner. After completing the first examination, reverse roles with the participant–observer and complete the second and third round of practice. Compare your techniques and findings and share helpful hints with each examiner. During the rehearsal and practice, feel free to use faculty guidance and validation. At the completion of this activity be prepared to discuss your experiences with faculty before or during the next class.

Although this learning activity is designed to focus primarily on skill development in the psychomotor domain, it is clear that students need to possess knowledge about how to use and place the stethoscope, how to execute the manual techniques necessary for palpation and percussion, how to find the normal range of results that are obtained from each assessment technique, and how to write a description of the findings with the correct terminology. In addition, students also need to demonstrate their willingness to engage in rehearsal and practice, a second-level affective domain response.

LEARNING ACTIVITIES TO PROMOTE CRITICAL THINKING

Bandman and Bandman (1995) and others define critical thinking and its application to nursing practice and education by describing key attributes of critical thinkers. They describe critical thinkers as having the following key attributes:

- Analytical
- Articulate and able to support their ideas
- Clear thinking
- Creative
- Fact-finding
- Logical
- Objective
- Open-minded
- Precise in their thinking
- Self-confident
- Truth seeking
- Unbiased
- Willing to reconsider

By designing and selecting learning activities that require overt active learning, faculty can stimulate critical thinking in their students. Approaches that contribute to the development of students' critical thinking skills include integrating thought-provoking questions into activities, using the Socratic or a focused questioning method, dividing the class into heterogeneous work groups, placing the primary emphasis on learning concepts rather than factual information, and having students share their reasoning processes. See Chapter 13 for information about how faculty can use writing and thinking exercises to stimulate students and to further develop their critical thinking skills.

CONSTRAINTS TO CHOOSING AND IMPLEMENTING LEARNING ACTIVITIES

Constraints to choosing and implementing learning activities may arise from faculty, students, time, and resources. Although it may not be possible to eliminate all constraints, by making a careful assessment of each source of constraint during the planning phases, faculty will be able to avoid many pitfalls. Faculty gain an appreciation of the benefits and limitations of any learning activity after implementing it, reflecting on how students responded, and assessing how the activity contributed to learning. Taking time to debrief themselves after an activity helps faculty to decide whether to repeat, revise, or delete the activity. Table 10-3 presents a summary of the sources of constraint in selecting and implementing learning activities.

Faculty Constraints

Some constraints in choosing and implementing learning activities arise from faculty. A faculty member's lack of experience in teaching in an academic

TABLE 10-3   Sources of Constraint in Choosing and Implementing Learning Activities

SOURCE	CONSTRAINT
Faculty	Faculty/student ratio
	Lack of experience
	Lack of knowledge of course content
	Lack of understanding of students' knowledge and skills
	Personal attributes:
	Personality
	Vocal qualities
Students	Distractions
	Inability to use equipment/technology
	Lack of prerequisite knowledge and skills
	Resistance to active participation
	Stress/anxiety
	Student–faculty ratio too large
Time	Inadequate for activity
	Inadequate for debriefing
Resources	Copyright restrictions
	Inadequate clinical or classroom facilities
	Inadequate funds
	Unavailable audiovisual equipment
	Unavailable electronic technology

setting or in teaching students at the course level assigned may present some difficulty when he or she is choosing and implementing learning activities. Faculty are more likely to select appropriate activities when they have a reasonable understanding of the cognitive abilities of their students and some familiarity with the knowledge base and previous school and life experiences that their students bring to the course. Overestimating or underestimating the abilities and experiences of students can undermine the intended value of the learning experience. Another pitfall faculty may encounter is the failure to adequately appreciate a student's inability to engage in an activity. This inability may be attributed to an activity that is too sophisticated or complex, or it may be due to the student's attitude toward or lack of motivation to engage in the activity.

Novice faculty, and even experienced faculty who are teaching a new course, may not possess a comfortable or adequate command of the content and processes required by the learning activity. In addition, they may not be comfortable in dealing with questions, problems, or issues that may arise during the activity. Even under the best of circumstances it is often difficult for faculty to fully appreciate the various perspectives that students may bring to the activity. Students may raise questions and issues that faculty may not have even remotely considered as related to the activity. Consulting with senior faculty who have taught the course or who have had experience teaching the same level of students before designing the learning activities can provide valuable input that can help to reduce the potential for difficulties. Because learning activities are student centered, faculty must not only be prepared to deal with any ambiguity that may arise but also be willing to be flexible, to go with the flow of the learning experience while taking advantage of the opportunity to learn from students how they process the experience. Feedback from students about the different ways they interpreted the learning activity, or certain elements of it, can be used as points of discussion and thus expand the learning experience.

Demands on students outside the classroom can complicate and put constraints on faculty. Retaining standards and rigor while providing appropriate academic expectations for students with numerous job and family demands makes teaching a challenge and can have major implications for pedagogy. Yoder and Saylor (2002) found that students expected to be challenged, implying a higher level of intellectual effort, yet class preparation was far below the expectations of faculty. Concerns of the educators included whether assignments were reasonable and whether the effort to reduce preparation time simply dilutes course expectations to an unacceptable level. Incorrect assumptions and mismatched expectations, which might be increased if there is cultural diversity in the classroom, between students and teachers can promote an academic challenge and provide a critical focus and direction to establishing better nursing education policy and research with these issues.

Faculty may have personal attributes that interfere with their ability to establish a climate that stimulates student interest, motivation, and engagement in learning activities. Having a soft or a poor-quality voice, talking too fast or too slow, or speaking in a monotone may make it difficult for students to attend to and follow verbal presentations. Faculty with a reserved or shy personality, or those with a matter-of-fact orientation, may be perceived by students as distant, aloof, or uncaring. Personal habits faculty may be unaware of may also be distracting for students and interfere with their ability to fully focus on the learning experience. Although students may be reluctant to share some of their perceptions about faculty personal attributes, inviting a colleague to attend a class can provide some helpful input that can be used to improve classroom performance.

Student Constraints

Student constraints may be due to the number of students enrolled in a course. There may be too many students to ensure that they all have the same or a comparable experience. The student–faculty ratio may make a particular activity too labor and time intensive.

Students may lack some of the prerequisite knowledge and skills required for an activity, knowledge and skills that faculty reasonably assumed that the students would possess. There are usually some students, regardless of the clarity of the activity and the directions, who fail to understand the activity or who are unable to connect parts of the activity with previous knowledge and experience. Some students are not skilled listeners and do not adequately follow directions.

Stress or anxiety may interfere with some students' ability to attend to and participate in an activity. Distractions such as mechanical noise in the classroom and noise from outside the building may also interfere with learning activities. Students working in groups may make enough noise to interfere with others working in proximity.

Resistance to participation in learning activities is another constraining force. Students socialized to a passive learning model may be resistant to engaging in some or all types of activities. Students may perceive learning activities as a form of busywork that has little or no meaning for them and not accept the activity as a meaningful experience.

Students may not have the skill or experience in using the resources, equipment, or electronic technology required for a learning activity. Although many types of computer equipment are easily and quickly learned, there are students who lack experience, skill, and comfort in using computers for any purpose.

Time Constraints

Time is an all too common constraint in teaching. Faculty must carefully weigh the tradeoffs between faculty-centered and student-centered activities when determining how to most effectively use class time. For all learning activities faculty must prioritize and then select the essential objectives or competencies and the related content and processes. Also, faculty must assess the complexity of the learning activity to ensure that it can be accomplished given the ability of the students and the allotted time.

For an activity to be of maximum value, adequate time needs to be allowed both for students to actively participate in the activity and for the debriefing that follows the completion of the activity. Although the need to debrief students after the activity depends on the nature of the activity, debriefing is an important part of learning, and it has several benefits for both students and faculty. It extends the learning process because students share what they did with their peers; it enables faculty to gain a more comprehensive perspective of the kinds of thinking processes students use; and it provides a window of opportunity for students to identify issues or problems that came up during the activity. Faculty can use this information as the basis for further discussion of issues and problems relevant to the students' immediate learning situation. Information gleaned from students about their difficulties with the directions, elements, or focus of the activity itself is useful to faculty when deciding whether to retain, revise, or delete the activity.

Resource Constraints

Resources may be another source of constraint. The resources used to support learning activities include clinical facilities; learning resource centers; physical examination rooms; classrooms; supplies and equipment; print materials; audiovisual equipment and programs such as films, videotapes, and audiotapes; computer-assisted instructional programs; and a variety of information technologies. The use of a particular learning activity or type of activity may not be possible because of a lack of the appropriate resources needed to implement the activity. For example, a clinical unit may not be able to accommodate the students; the type of clinical facility desired may not be available; classroom size or design may not be adequate; audiovisual equipment may be unavailable for the specific class day and time; or films, videotapes, or computer software may not be accessible because of heavy demand or lack of funds to acquire them. In addition, licensing or copyright restrictions may prohibit or limit faculty use of a particular resource.

Information technologies may not be available or they may be difficult to access during the desired time because of limited hardware or software or because of an unusually heavy demand and use during the desired time period. Although the number of students who have computers and modems at home continues to increase, large numbers still depend on the resources available at the academic setting.

Information technology, e-mail, and other electronic messaging and conferencing systems are useful tools that can be used as a vehicle for selected learning activities. Although faculty may inform students in advance of the course that skill and experience in using electronic technology are required, students often report that they are too busy to allocate the time to acquire the necessary training on their own time. In addition to time, money may also be a barrier. Some academic institutions charge students to learn how to use electronic messaging systems or computer software programs. Faculty who are committed to using some form of computer or electronic technology as a means of implementing one or more learning activities may find it necessary to schedule training sessions for students during class time.

EVALUATION OF LEARNING ACTIVITIES

Evaluation of teaching and learning is a continuous process for both faculty and students. Faculty need to be aware that in education two types of evaluation are commonly used: formative and summative (Bevis, 1989a; Worthen & Sanders, 1973). Selecting the appropriate type of evaluation for use at the appropriate time is important. Formative and summative evaluations are further discussed in Chapter 20.

Formative Evaluation

Formative evaluation is conducted while the teaching–learning process is unfolding. Faculty use formative evaluation (1) to appraise learning activities while they are developing and using them, (2) to assess student learning and ability to apply the content, and (3) to identify any difficulties that come up during the implementation.

Students use formative evaluation to appraise (1) the effectiveness of their learning strategies; (2) the extent to which they are grasping the knowledge, skills, and attitudes presented in the course; (3) the need for additional clarification of the material; and (4) the need for further study.

Clearly differentiating between learning and evaluation and allocating specific time for each purpose is essential. However, separating learning from evaluation does not mean that frequent formative assessment of student learning can be neglected. Collecting systematic verbal and written feedback from students is an integral and essential component of the teaching–learning process. These data enable faculty to monitor student progress and design appropriate strategies to improve student achievement.

When most students demonstrate problems in achieving the desired outcomes for a specific content topic, it may be necessary for faculty to select a different activity to present and reinforce the content. Faculty can use a variety of other strategies to facilitate student learning, such as giving supplemental assignments, organizing students with different levels of ability into learning groups, scheduling personal conferences with individuals or groups of students, or referring students to tutors. Students deserve to be informed about when they will be evaluated and the purpose of the evaluation. Because formative evaluation data can provide valuable feedback to students about their performance, faculty should frequently share these data in both verbal and written form with students.

Students often believe that they have little or no time to learn, experiment, and test the extent to which they have attained the expected objectives of the course before being required to demonstrate achievement for purposes of grading (Diekelmann, 1990). Students require time to learn and practice applying the knowledge, processes, skills, and attitudes before being required to demonstrate achievement for final evaluation.

Novice faculty can benefit by consulting mentors or senior colleagues to discover the content areas and processes that usually pose difficulty for students. This information can be used to shape the learning activities and determine the amount of time students need to attain the course objectives before being evaluated.

Summative Evaluation

Summative evaluation is conducted by faculty at the completion of the course and program; it is the final outcome. Faculty use summative evaluation to (1) appraise the students' learning outcomes, (2) determine the effectiveness of all the instructional strategies and learning activities used during the course, and (3) plan appropriate revisions to the planned learning activities of the course.

Because evaluation of learning should be done in the same manner in which students learned, the same types of learning activities that were used as part of the instructional strategies may also be used for the summative evaluation. Many types of learning activities, such as case studies, simulations, and audiovisual media, can also be included in an examination. Faculty may choose to use these types of learning activities for the complete examination or only part of it. For example, when faculty use case studies or simulations or other approaches designed to promote in-depth thinking and problem solving, they may prefer to test students by using short answer essay questions based on the content presented in a case study. Although short answer essay questions are an excellent testing method, grading them can be a labor-intensive activity, especially if there are a large number of students in the course. In this situation, one strategy that faculty may choose is to create an examination that combines traditional multiple choice items with a few essay questions.

Another useful strategy for handling the grading of essay examinations is to have students exchange examinations and grade each other's work, with faculty providing the criteria for the grading. In this model faculty may also choose to grade the graders on their ability to critically examine their peers' performance. Students must sign their names on the examination they are grading. This helps the grader to focus on the content of the examination rather than the person who wrote the examination, who may be a friend. If faculty wish to preserve the anonymity of students taking the examination, identification codes may be used rather than student names. When this strategy is used, separate points for graders are allocated to their examination score. Although this approach requires that more time be allocated for the examination, it provides students an opportunity to learn from others' work as they critically assess the quality of the responses.

A third strategy that serves to reduce the workload of grading essay examinations is to allow students to work in pairs or small groups. This strategy is sometimes used with a cooperative learning model.

Cooperative learning (Goodfellow, 1995; Johnson et al., 1991; Matthews et al., 1995) uses instructional strategies that structure the environment to encourage and promote students working actively together in small groups on academic tasks. These strategies are designed to maximize students' own and each others' learning. Research evidence indicates that cooperative learning increases students' achievement, creates positive relationships among students, and promotes a healthier psychological adjustment than learning in a competitive or individualistic mode.

Maximum benefits of cooperative learning are derived when learning groups are carefully designed and facilitated. Cooperative learning requires that group members (1) develop positive interdependence among themselves, (2) assume responsibility for promoting each other's learning, (3) assume individual responsibility and accountability for doing a fair share of the work, (4) know and use appropriate interpersonal and small group process skills, and (5) actively process how effectively they are working together.

SUMMARY

Selecting learning activities is an intentional, systematically planned effort that is time consuming. It requires attention to several important issues. Faculty must keep in mind that learning activities that require students' active engagement in their own learning have positive benefits for students and faculty. Within this context faculty must consider when to use structured or unstructured activities; whether learning activities are needed for critical learning experiences; how to appropriately match the objectives/competencies, learning domain, and domain level with the instructional materials and the learning activities; and how to design and incorporate formative and summative evaluation strategies.

In addition, faculty must determine how and where it is appropriate to integrate critical thinking skills, simulations, and technology into the activities. Using a set of principles for selecting learning experiences helps to ensure that the learning activities will maximize student learning. Faculty also need to be conscious of the sources of constraints that may interfere with choosing and implementing learning activities.

REFERENCES

AcheyCutts, P. (2002). Enriched environments enhance learning. *Ed Tech Online*. Retrieved on April 2, 2003, from http://edservices.aea7.k12.ia.us/edtech/classroom/brain/environment.html.

Bandman, E. L., & Bandman, B. (1995). *Critical thinking in nursing* (2nd ed.). Norwalk, CT: Appleton & Lange.

Bevis, E. O. (1989a). *Curriculum building in nursing: A process*. St. Louis: Mosby.

Bevis, E. O. (1989b). Teaching and learning: A practical commentary. In E. O. Bevis & J. Watson (Eds.), *Toward a caring curriculum: A new pedagogy for nursing* (pp. 217-259). New York: National League for Nursing.

Billings, D. M. (2002). What is e-learning? In D. Billings (Ed.), *Conversations in e-learning*. Pensacola, FL: Pohl Publishing.

Bloom, B. S. (Ed.). (1956). *Taxonomy of educational objectives. Handbook 1: Cognitive domain*. New York: Longman.

Bruner, J. (1977). *The process of education*. Cambridge, MA: Harvard University Press.

Chastain, R. (2002). Are nursing faculty members ready to integrate information technology into the curriculum? *Nursing Education Perspectives, 23*(4), 187-190.

Darr, L. R. (2000). Advanced cardiac life support education: a self-directed, scenario-based approach. *Journal of Continuing Education in Nursing, 31*(3), 116-120.

Dave, R. (1970). *Psychomotor levels in developing and writing objectives*. Tucson, AZ: Educational Innovators Press.

Davies, I. K. (1976). *Objectives in curriculum design*. New York: McGraw Hill.

Davis, B. G. (1993). *Tools for teaching*. San Francisco: Jossey-Bass.

DeYoung, S. (1990). *Teaching nursing*. Redwood City, CA: Addison-Wesley.

Dick, W., & Carey, L. (1985). *The systematic design of instruction* (2nd ed.). Glenview, IL: Scott, Foresman.

Diekelmann, N. (1990). Nursing education: Caring, dialogue and practice. *Journal of Nursing Education, 29*(7), 300-306.

Garrison, D. R., & Archey, W. (2000). *A transactional perspective on teaching and learning: A framework for adult and higher education.* Oxford: Pergamon.

Goodfellow, L. M. (1995). Cooperative learning strategies. *Nurse Educator, 20*(4), 26-29.

Halstead, J. (2002). How will my role change in teaching on the Web? In D. Billings, *Conversations in e-learning,* Pensacola, FL: Pohl Publishing.

Heidgerken, I. E. (1953). *Teaching in schools of nursing* (2nd ed.). Philadelphia: J. B. Lippincott.

Jeffries, P., Rew, S., & Cramer, J. (2002). A comparison of student-centered versus traditional method of teaching basic nursing skills in a learning laboratory. *Nursing Education Perspectives, 23*(1), 14-19.

Johnson, D. W., Johnson, R. T., & Smith, K. A. (1991). *Cooperative learning: Increasing college faculty instructional productivity.* ASHE-ERIC Higher Education Report No. 4. Washington, DC: The George Washington University, School of Education and Human Development.

Johnson, J., Zeriwic, J. & Theis, S. (1999). Clinical simulation laboratory: An adjunct to clinical teaching. *Nurse Educator, 24*(5), 37-41.

Krathwohl, D., Bloom, B., & Masia, B. (1964). *Taxonomy of educational objectives. Handbook II: Affective domain.* New York: Longman.

Matthews, R. S., Cooper, J. L., Davidson, N., & Hawkes, P. (1995). Building bridges between cooperative and collaborative learning. *Change, 27*(4), 35-40.

Menges, R. J. (1994). Teaching in the age of electronic information. In W. J. McKeachie (Ed.), *Teaching tips* (9th ed.). Lexington, MA: D.C. Health and Co.

Menges, R., & Austin, A. (2001). Teaching in higher education. In V. Richardson (Ed.), *Handbook on research on teaching* (4th ed., pp. 1122-1156). New York: Macmillan.

Muse, M. B. (1950). *Guiding learning experience.* New York: Macmillan.

Phoenix, C. (1986). Get them involved! Styles of high- and low-rated teachers. *College Teaching, 35*(1), 13-15.

Rauen, C. A. (2001). Using simulation to teach critical thinking skills: You can't just throw the book at them. *Critical Care Nursing Clinics of North America, 13*(1), 93-103.

Reilly, D. E. (1980). Behavioral objectives—evaluation in nursing. New York: Appleton-Century-Crofts.

Reilly, D. E., & Oermann, M. H. (1990). *Behavioral objectives: Evaluation nursing* (3rd ed.). New York: National League for Nursing.

Sell, G. R., & Lounsberry, B. (1997). Supporting curriculum development. In J. G. Gaff & J. Ratcliff & Associates (Eds.), *Handbook of the undergraduate curriculum* (pp. 661-681). San Francisco: Jossey-Bass.

Van Hoozer, H. L., Bratton, B. D., Ostome, P. M., Weinholt, D., Craft, M. J., Gjerde, C. L., & Albanese, M. A. (1987). *The teaching process: Theory and practice in nursing.* Norwalk, CT: Appleton-Century-Crofts.

Weimer, M. (1993). *Improving your classroom teaching.* Newbury Park, CA: Sage.

Weis, P. & Guyton-Simmons, J. (1998). A computer simulation for teaching critical thinking skills. *Nurse Educator, 23*(2), 30-33.

Worthen, B. R., & Sanders, J. R. (1973). *Educational evaluation: Theory and practice.* Belmont, CA: Charles A. Jones.

Yoder, M., & Saylor, C. (2002). Student and teacher roles: Mismatched expectations. *Nurse Educator, 27*(5), 201-203.

11

SERVICE LEARNING
DEVELOPING VALUES AND SOCIAL RESPONSIBILITY

Carla Mueller, PhD, RN, Barbara Norton, RN, MPH

Although the primary purposes of institutions of higher education are the imparting of subject matter and the development of academic skills, as many alumni reveal, much of what is learned in college is fleeting at best (Pascarella & Terenzini, 1991). However, what does endure, long after the college years are over, are the cognitive skills that have been developed, such as critical thinking, reflective judgment, and intellectual flexibility. These skills are tools that can be used by the individual in a variety of situations throughout a lifetime (Miller, 1995, p. 1). Institutions of higher education are therefore seeking opportunities for students to develop moral judgment, civic responsibility, cultural competence, and global awareness, in addition to the basic professional skills set forth in the curriculum. Service learning, a structured component of the curriculum in which students acquire social values through service to individuals, groups, or communities, is one way to provide opportunities for students to develop these values. Service offers opportunities for learning that cannot be obtained any other way. As such, a service experience may be one of the first truly meaningful acts in a student's life (Boyer, 1987). Service learning connects thought and feeling in a deliberate way, creating a context in which students can explore how they feel about what they are thinking, and what they think about how they feel (Ehrlich, 1995). As it does so, service learning becomes an integral part of students' education. The purpose of this chapter is to explain how service learning can contribute to these outcomes in nursing curricula.

SERVICE LEARNING

Service learning evolves from a philosophy of education that emphasizes active learning directed toward a goal of social responsibility. Service learning is not merely volunteerism, nor is it a substitute for a field experience or practicum that is a normal part of a course. In nursing education, service learning is not the same as a clinical experience because the focus of the learning is on meeting the needs of the host community rather than those of the academic or career program. Rather, service learning offers a way in which students can develop their own sense of civic responsibility and help to create a better world by contributing to national renewal.

Service learning is an educational experience in which students participate in a service activity that meets the community needs within the framework of a specific credit-bearing course. Service learning is "more of a program emphasis, representative of a set of educative, social and sometimes political values, rather than a discrete type of experiential education" (Stanton, 1990, p. 65). Service learning is also defined as a way of connecting academic learning with service; it provides concrete opportunities for students to learn new skills, think critically, and test new roles in situations that encourage risk taking and reward competence.

Often the terms *service learning* and *experiential learning* are used interchangeably; however, they are distinct entities. Experiential learning includes hands-on work and has learning work-related skills as its major goal. Traditional nursing clinical experiences are an example of experiential learning. In contrast, service learning involves work that meets actual community needs, has as one of its goals the fostering of "a sense of caring for others," and includes structured time for reflection (Bailey et al., 2002).

Service learning expands the learning environment for students and faculty. Service learning is population focused and therefore provides opportunities for students to act locally to solve social problems (Eads, 1994). Although a number of similarities are present, key differences exist between traditional learning and service learning (Richardson et al., 1996). These differences are summarized in Table 11-1.

Colleges and universities may perform service learning differently because of different institutional missions and traditions (Jacoby, 1996). Some universities embrace service learning as a philosophy, some as part of their spiritual mission. Others embrace service learning as part of a "commitment to citizenship,

TABLE 11-1   Differences Between Traditional Learning and Service Learning

	TRADITIONAL LEARNING	SERVICE LEARNING
Location	Classroom	Classroom, community
Teacher	Professor	Professor, preceptor/facilitator, patients
Learning	Writing	Writing
	Examinations	Examinations
	Passive	Active
	Authoritarian	Shared responsibility
	Structured	Reflective
	Compartmentalized	Expansive, integrative
	Cognitive	Cognitive and affective
	Short term	Short and long term
Reasoning	Deductive	Inductive
Evaluation	Professor	Professor, preceptor/facilitator, self-assessment by students

civic responsibility and participatory democracy, and still others ground their service learning programs in community partnerships" (Jacoby, 1996, p. 17).

Regardless of how universities embrace service learning, four cardinal components of service learning exist. Service learning must do the following (Jacoby, 1996; Shah & Glascoff, 1998):

1. Be experiential
2. Allow students to engage in activities that address human and community needs via structured opportunities for student learning and development
3. Be reflective
4. Embrace the concept of reciprocity between the learner and the person/organization being served

Service learning may be a separate course within the college curriculum or integrated as a thread throughout multiple courses. The trend is toward the latter. Faculty members intentionally and strategically plan to incorporate service learning experiences as part of a course. When service learning is integrated into existing courses, it is important that it is not added as an "additional" course requirement. Instead it should be a learning activity that replaces one or more learning activities previously used. Credit should be given for the learning and its relation to the course, not for the service alone. The service activity must match course content and enhance learning by allowing application of the theoretical principles taught in the classroom setting. Some colleges allow students to select an alternate learning activity if they do not wish to participate in service learning.

THEORETICAL FOUNDATIONS OF SERVICE LEARNING

Kolb's (1984) theory of experiential learning has been widely used as a theoretical basis for designing and analyzing service learning programs. Reflective observation about the experience is essential to the learning process. It links the concrete experience to abstract conceptualizations of that experience. Learning is increased when students are actively engaged in gaining knowledge through experiential problem solving and decision making (Dewey, 1933; Kolb, 1984; Miettinen, 2000). Use of reflection is built on the work of Kolb (1984) and Dewey (1916, 1933, 1938). In service learning, reflection is both a cognitive process (Kolb, 1984; Mezirow, 1990; Schon, 1983) and a structured learning activity (Silcox, 1994). Effective reflection fosters moral development and enhances moral decision making. Moral decisions involve an exercise of choice and a corresponding willingness to accept the responsibility for that choice (Gilligan, 1981).

Delve et al. (1990) developed a service learning model based on the theories of moral decision making and values clarification (Gilligan, 1982; Kohlberg, 1976). The model includes five phases of development: exploration, clarification, realization, activation, and internalization. It illustrates that service learning is developmental, providing students with an opportunity to move from charity to justice as they become more empathetic. Delve et al. (1990) believe that without that empathy, the student will not come to recognize the members of the patient population as valued individuals in the larger society and sources for new learning.

The pedagogy of service learning has powerful flexibility. It can be based on subject matter or learning process; it can connect theory and practice; it integrates several different approaches to knowledge and uses of knowledge; it encourages learning how to learn; and it can focus on a wide range of issues, problems, and interests (Pellietier, 1995).

OUTCOMES OF SERVICE LEARNING

Service learning in the curriculum provides opportunities for students to attain personal, professional, and curriculum goals. Service learning also contributes to the overall educational experience of the college or university and thus provides benefits to the institution as well.

Benefits to Students

A review of the literature on the outcomes of service learning reveals four themes: direct participation, self-knowledge, academic inquiry, and social impact (Bailey et al., 2002; Batchelder & Root, 1994; Battistoni, 1995; Callister & Hobbins-Garbett, 2000; Carter & Dunn, 2002; Cohen & Kinsey, 1994; Ehrlich, 1995; Fleischauer & Fleischauer, 1994; Giles & Eyler, 1994; Hales, 1997; Herman & Sassatelli, 2002; Kraft & Kielsmeier, 1995; Macy, 1994; Narsave et al., 2002; Pellietier, 1995; Redman & Clark, 2002; Schaffer & Peterson, 2001; Wills, 1992). Direct participation in the service learning activity assists with socialization into the profession, introduces new technical or professional skills, increases motivation to learn, and encourages self-directed learning (Bailey et al., 2002; Narsavage et al., 2002; Pellietier, 1995; Wills, 1992). Service learning has been found to provide a more thorough understanding of "self" and provides insight into personal strengths and weaknesses (Batchelder & Root, 1994; Ehrlich, 1995). It also has been found to contribute to the development of personal vision, moral sensitivity, clarification of values, and spirituality (Ehrlich, 1995; Fleischauer & Fleischauer, 1994; Hales, 1997; Macy, 1994). Service learning facilitates academic inquiry by connecting theory and practice, enhancing disciplinary understanding and understanding of complex material, bringing greater relevance to course material, and helping students to generalize their learning to new situations (Carter & Dunn, 2002; Cohen & Kinsey, 1994; Ehrlich, 1995; Hales, 1997; Kraft & Kielsmeier, 1995, Schaffer & Peterson, 2001; Williams, 1990). Service learning experiences also develop critical thinking (Battistoni, 1995; Callister & Hobbins-Garbett, 2000; Herman & Sassatelli, 2002), leadership, and professional skills (Giles & Eyler, 1994; Hales, 1997; Pellietier, 1995; Schaffer & Peterson, 2001; Wills, 1992). The social impact of service learning includes the development of civic responsibility, increased orientation to volunteerism, increased political/global awareness, development of cultural competence, and improved ethical decision making (Herman & Sassatelli, 2002; Kraft & Kielsmeier, 1995; Palmer & Savoie, 2001; Redman & Clark, 2002; Wills, 1992).

Institutional Benefits

Service learning also has institutional benefits. These include invigoration of the campus educational culture, development of a strong sense of campus community, increased institutional visibility, and enhanced appeal to potential donors (Cooper, 1993; Molledahl, 1994; Pellietier, 1995; Rehnke, 1995; Wills, 1992). Service learning invigorates the campus culture by increasing students' engagement in their own learning, revitalizing faculty, and allowing faculty to mesh service projects with research interests (Pellietier, 1995; Rehnke, 1995; Wills, 1992). The interdisciplinary nature of service learning helps the campus to regain a strong ethos of community, keeps students and faculty more engaged in the life of the college, and contributes to student retention (Hamner et al., 2002; Pellietier, 1995). Increased institutional visibility contributes to increased student recruitment by providing a visible link between the community and the institution and by providing a perception of access to higher education to community members who have not believed higher education to be within their reach (Cooper, 1993; Molledahl, 1994; Pellietier, 1995; Wills, 1992). Service learning enhances the institution's appeal to potential donors by providing a direct link between the college and the community and also appeals to donors interested in community service educational reform (Pellietier, 1995).

The mentoring environment that is created between students, faculty, staff, administration, and the broader community becomes a "complex ecology of higher education . . . that can provide knowledge, support, and inspiration" (Daloz et al., 1996). The new alliances formed between academic institutions and community service agencies/organizations eliminate or minimize the traditional separation between the "gown and the town." Cotton and Stanton (1990) indicated that the gap between gown and town is bridged by successful service learning programs that cultivate "a spirit of reciprocity, interdependence, and collaboration" (p. 101).

INTEGRATING SERVICE LEARNING INTO THE CURRICULUM

Integrating service learning experiences into the curriculum requires careful planning. The experience must be developed and resources acquired before the course is offered. Faculty development is key to success.

Planning Faculty Development

Planning for a change to service learning begins with faculty development that may be available from the academic institution, workshops, and independent study. These resources will help faculty obtain essential information about how to design and implement service learning. A few of the practical considerations involved in planning service learning include establishing good relationships with community agencies, identifying the types of experiences suitable for the course content, finding agency representative supervisors, structuring the types of activities, and scheduling the activity.

Preparation links the service learning activities to specific learning outcomes and prepares students to perform the activities. The service needs to be challenging, engaging, and meaningful to the students, and it must focus on meeting an actual community need that students can perceive as important and relevant to their own development.

Preparation also includes finding agencies for student placement. Students involved in service learning typically work in voluntary not-for-profit community or public tax-supported service agencies/organizations that provide services that meet people's actual needs. Agencies and programs are selected on the basis of their congruence with the academic program or course and student goals and objectives.

Faculty development provides an explanation of a new pedagogy for many and establishes a common definition and a sound knowledge base. Consultants can be an invaluable aid in this early development process. It is also helpful for faculty to make contact with faculty in other colleges to identify what others have been doing. The Internet can be a means of making contact with other faculty involved in service learning. LISTSERVs are available, and many sources of information are available on the Internet that list faculty involved in service learning. The Internet can also be a source of information about starting service learning programs, sample course descriptions, syllabi, LISTSERVs, funding resources, and best practices. Some of the most widely recognized Internet resources are the following:

http://www.compact.org (Campus Compact)
http://csf.colorado.edu/sl/ (Colorado Service-Learning Homepage)
http://www.cns.gov (Corporation for National and Community Service)
http://www.servicelearning.org (National Service-Learning Clearinghouse)
http://www.nslexchange.org/ (National Service-Learning Exchange)
http://www.studentsinservicetoamerica.org (Students in Service to America)

Faculty support is also important to cultivating success. Faculty can organize a faculty service learning committee or advisory board. This group could be an invaluable advocate of service learning as a teaching tool. The committee can establish faculty handbooks and guidelines for service learning courses, sponsor brown bag lunches on service learning for particular departments or collegewide, and organize faculty development opportunities regarding service learning pedagogy. This committee also encourages the development of interdisciplinary professional relationships and provides an avenue for sharing ideas, successes, and failures.

The goal of planning and faculty development is to work for sustainability of service learning throughout the curriculum. Funding for service learning can be obtained from the community, from grant funding, and often from the college or university itself. Although service learning is not expensive, it does require time for planning and course development and the personnel to make the arrangements. A number of colleges and universities have a service learning office or coordinator. Staff from this office provide assistance in structuring the program, identifying community partners, and placing students according to mutual needs.

Selecting Placement Sites

It is important to match the type of community organization and service with the institutional mission of the college when service learning experiences are being planned. Before making plans regarding service placements, faculty should conduct a community needs assessment and develop a resource inventory, either informally through personal and telephone contact or formally through surveys or needs assessments. Community agency staff are invaluable in determining where students are needed the most. Allowing community partners to control the identification of the service helps to ensure that projects meet agency needs. Involvement of agency staff in the planning process also helps educate community agencies about service learning. Community advisory boards often help ensure continual contact between agencies, students, faculty, and staff and ascertain evolving community needs.

Once placement sites have been determined and service learning projects are finalized, preceptors must be identified and dates for student orientation and initial meetings must be planned. Written project descriptions, contact information, and a schedule of initial meetings should be available for students on the first day of class. Organization before the start of the semester ensures that students get started on projects promptly and are likely to complete projects within the semester time limit.

Although careful planning prevents many problems, faculty members should be prepared for the unexpected. Occasionally the needs of community agencies change (e.g., because of funding cuts or receiving a grant), there may be conflicts between agencies' needs for services and students' schedules, or there may be dissatisfaction. Sources of dissatisfaction may include students' perception of inequality of time investment between groups, failure of the reality of the situation to match expectations, and problems in communication (Schaffer & Peterson, 2001). Faculty members may need to intervene to prevent the escalation of problems and to renegotiate expectations.

Planning Learning Activities

Service learning can be used as an experientially based pedagogy to bring excitement and vitality to the classroom, to assist community members in need while at the same time learning from them, and to provide students with information and experiences through which to engage in critical reflection about society's needs and one's responsibility to the community (Palmer & Savoie, 2001). Opportunities for service learning may be discovered from a number of sources. Faculty may identify appropriate situations for service learning from their own service activities in a wide variety of community agencies. Service opportunities may also be suggested by friends, colleagues, agency personnel, or students, or they may be found in the professional or secular literature. When faculty have identified potential service learning experiences that seem to be appropriate for the course, discussions and negotiations are held with the agency staff.

Legal issues also need to be considered when planning service activities. Any time a student performs service off campus in conjunction with coursework, liability issues can arise. Faculty should seek legal counsel from the college or university regarding activities with potential liability just as legal counsel is sought when contracts with clinical agencies are established.

Once service learning experiences have been planned students must be engaged. Faculty can use groups such as the student nurses association, student government, the student life office, and campus publicity mechanisms (e.g., newspaper, radio station, bulletin boards) to inform students about service learning. Often courses or service learning components of courses are open to students from a variety of disciplines, and faculty should distribute the course announcements widely. Service learning's best promoters are its own students, who attract other students by word of mouth.

Student activities are planned so that they relate to the course objectives and content (Kendall, 1990). Types of agencies and programs that could be used for nursing students engaged in service learning include state or county services for persons with different forms of impairment or disability, various types of health and health care facilities, social welfare agencies and daycare programs, Meals on Wheels, senior centers, youth services, civic leagues, drug education programs, and groups or committees related to some aspects of government. Community agencies offer many opportunities for students to collaborate with the agency to fulfill unmet needs. Some service experiences will involve assessment, others work in ongoing programs, and still others development and implementation of new programs or services. During the final phase of the service experience, students who have developed new programs should work with agency partners to establish plans for sustainability. Students should compile materials to facilitate this continuation.

SERVICE LEARNING IN THE NURSING CURRICULUM

The Pew Health Professions Commission (1998) identified service learning as a key competency for programs educating health professionals. Community-based service learning is increasingly being integrated into nursing courses (Callister & Hobbins-Garbett, 2000). Some of the service learning endeavors are part of a larger consortium. An example of this is the Community-Campus Partnerships for Health (CCPH), an independent, nonprofit organization that organized the Partners in Caring and Community: Service Learning in Nursing Education project. The Partners in Caring and Community project works with teams of nursing faculty and students and their community partners to facilitate the integration of service learning into nursing education curricula, increase the understanding and support for service learning in nursing education, and disseminate new knowledge and information about best practices and models of service learning and nursing education (CCPH, n.d.). The CCPH website *(http://futurehealth.ucsf.edu/ccph/pcc.html)* provides links to participatory institutions and a wide variety of information.

Examples of independent service learning projects from nursing programs across the nation include the following:

Yale University School of Nursing's linkage of service learning with health policy in graduate nursing education. Students spend the first half of the semester in the classroom learning background material and the second half of that semester and all of the following semester in a service learning experience. Past student placements include the Connecticut Women's Health Campaign, where the student coordinated a coalition of organizations and developed fact sheets to educate women and public officials on issues such as breast cancer legislation and access to health insurance, and the Connecticut Department of Health, where the status of the state's safety net providers was analyzed for the Commissioner of Health to assist in planning services and allocating public funds for health care (Cohen & Milone-Nuzzo, 2001).

Indiana University School of Nursing's collaboration with a sister city in Nicaragua to provide an international service learning course. Students were provided with information about the Nicaraguan culture before starting the experience. Activities included conducting a nutritional needs assessment; providing prenatal education for community health workers and lay midwives, with a special emphasis on nutrition; and supporting the relief efforts in refugee camps following Hurricane Mitch (Riner & Becklenburg, 2001).

The University of New Mexico Department of Nursing's elective in Community and Public Service. This course provides service learning experiences for nursing students while increasing their understanding of disenfranchised or special needs populations. Placement sites include a childcare center for homeless children, a senior citizen's program, a center serving teenage parents, a mission for homeless individuals, Habitat for Humanity, and Head Start (Hales, 1997).

The Ohio State University College of Nursing's clinical site for senior pediatric nursing students in the local Head Start schools based on service learning principles. This provides an opportunity for students to work with an underserved sector of society that has a variety of needs and challenges that are often different from their own. Students provide health and developmental screenings, create handouts for parents, assess the social behavior of children, read safety storybooks to the children, and assist with classroom activities (Kulewicz, 2001).

Nebraska Methodist College Department of Nursing's faith-based partnership with Catholic Charities in Omaha. Several Catholic Charities programs were targeted for service experiences, including an emergency shelter for battered women and their children, an addiction recovery treatment center for economically disadvantaged individuals, food pantries, and an inner-city school counseling service. Initially the Department of Nursing focused on students' ability to apply theoretical knowledge during the service experience. However, Herman and Sassatelli (2002) report that as the program evolved, it embraced Brackley's (1988) challenge to have the "courage not to turn away from the eyes of the poor, but to allow them to break our hearts and shatter our world" (p. 38). They also incorporated Dorr's (1993) emphasis on the importance of not only feeling for economically disadvantaged individuals but also discovering what it means to be with them. Faculty and students found that companionship with economically disadvantaged individuals during the service experience encouraged understanding of what it means to be humanly weak and powerless (Herman & Sassetelli, 2002).

School of Nursing at the University of Colorado Health Sciences Center. Faculty extended the reach of their service learning initiative to include distance education students by reformulating the course in a Web-based format, with the materials available online (Redman & Clark, 2002). An asynchronous forum allows discussions with opportunities for reflection. Descriptions of agencies and service projects used by on-campus students are posted online to help distance education students find comparable experiences within their own community. Faculty members work collaboratively with students to finalize arrangements with those agencies.

Incorporating Reflection

Reflection is a critical and an essential aspect of service learning that further differentiates it from volunteerism, community service activities, and nursing students' clinical experiences (Hatcher & Bringle, 1995; Kendall, 1990). Reflection is an active, persistent, thoughtful, and intentional consideration of the service activity. Reflection must include the student's behavior, practice, and achievement. Within the reflective process, students must respond to basic questions, such as What am I doing? Why am I doing it? and What am I learning? and they should critically examine their actions, feelings, and thoughts. During this examination and while responding to the questions posed, students contemplate, think, reason, and speculate about their service experiences (Fertman, 1994).

Reflection is a learning tool that serves to maximize students' highly individualized learning experiences by linking the service experiences with the learning objectives established for the course and curriculum. Reflection combines cognitive and affective activities in a way that bridges the gap between the service experience and the course.

Reflection also provides opportunities for students to improve their self-assessment skills and have insights that help build on their strengths. Because reflection and self-assessment are skills that require development, many students new to service learning find faculty facilitation during reflection activities helpful (Elam et al., 2002).

Faculty responsibilities include designing reflection activities, coaching students during reflection, monitoring students' reflections, and providing feedback (Rama, 2001). The Service Reflection Toolkit developed by Northwest Service Academy is available on the Internet *(http://www.studentsinservice-toamerica.org/tools_resources/docs/nwtoolkit.pdf)* and provides a collection of reflection activities that faculty may find valuable. Faculty will also find a wealth of other information on reflection activities available on the Web.

Reflection is most effective when it is continuous, connected, contextual, and challenging (Eyler et al., 1996; Williams, 1990). Continuous reflection involves reflection before, during, and after the service learning experience. Connecting service with classroom learning assists students to develop a conceptual framework for their service project and to apply concepts and theories learned in class to the experience. Reflection must be appropriate for the context and setting of the experience. Some service learning experiences lend themselves to formal methods of reflection, such as written papers, whereas others are best suited to informal discussions. Whether formal or information methods are used, reflection should challenge students to think in new ways, question their assumptions, and formulate new understandings and new ways of problem solving (Rama, 2001).

Including service partners in the reflective dialogue enhances communication and increases the depth and breadth of learning. Without an emphasis on dialogue between individuals and community partners, reflection becomes one sided, focusing on the isolated views and perceptions of the individual student without coming to an understanding of each person's perspective (Noddings, 1992; Rama, 2001).

One common approach to stimulate reflection is to have students keep a journal or engage in directed writing that faculty read and respond to frequently throughout the course. Journals allow students to record thoughts, observations, feelings, activities, questions, and problems encountered and solved during the service learning experience. If students are working on a service learning project as a team, a team journal can be used to promote interaction between team members on project-related issues and to introduce students to different perspectives on the project (Rama, 2001).

Portfolios can be developed to organize materials related to the service learning project and document accomplishments and learning outcomes. Other reflective activities include small group discussions and presentations that relate the service experience to classroom concepts, introduce students to different perspectives, and challenge them to think critically about the service experience. It is helpful for faculty to pose a few questions to guide the discussion, but students should also be allowed to freely discuss and reflect on ideas and issues. In such discussions students often disclose expectations and myths about the service experience. Themes that may emerge during reflections include social analysis of community needs and the importance of civic responsibility (Bailey et al., 2002). A final reflective paper based on the writing done during the semester provides a comprehensive description of students' learning (Hatcher & Bringle, 1995).

Bringle and Hatcher's (1996) guidelines help clarify the nature of effective reflection activities in a service learning course. Effective reflection activities do the following:

1. Link the service learning experiences to the learning objectives
2. Are designed, structured, and guided by faculty
3. Are planned so that they occur across the span of service learning experience
4. Permit faculty feedback and assessment of progress and learning
5. Foster the clarification and exploration of values

Evaluation

After the completion of service learning, faculty should evaluate student outcomes, the usefulness of the service learning experience, and the contribution of the experience to overall curriculum goals. Evaluation of students' achievement is based on the students' learning and not merely on their experience or participation in the service activities. Faculty, the agency supervisor, and students' self-assessment provide the evaluation data.

Many faculty administer preservice and postservice surveys that measure students' attitudes toward community service and civic responsibility and toward their coursework. Such instruments not only help faculty evaluate their students and assess the usefulness of service learning but also help students see how much they have learned and how their attitudes may have changed because of their service learning experience. In addition to the short-term course evaluation, a systematic long-term follow-up of students helps to determine any additional learning that may have occurred after the course is completed.

Challenges

Some of the challenges to implementing service learning result from ordinary budgetary constraints in higher education (Palmer & Savoie, 2001). Multiple departments and programs compete for limited resources. Those beginning a service learning initiative may need to search for external funding sources and rely on the goodwill of faculty members willing to spend extra time learning about service learning and then incorporating service learning into their courses without extra compensation.

Institutions that lack a dedicated service learning office may struggle with organization and effective evaluation strategies. When funding issues prevent the establishment of a service learning office, a service learning council composed of faculty members from each department on campus can provide direction for faculty development, coordinate student learning activities with community agencies, evaluate service learning experiences, and facilitate the sharing of information (Palmer & Savoie, 2001).

Convincing faculty members to adopt service learning as an effective pedagogical device can also be a challenge. This resistance is understandable because of the time and effort involved in incorporating service learning into courses. Faculty members involved in service learning often serve as the best change agents as they extol the benefits of service learning, including increased student engagement in the learning process and increased sense of collegiality because of their intradisciplinary and interdisciplinary activities (Palmer & Savoie, 2001).

Challenges encountered by faculty include time constraints; students' commitments to work and family; and students', faculty's, and community partners' heavy workloads. Community partners may struggle with orienting new students each semester and the lack of students during summer break (Holloway, 2002; Mayne & Glascoff, 2002). Several universities reported designing experiences lasting more than one semester or encouraging students taking multiple courses with service learning components to remain at the same community agency to increase continuity (Cohen & Milone-Nuzzo, 2001; Holloway, 2002).

SUMMARY

Service learning is not new. However, it has been recently revived on college campuses and within nursing curricula. Nursing faculty have the opportunity to be leaders on their campus and enhance learning through the integration of a service learning experience in the curriculum. Service learning experiences have the benefits of increasing retention of academic material and fostering global awareness and a sense of social responsibility within the participants. Service learning is a win–win situation for the college, the students, the community agency, and the patients.

REFERENCES

Bailey, P. A., Carpenter, D. R., & Harrington, P. (2002). Theoretical foundations of service-learning in nursing education. *Journal of Nursing Education, 41*(10), 433-436.

Batchelder, T. H., & Root, S. (1994). Effects of an undergraduate program to integrate academic learning and service: Cognitive, prosocial cognitive, and identity outcomes. *Journal of Adolescence, 17*(4), 341-355.

Battistoni, R. (1995). Service learning, diversity, and the liberal arts curriculum. *Liberal Education, 81*(1), 30-35.

Boyer, E. (1987). *College: The undergraduate experience in America.* Princeton, NJ: The Carnegie Foundation for the Advancement of Teaching.

Brackley, D. S. J. (1988). Downward mobility: Social implications of St. Ignatius's two standards in studies of spirituality of Jesuits. *Studies in Spirituality of Jesuits, 20*(1), 38.

Bringle, R. G., & Hatcher, J. A. (1996). Implementing service learning in higher education. *Journal of Higher Education, 67*(2), 221-239.

Callister, L. C., & Hobbins-Garbett, D. (2000). Enter to learn, go forth to serve: Service learning in nursing education. *Journal of Professional Nursing, 16*(3), 177-183.

Carter, J., & Dunn, B. (2002). Educational innovations. A service-learning partnership for enhanced diabetes management. *Journal of Nursing Education, 41*(10), 450-452.

Cohen, J., & Kinsey, D. F. (1994). "Doing good" and scholarship: A service-learning study. *Journalism Educator, 48*(4), 4-14.

Cohen, S. S., & Milone-Nuzzo, P. (2001). Advancing health policy in nursing education through service learning. *Advances in Nursing Science, 23*(3), 28-40.

Community-Campus Partnerships for Health (CCPH), Partners in Caring and Community. (n.d.). *Service-learning in nursing education.* Retrieved June 19, 2003, from http://futurehealth.ucsf.edu/ccph/pcc.html

Cooper, J. (1993). Developing community partnerships through service learning programs. *Campus Activities Programming, 26*(1), 27-31.

Cotton, D., & Stanton, T. K. (1990). Joining campus and community through service learning. In C. I. Delve, S. D. Mintz, & G. M. Stewart (Eds.), *Community service as values education: New directions for student services.* San Francisco: Jossey-Bass.

Daloz, L. A., Keen, C. H., Keen, J. P., & Parks, S. D. (1996). Lives of commitment. *Change, 28*(3), 11-15.

Delve, C. I., Mintz, S. D., & Stewart, G. M. (1990). Promoting values development through community service: A design. *New Directions for Student Services, 50*(2), 7-29.

Dewey, J. (1916). *Democracy and education.* New York: Macmillan.

Dewey, J. (1933). *How we think.* Boston: Heath.

Dewey, J. (1938). *Experience and education.* New York: Macmillan.

Dorr, D. (1993). *Options for the poor: A hundred years of Vatican social teaching.* Maryknoll, NY: Orbis Books.

Eads, S. E. (1994). The value of service learning in higher education. In R. J. Kraft & M. Swadner (Eds.), *Building community: Service learning in the academic disciplines* (pp. 35-40). Denver: Colorado Campus Compact.

Ehrlich, T. (1995, March). Taking service seriously. *AAHE Bulletin, 47*(7), 8-10.

Elam, C. L., Musick, D. W., Sauer, M. J., & Skelton, J. (2002). How we implemented a service-learning elective. *Medical Teacher, 24*(3), 249-253.

Eyler, J., Giles, D. E., & Schmiede, A. (1996). *A practitioner's guide to reflection in service learning: Student voices and reflections.* A technical assistance project funded by the Corporation for National Service. Nashville, TN: Vanderbilt University.

Fertman, C. L. (1994). *Service learning for all students.* Bloomington, IN: Phi Delta Kappa Educational Foundation.

Fleischauer, J. P., & Fleischauer, J. F. (1994). College credit for community service: A "win-win" situation. *Journal of Experiential Education, 17*(3), 41-44.

Giles, D. E., & Eyler, J. (1994). The impact of a college community service laboratory on students' personal, social, and cognitive outcomes. *Journal of Adolescence, 17*(4), 327-339.

Gilligan, C. (1981). Moral development in the college years. In A. Chickering (Ed.), *The modern American college.* San Francisco: Jossey-Bass.

Gilligan, C. (1982). *In a different voice: Psychological theory and women's development.* Cambridge, MA: Harvard University Press.

Hales, A. (1997). Service-learning within the nursing curriculum. *Nurse Educator, 22*(2), 15-18.

Hamner, J. B., Wilder, B., Avery, G., & Byrd, L. (2002). Community-based service learning in the engaged university. *Nursing Outlook, 50*(2), 67-71.

Hatcher, J. A., & Bringle, R. G. (1995). *Reflection: Bridging the gap between service and learning.* Unpublished manuscript, Indianapolis, IN: Indiana University-Purdue University-Indianapolis.

Herman, C. & Sassatelli, J. (2002). DARING to reach the heartland: A collaborative faith-based partnership in nursing education. *Journal of Nursing Education, 41*(10), 443-445.

Holloway, A. S. (2002). Educational innovations. Service-learning in community college nursing education. *Journal of Nursing Education, 41*(10), 440-442.

Jacoby, B. (1996). *Service-learning in higher education: Concepts and practices.* San Francisco: Jossey-Bass.

Kendall, J. C. (1990). *Combining service and learning: A resource book for community and public service* (Vol. 1). Raleigh, NC: National Society for Internships and Experiential Education.

Kohlberg, L. (1976). Moral stages and moralization: The cognitive-developmental approach. In T. Lickona (Ed.), *Moral development and behavior: Theory, research and social issues.* New York: Holt, Rinehart & Winston.

Kolb, D. A. (1984). *Experiential learning: Experience as the source of learning and development.* Englewood Cliffs, NJ: Prentice Hall.

Kraft, R. J., & Kielsmeier, J. (Eds.). (1995). *Experiential learning in schools and higher education.* Boulder, CO: Association for Experiential Education.

Kulewicz, S. J. (2001). Service learning: Head Start and a baccalaureate nursing curriculum working together. *Pediatric Nursing, 27*(1), 27-43.

Macy, J. E. (1994). A model for service learning: Values development for higher education. *Campus Activities Programming, 27*(4), 62, 64-69.

Mayne, L., & Glascoff, M. (2002). Service learning: Preparing a health care workforce for the next century. *Nurse Educator, 27*(4), 191-194.

Mezirow, J. (1990). How critical reflection triggers transformative learning. In J. Mezirow (Ed.), *Fostering critical reflection in adulthood: A guide to transformative and emancipatory learning.* San Francisco: Jossey-Bass.

Miettinen, R. (2000). The concept of experiential learning and John Dewey's theory of reflective thought and action. *International Journal of Lifelong Education, 19,* 54-73.

Miller, S. L. (1995). *Volunteerism, community service & service learning on Catholic campuses.* Paper presented at the Association of Catholic Colleges and Universities conference, St. Paul, MN, August 3-6, 1995.

Molledahl, A. K. (1994, Winter). Student volunteers live out Catholic mandate of service. *St. Thomas,* 27-30.

Narsavage, G. L., Lindell, D., Chen, Y., Savrin, C., & Duffy, E. (2002). A community engagement initiative: Service-learning in graduate nursing education. *Journal of Nursing Education, 41*(10), 457-461.

Noddings, N. (1992). *The challenge to care in schools: An alternative approach to education.* New York: Teachers College Press.

Palmer, C. E., & Savoie, E. J. (2001). Service learning: A conceptual overview. In G. P. Poirrier (Ed.), *Service learning: Curricular applications in nursing.* Boston: Jones and Bartlett.

Pascarella, E. T., & Terenzini, P. T. (1991). *How college affects students: Findings and insights from twenty years of research.* San Francisco: Jossey-Bass.

Pellietier, S. (1995, April). The quiet power of service learning: Report from the national institute on learning and service. *The Independent, 95*(4), 7-10.

Pew Health Professions Commission. (1998). *Recreating health professional practice for a new century.* San Francisco: The Center for Health Professions.

Rama, D. V. (2001). *Using structured reflection to enhance learning from service.* Retrieved June 19, 2003, from http://www.compact.org/disciplines/reflection

Redman, R. W., & Clark, L. (2002). Educational innovations. Service learning as a model for integrating social justice in the nursing curriculum. *Journal of Nursing Education, 41*(10), 446-449.

Rehnke, M. A. F. (1995). Teaching and learning: Why should colleges encourage community service learning? *The Independent, 95*(2), 6.

Richardson, B., Billings, D. M., & Martin, J. S. (1996). *Service learning as a pedagogy for community-based nursing education.* Poster presented at the NLN-CRNE 13th Conference on Research in Nursing Education, San Antonio, TX, January 10-13, 1996.

Riner, M. E., & Becklenberg, A. (2001). Partnering with a sister city organization for an international service-learning experience. *Journal of Transcultural Nursing, 12*(3), 234-240.

Schaffer, M. A., & Peterson, S. J. (2001). Teaching undergraduate research and group leadership skills through service learning projects. In G. P. Poirrier (Ed.), *Service learning: Curricular applications in nursing.* Boston: Jones and Bartlett.

Schon, D. A. (1983). *The reflective practitioner: How professionals think in action.* New York: Basic Books.

Shah, N., & Glascoff, M. (1998). The community as classroom: Service learning in Tillery, North Carolina. In J. Norbeck, C. Connelly, & J. Koerner (Eds.), *Caring and community: Concepts and models for service-learning in nursing* (pp. 111-118). Washington DC: American Association for Higher Education.

Silcox, H. C. (1994). *A how to guide to reflection: Adding cognitive learning to community service programs.* Holland, PA: Brighton Press.

Stanton, T. K. (1990). Service learning: Groping toward a definition. In *Combining service and learning: A resource book for community and public service* (Vol. 1). Raleigh, NC: National Society for Internships and Experiential Education.

Williams, R. (1990). The impact of field education on student development: Research findings. In J. C. Kendall & Associates (Eds.), *Combining service and learning: A resource book for community and public service* (Vol. 1, pp. 130-147). Raleigh, NC: National Society for Internships and Experiential Education.

Wills, J. (1992). Service: On campus and in the curriculum. *Educational Record, 73*(2), 32-36.

UNIT III

TEACHING AND LEARNING

12

FROM TEACHING TO LEARNING
THEORETICAL FOUNDATIONS

Melissa Vandeveer, PhD, RN, PNP, Barbara Norton, RN, MPH

Teaching and learning are dynamic processes. Recent literature on learning suggests a paradigm shift away from an emphasis on the teacher and teaching to an emphasis on the learner and learning. This shift places the purpose of the educational enterprise on the end results of the process by which learning occurs.

The learning paradigm, as opposed to the instructional paradigm, "frames learning holistically, recognizing that the chief agent in the process is the learner" (Barr & Tagg, 1995, p. 21). Within this process, faculty are responsible for "creating environments and experiences that bring students to discover and construct knowledge for themselves" (Barr & Tagg, 1995, p. 15). In the learning paradigm, the learning environment and learning experiences are learner centered and learner controlled. In contrast, the instructional paradigm positions the faculty as the chief controlling agent providing instruction with the expectation of transferring knowledge to students. Faculty perceive students and students see themselves as passive receivers, taking in information and then recalling it during examinations.

The purposes of this chapter are to (1) differentiate between the processes of teaching and learning, (2) explore the dimensions of the teaching–learning process, and (3) provide an overview of selected learning theories and pedagogical or educational frameworks that can be used to guide faculty and learners in their quest to discover nursing knowledge.

TEACHING

Teaching is a complex and abstract concept that has several definitions. Teaching is a system of directed and deliberate actions that are intended to induce learning through a series of directed activities designed to induce learning (Heidgerken, 1953; Hyman, 1974). Bevis (1989a) defined teaching as an art and science in which the content is structured and the processes used enable student learning. For Bevis (1989a), teaching includes determining the objectives, arranging the instructional materials, creating the learning activities, and evaluating student learning. However, Bevis (1989c) addressed the need for teachers to restructure their perception of the teaching role from one that focuses on establishing the climate, structure, and teaching role to one that focuses on establishing the climate, structure, and dialogues that engage students' intellectual processes. This redirected focus is necessary so that students will be able to find patterns that can eventually be used as their prototypes for clinical practice. Intellectual engagement is promoted through the use of questions that direct students to read, observe, analyze, and reflect on the care of patients. Within this context, teachers are also involved in nurturing students, ethical ideals, caring, creativity, curiosity, assertiveness, and dialogue.

Davis (1993) also viewed teaching as a science and art. In nursing education the science aspect of teaching is based in a body of knowledge derived from the theories and research from natural and social science disciplines, such as microbiology, anatomy, physiology, anthropology, psychology, sociology, and speech communication. In addressing the art aspect of teaching, Eisner (1983) used the analogy of an orchestra conductor for the teacher because conductors and teachers must use a wide variety of skills while making judgments about complex issues that arise while conducting or teaching. The teacher and conductor must be prepared to deal creatively with unexpected events. For example, although the conductor and teacher are knowledgeable about the musical score and content for a given session, both persons must provide appropriate guidance, attend to the responses from the participating members, maintain and adjust the desired pace, make every effort to evoke the best responses, and be flexible and creative when the members have problems producing the desired effect.

LEARNING

In general, learning is considered a change in a person that has been caused by experience (Slavin, 1988). Learning is a process of understanding, clarifying, and applying the meanings of the knowledge acquired. Furthermore, learning is the exploration, discovery, refinement, and extension of the learner's meanings of the knowledge (Heidgerken, 1953). Learning occurs when an individual's behavior or knowledge changes.

Learning has also been defined from the perspectives of two major bodies of learning theory: behaviorism and cognitivism. The behavioristic perspective views learning as a change in observable behavior or performance resulting from some external reinforcers that stimulate the change. To be considered learning, a change in performance must come about as a result of the learner's interaction with the environment (Driscoll, 1994). In contrast, the cognitive perspective views learning as occurring when a new experience alters some unobservable mental processes that may or may not be manifested by a change in behavior or performance.

Bevis (1988) proposed that the distinction between training and education is essential for the development of curriculum and indicated six types of learning (Box 12-1). The first three types of learning are associated with technical aspects and may be observed. The last three are associated with mental processes that may or may not produce an observable change.

> **Box 12-1**
> **SIX TYPES OF LEARNING**
>
> Directive learning
> Item learning
> Rational learning
> Contextual learning
> Inquiry learning
> Syntactical learning
>
> From Bevis, E. O. (1988). New directions for a new age. In *Curriculum revolution: Mandate for change* (pp. 27-52). New York: National League for Nursing.

Learning is self-active; it can be accomplished only by the learner. Learning is influenced by a person's profile of intelligences (Gardner, 1983), background, and experience; by the type of learning activities and the degrees of participation in the teaching–learning situation (Barr & Tagg, 1995); and by the power structure that dictates what knowledge is valid (Freire, 1971).

TEACHING–LEARNING PROCESS

The teaching–learning process or transaction is a complex cooperative and personal relationship between faculty and students. When viewed from the perspective of the "learning paradigm" rather than the "instructional paradigm," the teaching–learning process is a personal interactive relationship that extends beyond the subject matter. Within the interactive relationship faculty relate to students with dignity and respect, with the expectation that students will be supported and stimulated to develop intellectual integrity and independent judgment (Hyman, 1974). The roles of the teacher are facilitator, guide, coach, and mentor acting in partnership with students. The student roles become those of learner inquirer and seeker of knowledge within an active participative student–faculty relationship.

In a humanistic model both the faculty, as senior learner, and student, as junior learner, are engaged in the teaching–learning process (Rogers, 1969). According to Diekelmann (1989), both teacher and learner engage in a transformed relationship as a result of meaningful dialogue with one another. Shared responsibility and an egalitarian relationship between student and teacher are also key components of feminist pedagogy (Wheeler & Chinn, 1989).

Bevis (1988) identified the purpose of nursing education as twofold: to ensure safety and to provide the climate, structure, and dialogue that promote praxis. The roles associated with these purposes include raising questions; nurturing creative drive, caring, assertiveness, and ethics; designing ways to engage mental processes; and interacting with students as persons of worth, dignity, intelligence, and high scholarly standards.

The four steps of the teaching–learning process are assessment, planning, implementation, and evaluation. The process is circular, with each step interacting with the preceding and subsequent step.

Assessment

Assessment has three major components: the curricular attributes, the faculty attributes, and the student attributes. The program and course objectives, critical learning experiences, and learning outcomes must be thoughtfully examined. These curricular components provide the foundation for identifying and preparing the appropriate content that is to be taught.

Faculty also need to appraise their own attributes, including their level of content knowledge, their philosophy and attitudes about teaching, and the instructional skills they already possess and those they want to develop. Faculty should be well informed about various theories of learning and other theories relevant for teaching and learning. Appropriate theories relevant to learning are used as a framework to design the teaching–learning process.

Students' personal attributes that are particularly relevant are those associated with successful learning. Student attributes having significant bearing on the decisions made for the entire teaching–learning process include the students' entry knowledge and skills, cognitive abilities, learning styles, motivation to achieve, study habits, readiness to learn the content, and preference for instructional methods (Snow & Peterson, 1980).

Data about students' personal attributes can be obtained from various sources. Students' entry knowledge and skills can be obtained from a brief review of the course materials and texts used for prerequisite courses; this helps to establish reasonable expectations of the students. Informal discussions with faculty and students are another excellent source of entry-level information. During the first or second class meeting, students' interest in the course and content and their perception of the class's relationship with previous and concurrent courses can be elicited through class discussion. Students can also be asked about individual skills, abilities, and personal gifts that have not been directly associated with their formal education in a nursing program. This type of discussion often stimulates a lively interaction and helps students to become aware of faculty interest in the student as a whole person. Individual learning styles and preferences can also be elicited. See Chapter 2 for further discussion on assessment of student learning styles.

Planning

Assessment data are used as a foundation for instructional planning. Instructional plans are essential for good teaching; plans serve to help faculty better prepare to meet their teaching responsibilities. Instructional plans can be thought of as maps developed at the course, unit, and lesson level.

Instructional planning includes selecting and organizing the appropriate and essential content in a logical and meaningful sequence, with attention given to the appropriate delineation of the important relationships between facts, concepts, and principles. Planning also includes selecting the instructional strategies and designing all of the learning activities. Developing a map of all of the lesson plans before the course begins is beneficial because it helps to ensure that the content will be adequately addressed and allows faculty to examine the variety of instructional strategies and learning activities to be used throughout the course. See Chapter 10 for further discussion about planning learning experiences and developing instructional plans.

Implementation

To enhance student achievement, faculty should be flexible when adapting and modifying preselected instructional strategies or when implementing the predesigned lesson plan. Students' verbal and nonverbal responses during the lesson usually provide cues that indicate a need for some further explanation, clarification, or additional practice in applying the content. The common saying, "There is the lesson you planned to give, the lesson you gave, and the lesson you wished you had given" provides some insight into the need for flexibility and an awareness of recognizing that the practice of teaching is an ever-evolving process.

Evaluation

Evaluation is the final step of an iterative teaching–learning model. Formative and summative evaluations are two common forms of evaluation used during instruction. Formative evaluation is used to determine student progress throughout the course and is often used during a class session. Informal strategies such as questions, discussion, and feedback about student participation and success in attaining the objectives of the learning activities provide faculty with valuable information about student comprehension and achievement during the lesson. Having students participate at the end of class in constructing a summary of the key points of the lesson also provides valuable information. Formative evaluation strategies can be considered diagnostic tools in that they help faculty to focus on difficulties students are having in attaining the learning outcomes and provide opportunities for corrective interventions designed to further facilitate learning (see Chapter 21).

Summative evaluation is conducted at the end of a course and is used to determine the extent to which students have achieved the desired learning outcomes. Strategies used for summative evaluation include multiple choice, essay, and short answer examinations; simulations; case studies; and formal papers. Faculty may choose to use the results of a combination of formative and summative evaluation data as the basis for assigning student grades.

The formative and summative evaluation strategies selected to determine student learning need to be consistent with the approaches used during the instructional strategies and learning activities. For additional information on evaluation and evaluation strategies see Unit V.

LEARNING THEORIES AND EDUCATIONAL FRAMEWORKS/PHILOSOPHIES

Learning theories and educational frameworks/philosophies provide the structure that guides the selection of faculty-centered instructional strategies and student-centered learning activities. Faculty's beliefs about learning provide the assumptions that underlie the approaches used in their teaching. Being cognizant of various theories is a prerequisite to effective teaching. Experienced and novice faculty are challenged to select theories that best support the school philosophy and at the same time complement individual teaching preferences.

Learning theories focus on how people learn, whereas educational frameworks/philosophies focus on identifying the methods that will provide students with the conditions that are most likely to facilitate attainment of the learning outcomes (Reigeluth, 1983). As faculty shift the emphasis from teaching to learning, educational frameworks may used to enhance the faculty-facilitated learning environment (Barr & Tagg, 1995).

Discussion of learning theories and educational frameworks/philosophies is organized in the following manner. After a brief overview of each theory or framework, additional information is presented from the perspectives of the basic premise, the setting or climate in which the theory or framework may be used, the role of the faculty, the role of the student, some of the advantages and disadvantages associated with theory or framework, and application. Summaries of the premises for the learning theories and educational frameworks/philosophies are presented in Box 12-2 and Table 12-1, respectively.

Learning theories and frameworks are descriptive in that they focus on and describe the processes used to bring about changes in either the way in which students perform or the way in which they understand or organize elements in their environment. Theories of learning include sets of concepts of psychological variables that are presented as laws or principles about learning. Theories of learning can be used as prescriptions that provide a focus for creating an environment and conditions in which the instruction will occur (Driscoll, 1994).

Psychologists have developed two principal types of learning theory—behavioral and cognitive—to explain how people learn. In addition to the cognitive theories, educators and counselors are using cognitive development

---

Box 12-2
PREMISES OF LEARNING THEORIES

- **Behavioral:** All behavior is learned and can be shaped and rewarded to attain desired ends.
- **Cognitive:** Conditions of learning influence acquisition and retention by modifying existing cognitive structures. Assimilation, accommodation, and construction of knowledge are basic processes in learning.
- **Cognitive development:** Development is sequential and progresses in an uneven and interrupted manner through several identifiable phases.
- **Cognitive development: sociocultural historical influences:** Learning is interactive and occurs in a social, historical context. Knowledge, ideas, attitudes, and values are developed as a result of relationships with people.
- **Multiple intelligences:** Human beings have unique profiles composed of varying degrees of eight and one half research-based intelligences.

theories because they focus on the ways in which thought processes develop over time and the influence those processes have on other dimensions of personality development (Widick & Simpson, 1978). Adult education and humanistic theories are also commonly used in educational programs. There is no single behavioral, cognitive, cognitive development, adult education, or humanistic theory; variations exist for each type of theory.

The learning theories discussed are behavioral, cognitive (including information processing, constructivism, and assimilation), cognitive development, cognitive development: sociocultural historical influences, and multiple intelligences (MI).

BEHAVIORAL LEARNING THEORIES

Ivan Pavlov and Edward Thorndike established the roots for behaviorism in the late nineteenth century with their systematic scientific investigation of how animals and human beings learn (Hilgard & Bower, 1966). The work of these men provided the basis for what became known as *behaviorist psychology.* Pavlov and Thorndike associated behavior with physical reflexes (Hilgard & Bower, 1966). However, Thorndike believed that the behavior was in response to rewards or reinforcements; he called this the *Law of Effect.* The focus of their research later became known as *stimulus–response theory.*

Skinner's principles of operant conditioning focus on arranging consequences for learner behavior (Slavin, 1988). Skinner suggested a different type of behavior associated with learning that he named *operant behaviors.* Operant behaviors are a person's responses that act on the environment as an immediate response to the consequence resulting from the behavior. A behavior is strengthened or weakened in response to positive or negative consequences. Positive consequences are referred to as *reinforcers* because they strengthen or increase the frequency of behaviors, whereas negative consequences weaken the behavior by not reinforcing it (Skinner, 1953; Slavin, 1988).

Complex behaviors are acquired by shaping through providing reinforcement. Reinforcement is an essential condition for learning because reinforced responses are remembered. Skinner defined learning as a process of behavioral change. A learning act consists of discrimination stimulus, learner response, and a consequence. Skinner's early work focused on behaviorism but later moved toward cognitivism.

Although all behaviorists do not have the same framework for their theories, there are some fundamental similarities in that they all look for behavioral change in the learner and define learning as permanent change in behavior. In addition, they all place great importance on the external environment as a main element in controlling what people learn (Dembo, 1988).

Since the 1950s the principles of behaviorism have been incorporated into the widely promulgated work of several renown educators. Tyler (1949) addressed the psychology of learning, the learning setting, and learning conditions and presented a model for writing behavioral objectives. Bloom et al. (1956) compiled a taxonomy of the cognitive domain incorporating the use of action verbs to differentiate levels of cognition. Mager (1962) developed a model for writing highly prescriptive behavioral objectives that consist of three components: specification of the behavior to be acquired, conditions under which the behavior is to be demonstrated, and the criteria for how well the behavior is to be performed.

The prominent nurse educators of the 1970s and 1980s who adopted the behavioristic paradigm into their works include Bevis (1973, 1978, 1982, 1989a), deTornyay (1971, 1982), deTornyay and Thompson (1987), Reilly (1975, 1980), and Reilly and Oermann (1990). As a result of these publications, programs in nursing education once made extensive use of the principles of behaviorism.

Premise

All behavior is learned; it can be shaped and rewarded to achieve appropriate and desired ends. Learning results from a process of attaching one element of learning to another in an environment in which external reinforcement stimulates a change in behavior (Grippin & Peters, 1984).

Setting/Climate

Behavioristic principles are used in classrooms, clinical settings, and learning resource centers in which the faculty design and control highly structured learning environments.

Role of Faculty

Faculty dominate the highly structured learning environment and perform as an authority, dispensing knowledge and wisdom while exercising control of the learning experiences. Formal control of the learning situation is clearly established by creating all of the favorable conditions required for learning., by providing all of the content and audiovisual media to be used, and by determining the time allowed for instruction and practice, as well as for breaks. Stimuli to which students are to respond are carefully selected. Learning occurs in an environment that consists of clearly established learning objectives and highly structured learning experiences in which student behavior is intentionally shaped and managed by faculty's cues, prompts, directions, and redirections.

Faculty establish a positive learning climate by responding to student success with a previously determined system of positive reinforcers (rewards) to shape behavior. The desired learner behavior or correct performance is reinforced by tangible rewards, such as praise or bonuses, whereas an absence of the desired behaviors, lack of achievement, or deviant behavior is ignored. Faculty's focus is on what the student is doing correctly rather than on what is being done incorrectly. Achievement is monitored by looking for behavior patterns demonstrated over a period.

Role of Student

Students follow faculty's directions and use the behavioral objectives as a prescription for what is to be learned. Students work to achieve and demonstrate the desired behavior as determined by faculty and plan the time needed to practice as much as necessary to attain the desired behavior. Student motivation for achievement is obtained from the tangible rewards that reinforce the desired behavior.

Advantages

Faculty find that behaviorist principles are very appropriate for highly structured situations in which the objectives can be clearly established in a step-by-step sequence and the desired behavior can be defined, quickly learned, and observed. Behaviorist principles are particularly useful for skills training in which the steps and sequences can be clearly delineated and observed.

Disadvantages

The organization of instruction is dominated and directed by behavioral objectives and learning outcomes that can be specified, observed, and measured. Common criticisms of the behavioristic model for instruction are that it is mechanistic and decreases or minimizes student involvement in learning. Less visible and unobservable processes involved in complex mental processes, such as concept formation, problem solving, and critical thinking, are not deemed appropriate in the behavioristic paradigm. Romyn (2001) challenges such criticism with the claim that a professional shift in value orientation from one of learning outcomes based on a behaviorist paradigm to social change based on an emancipatory paradigm is the foundation of this criticism. In the emancipatory or interpretive pedagogies the egalitarian, shared responsibility for learning replaces fixed, directive outcome objectives with meaningful dialogue (Tanner, 1990). Romyn (2001) suggests an inclusive approach in which both emancipatory and behaviorist paradigms are available to nursing education and practice is the solution to this criticism.

Students vary in response to clearly defined steps presented in a highly structured learning situation. Some students prefer to explore and discover their own ideas outside of a highly structured and directive environment.

Application

The instructional focus is on the stimuli that lead to the desired behaviors; the existing classroom climate needs to be analyzed and changed if necessary to develop a positive classroom climate. If the climate is one in which behaviors or attitudes about learning are negative, faculty can change the climate by responding to and emphasizing only student successes rather than pointing out what students are doing incorrectly. Other positive reinforcer approaches include calling the class's attention to and praising students who made correct responses, writing positive comments on written work, and enlisting students with correct responses to serve as peer tutors for students who did not respond correctly. Serving as a peer tutor enhances self esteem and stimulates students to continue their efforts to perform well.

Determining the type of positive student behaviors to receive reinforcement and appraising the students' responses to the reinforcer help faculty to develop other effective tangible reinforcers. In addition to faculty's list of tangible reinforcers, students can provide suggestions for reinforcers they would appreciate and respond to positively.

COGNITIVE LEARNING THEORIES

The initial focus on the cognitive aspects of learning is attributed to the work of the gestalt psychologists during the early 1900s. *Gestalt,* a German word, means "patterns" or "configurations." Gestalt psychologists emphasized perception, and learning was interpreted in terms of perceptual principles of organization. Gestalt psychologists believe that people respond to whole situations or patterns rather than parts (Shuell, 1986).

Insight is an important concept in Gestalt psychology. Insight is often referred to as the "aha" phenomenon. Insight is primarily a matter of perception that is explained as a procedure of mental trial and error that results in a solution. When a person's perceptual field is disorganized, order is imposed by restructuring problems into a better gestalt (pattern); the restructuring may occur through a process of trial and error (Dembo, 1988). Lewin (1951) believed that because human beings have a basic need to bring order to the situation, the motivation to learn is stimulated by the ambiguity perceived in the situation.

During the 1960s criticism of the limitations of behaviorism as a system for explaining learning led to the development of other theoretical formulations in cognitive and developmental psychology that focused on how people learn. Cognitive psychology has several perspectives and approaches that try to explain particular aspects of human behavior (Weinstein & Meyer, 1991).

Cognitive theorists focus on and emphasize the mental processes and knowledge structure that can be inferred from behavioral indices. Cognitive learning theorists are concerned with the mental processes and activities that mediate the relationship between stimulus and response; the learner selects from stimuli in the environment according to his or her own internal structures (Grippin & Peters, 1984; Slavin, 1988).

Cognitive theorists seek the factors that explain complex learning; they are concerned with meaning rather than behavior. In cognitive systems of learning, behavior is not automatically strengthened by reinforcers; the reinforcers provide affective and instructional information. The specific focus is on mental processes that include perception, thinking, knowledge representation, and memory, with emphasis on understanding and acquisition of knowledge and not merely on acquiring a new behavior or learning how to perform a task.

Cognitive theories define learning as an active, cumulative, constructive process that is goal oriented and dependent on the learner's mental activities (Shuell, 1986; Wittrock, 1978). Learning is an internal event in which modification of the existing internal representations of knowledge occurs. Learning is processing information; it is experiential and formed by a person's experience of the consequences.

In cognitive models of learning, students have active rather than passive roles in the instruction and a new responsibility for learning. A transfer of information from faculty to student does not automatically result in learning; students must discover meaning by using information-processing strategies, memories, and attentional and motivational mechanisms to organize and understand it (Wittrock, 1978).

Some authors associated with cognitive learning theory are Anderson (1980, 1985), Ausubel (1960, 1978), Ausubel and Robinson (1969), Ausubel et al. (1968), Piaget (1970a, 1970b, 1973), Rumelhart and Ortony (1977), Shuell (1986), Tulving (1972, 1985), and Wittrock (1977, 1978, 1986).

Information-Processing Theories

Information-processing theories emerged during 1970s; they focus on describing the way information is tracked, the sequences of mental operations, and the results of the operations (Anderson, 1980). A computer model provides the basis on which the theories were developed. The primary focus of information processing investigations is the various ways in which individuals perceive, organize, and remember large amounts of information.

In the information-processing theory, memory is viewed as a complex organized system. Memory selects the sensory data to be processed and transforms the data into meaningful information before storing it for later use. Information is processed through three components of the memory system: the sensory register, short-term memory, and long-term memory. The sensory register receives stimuli from visual and auditory information from the physical environment; only some of these data are retained for further processing. Information that is retained then enters the short-term (working) memory, where it is either forgotten or encoded into some meaningful form. Short-term memory is believed to be brief (a few seconds) and to have a limited capacity of six to seven items (the capacity can be enlarged by chunking related items). Some of the information may be quickly used and not further processed for transfer to the third component, long-term memory. Rehearsal of the information is important for retention in short-term memory and helps it to persist long enough to move to long-term memory (Atkinson & Shiffrin, 1968; Norman, 1970, 1989; Simon, 1980).

The capacity for long-term memory or for permanent storage of information is believed to be limitless. Information in long-term memory may be moved from short-term memory even while new information is being received from the environment. Information in long-term memory is stored in a complex system of nodes that are interrelated through learning. A node has one information item or a cluster of related items. In the event that some elements in a cluster are activated, all elements are likely to be activated.

Long-term memory has at least three parts—episodic, semantic, and procedural—all of which are organized differently (Tulving, 1972, 1985). Episodic memory contains the memories of personal experiences. Semantic memory is organized into networks that have connected ideas or relationships that are referred to as *schemata* (Anderson, 1985), which hold meaningful information. Schemata are packages of knowledge that include different concepts that are organized into larger groups in an outline form (Rumelhart, 1981). Procedural memory is where the ability to do a task or skill resides.

Constructivism

Constructivism, a psychology of learning theory, is based on the work of Piaget (1970a, 1970b, 1973) and Vygotsky (1986). Constructivism theory holds that learning is development (Fosnot, 1996) and that assimilation, accommodation, and construction are the basic operating processes in learning. A learner constructs new knowledge by building on an internal representation of existing knowledge through a personal interpretation of experience. Constructivists assume that learners construct knowledge in an attempt to make sense of their experiences and that learners are active in seeking meaning. Constructive processes operate in all types of learning; learners form, elaborate, and test their mental structures until they get one that is satisfactory to them. In the constructivist paradigm, knowledge representation is open to change as new knowledge structures are added to the existing foundational structure and connections (Reigeluth, 1983; Walton, 1996). Piaget's (1970a, 1970b, 1973) theory of cognitive development introduced the notion of knowledge construction. Wittrock's generative learning theory (1977, 1978, 1986) and the works of Ausubel and colleagues (Ausubel, 1978; Ausubel & Robinson, 1969; Ausubel et al., 1968) also fit within the constructivist paradigm.

Assimilation Theory

Ausubel and colleagues (Ausubel, 1978; Ausubel & Robinson, 1969; Ausubel et al., 1968) developed assimilation theory to describe meaningful learning processes involved in assimilating old meanings with the new meanings that form a more highly differentiated cognitive structure. Cognitive structure refers to a person's store of information. Cognitive structure provides an overall framework that incorporates new knowledge, and it is a prerequisite to meaningful learning. Ausubel (1978) held that prior knowledge is the most significant factor in determining the occurrence of new learning.

Ausubel and Robinson (1969) and Ausubel (1978) held that a learner may incorporate received information by either a meaningful or rote approach and that the information can be learned by one of two methods: reception or discovery. In the rote reception method learning is acquired by memorization, whereas in the meaningful reception method learning results from information that is logically organized and presented to the learner in a final form. This information is then integrated into the learner's own existing cognitive structure.

Meaningful learning can be attained only if (1) the learner has a mental set to learn the task in a meaningful way, (2) the task has a logical meaning, and (3) specific and relevant concepts in the learner's cognitive structures can interact with the new material (Ausubel, 1978).

Ausubel (1960) and Ausubel and Robinson (1969) proposed the use of different aids to facilitate students' learning processes. Aids help students to fit new material into existing cognitive or affective structures. One aid is prompting learners about what they already know by questioning, giving, and asking for examples and recalling their existing knowledge for them and showing how it relates to points presented in an explicit introductory example. Another aid is the use of advanced organizers. Advanced organizers are process-oriented introductory presentations that emphasize the context for the content; they are developed at a higher level of abstraction and are presented before students engage in the learning task. Advanced organizers provide a broad conceptual framework that students can use to gain clarity about the subsequent material. Advanced organizers may consist of verbal or written prose or a visual presentation (Ausubel & Robinson, 1969; Hartley, 1976; Mayer, 1979).

Premise

In cognitive learning theory the conditions of learning primarily influence the meaningful acquisition and retention of ideas and information by modifying the existing cognitive structure. Learning involves perceptual reorganization because individuals respond to meaningful wholes. Analysis begins with the situation as a whole, from which the component parts are differentiated.

Setting/Climate

Cognitive theories can be applied in any formal or informal academic setting and in continuing education classes. The climate must allow for time and flexibility so that the learner can experience and make meaning of that which is to be learned.

Role of Faculty

Emphasis is on designing an active, constructive, and goal-directed learning environment appropriate for the students' cognitive abilities. Faculty relinquish some control of the learning situation to the students and actively involve students in assessing what they have learned. Creating a rich, real world context in the classroom facilitates students' learning constructive processes that can be applied outside the classroom. It is important for students to have the opportunity to construct knowledge for themselves; group discussions of topics that involve a number of different variables enhances knowledge construction.

A primary focus is on changing the learners by modeling and encouraging the use of appropriate teaching strategies. Understanding how students process information helps faculty in selecting and implementing teaching strategies. Using think-aloud protocols, which is the process of having students verbalize their thinking while they are thinking, helps faculty to gain some understanding of how students are processing information (Corcoran et al., 1988; Muth et al., 1988).

Using an introduction with an advanced organizer before actually beginning a lesson helps faculty to prepare students for the subsequent learning experience (Ausubel, 1960). An advanced organizer includes only broad concepts presented in a hierarchical order; following this presentation with some discussion of the interrelationships between the topics helps students to see linkages and patterns. An advanced organizer does not contain specific content material that is to be learned.

Faculty's selecting other appropriate instructional strategies and learning activities will assist students in assimilating and accommodating new information. For example, concept mapping, sometimes referred to as mind mapping, is a strategy based on Ausubel's assimilation theory (Ausubel & Robinson, 1969; Ausubel et al., 1968). Concept mapping has been shown to be effective in helping students assimilate and accommodate the concepts (Novak et al., 1983; Rooda, 1994).

McKeachie (1980) recommended that faculty relate new information to students' existing cognitive structure. Faculty often discover that students know more than they think they do; students may need some prompting and cues to recognize that the new information being presented is a variation or extension of something they have previously learned and applied. Auditory and visual cues help students to activate and connect what has been previously learned to the new knowledge.

Faculty can create an organizational structure for the content, such as cause and effect, time sequence, parallel organization, phenomenon to theory to evidence, problem to solution, pros versus cons to resolution, familiar to unfamiliar, and concepts to application. Faculty should also present a prototype model and to make every effort to ensure that students understand it before progressing to new concepts (Norman, 1989).

Faculty's limiting the number of elements presented at one time to the six or seven that can be contained in short-term memory and helping students rehearse the information is beneficial; this tactic facilitates learning and retention. Providing examples of concepts and asking students for additional examples from their own perspective encourage concept development and learning. Presenting a prototype model and making every effort to ensure that students understand it before progressing on to some new concepts are important. The use of periodic summaries and reiteration of the relationships between the concepts is also beneficial. In addition, faculty can provide some suggestions to students about ways to improve their learning strategies. For example, using mental elaboration, attending to verbal and visual cues, and drawing pictures and diagrams can help stimulate imagery of old and new information (Wittrock, 1978).

Role of Student

Students have the responsibility to assume some control of the learning situation and their own learning. They become actively engaged in the instruction and the learning process. This engagement occurs when they are cognitively interacting with the subject matter. Concentrating and thinking about the content, making relationships between the concepts and principles, completing assignments, participating in learning activities, asking questions, seeking clarification, giving examples from their own experiences, and interacting in dialogues with faculty and peers are some examples of active engagement in learning.

Passively receiving information from faculty or instructional materials does not automatically result in learning; students must discover the meaning by using information-processing strategies, memories, and attentional and motivational mechanisms to organize and understand information (Wittrock, 1978). Students may discover the meaning of information by presenting analogies, using and describing prior knowledge and experiences, and having dialogues with faculty and peers about real-life situations that require application of the content. With faculty and peer support, students can acquire an increased self-awareness about what is known and become aware of how the new knowledge fits into their existing knowledge structure. Reflection, an intentional retrospective process focused on the meaning of the content and the learning experiences, is a process students can use to enhance and extend their learning.

Advantages

Cognitive learning theories provide some specific direction to faculty about instructional approaches. Cognitive instructional approaches are expected to enhance retention of concepts and relationships between concepts and promote improved problem solving and critical thinking. Students' prior knowledge is valued and used as the basis for acquiring new knowledge. Students may sense more ownership of their learning and feel an increase in their self-esteem as a learner while being able to see the real world relevance of their newly acquired knowledge. Learning may become more effective and efficient when students develop schemata and improve their ability to make more extensive linkages between their schemata.

Disadvantages

Faculty may be unable to relinquish some control of learners, as well as be unwilling and uncomfortable in supporting and coping with students' and colleagues' reactions to students' increased responsibility for learning. The use of cognitive approaches may require some reduction in the amount of content for which learners will be held accountable so that their learning has more meaning and depth.

Application

The key to learning in the cognitivists' paradigm is the use of cognitive apprenticeship, reflection on the collaboration required in real-life problem solving, and the use of tools available in the problem situation. In the learning paradigm faculty create the learning environments and experiences that assist students to move toward discovering and constructing knowledge for themselves (Barr & Tagg, 1995; Bevis, 1989c).

Concept mapping (Rooda, 1994) and problem-based learning (Heliker, 1994; van Niekerk & van Aswegen, 1993) are examples of instructional approaches that incorporate principles derived from cognitive theories. The use of journals for didactic and clinical courses enables students to take the time to reflect on and describe their own learning; journals also provide faculty opportunities to communicate with students through writing.

COGNITIVE DEVELOPMENT THEORIES

Cognitive development theories provide a practical model of the student and present ways in which the organization and structure of instruction can be designed to accommodate the students' readiness to learn (Widick & Simpson,

1978). Cognitive development occurs in sequential, predictable stages; in each stage aspects of the previous stage are expanded.

Perry's model of intellectual and ethical development of college students is presented here because it has received increased attention in the nursing education literature. Perry (1970) and his associates developed the model based on the results of a study of undergraduate students who volunteered to report on their college experiences. The study sample included men at Harvard and women at Radcliffe; the students were interviewed at the end of each academic year for a period of 4 years during the late 1950s and early 1960s (Perry, 1970). Analysis of the interview data revealed dominant themes with regard to students' orientation to authority; the nature of knowledge; and other themes such as simplicity versus complexity, good versus bad, right versus wrong, orientation to responsibility, reasoning, open versus closed mental perspective, rationale for differences of views, and concreteness versus abstractness (Perry, 1970, 1981; Valiga, 1988).

Perry organized the phenomenological themes into nine positions that were further categorized into four broad categories: dualism, multiplicity, relativism, and commitment. Students progress through the positions in each of these categories in a sequential manner demonstrating specific intellectual skills and values. At any point in time, however, further development may be halted or suspended. Growth is usually not linear and usually occurs in fluctuating surges (Perry, 1970, 1981).

In the two positions of dualism, students view knowledge and values with the assumption that all knowledge can be either right or wrong; learning consists of finding and knowing the right answers. Progress to the category is indicated by students having some ability to accept the legitimacy of diversity and uncertainty with their own explanations that the authority has not yet found the answers. Perry (1970, 1981) referred to this latter stage as multiplicity.

The two positions of relativism begin with movement to accept that views of right and wrong and good and bad are not sufficient to deal with real-life situations. Continued progress in development is demonstrated by the recognition that knowledge is contextual, uncertain, and relative. Students develop the ability to abstract and weigh information to problem solve in specific situations. Perry considered that the progression of cognitive development that occurs between the stages of the legitimacy of uncertainty and the acceptance that knowledge is contextual is a revolutionary change in cognitive restructuring. This stage is necessary for students to fully engage in critical thinking activities (McGovern & Valiga, 1997).

The last category in this model is marked by the students' understanding that making a commitment is necessary to become oriented to a world of relativism. At this stage "commitment is foreseen as the resolution of the problems of relativism, but it has not yet been experienced" (Perry, 1970, p. 137). In commitment, continued cognitive development focuses on the affective domain. Responsibility is the theme in this phase of development. Progression is through phases of initial commitment, orientation in implications of commitment, and developing commitment. Students reveal the ability to take a risk by making an initial commitment in some particular area. Movement to this phase involves realization of the implications of what the experience of commitment means in terms of responsibility. Here students affirm their identity and accept the reality that commitment is a continuing experience that is revealed through a personal lifestyle.

Research findings from studies in which Perry's model was used have particular relevance for nursing education because of the responsibility faculty have for preparing graduates who need highly developed critical thinking skills and the ability to deal with uncertainty if they are to provide care in an increasingly complex society and health care system.

Valiga (1988) summarized several variables identified through research with Perry's model that relate to cognitive development. Variables that pertain to the student include age, sex, socioeconomic status, verbal fluency, size of the student's hometown population, educational motivation, and learning style preference. Variables related to the development and implementation of the curriculum and courses include the subject matter discipline of the curriculum, the amount of structure and flexibility, the degree of challenge and support given, the types of course assignments, the nature of student–peer interactions, the openness of student–faculty relationships, and the degree of fit between the students' positions in the Perry model and the learning environment.

Frisch (1990) reported on the results of Collins' (1981) study that revealed that baccalaureate nursing students functioned in the dualistic stage. Frisch's (1987) study of junior baccalaureate nursing students revealed that most students operated at the end of the dualistic stage, whereas only one had attained multiplicity, which occurs at the beginning of the relativism stage. Frisch (1990) noted that these findings are consistent with studies conducted on other college students. Valiga (1988) reported her study results on a sample of 123 nursing students. At the beginning and at the end of the academic year most of the students were at the dualistic stage. Although some showed no change, a few gained almost two positions, moving them into the relativism stage. Positive gains in cognitive development were found by Zorn (1995) and Frisch (1990) with some students who had an international learning experience in Mexico.

Premise

Cognitive development progresses in a sequential but fluctuating manner. Growth begins with a narrow, absolute, right versus wrong view of the world; it moves to further development, in which knowledge and values are perceived as contextual and relative, and finally to the stage in which a responsible commitment is made to establish a personal identity in a pluralistic world.

Setting/Climate

Perry's model is appropriate for generic undergraduate and RN to BSN and RN to MSN mobility students enrolled in undergraduate programs. The climate is one in which the student's cognitive development is considered.

Role of Faculty

Implementing a cognitive development model requires that faculty give attention to the cognitive and interpersonal characteristics of the students who will actually be in the classes rather than focus only on increasing the subject matter content. Guardo (1986) contended that faculty design curriculum for imaginary students with little or no regard for their cognitive and interpersonal characteristics. Information about the students may be collected at the time of entry into the program or at the beginning of a semester or course. Data such as age; sex; socioeconomic status; verbal fluency; and the type and composition of students' hometown, educational motivation, learning style preference, and life experiences can be elicited through informal conversation. These conversations will also facilitate development of a closer student–faculty relationship and begin the trust-building process.

Developing open, honest, and supportive partnership with students within the context of challenging experiences promotes intellectual development. Open discussions that reveal the faculty's own sense of uncertainty helps to legitimize students' own sense of uncertainty.

Role of Student

Students must be willing to be socialized to the college experience and risk entering into new experiences with others whose background and views are different from their own. Having an open and receptive attitude and a disposition to become comfortable in revealing aspects of the self is important. Students' being aware of the importance of their active participation in new and challenging experiences that will stretch their cognitive abilities is beneficial for their development. Students can also expect that progression through school will bring increased intellectual demands, higher faculty expectations, and some disruptions in their sense of certainty about their world.

Advantages

The use of Perry's model offers faculty opportunities for further personal and professional development and increased satisfaction in relationships with students, as well as satisfaction about their students' progressing cognitive development. The increased use of a variety of instructional strategies encourages faculty creativity and has the potential for energizing teaching.

Students who progress into different developmental positions experience increased sophistication in their view of the world; they can expect to receive rewards for improved cognitive ability and look forward to a more challenging and stimulating life.

Disadvantages

Faculty who are interested in using Perry's model for curriculum, course, and instructional development will need to study the model and related materials to become knowledgeable about the different positions and divisions of the model. Although this study takes time, it is essential before attempting to implement this model in the curriculum, courses, and instructional strategies.

Faculty may find it difficult to find time for informal interactions with students outside of the classroom.

Program design and course materials will need significant revision. Frustrations may arise as the demands on faculty time increase when planning and evaluating the new course requirements. Furthermore, for various reasons colleagues may resist or be reluctant to consider using the model for curricular and course development. Faculty who chose to implement the model in their own course may find weak support from colleagues.

Students who are unwilling to accept the challenge of cognitive development may be resistive and adopt a negative attitude about the amount of time and effort required to meet the program and course objectives. The intellectual challenges presented in activities suggested by the Perry model may increase the stress students experience.

Application

Valiga (1988) recommended that faculty design curricula that require students to have organized experiences with other students who have alternative ways of thinking, reasoning, and viewing the world. These experiences should be introduced during the freshman year. In addition, requiring courses in different disciplines that provide gradual degrees of complexity should be part of the curricular design.

Other instructional and evaluation strategies suggested include instructional strategies that minimize the use of lecture and promote faculty–student interactions and student-to-student interactions. Role play, debate, discussion, frequent use of questioning, and use of materials that present opposing opinions and positions are appropriate. Evaluation strategies should include essay examinations, position and reaction papers, projects, and journals, with less frequent use of multiple choice examinations. Allowing students choices in some content areas and assignments facilitates development (Valiga, 1988).

Hodges (1996) described how she developed a model for journal writing for RN to BSN students. The model incorporated concepts from Knowles' model of adult education, Perry's model of intellectual development, and qualitative research on women's ways of knowing. The model progresses through four levels: dualism, multiplicity, relativism, and commitment. Colucciello (1988) also recommended the use of Perry's model as a way to create a powerful learning environment after she found students operating at the dualistic stage of conceptualization. Colucciello (1988) identified several instructional strategies and learning activities that are consistent with those already described. She concluded that powerful learning environments are essential if faculty are to prepare graduates to achieve a professional career rather than functioning at the technical level.

McGovern and Valiga (1997), using Perry's model, report the use of developmental instructional strategies to promote cognitive change in freshman nursing students. They used interactive teaching strategies in the classroom to provide diversity in learning experiences, integrate previously learned information, and encourage the use of active learning strategies such as group projects. Although students were at lower levels of cognitive development, they did show cognitive growth.

Lessons about implementing Perry's model can be found in other disciplines. For example, Thoma (1993) has described how he developed instructional strategies in an economics course that specifically focus transitions from dualism through relativism. Ward (1992) used the Perry model as a framework for developing writing exercises in a legal environmental course.

COGNITIVE DEVELOPMENT: SOCIOCULTURAL HISTORICAL INFLUENCES

An emphasis on the social nature and thus the cultural influences on the expressions of cognitive development were central to the research and subsequent theories attributed to Lev Vygotsky, a Russian psychologist (Newman & Holzman, 1993; Van der Veer & Valsiner, 1994; Wertsch, 1985). While acknowledging a biological base to the human development potential and recognizing cognitive learning theory such as that suggested by Piaget, Vygotsky contributes as key concepts (1) cognitive self-instruction, (2) assisted learning, and (3) the zone of proximal development.

Cognitive self-instruction through language begins in early childhood and was recognized by Piaget as egocentric. Vygotsky (1986) recognized a process between word and thought with the thought being more dynamic and never completely expressed in word. The child and beginning learner may use self-talk to mature the thought, eventually not only mastering the thought but also going beyond the basic understanding to create the new and more complex. (Ratner, 1991).

Assisted learning requires that a senior learner (adult, teacher) provide the learner with the necessary support to allow the learner to eventually solve the problem. The senior learner gradually diminishes instruction as the student gains independence. Support includes clues, affirmation, reducing the problem to steps, role modeling, and giving examples.

Real learning occurs in the zone of proximal development (ZPD). This is the point at which the learner cannot solve the problem alone but has the potential to succeed and can do so with assistance. The teacher/facilitator must understand what the learner has mastered and what comes next. Unlike for Piaget, who viewed development from a separatist perspective, for Vygotsky both the mastered and the to be mastered are heavily influenced by sociocultural exposure (Newman & Holtzman, 1993).

Premise

Learning is interactive and occurs in a social, historical context. Knowledge, ideas, attitudes, and values are developed as a result of relationships with people.

Setting/Climate

Interactive learning can be used in the classroom, online, and in the clinical setting.

Role of Faculty

To facilitate further learning nursing faculty can recognize learners' zones of proximal development and provide assistance through encouragement, affirmation, role modeling, and the breakdown of steps. As nursing education increasingly addresses the positive aspects of cultural differences, faculty may enjoy the challenge of recognizing student differences in learning as a result of individual sociocultural exposure.

Role of Student

Students may benefit from recognizing and honoring their unique matured cognitive attributes and their contributions to the specialized profession of nursing. Self-recognition of the expected need for assistance in a developmental and historical sense can alleviate the stress experienced by the novice learner.

Advantages

Faculty can recognize learners as having unique cognitive skills influenced by a social and cultural history. Students can learn to appreciate differences in peers in an environment in which the teacher is sensitive to sociocultural differences. Such differences can translate into a greater understanding of the patient in the nurse–patient relationship.

Disadvantages

Faculty may not have enough time to evaluate the social and cultural context individual learners bring to advanced learning, and therefore it may be difficult for faculty to provide unique or specific assistance. Faculty may resort to general appreciation and a broad application of theory and not be able to capture individual student contributions.

Application

Faculty can encourage student identification of the sociocultural nature of their previous learning through personal reflection, storytelling, and comparisons between textbook or clinical examples and their own experience. Encouraging students to communicate in their own voice in both written and in oral presentations can serve to both illuminate and enrich individual and peer learning.

MULTIPLE INTELLIGENCES

Howard Gardner (1983) challenged the classical view of intelligence and posited a plurality of intellects. The idea of multiple intelligences (MI) began with a preliminary list of seven constructs. As a result of ongoing empirical research the list has expanded to eight and one half. Intelligence is defined by Gardner (1999) as a biopsychological potential specific to the species. Gardner considers the intelligences to be raw, biological potentials that work together to solve problems and lead individuals to vocations, avocations, and cultural end states. The theory suggests that individuals differ in the intelligence profiles they are born with and that profiles work in harmony, changing as influenced by experience and learning throughout life.

The original seven intelligences are bodily-kinesthetic, visual-spatial, verbal-linguistic, logical-mathematical, musical-rhythmic, interpersonal, and intrapersonal (Gardner, 1983). The eighth intelligence is naturalist. Another intelligence, existential, is now considered number eight and one half (Gardner, 1999, 2003). The one/half assignment to existential intelligence by Gardner (1999) is in recognition of the possible overlap or confounding existence of yet another intelligence: spiritual intelligence.

Bodily kinesthetic intelligence is the ability to solve problems or create using the body. The person who is agile and especially skilled in bodily movement may become notable as a dancer or a surgeon, exhibiting fine and gross motor control. Visual-spatial intelligence is observed in people who enjoy learning through charts, graphs, maps, and drawings and who draw on their ability to maneuver in a spatial world. Sailors, engineers, sculptors, and painters draw on visual-spatial intelligence. Persons with high-profile verbal-linguistic skills (intelligence) demonstrate strength in the language arts: speaking, writing, reading, and listening. Poetry is a highly skilled product of verbal-linguistic skill. Logical-mathematical intelligence is just what the name implies—logical and mathematical skill—and is probably the skill studied by Jean Piaget (Gardner, 1983, 1993), who thought he was studying all intelligences. Musical-rhythmic intelligence is the gift possessed by those who learn through songs, patterns, rhythms, and musical expression. These people are sensitive to pitch, melody, rhythm, and tone. Two forms of personal intelligence are included in the MI list. The first is interpersonal intelligence, which is the ability to be "people smart." The people smart person is a good listener and communicator and is likely to be an exceptionally good salesperson, politician, teacher, or clinician. The second is intrapersonal intelligence, which is the ability to turn inward. The person with intrapersonal intelligence has the capacity to access his or her own emotions and is in touch with feelings, ideas, and values as a means to understanding self and others. The eighth intelligence is naturalist. Persons who identify and classify demonstrate naturalist expertise. Although it was initially identified as those skills associated with the recognition of flora and fauna in the environment, other classification patterns (e.g., mechanistic sounds such as car engines and heart sounds, artistic styles and behaviors) are thought to tap the naturalist intelligence. Existential intelligence (intelligence eight and one half) is the capacity to identify oneself in relation to the infinitesimal, to ponder the meaning of life and death, to experience love, and to immerse oneself in a work of art—in other words, the species potential to engage in transcendental concerns (Gardner, 1993, 1999, 2003).

Premise

Every human being has a unique intelligence profile, expressing the intelligences in varying degrees. Although in any one person one or more of the intelligences may be demonstrated at a higher operant level than the others, it is in the working together of the intelligences that a person solves problems and interacts with the environment.

Setting/Climate

The setting is basically within each individual student and teacher. Problems and solutions can be addressed and demonstrated in the formal classroom, in the clinical setting, and through the use of technology.

Role of Faculty

The relationship between the constructs identified in the eight and one half intelligences identified by Gardner (1985) and the profession of nursing is evident. Qualities identified in all of the categories can contribute to an optimal patient encounter in a practice profession such as nursing. Because most intelligence tests tap only the logical-mathematical and verbal-linguistic intelligences, students enter nursing with documentation that only partially identifies preparation for nursing. Faculty have the opportunity, using the MI theory, to focus on each student's unique profile and to use students' strengths to enhance contributions to practice and the profession. The MI theory is not a prescriptive theory. Application in educational settings is left to faculty to develop, test, and refine. In this explanatory theory nursing faculty may enjoy the discovery of untested, undocumented yet affirmed abilities in students, as well as in themselves, that contribute to nursing.

Role of Student

The student can use the MI theory for self-evaluation and for the evaluation of others. Because there is no hierarchy in the MI theory, no intelligence is thought to be of higher value than any other. The student may enjoy the recognition of untested, undocumented yet affirmed abilities that can contribute to their success in nursing. Students can find direction for within-nursing vocations, as well as other social choices, by giving attention to their personal profile.

Advantages

A broader, more comprehensive view of the intelligences nurses, students, faculty, and other health care professionals bring to the learning encounter can contribute to greater understanding of potential nursing interaction. The complexity of MI and individual profiles mirrors the complexity of holistic nursing. Specific and broadened attention to course and clinical learning goals relative to the constructs in the MI theory may contribute to greater student success and satisfying professional performance.

Disadvantages

The MI theory is not prescriptive. Direct use of the theory may require changes across the curriculum, study of the theory, and identification of a specific application in nursing. Adult students who have developed through a traditional primary and secondary school curriculum followed by a focus on the sciences in their professional education may not have had the opportunity to develop intelligences in which they have great strength and that could be of service in their nursing career. This is not a disadvantage of the theory but of its application at the postsecondary level.

Application

Although not a prescriptive theory, MI provides a framework for understanding intelligence that can benefit both students and teachers. Teachers can empower students to recognize their own unique gifts to the nursing encounter by acknowledging profiles of problem-solving abilities that consider more than the narrow range of verbal-linguistic and logical-mathematical abilities traditionally associated with intelligence quotient (IQ) testing. The development of teaching strategies to complement all MI categories would be of benefit to nursing.

EDUCATIONAL FRAMEWORKS/PHILOSOPHIES

In addition to behavioral and cognitive learning theories and cognitive developmental theories, nursing faculty have recently used other frameworks, such as adult education models and interpretive pedagogies, to guide the development of the curriculum and the teaching–learning process. These educational frameworks tend to assist faculty in adjusting students' attitude and the environment to facilitate learning. The interpretive pedagogies discussed are critical, feminist, postmodern, and phenomenological. Nursing faculty have advanced concepts inherent in, or applicable to, the interpretive pedagogies that include caring, patterns of knowing, and narrative pedagogy. Table 12-1 indicates the educational frameworks/philosophies and premises discussed in following sections.

ADULT EDUCATION THEORY

Andragogy is the term used to refer to the education of adults; it is used in contrast to *pedagogy,* the term used for the education of children. Knowles (1980) defined andragogy as "the art and science of helping adults learn" (p. 43). From a psychological perspective, adults are persons with a self-concept of

TABLE 12-1 Premises of Educational Frameworks/Philosophies

FRAMEWORKS	PREMISE
Adult education	Adults are self-directed and problem centered and need to learn useful information
Caring	Education consists of an integration of humanistic–existential, phenomenological, feminist, and caring ideologies.
Critical	The liberation of thought occurs through analysis of power and relationships within social structure information.
Feminism	Intellectual growth, activism, and empowerment can change injustice and inequity for all persons.
Humanism	Education motivates the development of human potential.
Narrative pedagogy	A practical discourse using nine themes allows knowledge gained through experiences of teachers, students, and clinicians to direct nursing education.
Phenomenology	Understanding the hows and ways humans experience and perceive events that result in learning.
Postmodern discourse	Truth is related to specific context and is constantly being constructed.

being self-directing and being responsible for their own life (Knowles, 1990). Cross (1981) proposed that learners who are adults should be conceptualized from a developmental perspective that includes the physical, psychological, and sociological aspects of the learner.

Knowles (1980) described adult learners as persons who do best when asked to use their experience and apply new knowledge to solve real-life problems. Adult learners' motivation to learn is more pragmatic and problem centered than younger learners. The basic assumptions about adult learners are that they are increasingly self-directed and have experiences that serve as a rich resource for their own and others' learning. Their readiness to learn develops from life tasks and problems, and their orientation to learning is task or problem centered. Adult learners' motivation is internal; it arises from their curiosity (Knowles, 1990).

The following five additional characteristics of adult learners have been described by Jackson and Caffarella (1994):

1. Adults have more and different types of life experiences that are organized differently from those of children.
2. Adults have preferred differences in personal learning style.
3. Adults are more likely to prefer being actively involved in the learning process.
4. Adults desire to be connected to and supportive of each other in the learning process.
5. Adults have individual responsibilities and life situations that provide a social context that affects their learning.

Adults make a commitment to learning when the learning goals are perceived as immediately useful and realistic and as important and relevant to their personal, professional, and career needs. The learning behaviors of adults are shaped by past experiences; their maturity and life experiences provide them with insights and the ability to see relationships.

Some contemporary authors associated with adult learning are Caffarella and Barnett (1994); Cross (1981); Galbraith (1991a, 1991b); Hiemestra and Sisco (1990); Knowles (1980, 1984, 1986, 1990); Merriam and Caffarella (1991); and Schon (1983).

Premise

Adults are not content centered; adults are self-directed and problem centered, and they need and want to learn useful information that can be readily adapted. Adults need a climate that enables them to assume responsibility for their learning.

Setting/Climate

The learning setting is unique for each individual; it becomes individualized and personalized. Adult education takes place in formal and informal classrooms in which academic courses, continuing education, self-development, and personal enrichment courses are presented. Opportunities to teach based on adult learning methods are increasing in nursing education in traditional classroom settings, in distance learning, and in other settings where staff development and continuing education occur. Learning opportunities are becoming increasingly available in the home and workplace through the use of audiovisual media and computer technology. Social interaction in the learning environment is important, and opportunities for social interaction are available with distance learning through computer technology.

Role of Faculty

Because adults fear failure, faculty must create a relaxed, psychologically safe environment while developing a climate of trust and mutual respect that will facilitate student empowerment. Faculty facilitate, guide, or coach adult learners. Courses that rely heavily on pedagogical teaching strategies must be modified to meet the needs of adult learners.

Although faculty assume responsibility for being the content expert, a collaborative relationship and use of the democratic process are essential with adult learners. As content experts, faculty need to design learning activities that are as close as possible to the actual practice they represent so that learning transfer becomes a reality. The activities should stimulate and encourage reflection on past and current experiences and be sequenced according to the learners' needs. Faculty attend to adult learners' needs and concerns as legitimate and important components of the learning process; this helps to ensure that their learning experiences are maximized.

Course materials are sequenced according to learner readiness. Learning plans are actually learning contracts established with learners. Learning contracts are often used with adult learners in formal academic classrooms and staff development. Contracts are developed collaboratively and should specify the knowledge, skills, attitudes, and values students will acquire; the means by which students will attain the objectives; the criteria and evidence by which they will be judged; and the date for completion of the work (Knowles, 1980). Learning contracts allow students some control when they are given the option to select their learning experiences.

Learning activities should include independent study and inquiry projects that focus on inquiry and experiential techniques (Caffarella & Barnett, 1994). Field-based experiences such as internships and practicum assignments provide experiential learning. Reflective journals, critical incidents, and portfolios are other types of activities that allow adult learners to introduce their past and current experiences into the content of the learning events (see Chapters 10 and 13). These activities also help learners make sense of their life experiences, providing added incentive to learn (Caffarella & Barnett, 1994).

The use of adult learning principles is actually a constructivist instructional model because consideration is given to how previously learned knowledge and experience influence new learning. Teaching adult learners is a reflective practice in which faculty stimulate learners to develop, from a single experience, new ideas and ways of thinking through an internal dialogue. In reflective practice the process is to bring forth past events to a conscious level and then determine some appropriate ways to think, feel, and behave in the future (Brookfield, 1995; Schon, 1983). Within the context of the content, faculty help learners use their experience, intuition, and trial-and-error thinking to define, solve, or rethink a particular problem or issue (Schon, 1983).

Evaluation is shared with the students and peers; students should have some options for selecting the tools or approaches. The basis for the judgment of performance is criterion referenced, not norm referenced. Students collect evidence that is validated by peers and facilitators.

Role of Student

Students must be able, with support from faculty and peers, to determine their own learning needs and work collaboratively in negotiating their learning experiences. Self-directedness and the ability to pace learning and monitor progress toward completion of goals are essential attributes of adult learners.

Advantages

Faculty using adult learning principles assume very different roles in using a process structure for the course experiences in which students are provided considerable freedom and responsibility. The use of adult learning principles actively involves students and stimulates the use of a broader variety of resources as students work collaboratively with others to achieve their personal learning objectives. Box 12-3 identifies the teaching and learning principles associated with Knowles' adult learning model.

Box 12-3
ADULT TEACHING AND LEARNING PRINCIPLES BASED ON KNOWLES' MODEL OF ADULT LEARNING

---

1. Faculty
   a. Relate to learners with value and respect for their feelings and ideas
   b. Create a comfortable psychological and physical environment that facilitates learning
   c. Involve learners in assessing and determining their learning needs
   d. Collaborate with learners in planning the course content and the instructional strategies
   e. Help learners to make maximum use of their own experiences within the learning process
   f. Assist learners in developing their learning contracts
   g. Assist learners in developing strategies to meet their learning objectives
   h. Assist learners in identifying the resources to help meet their learning objectives
   i. Assist learners in developing their learning activities
   j. Assist learners in implementing their learning strategies
   k. Encourage participation in cooperative activities with other learners
   l. Introduce learners to new opportunities for self-fulfillment
   m. Assist learners in developing their plan for self-, peer, and faculty evaluation
2. Learners
   a. Accept responsibility for collaborating in the planning of their experiences
   b. Adopt goals of learning experiences as their goals
   c. Actively participate in the learning experience
   d. Pace their own learning
   e. Participate in monitoring their own progress

Students' ability to be self-directed is increased, their sense of accountability is increased, and their motivation for learning is maximized. Adult learners are able to find their own level of comfort within their learning experiences. The means for systematic feedback from faculty is established in collaboration with faculty (Knowles, 1980).

Disadvantages

The roles and responsibilities of faculty as facilitators and mentors in the learning process should be clearly described and explained (Knowles, 1980). Adult learning principles generate more ambiguous learning directives than those experienced in a traditional classroom; therefore participants may not be comfortable with the requirement that they establish their own learning needs and objectives. Students who lack experience in the domains or topics of the course or lesson may not be able or willing to actively participate. The absence of a highly structured experience may be disconcerting and stressful. The demands of an adult learning model may require that students change their attitudes and beliefs about learning. Some of these difficulties may be overcome by the way in which faculty attend and respond to the affective aspects presented by individual students during learning experiences. It may be possible to move dependent learners toward independence by involving them in group learning activities and peer support groups and providing overt praise for their independent activities. In addition, faculty may choose to use class time to discuss adult learning styles and preferences. Giving attention to students' personal concerns in a caring and supportive manner may help to improve their comfort level.

Adult learning methods are not necessarily suitable for all adult learning situations; they may be inappropriate for courses in which the content is totally unfamiliar to the learners and for courses that focus on interpersonal skills, group dynamics, or psychomotor skill development.

Application

Opportunities to use adult learning methods are increasing in nursing education in traditional classroom settings. Adult learning methods are also appropriate for courses in nursing mobility programs (e.g., baccalaureate degree completion nursing programs designed for LPN or RN students; RN to MSN students). Hodges (1996) developed a model for journal writing in which she used principles of adult learning. The model was developed for use with RN to BSN students for the purpose of assisting students to develop writing and critical thinking skills and to assist in their "social, cognitive and professional development" (p. 137).

Adult learning theory can also be applied in clinical practice because nurses are becoming more actively involved in teaching adult patients and clients in acute care, long-term care, and various community settings about self-care practices and about interventions for health promotion and disease prevention. Nurses must understand and incorporate principles of adult education when teaching patients and clients.

HUMANISM

Humanism has been used as an approach to education. Sometimes referred to as the human potential movement, humanism became an important force during the 1970s, although its early beginnings are attributed to Maslow's *Motivation and Personality,* published in 1954. Humanistic psychologists, building on Maslow's work (1954, 1962), refer to themselves as the "third force" psychologists. Third force psychologists have been concerned with the study and development of self-actualizing or fully functioning persons. The use of these descriptors is associated with Maslow (1954, 1962) and Rogers (1954, 1961, 1969).

The humanistic approach to education was developed as a strong reaction to the excessive use of drill and practice that had been common in education (Holt, 1964). Humanistic education is considered a successor to John Dewey's (1916, 1938, 1939) progressive movement in the early 1900s. Humanistic psychologists are primarily concerned with motivating students for growth toward becoming self-actualized. Individual behavior is described according to the person rather than the observer.

Humanistic education has been defined as a "commitment to educational practice in which all facets of the teaching–learning process give major emphasis to the freedom, value, worth, dignity and integrity of persons" (Combs, 1981, p. 446). Learn (1990) indicated that humanism in education is both a philosophy and a "practice-oriented program of education for professional nurses" (p. 235). Humanistic education focuses more on the affective outcomes of education, with helping students learn how to learn and promoting creativity and human potential as its primary concerns (Glasser, 1969; Rogers, 1961, 1969). Rogers (1961) conceptualized the notion of student-centered teaching. The humanistic approach supports and promotes the dignity of the individual, values students' feelings, and promotes the development of a humanistic perspective toward others.

Educators adopting this approach use learning experiences that emphasize the affective aspects of development, promoting the students' sense of responsibility, cooperation, and mutual respect. Honesty and caring are considered equally important as the learning goals that focus on the cognitive and psychomotor domains (Slavin, 1988). Traditional forms of evaluation of learning such as letter grades and standardized examinations are inconsistent with the philosophy of humanistic education. Learning is defined as a process of developing one's own potential with the goal of becoming a self-actualized person. Proponents of the humanistic movement in education include Combs (1959, 1981, 1994), Glasser (1969), Kohlberg (1984), Learn (1990), Leininger (1978), Maslow (1954, 1962), and Rogers (1961, 1969).

Premise

Education motivates students to develop their human potential so that they can progress toward self-actualization.

Setting/Climate

Humanistic education is appropriate for a formal or an informal setting and involves a climate in which there is recognition and valuing of individual freedom and worth. It may be the framework for traditional academic courses, continuing education courses, staff development programs, and personal development seminars and courses.

Role of Faculty

Faculty create an educational environment that fosters and promotes self-development by establishing an informal and relaxed climate. This can be accomplished by taking about 15 minutes at the beginning of the first few classes to use "icebreaker" strategies that invite students to mingle and become acquainted with each other and the teacher. For example, students can be asked to complete a 5×8 index card with their name and some personal information, such as a list of three things they like most and three things they like least, and wear it as a nametag for several class periods. This allows students to find out about each other and helps students and faculty remember each others' name.

One way to help students learn the behaviors consistent with the humanistic movement is through modeling. Faculty can consistently model the desired behaviors and attitudes that are integral components of humanistic education; some of these behaviors include being a caring, empathetic person and demonstrating genuineness while being consistently respectful of self and others. Faculty's recognition of themselves as a colearner in educational transactions encourages more egalitarian student–teacher relationships.

Faculty help students recognize and develop their own unique potential by facilitating their growth process. This may be facilitated by praising students' positive behaviors, asking students to draw on and share their own experiences, asking questions that enable students to contribute to discussions, and elaborating on students' responses and questions.

Prepared lessons are rarely presented to the whole class; instructional time is spent working with individuals or small groups. Faculty or student-created case studies studies promote self-directed experiences. Faculty develop learning contracts with students to allow them to negotiate their own objectives and pace their own learning. A strong focus is on the frequent use of open-ended activities in which students find their own information; make decisions; solve problems; and create their own, rather than required, products (Slavin, 1988). Selective and appropriate field trips allow students to explore and learn from real-life settings.

Role of Students

Students are responsible for their own learning and determine their own needs, goals, and objectives and conduct self-evaluations. Students become actively engaged in the learning process, assume responsibility, are open to discussion, and are able to use reflection and introspection. In addition, students adopt the respectful and caring behaviors modeled by faculty.

Advantages

Humanistic education focuses on honesty, integrity, manners, respect for the rights of others, caring, and accepting responsibility for self-development; these are important ethical and moral dimensions. Faculty and students are able to draw on prior school and life learning experiences. The environment provides opportunities to maximize use of the "teachable moment." Students are actively engaged in all aspects of the learning experiences.

Disadvantages

Direction by faculty is necessary to ensure that all domains of learning (cognitive, affective and psychomotor) are adequately addressed. Although self-evaluation is key to humanistic growth, teachers must maintain responsibility in verifying clinical competence and content mastery (Learn, 1990).

Application

The humanistic approach to education is appropriate for courses in the social sciences and humanities, as well as for teaching communication skills, interpersonal dynamics, and group dynamics. The approach is also appropriate for courses in which the goal is to teach approaches to problem solving and different points of view (Slavin, 1988). The general precepts of humanistic education are relevant to all forms of formal and informal educational experiences.

INTERPRETIVE PEDAGOGIES: CRITICAL, FEMINIST, POSTMODERN, AND PHENOMENOLOGICAL THEORIES

The interpretive pedagogies focus on exploring, deconstructing, and critiquing experiences. They embrace multiple epistemologies, ways of knowing, and practices of thinking (Diekelmann, 2001). The interpretive pedagogies are methods to use when the educational emphasis is understanding or appreciating the nature of experience. The interpretive pedagogies empower the student, decenter authority, encourage social action, and construct new knowledge.

Critical Pedagogy

Critical pedagogy guides the learner to discover practices that oppress and silence people (Hartrick, 1998). The commitment is to social action, community building, and collective good. Critical pedagogy is based on the critical theory and work of Paulo Freire (1971). Freire, a Brazilian educator and theorist, posited that those in power for the purpose of marginalizing the masses maintain oppressive social reality. For Freire the purpose of education was to encourage conscious understanding of the oppressive context to eliminate domination. The ultimate goal is social transformation through the liberation of thought.

Education as an act of freedom is first the analysis of one's own experiences within ongoing relationships with power, giving meaning and expression to one's own needs and voice for the purpose of self-empowerment and social empowerment. Naming one's own experience, therefore, is the beginning of understanding the political nature of the limits and possibilities that make up the larger society (Freire and Macedo, 1987). Teachers, nurses, students, and patients all have experiences and relationships with power and can be situated in marginalized positions. These marginalized positions are to be discovered, understood, and analyzed for the purpose of eliminating oppression.

The concept of marginalization was expanded on in nursing and proposed by Hall et al. (1994) as a guiding concept for valuing diversity in nursing knowledge. The concept has relevance to all of the interpretive pedagogies, as well as the strategies related to cultural competence. Marginalized people are vulnerable within the health care system as result of discrimination, environmental dangers, severe illness, trauma, and restricted access to health care (Hall, 1999). A discussion of marginalization and seven properties with associated risks and resilience can be found in Hall et al. (1994) and Hall (1999). The seven properties are intermediacy, differentiation, power, secrecy, reflectiveness, voice, and liminality.

Premise

Critical pedagogy is the liberation of thought through analysis of power and relationships within social structure. Opportunity exists, through critical social examination, for education to give meaning and expression to self and social empowerment (Freire and Macedo, 1987).

Setting/Climate

Critical pedagogy can be used in any climate in which it is desirable to focus and understand people or groups of people who are marginalized through the formal and informal educational experience. Analysis is appropriate for students, teachers, and patients as individuals or populations.

Role of Faculty

Faculty identify and accept student identification of literature, issues, and clinical examples that relate to the course content and are amenable to critical review. Faculty decenter authority and empower students (Ironside, 2001). Faculty accept the power shift with an examination of values and position of self in the sociopolitical structure. Assignments constructed around the properties of marginalization can guide greater understanding of risks and resilience in vulnerable populations.

In the clinical setting, faculty support student identification of injustices and imbalances in power and guide analysis of issues and support action for change. Learning issues come from the field of faculty, student, and patient experiences.

Role of Student

Students are challenged to understand themselves and others relative to sociopolitical power. Responsibility to accept empowerment requires self-direction and the examination of values and the position of self in the sociopolitical structure.

Advantages

Personal and professional growth are made possible through critical examination of social power structures between and among faculty, students, patients, education, and health care systems. The potential exists for interrupting systems of oppression.

Disadvantages

The nature of critical social examination exposes the individual to the realization of a position or relative power or powerlessness within a system(s). This realization can be personally meaningful and emancipating or can produce a painful realization. The educational climate must be appropriate and supportive for all contingent realizations.

Application

Depending on the course content, any or all of the following power structures and relationships may be identified for critical review in nursing curricula: individuals or populations of patients and health care systems; local, state, and federal governments; student–faculty and faculty–administration relationships; and nursing schools in relationship to accrediting agencies. Assignments that address issues can include a deconstruction of the issue relative to the identification of stakeholders and power structures. Support for action for change is possible through written assignments, field trips, and experience with professional lobbyist organizations and organizations that support change.

Feminist Pedagogy

Feminist pedagogy is associated with critical pedagogy in that the approach is a commitment to overcoming oppression but with a focus on gender. The challenge is to embrace inclusiveness, cooperation, collaboration, multiple ways of knowing, and collective action in learning.

Feminism is described as an ideology of beliefs and values about women and relationships of gender (Boughn & Wang, 1994; Morse, 1995). The life, work, and writings of early leaders in professional nursing, such as Nightingale, Wald, and Sanger, demonstrate feminist perspectives (Chinn & Wheeler, 1985). Nursing and feminist theory are interrelated because they both have central beliefs that reflect a reverence for life and respect for the uniqueness of each individual (Chinn & Wheeler, 1985).

Feminist pedagogy is based on the assumptions that traditional models of education do not meet all of the educational needs of women and that "education must serve as a means for individual development and social change in order to meet those needs" (Hayes, 1989, p. 56). Boughn (1991) indicated that nursing curricula are beginning to incorporate a feminist perspective as a way to focus on gender issues pertinent to the roles of women as consumers of health care services and as providers of that care.

According to Chinn and Wheeler (1985), the feminist approach values all persons regardless of gender and has a goal of bringing an end to the dehumanizing polarizations that have traditionally existed. The long history of oppression in nursing has been revealed through the absence of autonomy in practice, lack of professional power, inadequate social status, and income inequities (Boughn & Wang, 1994). Benefits from using a feminist theory in nursing education are viewed as being consistent with professional nursing values; some of these include heightened self-awareness, independence, and empowerment (Beck, 1995; Boughn, 1991; Boughn & Wang, 1994; Ruffing-Rahal, 1992).

Boughn (1991) believes that feminist theory provides a basis for restructuring nursing education. Chinn (1989b) indicated that a more complete understanding of nursing's patterns of knowing can be achieved through the contributions of feminist thought.

From the feminist perspective the caring aspect of nursing should focus on care of self and patients. Care of self includes behaving autonomously, having high self-esteem, understanding power and its use, holding a commitment to other nurses, and advocating for patients served (Boughn, 1991). Feminism is considered to be "a personal, philosophical and political means for analyzing the realities of women's lives as lived in patriarchal systems" (Chinn & Wheeler, 1985, p. 77). Ruffing-Rahal (1992) viewed feminism as an ideology that can change nursing's caring ethic into a political agenda that promotes social justice for the people served; feminism also has the potential for changing professional nursing into a worldwide network of competent, caring, and activist healers.

Premise

In feminist pedagogy the commitment is the emancipation of women (Ironside, 2001). It provides a framework that promotes and enables the development of intellectual growth, activism, and empowerment in nursing (Ruffing-Rahal, 1992).

Setting/Climate

Feminist theory may be used in any setting that provides formal and informal learning experiences for nurses. The theory has relevance for nursing education in all courses. Many of the concepts and principles may used when emphasizing group dynamics, interpersonal relationships, power and authority, and the understanding of personal meaning. The application of feminist theory may be useful for continuing education, staff development, and personal growth programs.

Role of Faculty

Faculty strive to foster partnerships with and among students, reducing traditional barriers between faculty and students. The feminist teacher exposes gender bias and oppression in education and health care. Instructional strategies and learning activities that encourage, facilitate, and support students' development in terms of personal autonomy, independence, assertiveness, and sense of achievement should be selected. Insofar as is possible, a course should be structured to allow students to select some of the content and to propose topics or issues that they will address, as well as to revise or omit topics.

Formative and summative evaluations are a collection of information obtained from students' self-evaluations combined with evaluations from faculty and peers (Boughn & Wang, 1994). A desired outcome of students' learning experiences is that they develop positive attitudes and behaviors for all women and nurses. Another desired outcome is that students understand and endorse professional nursing organizations to advance professional nursing (Boughn, 1991).

Role of Students

Students become actively engaged in the course and willing to accept responsibility for contributing to discussions and participating in consensus building. Students listen and talk while sharing life experiences, engage in introspection, support their peers, and become comfortable in relating to the faculty as colleagues rather than as authority figures.

Advantages

The use of feminist theory and methods is described as promoting positive benefits for both male and female nursing students. The potential exists for significant change in the sociopolitical arena with the empowerment of professional nursing. Empowerment of professional nursing has the potential for revolutionizing the way in which men and women live their life and for initiating and sustaining major changes in the practice of nursing within the health care delivery system.

Disadvantages

Feminism is perceived by many as an emotional issue because it challenges the basic structure of a worldwide societal view (Chinn & Wheeler, 1985). Despite the feminist position that both male and female students can benefit from learning nursing from the feminist perspective, some male and female faculty and students may struggle with the ideology because it is not in accord with their own beliefs or construct of reality.

Application

Feminism upholds personal lived experience as the content for analysis in research investigations (Belenky et al., 1986). Chinn (1989a) presented a detailed description of a prototype course with the pedagogical strategies and feminist philosophy she developed as a way of assisting others who are interested in integrating a feminist philosophy into their teaching. The research method or the findings of lived experiences can be used as part of a course's content. Feminist theory and methods have been used in some undergraduate and graduate courses (Ruffing-Rahal, 1992; Walton, 1996). Boughn (1991) described using the feminist perspective in an elective course on women's health for junior and senior level baccalaureate nursing and nonnursing students. Teaching women's health can be influenced by feminist values and beliefs (Morse, 1995). A feminist perspective also has been used in conjunction with a model for cooperative learning in a baccalaureate course on professional nursing for male and female RN students (Beck, 1995). Hodges (1996) used feminist theory as a partial framework for developing a model for journal writing for RN to BSN students.

Postmodern Discourse

The postmodern position is that of multiple meanings of reality. It rejects the meta-narrative in favor of recognizing what is "real" as that which is socially constructed within specific contexts (Hall, 1999). The postmodernist will keep everything in process, avoiding the power and domination of one central truth (Traynor, 1997).

The deconstruction of the rules and principles of education and practice clarifies who is served by the rules and principles, drawing attention to the changing, fragmented, and political nature of difference, of knowledge, and of the uses of knowledge. Thus the historic, social, cultural, and fluid construction of knowledge is exposed (Ironside, 2001). Deconstruction allows the student and teacher to review how knowledge is both possible and problematic (Escolano, 1996; Traynor, 1997).

Premise

The specific context is essential in understanding what is real (true). Truth is constantly being constructed and is in process.

Setting/Climate

The application of postmodern thinking is appropriate in climates in which ambiguity is possible and concrete application of knowledge is not required. It is useful for beginning level students to understand context-specific reality and essential for advanced students to evaluate and prepare for changing perceptions in themselves, patients, and the profession.

Role of Faculty

Faculty work with students to develop an appreciation of the multiple ways of understanding socially constructed systems in health care and education. While in the deconstruction mode faculty must resist jumping to conclusions and instead support the idea of multiple realities, yet they must work in a system(s) in which rules, regulations, and single truths are clearly established.

Role of Student

Students learn a method of analysis that exposes a stated position, rule, policy, or truth and become familiar and comfortable working with the notion of multiple changing truths. In a learning environment with rules and expectations, motives and rationales are examined.

Advantages

Postmodern approaches serve to expose multiple truths in socially structured educational and health care climates, with the expectation of a single or better truth and the requirements for actions based on set principles. Personal and professional growth is enhanced through academic examination of changing truths.

Disadvantages

Postmodernism has been critiqued for its lack of practical application (Ironside, 2001; Kaufmann, 2000). There is scant documentation on how to apply the theory in concrete terms. Postmodern theory, including deconstruction, provides no results, no conclusion, and no final decision on which to base a nursing action. The application of postmodern thought is theoretical.

Application

A postmodern approach is desirable in an academic situation in which faculty wish to deconstruct a situation to illustrate how subjects, individuals, ideologies, and relationships all hold different and multiple positions in society (Giroux and McLaren, 1992). Deconstruction exercises may be used to encourage pluralistic appreciation. Examples can be found in any clinical and educational setting or situation.

Phenomenology

Phenomenology is a philosophy and a qualitative research method nurse scholars use to study the lived human experience. It is an inductive, descriptive approach used to explain the phenomenon of the human experience (Omery, 1983). Van Manen (1990) wrote that "phenomenology is, on the one hand, a description of the lived-through quality of lived experience, and on the other hand, description of meaning of the expressions of lived experience" (p. 25). Phenomenology has been used by philosophers such as Heidegger (1962) and Merleau-Ponty (1962).

Phenomenology is a research method that "acknowledges and values the meanings people ascribe to their own existence" (Taylor, 1993, p. 173). Phenomenology is concerned with communicating understandings of meanings of phenomena and offers multiple approaches to examine problems at any system level. It involves reflection and discourse through a dialogue of language and experience of caring about phenomena from which meanings are transformed into themes that capture the phenomenon that one is trying to understand (Van Manen, 1990). When applied in nursing education and clinical practice, phenomenology can be used to gain some understanding of the phenomena that are the focus of nursing in clinical practice. The phenomenon of concern of nursing includes nurses themselves as students and practitioners and, of course, their patients. The concerns include, but are not limited to, human experiences such as pain, suffering, loss, grief, and hope (Taylor, 1993).

Phenomenology offers a way to describe the nature of nursing practice in actual practice settings; it is a flexible and fluid pedagogy that is situated in the entire universe of professional nursing as viewed through a holistic lens. This view enables perception of the gestalt of the lived experience of nurses and patients. The physical and social environments merge into a personal, intimate, and holistic experience. A phenomenological approach establishes a view that shifts the focus from a technical skills orientation to one that is concerned with the whole human being.

Phenomenology restructures the relationship between knowledge and skill because of the holistic view of the phenomena of interest in the human being. The themes elicited in the phenomenological approach become the pedagogy (Van Manen, 1990). Faculty can integrate themes elicited through phenomenology into the appropriate content portion taught in the classroom. Students can be shown how to expand their databases to include aspects of the lived experiences of patients with specific health problems or concerns and integrate this type of knowledge into case studies. Case studies are a useful instructional strategy and learning activity through which various layers of the meaning of the phenomena pertaining to patients' experiences may be extracted (Boyd, 1988).

Phenomenology has been used by nurse scholars such as Benner (1983, 1984, 1985), Benner and Tanner (1987), Benner and Wrubel (1989), Bevis (1989b), Diekelmann (1988, 1989), Kondora (1993), Paterson and Zderad (1976), Tanner (1987), and Tanner et al. (1993).

Premise

The goal of phenomenology is to understand human experience—the hows and ways events are experienced. Phenomenology informs "the discipline of nursing about phenomena of concern to it" (Taylor, 1993).

Setting/Climate

Phenomenology can be used in the classroom; in clinical practice; and in any other situation in which patients, nurses, and nursing students are the phenomena of interest. Both the beginning and the more advanced student can learn from this inductive approach to what is relevant. The beginning student will have an opportunity to be impressed with the power of the theory and the more advanced student will have the option of assimilating new information into existing constructs.

Role of Faculty

Faculty select phenomena from professional literature that is relevant to the course content and explore them in the classroom. Faculty can also demonstrate ways in which aspects of a patient's or nurse's lived experience can be elicited through the use of open-ended and probing questions. Guest speakers may enhance classroom learning experience by sharing their own personal knowledge of the lived experience of patients or themselves.

In clinical practice settings expert nurse clinicians assume the primary instructional role; if the expert clinician is other than the faculty member, the faculty member assumes a secondary role. Control of the agenda and learning experiences is left to students and to the expert clinicians. Faculty guide and show students how to learn from the expert clinician. Faculty assume responsibility for identifying, negotiating, and collaborating with the expert clinicians who guide and mentor students' learning experiences in clinical practice. In addition, faculty initiate discussion and debate, offer critiques without judgments, and guide the agenda without controlling it. Faculty become listeners and responders and enter into dialogues with students. The climate provides opportunities for students to become empowered.

Role of Student

The role of students varies according to the level of exposure to the issue or subject of interest. Students assume an active role in making meaning out of information. Students must be self-directive in seeking out what they want and need to learn from the expert clinician or faculty.

Advantages

Faculty and students have unique opportunities to gain knowledge and learn new skills from all subjects. Patients, expert clinicians, students, and faculty all have a story to unfold. Phenomenology clearly acknowledges the value of the students in making meaning out of stories while promoting trust, creativity, and inquiry. These learning experiences have the potential for promoting a more in-depth understanding and enhancing the caring aspects of students' clinical practice.

Disadvantages

Faculty must have an understanding of phenomenology and some knowledge of the phenomenological themes that have been elicited through clinical practice and research. When serving in a secondary role in the teaching–learning process, faculty must be willing to relinquish considerable control and power in the classroom to the students and in the clinical setting to the clinician.

Students must assume the primary responsibility for their own learning and seek understanding of the lived experience of others along with the tasks of nursing that often are the focus of the beginner.

Application

The anecdotal phenomena from which faculty and student may draw are unlimited. Bevis (1988) suggests the following: the nurse–patient relationship, the patient and his or her circumstance as object, the nurse (self) as object, the vicarious experience, the patient's description of his or her experience, and the nurse's and patient's indirect expressions. Bevis (1988) also suggests expanded database formats, clarified nursing perspectives, nursing prose, logs, case studies, anecdotal recordings, dialogue, fictional and autobiographical accounts of experience, responses to art, and artistic expression.

Patterns of Knowing in Nursing

Carper (1978) proposed four patterns of knowing in nursing as a typology of knowledge forms: empirics, aesthetics, personal knowledge, and moral knowledge. Empirics is the science of nursing: the systematic collection of facts, laws, and theories for the purpose of describing, explaining, and predicting phenomena of concern to nursing. Since 1950 the increasing emphasis on establishing a science of nursing has been generally associated with empirical knowledge as discovered through logical positivistic methods. In contrast, the aesthetic pattern of knowing involves creation and subjective expression of imagined possibilities. The knowledge gained by subjective means is specific and unique and associated, by Carper, with the experience of helping and the concept of nursing the whole patient. Personal knowledge is an interpersonal process and involves interactions, relationships, and transactions between the nurse and patient. The resulting nurse–patient relationship is authentic and personal within a process of becoming. The fourth and final pattern of knowing is the moral component, which focuses on matters of obligation or what ought to be done. It goes beyond knowing the norms or ethical codes of the discipline and is based on specific, concrete situations. Carper suggested that the application of the fundamental patterns of knowing addresses new, developing, and unsolved problems that reference the structure of the discipline and its changing, developing nature. Jacobs-Kramer and Chinn (1988) expanded on Carper's typology with descriptions of developmental processes and product outcomes, expressions of the patterns and process context for assessing knowledge associated with the pattern. They assert that all knowledge patterns must be integrated into the "art-act" of nursing to facilitate clinical choices and dynamic meaning.

Premise

Nursing knowledge is more than that which is discovered through the scientific method. Patterns of knowing provide the nursing professional in practice, education, and research with new means to understand meaning in context to a specific situation.

Setting/Climate

An emphasis on all or select patterns is possible in any nursing clinical or academic setting.

Role of Faculty

Emphasis is on the development of student consciousness of the four patterns through study and application. Faculty focus on the development of the individual patterns, with a goal of total patient consideration. The nature of the aesthetic, personal knowledge and moral patterns necessitates that faculty seek to understand their own personal understanding and experience for the purpose of role modeling the theory.

Role of Student

Students must broaden their understanding of their own personal beliefs to engage in total patient care based on all four patterns of knowing. Some students will be stronger in some areas than in others (similar to Gardner's [1999] MI theory) and will need to seek assistance to apply the theory completely.

Advantages

Carper (1978) provided leadership in articulating the art of nursing and therefore much more than a profession based on knowledge discovered through the scientific method. By introducing empirics, aesthetics, personal knowledge, and moral patterns of knowledge, she effectively legitimized the art of holistic nursing.

Disadvantages

In today's nursing education climate faculty desiring to embrace the patterns of knowing in a curriculum may find it difficult to balance learning opportunities in the art of nursing patterns with those in empirical knowledge, which is the focus of licensure and accreditation.

Application

The use of the patterns of knowing will require that faculty embrace the concepts as central to a school or program philosophy. The curriculum framework must be designed to include the patterns of knowing and ensure learning opportunities. Seminars, postconferences, and care plan discussions may be designed around the four patterns as a means of valuing each pattern contribution. Opportunities to discuss all patterns relative to clinical experiences can be afforded in clinical, postconference, and classroom environments. Specific assignments can be designed to focus of each of the patterns.

Narrative Pedagogy

Narrative pedagogy is a research-based alternative for reforming nursing education and uses conventional, phenomenological, critical, and feminist pedagogies. Narrative pedagogy is the application of these pedagogies, along with postmodern discourses in nursing education. A 12-year study produced nine themes from interview texts obtained from teachers, students, and clinicians (Diekelmann, 2001). The experience of learning and teaching is articulated in the common and shared experiences of what is really important in nursing education. The Concernful Practices of Schooling Learning Teaching outlined by Diekelmann (2001, p. 57) are as follows:

- *Gathering:* Bringing in and calling forth
- *Creating places:* Keeping open a future of possibilities
- *Assembling:* Constructing and cultivating
- *Staying:* Knowing and connecting
- *Caring:* Engendering community
- *Interpreting:* Unlearning and becoming
- *Presencing:* Attending and being open
- *Preserving:* Reading, writing, thinking, and dialogue
- *Questioning:* Meaning and making visible

Narrative pedagogy is a commitment to practical discourse in which knowledge gained through the experiences of teachers, students, and clinicians can be used to reform nursing education. It is the collective interpretation of common experience that encourages shared learning.

Premise

Narrative pedagogy is the dialogue and debate among and between teachers, students, and clinicians that questions both what is concealed and what is revealed. The nine themes listed earlier exemplify Concernful Practices of Schooling Learning Teaching.

Setting/Climate

The Concernful Practices are applicable in any setting and offer a climate of productive dialogue among and between clinicians, teachers, and students.

Role of Faculty

Faculty must develop an understanding and skill in using the nine themes of Concernful Practices to expose the hidden understandings and provoke new possibilities in nursing education. Faculty must also understand the nature of the interpretive pedagogies in contrast to and along with conventional pedagogy. Faculty will likely engage in personal and professional introspection because the nine Concernful Practices will illuminate both positive and negative attributes.

Role of Student

Students share the responsibility for discourse and deconstruction with clinicians and faculty.

Advantages

Narrative pedagogy gathers and explores contemporary successes and failures in nursing education. It uses all pedagogies and creates new possibilities for schooling, teaching, and learning that not only meld the conventional and interpretive pedagogies but also move beyond the issues of power, critique, and deconstruction (Diekelmann, 2001).

Disadvantages

Narrative pedagogy represents a new frontier in nursing education and currently relies on the theoretical understanding of the concepts and theories leading up to the discovery of the nine themes.

Application

Faculty construct activities for content and skills acquisition through encouraging meaning making in students relative to stories about experience. Through listening and responding to stories and personal perceptions knowledge is developed in context. Questions around stories enact narrative pedagogy as a means for shifting thinking from what is known to what is important and needs to be known.

Caring

Watson (1989) indicated that "the ethic of caring provides an expanded context for nursing education by calling upon the highest ethical self in the process of an evolving consciousness" (p. 53). The caring curriculum movement refers to a reconceptualization of nursing education that has been presented as a "curriculum revolution." The movement has been extensively described by Bevis (1988, 1989a, 1989b, 1990, 1993), Bevis and Murray (1990), Diekelmann (1988, 1989), Munhall (1988), Tanner (1988), and Watson (1988). The caring curriculum model integrates the pioneering work of Bevis (1989a), Leininger (1981), Murray (1989), Watson (1988), and others who believe that caring represents the moral ideal and central essential core of nursing (Bevis, 1989b).

The model integrates, within a human science orientation, concepts and principles drawn from the humanistic–existentialist perspective and feminist philosophy, as well as from phenomenology (Bevis, 1990). Benner's work (1983, 1984, 1985), presented in several publications (Benner & Tanner, 1987; Benner & Wrubel, 1989; Benner et al., 1992), about novice to expert clinical practice is considered an important model for educative experiences. Although no specific component focuses on cognitive learning theories, the concept of constructivism is an integral part of the caring curriculum model. Symonds (1990) advocated that a feminist philosophy and principles become an integral part of a new model for nursing education. Diekelmann (1989) suggested that faculty engage in hermeneutic inquiry as a way of assisting students to gain new meanings for their clinical practice.

The caring movement mandates significant changes in the design and implementation of nursing curriculum; this directive is based, in part, on the rationale that nursing education thus far has not been successful in advancing nursing as a professional discipline (Bevis, 1988, 1989c). Advocates for the movement assert that the behavioristic learning model used in nursing education since the 1950s is more suitable for industrial training than for a professional educative experience (Bevis, 1988, 1993; Diekelmann, 1988).

Valiga (1988) indicated that evidence supports a lack of progress in nursing education and a lack of any significant change in the cognitive development of students. In addition, social forces associated with the increasingly complex and multifaceted nursing roles needed to meet the health care needs of a diverse multicultural society require well-educated and well-trained nurses who are highly skilled scholar–clinicians.

The goal of the caring curriculum is to create an educational experience in nursing that is more in accord with true education and consistent with the professional nursing philosophy and values that are an integral part of contemporary nursing practice, research, and education. Bevis (1988, 1990) and Bevis and Murray (1990) described the caring curriculum model as providing education for professional nursing that emphasizes analytical, problem-solving, and critical thinking skills.

Content and student learning experiences must be based on the science of human caring and grounded in and derived from the actual reality of lived experience as ascertained from phenomenology rather than merely the content that nurse educators have traditionally taught or the content as they believe it should be. Although theory traditionally has been taught to inform practice, in the new models theory and practice are viewed as informing each other. A restructured focus of learning is based in clinical practice and uses content as the substance to actively involve students in scholarly endeavors (Bevis, 1988).

Premise

Curriculum is based on the integration of humanistic–existential, phenomenological, feminist, and caring ideologies (Bevis, 1990). The educative experience requires caring faculty–student relationships.

Setting/Climate

The caring curriculum model can be implemented in any setting that encourages an interactive relationship between faculty and students.

Role of Faculty

Faculty implementing a caring curriculum work to discover ways to eliminate adversarial relationships with students (Diekelmann, 1989); faculty also strive to maintain open, honest, caring, and supportive relationships. It is within this context that faculty create a climate and structure that promotes the desired learning environment. Faculty develop and model the spirit of inquiry that helps students to develop maturity in their learning and cognitive abilities. Students are guided as they examine information, concepts, and principles and struggle with uncertainty (Bevis, 1989d). The content selected is basic to what is needed in accord with the program's philosophy and desired graduate outcomes. Although the primary content may be presented as information, faculty focus their efforts on helping students see beyond the information to discern the underlying assumptions (Bevis, 1989c).

To provide students with an in-depth educative learning experience, faculty function in different roles and become experts in learning and in the subject matter. Frequent use of instructional strategies that facilitate active learning, such as the use of questioning and dialogue, is important. Faculty-initiated dialogues with students focus on developing the attributes of intellectual curiosity, caring, caring roles, ethical ideals, and assertiveness (Bevis, 1988). Dialogues occur within the context of a spirit of inquiry and should stimulate and enhance faculty and student learning as meanings of the content are explored.

The use of lecture as an instructional strategy is minimized; instead, faculty use instructional strategies such as role play, debate, discussion, questioning, and case studies (see Chapter 13). Exploration of the cases of actual lived experiences of patients cared for by expert nurses rather than constructed case studies allows examination of the real-life complexities encountered in nursing practice. This approach enables faculty to find out how students develop meanings for their practice (Bevis, 1989c). In addition, instructional materials that present opposing or different points of view and different ways of doing things expand students' cognitive development (Bevis, 1989d).

Tools for evaluating learning, such as essay examinations, position and reaction papers, reflective journals, and projects that involve active student participation, are used because they are consistent with the teaching and learning strategies (Bevis, 1989d). (See Chapters 21 and 23 for further information about the evaluation of learning outcomes.)

Role of Student

Students adopt different learning styles that include assuming responsibility for active learning and seeking support and guidance from faculty. It is important that students shift their conception of faculty as authority figures to that of colleagues in the learning enterprise because students are expected to function as active participants in the decision-making structure. Flexibility, tolerance for ambiguity, the ability to manage diversity and conflicts, and the ability to organize their own knowledge and experiences are additional student characteristics considered to be essential for learning within the caring curriculum paradigm (Valiga, 1988).

Advantages

Faculty gain new and challenging opportunities to engage in the scholarship of teaching as they become knowledgeable about and able to apply new theoretical models in curriculum development and instructional strategies. They also have increased opportunities to use creativity and problem solving to deal with instructional issues and improve the way in which students are taught.

Changes in faculty's relationship with students promote an energized climate in which faculty become allies with students. Students' active engagement in the teaching–learning process allows more opportunities for faculty to observe increases in students' self-esteem, self-confidence, and competence. Students experience an increase in their internal motivation and sense of responsibility. Opportunities to observe students' increased intellectual growth and commitment to professional nursing should provide more personal satisfaction to faculty. Furthermore, the status of professional nursing is enhanced as nurses in clinical practice demonstrate higher levels of competence.

Disadvantages

Implementation of the caring curriculum model is a labor-intensive and time-consuming process that includes advanced long-term planning for curriculum redesign, creation of new instructional strategies, and development of faculty. The model may not be feasible for courses or programs with large enrollments because of the demands placed on faculty and students for new teaching–learning behaviors. Development of these new behaviors involves trust and socialization to instructional approaches that are different from the traditional behavioristic model. The shift to a student-centered and learning-centered focus from a teacher-centered focus is challenging for both faculty and students. Faculty should expect and be prepared to provide more support to students as they adapt to this new approach to learning. Students need to have attained a level of cognitive development that enables them to shift from the behavioral model.

Application

Heliker (1994) suggested that problem-based learning has many features that are consistent with the goals and elements presented in caring curriculum models. Content should be substantive and based on the reality of actual clinical practice so that practice and theory inform each other. Small groups of students can dialogue cooperatively about real cases of the lived experience of patients, and questions designed to initiate and stimulate inquiry for each paradigm case can guide the dialogues.

SUMMARY

The central focus of the educational experience is the learner as active participant in transaction with the teacher. Students are given considerable control over the development of learning experiences, and they construct and create knowledge. Faculty assume a primary role as designers of the learning environment and learning experiences in a shared governance approach with students and others contributing to the learning climate.

The learning theories and frameworks presented in this chapter provide a guide for faculty to use within the four steps of the teaching–learning process. Each theory or framework has varying degrees of usefulness depending on the faculty's philosophy about teaching; the philosophy that guides the curriculum; the setting and climate in which the teaching is to occur; student characteristics; and the purpose, nature, and content of the course. Within these contextual variables, faculty need to weigh the advantages and disadvantages of each theory or framework and select those that are most appropriate.

Recent literature in education and nursing education indicate that the current and future emphasis in the learning paradigm is and will be on having learners construct and create knowledge while faculty serve as designers, facilitators, coaches, guides, and mentors. For most learning experiences in higher education and for nursing in particular, behavioristic principles have limited relevance. Current and emerging concepts and principles in cognitive, humanistic, and adult learning theories and Perry's model for intellectual and cognitive development, as well as those included in the interpretive pedagogies, patterns of knowing, narrative pedagogies, and caring, are consistent with the thrust of the learning paradigm in which faculty create the environment and learning experiences and the learner has the central role and assumes control (Barr & Tagg, 1995).

REFERENCES

Anderson, J. R. (1980). *Cognitive psychology and its implications.* San Francisco: W. H. Freeman.

Anderson, J. R. (1985). *Cognitive psychology and its implications* (2nd ed.). San Francisco: W. H. Freeman.

Atkinson, J. R., & Shiffrin, R. M. (1968). Human memory: A proposed system and its control processes. In K. W. Spence & J. T. Spence (Eds.), *The psychology of learning and motivation: Advances in research and theory* (Vol. 2, pp. 89-115). New York: Academic Press.

Ausubel, D. P. (1960). The use of advanced organizers in the learning and retention of meaningful verbal material. *Journal of Educational Psychology, 51,* 267-272.

Ausubel, D. P. (1978). *Educational psychology: A cognitive view* (2nd ed.). New York: Holt, Rinehart & Winston.

Ausubel, D. P., Novak, J. D., & Hanesian, H. (1968). *Educational psychology: A cognitive view.* New York: Holt, Rinehart & Winston.

Ausubel, D. P., & Robinson, F. G. (1969). *School learning: An introduction to educational psychology.* New York: Holt, Rinehart & Winston.

Barr, R. B., & Tagg, J. (1995). From teaching to learning. *Change, 27*(6), 13-25.

Beck, S. E. (1995). Cooperative learning and feminist pedagogy: A model for classroom instruction in nursing education. *Journal of Nursing Education, 34*(5), 222-227.

Belenky, M. F., Clinchy, B. M., Goldberger, N. R., & Tarule, J. M. (1986). *Women's ways of knowing.* New York: Basic Books.

Benner, P. (1983). Uncovering the knowledge embedded in clinical practice. *Image, 15*(2), 36-41.

Benner, P. (1984). *From novice to expert.* Menlo Park, CA: Addison-Wesley.

Benner, P. (1985). Quality of life: A phenomenological perspective on explanation, prediction, and understanding in nursing science. *Advances in Nursing Science, 8*(1), 1-14.

Benner, P., & Tanner, C. (1987). Clinical judgment: How expert nurse uses intuition. *American Journal of Nursing, 87*(1), 23-31.

Benner, P., Tanner, C., & Chesla, C. (1992). From beginner to expert: Gaining a differentiated world in critical care nursing. *Advances in Nursing Science, 14*(3), 13-28.

Benner, P., & Wrubel, J. (1989). *The primacy of caring: Stress and coping in health and illness.* Menlo Park, CA: Addison-Wesley.

Bevis, E. O. (1973). *Curriculum building in nursing: A process.* St. Louis: Mosby.

Bevis, E. O. (1978). *Curriculum building in nursing: A process* (2nd ed.). St. Louis: Mosby.

Bevis, E. O. (1982). *Curriculum building in nursing: A process* (3rd ed.). St. Louis: Mosby.

Bevis, E. O. (1988). New directions for a new age. In *Curriculum revolution: Mandate for change* (pp. 27-52). New York: National League for Nursing.

Bevis, E. O. (1989a). *Curriculum building in nursing: A process* (3rd ed.). New York: National League for Nursing.

Bevis, E. O. (1989b). The curriculum consequences. In *Curriculum revolution: Reconceptualizing nursing education* (pp. 115-134). New York: National League for Nursing.

Bevis, E. O. (1989c). Teaching and learning: The key to education and professionalism. In E. O. Bevis & J. Watson, *Toward a caring curriculum* (pp. 153-188). New York: National League for Nursing.

Bevis, E. O. (1989d). Teaching and learning: A practical commentary. In E. O. Bevis & J. Watson, *Toward a caring curriculum* (pp. 217-259). New York: National League for Nursing.

Bevis, E. O. (1990). Has the curriculum become the new religion? In *Curriculum revolution: Redefining the student-teacher relationship* (pp. 57-66). New York: National League for Nursing.

Bevis, E. O. (1993). All in all it was a pretty good funeral. *Journal of Nursing Education, 32*(2), 101-105.

Bevis, E. O., & Murray, J. P. (1990). The essence of the curriculum revolution: Emancipatory teaching. *Journal of Nursing Education, 29*(7), 326-331.

Bevis E. O., & Watson, J. *Toward a caring curriculum* (pp. 153-188). New York: National League for Nursing.

Bloom, B. S., Englehart, M. D., Furst, E. J., Hill, W. H., & Krawthwhol, D. R. (1956). *Taxonomy of educational objectives: Handbook 1, Cognitive domain.* New York: David McKay.

Boughn, S. (1991). A women's health course with a feminist perspective: Learning to care for and empower ourselves. *Nursing & Health Care, 12*(2), 76-80.

Boughn, S., & Wang, H. (1994). Introducing a feminist perspective to nursing curricula: A quantitative study. *Journal of Nursing Education, 33*(3), 112-117.

Boyd, C. O. (1988). Phenomenology: A foundation for nursing curriculum. In *Curriculum revolution: Mandate for change* (pp. 65-87). New York: National League for Nursing.

Brookfield, S. D. (1995). *Becoming a critically reflective teacher.* San Francisco: Jossey-Bass.

Caffarella, R. S., & Barnett, B. G. (1994). Characteristics of adult learners and foundations of experiential learning. In L. Jackson & R. S. Caffarella (Eds.), *Experiential learning: A new approach* (pp. 29-44). San Francisco: Jossey-Bass.

Carper, B. (1978). Fundamental patterns of knowing. *Advances in Nursing Science, 1*(1), 13-23.

Chinn, P. L. (1989a). Feminist pedagogy in nursing education. In *Curriculum revolution: Reconceptualizing nursing education* (pp. 9-24). New York: National League for Nursing.

Chinn, P. L. (1989b). Nursing patterns of knowing and feminist thought. *Nursing & Health Care, 10*(2), 71-75.

Chinn, P. L., & Wheeler, C. E. (1985). Feminism and nursing. *Nursing Outlook, 33*(2), 74-77.

Collins, M. S. (1981). *An investigation of the development of professional commitment in baccalaureate nursing students.* Unpublished doctoral dissertation. Syracuse University.

Colucciello, M. L. (1988). Creating powerful learning environments. *Nursing Connections, 1*(2), 23-33.

Combs, A. W. (1959). *Individual behavior: A perceptual approach to behavior* (Rev. ed.). New York: Harper.

Combs, A. W. (1981). Humanistic education: Too tender for a tough world? *Phi Delta Kappa, 62*(6), 446-449.

Combs, A. W. (1994). *Helping relationships: Basic concepts for helping professions* (4th ed.). Boston: Allyn & Bacon.

Corcoran, S., Narayan, S., & Moreland, H. (1988). Thinking aloud: A strategy to improve clinical decision making. *Heart & Lung, 77*(5), 463-468.

Cross, K. P. (1981). *Adults as learners: Increasing participation and facilitating learning.* San Francisco: Jossey-Bass.

Davis, J. R. (1993). *Better teaching, more learning: Strategies for success in postsecondary settings.* Phoenix: Oryx Press.

Dembo, M. H. (1988). *Teaching for learning: Applying educational psychology in the classroom* (3rd ed.). Santa Monica, CA: Goodyear.

deTornyay, R. (1971). *Strategies for teaching nursing.* New York: Wiley.

deTornyay, R. (1982). *Strategies for teaching nursing* (2nd ed.). New York: Wiley.

deTornyay, R., & Thompson, M. (1987). *Strategies for teaching nursing* (3rd ed.). New York: Wiley.

Dewey, J. (1916). *Democracy and education.* New York: Macmillan.

Dewey, J. (1938). *Education and experience.* New York: Macmillan.

Dewey, J. (1939). *Freedom and culture.* New York: G. P. Putnam Sons.

Diekelmann, N. L. (1988). Curriculum revolution: A theoretical and philosophical mandate for change. In *Curriculum revolution: Mandate for change* (pp. 137-157). New York: National League for Nursing.

Diekelmann, N. L. (1989). The nursing curriculum: Lived experiences of students. In *Curriculum revolution: Reconceptualizing nursing education* (pp. 25-41). New York: National League for Nursing.

Diekelmann, N. (2001). Narrative pedagogy: Heideggerian hermeneutical analysis of lived experiences of students, teachers, and clinicians. *Advances in Nursing Science, 23*(3), 53-71.

Driscoll, M. P. (1994). *Psychology of learning for instruction.* Boston: Allyn & Bacon.

Eisner, E. (1983, January). The art and craft of teaching. *Educational Leadership*, p. 10.

Escolano, A. (1996). Postmodernity or high modernity? Emerging approaches in the new history of education. *Paedagogica Historica 32*(2), 325-331.

Fosnot, C. T. (1996). *Constructivism: Theory, perspectives and practice.* New York: Teachers College Press.

Freire, P. (1971). *Pedagogy of the oppressed.* Translated by M. B. Ramos. New York: Continuum.

Freire, P. & Macedo, D. (1987). *Learning: Reading the word and the world.* Westport, CT: Greenwood Publishing Group.

Frisch, N. C. (1987). Value analysis: a method for teaching nursing ethics and promoting the moral development of students. *Journal of Nursing Education 26*(8), 328-332.

Frisch, N. C. (1990). An international nursing student exchange program: An educational experience that enhanced student cognitive development. *Journal of Nursing Education, 29*(1), 10-12.

Galbraith, M. W. (1991a). *Adult learning methods.* Malabar, FL: Krieger.

Galbraith, M. W. (1991b). *Facilitating adult learning: A transactional process.* Malabar, FL: Krieger.

Gardner, H. (1983). *Frames of mind.* New York: Basic Books.

Gardner, H. (1985). *The minds' new science.* New York: Basic Books.

Gardner, H. (1993). *Multiple intelligences: The theory in practice.* New York: Basic Books.

Gardner, H. (1999). *Intelligence reframed: Multiple intelligences for the 21st century.* New York: Basic Books.

Gardner, H. (2003, April). *Multiple intelligences after twenty years.* Paper presented at the American Educational Research Association, Chicago, IL.

Giroux, H., & McLaren, P. (1992). Writing from the margins: Geographies of identity, pedagogy, and power. *Journal of Education, 174*, 7-30.

Glasser, W. L. (1969). *Schools without failure.* New York: Harper & Row.

Grippin, P., & Peters, S. (1984). *Learning theory and learning outcomes.* Lanham, MD: University Press of America.

Guardo, C. J. (1986). Designing curricula for imaginary students. *Liberal Education, 72*(3), 213-219.

Hall, J.M. (1999). Marginalization revisited: Critical, postmodern, and liberation perspectives. *Advances in Nursing Science, 22*(1), 88-102.

Hall, J. M., Stevens, P. E. & Meleis, A. I. (1994). Marginalization: A guiding concept for valuing diversity in nursing knowledge development. *Advances in Nursing Science 16*(4), 23-41.

Hartley, J. (1976, Spring). Preinstructional strategies: The role of pretests, behavioral objectives, overviews and advanced organizers. *Review of Educational Research, 46*(2), 239-265.

Hartrick, G. (1998). A critical pedagogy for family nursing. *Journal of Nursing Education, 37*(2) 80-84.

Hayes, E. R. (1989). Insights from women's experience for teaching and learning. In E. R. Hayes (Ed.), *Effective teaching styles: New directions for adult and continuing education* (p. 43). San Francisco: Jossey-Bass.

Heidegger, M. (1962). *Being and time.* Translated by J. Macquarrie & E. Robinson. New York: Harper & Row.

Heidgerken, I. E. (1953). *Teaching in schools of nursing* (2nd ed.). Philadelphia: J. B. Lippincott.

Heliker, D. (1994). Meeting the challenge of the curriculum revolution: Problem-based learning in nursing education. *Journal of Nursing Education, 33*(1), 45-47.

Hiemestra, R., & Sisco, B. (1990). *Individualizing instruction.* San Francisco: Jossey-Bass.

Hilgard, E. R., & Bower, G. H. (1966). *Theories of learning.* New York: Appleton-Century-Crofts.

Hodges, H. F. (1996). Journal writing as a mode of thinking for RN-BSN students: A leveled approach to learning to listen to self and others. *Journal of Nursing Education, 35*(3), 137-141.

Holt, J. (1964). *How children fail.* New York: Pitman.

Hyman, R. T. (1974). *Ways of teaching* (2nd ed.). Philadelphia: J. B. Lippincott.

Ironside, P.M. (2001). Creating a research base for nursing education: An interpretive review of conventional, critical, feminist, postmodern, and phenomenologic pedagogies. *Advances in Nursing Science, 23*(3), 72-87

Jackson, L., & Caffarella, R. S. (1994). *Experiential learning: A new approach.* San Francisco: Jossey-Bass.

Jacobs-Kramer, M., & Chinn, P. (1988). Perspectives on knowing: A model of nursing knowledge. *Scholarly Inquiry for Nursing Practice: An International Journal, 2,* 129-139.

Kaufmann, J. (2000). Reading counter-hegemonic practices through a postmodern lens. *International Journal of Lifelong Education, 19*(5), 430-447.

Knowles, M. S. (1980). *The modern practice of adult education.* Chicago: Follett.

Knowles, M. S. (1984). *The adult learner: A neglected species* (3rd ed.). Houston: Gulf.

Knowles, M. S. (1986). *Using learning contracts.* San Francisco: Jossey-Bass.

Knowles, M. S. (1990). *The adult learner: A neglected species* (4th ed.). Houston: Gulf.

Kohlberg, L. (1984). *The psychology of moral development: The nature and validity of moral stages.* San Francisco: Harper & Row.

Kondora, L. L. (1993). A Heideggerian hermeneutical analysis of survivors of incest. *Image, 25*(1), 11-16.

Learn, C. D. (1990). The moral dimension: Humanism in education. In M. Leininger & J. Watson (Eds.), *The caring imperative in education.* New York: National League for Nursing.

Leininger, M. (1978). *Transcultural nursing: Concepts, theories and practice.* New York: Wiley.

Leininger, M. (Ed.). (1981). *Caring: An essential human need.* Thorofare, NJ: Charles B. Slack.

Lewin, K. (1951). *Field theory in social science.* New York: Harper & Row.

Mager, R. F. (1962). *Preparing instructional objectives.* Palo Alto, CA: Fearon Publishers.

Maslow, A. (1954). *Motivation and personality.* New York: Harper & Row.

Maslow, A. (1962). *Toward a psychology of being.* Princeton, NJ: D. Van Nostrand.

Mayer, R. E. (1979). Twenty years of research on advanced organizer: Assimilation theory is still the best predictor of results. *Instructional Science, 8,* 133-167.

McGovern, M., & Valiga, T. M. (1997). Promoting the cognitive development of freshman nursing students. *Journal of Nursing Education, 36*(1), 29-35.

McKeachie, W. J. (1980). Improving lectures by understanding students' information processing. In W. J. McKeachie (Ed.), *Learning, cognition and college teaching.* San Francisco: Jossey-Bass.

Merleau-Ponty, M. (1962). *Phenomenology of perception.* Translated by C. Smith. New York: Humanities Press.

Merriam, S. B., & Caffarella, R. S. (1991). *Learning in adulthood: A comprehensive guide.* San Francisco: Jossey-Bass.

Morse, G. G. (1995). Reframing women's health in nursing education: A feminist approach. *Nursing Outlook, 43*(6), 273-277.

Munhall, P. L. (1988). Curriculum revolution: A social mandate for change. In *Curriculum revolution: Mandate for change.* New York: National League for Nursing.

Murray, J. (1989). *Developing criteria to support new curriculum models for doctoral education in nursing.* Unpublished doctoral dissertation, University of Georgia.

Muth, K. D., Britton, B. K., Glynn, S. M., & Graves, M. F. (1988). Thinking aloud while studying text: Rehearsing key ideas. *Journal of Educational Psychology, 80,* 315-318.

Newman, F., Holzman, L. (1993). *Lev Vygotsky: Revolutionalry scientist.* London: Routledge

Norman, D. A. (Ed.) (1970). *Models of human memory* (pp. 1-15). New York: Academic Press.

Norman, D. A. (1989). What goes on in the mind of the learner. In W. J. McKeachie (Ed.), *Learning, cognition and college teaching.* San Francisco: Jossey-Bass.

Novak, J. D., Gowin, D. B., & Johansen, G. T. (1983). The use of concept mapping and knowledge vis-à-vis mapping with junior high school science students. *Science Education, 67*(5), 625-645.

Omery, A. (1983). Phenomenology: A method for nursing research. *Advances in Nursing Science, 5*(2), 49-63.

Paterson, J., & Zderad, L. (1976). *Humanistic nursing.* New York: Wiley.

Perry, W. G. (1970). *Forms of intellectual and ethical development in the college years: A scheme.* New York: Rinehart & Winston.

Perry, W. G. (1981). Forms of cognitive and ethical growth: The making of meaning. In A. W. Chickering and Associates, *The modern American college: Responding to the new realities of diverse students and a changing society* (pp. 76-116). San Francisco: Jossey-Bass.

Piaget, J. (1970a). Piaget's theory. In P. H. Musen (Ed.), *Carmichael's manual of psychology* (pp. 703-752). New York: Wiley.

Piaget, J. (1970b). *Structuralism.* New York: Basic Books.

Piaget, J. (1973). *To understand is to invent: The future of education.* New York: Grossman.

Ratner, C. (1991). *Vygotsky's sociohistorical psychology and its contemporary applications.* New York: Plenum

Reigeluth, C. M. (1983). Instructional design: What is it and why is it? In C. M. Reigeluth (Ed.), *Instructional-design theories and models: An overview of their current status.* Hillsdale, NJ: Erlbaum.

Reilly, D. E. (1975). *Behavioral objectives in nursing evaluation of learner attainment.* New York: Appleton-Century-Crofts.

Reilly, D. E. (1980). *Behavioral objectives: Evaluation in nursing* (2nd ed.). New York: Appleton-Century-Crofts.

Reilly, D. E., & Oermann, M. H. (1990). *Behavioral objectives: Evaluation in nursing* (3rd ed.). New York: National League for Nursing.

Rogers, C. R. (1954). *Client-centered therapy.* Boston: Houghton Mifflin.

Rogers, C. R. (1961). *On becoming a person.* Boston: Houghton Mifflin.

Rogers, C. R. (1969). *Freedom to learn.* Columbus, OH: Charles E. Merrill.

Romyn, D. R. (2001). Disavowal of the behaviorist paradigm in nursing education: What makes it so difficult to unseat? *Advances in Nursing Science, 23*(3) 1-10.

Rooda, L. A. (1994). Effects of mind mapping on student achievement in a nursing research course. *Nurse Educator, 19*(6), 25-27.

Ruffing-Rahal, M. A. (1992). Incorporating feminism into the graduate curriculum. *Journal of Nursing Education, 31*(6), 247-252.

Rumelhart, D. E. (1981). *Understanding understanding.* La Jolla, CA: University of California, San Diego, Center for Human Information Process.

Rumelhart, D. E., & Ortony, A. (1977). The representation of knowledge in memory. In R. C. Anderson, R. J. Spiro, & W. E. Montague (Eds.), *Schooling and the acquisition of knowledge* (pp. 99-135). Hillsdale, NJ: Erlbaum.

Schon, D. (1983). *The reflective practitioner: How professionals think in action.* New York: Basic Books.

Shuell, T. J. (1986). Cognitive conceptions of learning. *Review of Educational Research, 56*(4), 411-436.

Simon, H. A. (1980). Information processing models of cognition. *Annual Review of Psychology, 30*, 363-396.

Skinner, B. F. (1953). *Science and human behavior.* New York: Macmillan.

Slavin, R. E. (1988). *Educational psychology: Theory into practice* (2nd ed.). Englewood Cliffs, NJ: Prentice Hall.

Snow, R. E., & Peterson, P. L. (1980). Recognizing differences in student aptitudes. In W. J. McKeachie (Ed.), *Learning, cognition, and college teaching.* San Francisco: Jossey-Bass.

Symonds, J. M. (1990). Revolutionizing the student-teacher relationship. In *Curriculum revolution: Redefining the student-teacher relationship* (pp. 47-55). New York: National League for Nursing.

Tanner, C. (1987). Teaching clinical judgment. In J. Fitzpatrick & R. T. Taunton (Eds.), *Annual Review of Nursing Research* (Vol. 5). New York: Springer.

Tanner, C. (1988). Curriculum revolution: The practice mandate. *Nursing & Health Care, 9*(8), 427-430.

Tanner, C. A. (1990). Reflections on the curriculum revolution. *Journal of Nursing Education, 29*(7), 295-299.

Tanner, C., Benner, P., Chesla, C., & Gordon, D. R. (1993). The phenomenology of knowing the patient. *Image, 25*(4), 273-280.

Taylor, B. (1993). Phenomenology: A way to understanding nursing practice. *International Journal of Nursing Studies, 30*(2), 171-179.

Thoma, G. A. (1993). The Perry framework and tactics for teaching critical thinking in economics. *Journal of Economic Education, 24*(2), 128-136.

Traynor, M. (1997). Postmodern research: No grounding or privilege, just free floating trouble making. *Nursing Inquiry, 4*(2), 99-107

Tulving, E. (1972). Episodic and semantic memory. In E. Tulving & W. Donaldson (Eds.), *Organization of memory.* New York: Academic Press.

Tulving, E. (1985). How many memory systems are there? *American Psychologist, 40,* 385-398.

Tyler, R. W. (1949). *Basic principles of curriculum and instruction.* Chicago: University of Chicago Press.

Valiga, T. M. (1988). Curriculum outcomes and cognitive development: New perspectives for nursing education. In *Curriculum revolution: Mandate for change* (pp. 177-200). New York: National League for Nursing.

Van der Veer, R., & Valsiner, J. (Eds.). (1994). *The Vygotsky reader.* Oxford: Blackwell

Van Manen, M. (1990). *Researching lived experience: Human science for an action sensitive pedagogy.* London, Ontario: State University of New York Press.

van Niekerk, K., & van Aswegen, E. (1993). Implementing problem-based learning in nursing. *Nursing RSA Verpleging, 8*(5), 37-41.

Vygotsky, L. (1986). *Thought and language.* Cambridge, MA: MIT Press. (Original work published in 1962.)

Walton, J. C. (1996). The changing environment: New challenges for nursing education. *Journal of Nursing Education, 35*(9), 400-405.

Ward, P. C. (1992). Two legal environment writing exercises following the Perry scheme of cognitive development. *The Journal of Legal Studies Education, 10*(1), 87.

Watson, J. (1988). Human caring as moral context for nursing education. *Nursing & Health Care, 9*(8), 423-425.

Watson, J. (1989). Transformative thinking and a caring curriculum. In E. O. Bevis & J. Watson, *Toward a caring curriculum: A new pedagogy for nursing* (pp. 51-60). New York: National League for Nursing.

Weinstein, C. E., & Meyer, D. K. (1991, Spring). Cognitive learning strategies and college teaching. In R. J. Menges & M. D. Svinicki (Eds.), *New directions for teaching and learning: College teaching: From theory to practice* (Vol. 45, pp. 15-25). San Francisco: Jossey-Bass.

Wertsch, J. V. (1985). *Vygotsky and the social formation of mind.* Cambridge, MA: Harvard University

Wheeler, C., & Chinn, P. (1989). *Peace and power: A handbook of feminist process* (2nd ed.). New York: National League for Nursing.

Widick, C., & Simpson, D. (1978). Developmental concepts in college instruction. In C. A. Parker (Ed.), *Encouraging development in college student* (pp. 227-259). Minneapolis: University of Minnesota Press.

Wittrock, M. C. (1977). Learning as a generative process. In M. C. Wittrock (Ed.), *Learning and instruction* (pp. 621-631). Berkeley, CA: McCrutchan.

Wittrock, M. C. (1978). Education and the cognitive processes of the brain. In J. S. Chall & A. F. Minsky (Eds.), *The seventy-seventh yearbook of the National Society for the Study of Education, Part II.* Chicago: University of Chicago Press.

Wittrock, M. C. (1986). Students' thought processes. In M. C. Wittrock (Ed.), *Handbook of research on teaching* (3rd ed., pp. 297-314). New York: Macmillan.

Zorn, C. R. (1995). An analysis of the impact of participation in an international study program on the cognitive development of senior nursing students. *Journal of Nursing Education, 34*(2), 67-70.

13

STRATEGIES TO PROMOTE CRITICAL THINKING AND ACTIVE LEARNING

Connie J. Rowles, DSN, RN, CNAA, Carole Brigham, EdD, RN

Nursing faculty spend a considerable amount of their time planning experiences to facilitate student learning. The selection of teaching strategies and learning experiences has been traditionally governed by behavioral objectives. However, nursing education has been undergoing a major revolution, with attention focused on how to teach students to think critically. Therefore nurse educators are continually reexamining the "best" way to teach and to empower students for learning. The purpose of this chapter is to identify strategies students and faculty can use to promote learning. The chapter begins with a discussion of critical thinking as the basis for any strategy and goes on to explain how to develop effective learning experiences. The chapter concludes with a description of a variety of teaching strategies. Each strategy is presented with a discussion of its use, its advantages and disadvantages, and tips for making the learning experience interactive and meaningful.

CRITICAL THINKING AND ACTIVE LEARNING

Thinking, reflective thinking, and critical thinking have been topics of discussion among educators for many years (Bandman & Bandman, 1995; Brookfield, 1987, 1995; Dewey, 1933; Facione, 1990; Halpern & Associates, 1994; Hunkins, 1985; Kurfiss, 1988; McPeck, 1981; Norris & Ennis, 1989; Paul, 1995; Perry, 1970; Siegel, 1980; Watson & Glaser, 1984). Although there are many definitions of critical thinking, this chapter focuses on the ideal critical thinker and the related cognitive skills.

The Ideal Critical Thinker Defined

Most experts agree that if an individual is a critical thinker, he or she not only has well-developed critical thinking skills but also exhibits what are variously described as a disposition, attitude, or traits of a critical thinker (Baron & Sternberg, 1986; Facione et al., 1994; Ford & Profetto-McGrath, 1994;

Kataoka-Yahiro & Saylor, 1994; Paul, 1995; Pless & Clayton, 1993; Watson & Glaser, 1984).

This chapter uses Facione's definition (1990) of an ideal critical thinker. This description was derived by a consensus of experts in critical thinking who participated in a Delphi study. The panel of experts included "46 scholars, educators and leading figures in critical thinking theory and critical thinking assessment research" (p. 34). The experts essentially agreed that

> The ideal critical thinker is habitually inquisitive, well-informed, trustful of reason, open-minded, flexible, fair-minded in evaluation, honest in facing personal biases, prudent in making judgments, willing to reconsider, clear about issues, orderly in complex matters, diligent in seeking relevant information, reasonable in the selection of criteria, focused in inquiry, and persistent in seeking results which are as precise as the subject and the circumstances of inquiry permit. (p. 3)

Facione et al. (1994) suggest that the Delphi study description of an ideal critical thinker describes a nurse with ideal clinical judgment.

Cognitive skills (subskills) of critical thinking were also delineated in Facione's Delphi study (1990). These include the cognitive skills and subskills of *analysis* (examining ideas, identifying arguments, analyzing arguments), *evaluation* (assessing claims, assessing arguments), *inference* (querying evidence, conjecturing alternatives, drawing conclusions), *interpretation* (categorizing, decoding significance, clarifying meaning), *explanation* (stating results, justifying procedures, presenting arguments), and *self-regulation* (self-examination and self-correction) (Facione, 1990).

Critical Thinking in Nursing and Nursing Education

Considering the discussion on the ideal critical thinker, critical thinking skills, and disposition, it is argued that nurses need a high level of critical thinking skills and a critical thinking disposition. Nurses encounter multiple patients with the same health care needs; however, each patient responds to those needs differently. Therefore nurses are required to use their holistic nursing knowledge base to think through each situation to provide individualized, effective care rather than simply following routine procedures.

Jones and Brown (1993) believe that nursing is practiced in complex environments with humans, who are complex beings. Technological advances and a knowledge explosion have also changed the face of health care. Thinking skills of the nurse become more important than the ability to perform the associated psychomotor skills. Case (1994) discussed the changing arenas for decision making as being not only at the bedside but also in quality assurance processes, delegation activities, shared governance, and management and executive roles. As health care reform extends patient care from the predominantly structured inpatient arena to the more unstructured outpatient or community arenas, critical thinking skills and empowerment become even more important.

Carlson-Catalano (1992), in discussing empowering nurses, believed that traditional curricula encourage students to be obedient, dependent, and fearful in caring for patients. She suggests that nurses in professional practice should be empowered and that students need to be treated as valued members of the profession. She offers analytic nursing, change activities, collegiality, and sponsorship as strategies for empowering nurses. These strategies would be addressed if nursing faculty adopted the principles of critical thinking as the foundation for practice.

Students must develop higher-order thinking skills. Brigham (1993) contends that faculty need to assist students to recognize how systems respond to specific health problems. Students need to know what nursing measures will be needed when they read laboratory reports with abnormal results; they do not need to memorize normal laboratory values. Jones and Brown (1991) argue that nurse educators can no longer convey facts to nursing students. "There are far too many facts, but there are far too many facts which become erroneous over time" (Jones & Brown, 1991, p. 533). Miller (1992) concurs:

> More emphasis should be given to the mental processes students engage in as they solve nursing problems and less given to simply identifying the correct answer. Focusing on making clinical inferences from given data, recognizing unstated assumptions, deductive reasoning, weighing of evidence and distinguishing between weak and strong arguments emphasizes the importance of the processes of thinking. (p. 1406)

Scheffer and Rubenfeld (2000) conducted a Delphi study to develop a consensus statement about critical thinking in nursing education. A panel of 55 experts from nine different countries determined that

> Critical thinking in nursing is an essential component of professional accountability and quality nursing care. Critical thinkers in nursing exhibit theses habits of the mind: confidence, contextual perspective, creativity, flexibility, inquisitiveness, intellectual integrity, intuition, open-mindedness, perseverance, and reflection. Critical thinkers in nursing practice [possess] the cognitive skills of analyzing, applying standards, discriminating, information seeking, logical reasoning, predicting and transforming knowledge. (p. 357)

In summary, Jackson (1995) states, "Every patient deserves caregivers who think critically. . . . The ability to think critically can be empowering. Practitioners must commit to a struggle of balancing an explosion of objective and intuitive information in an explosive health care environment" (p. 187). Therefore nurse educators are challenged to help students develop necessary critical thinking skills as the students progress through the curriculum.

Roles of Faculty and Students in Developing Critical Thinking Skills

The development of students' critical thinking skills and dispositions requires faculty to reconsider their philosophy of teaching. The faculty-dominated classroom is not conducive to development of critical thinking. It is the responsibility of faculty to think about the roles of the teacher and student, as well as to create an environment that empowers students. Transmitting information through rote lecture to students does not guarantee learning. Students must be actively engaged with the information for it to be transformed into knowledge. Lesson plans *must* be designed to foster the development of critical thinking skills (cognitive) and a critical thinking disposition (affective) as students *engage* with the theoretical, affective, and psychomotor content that is nursing. Students must become empathetic, empowered, and able to critically think about every situation if they are to succeed in nursing (Bevis, 1993; Ford & Profetto-McGrath, 1994).

Faculty Roles

Faculty must become facilitators of learning rather than teachers of content (Bevis, 1993; Brigham, 1993; Brookfield, 1995; Creedy et al., 1992; Jones & Brown, 1993). Ford and Profetto-McGrath (1994) believe that the teacher-student relationship must become a "working with" relationship—an egalitarian relationship. Burns and Egan (1994) suggest that faculty should demonstrate critical thinking as content is presented. For example, when teaching content such as medical acidosis and alkalosis, faculty could demonstrate their own problem-solving skills by thinking aloud as they discuss a relevant case study. Students should think aloud while interacting with the content so that faculty can identify inappropriate thinking processes and provide immediate constructive feedback.

Creedy et al. (1992) propose that faculty can empower students by valuing their contributions, encouraging expression of their opinions, exploring mistakes objectively without demeaning the students, and promoting risk taking. Brookfield (1987) cites the following principles that will facilitate students to think critically:

- "Affirm the critical thinkers' self-worth" (p. 72)
- "Listen attentively to critical thinkers" (p. 73)
- "Show that you support critical thinkers' efforts" (p. 74)
- "Reflect and mirror critical thinkers' ideas and actions" (p. 75)
- "Motivate people to think critically" (p. 76)
- "Regularly evaluate progress" (p. 78)
- "Help critical thinkers create networks" (p. 79)
- "Be critical teachers" (p. 80)
- "Model critical thinking" (p. 85)

Thus according to Brookfield (1987), the facilitator of learning must enter into an egalitarian relationship to support the learners' attempts to engage in critical thinking. Faculty can only provide learning experiences for students; faculty cannot teach (impart knowledge); they can only share their knowledge. Students must transform the content into their own knowledge.

Student Roles

Learning to think critically requires active student participation (Meyers, 1986); students must become active creators of their own knowledge (Creedy et al., 1992). At this time, it can be assumed most students have come from faculty-dominated classrooms in which the students have been the recipients of endless amounts of facts to be memorized and recalled for examinations (Valiga, 1983). Students have probably not been asked to apply those facts to real-life situations. Therefore students will have to be assisted with the transition from the passive to active learner role. Faculty need to create a risk-free environment that is conducive to active student participation. The discussion later in this chapter related to creation of an anticipatory set serves as an example of helping students to make the transition from passive to active learners. Repeated encounters with active learning situations are needed before students can become comfortable with the active learner role.

Active learners must come to class prepared. They cannot rely on the faculty to tell them what they need to know. "Preclass written assignments, study guides, quizzes and short in-class writings" (Brigham, 1993, p. 52) are effective in stimulating students to come to class prepared to engage with the content while interacting with faculty and fellow students in planned learning activities.

Classroom Environment for the Development of Critical Thinking Skills

The classroom environment changes when the principles of critical thinking are adopted. Active learning can be a very threatening situation. Faculty must create a risk-free environment that allows students to explore the content, make mistakes, reflect on the content, associate the content with experience, and transform the content into knowledge (McCabe, 1992).

Brigham (1993) suggests that faculty set the stage by sharing that their philosophy of teaching is to enhance critical thinking. This should be done during the time students are being introduced to the course. Students need to know that learning experiences have been designed for them to actively engage with the information and with each other while faculty facilitate the activities and learning process. Students must understand that through the interactions, information will be converted into knowledge (Bevis, 1993).

Classroom environments should establish a sense of connection between faculty and students and among students themselves. Students should understand that neither faculty nor students have all the answers and that no one answer is correct in all situations. Open discussion and student willingness to take risks should be supported while faculty guide the group toward the preestablished learning outcome.

Students need to be aware that there are conflicting ideas about some concepts. Faculty at some schools of nursing do not adopt a specific textbook for their courses; rather, the bookstore stocks appropriate textbooks by different authors, and students select the textbook they would like to use. This particular idea is intriguing because it certainly provides a basis for discussion of information from multiple points of view. When contradictions are found, it helps students recognize that the written word should be questioned.

The physical component of the classroom is important; however, any classroom can be conducive to active student learning. Students should be able to make eye contact with each other and with faculty. MacIntosh (1995) suggests rearranging chairs into small or large circles. Faculty can be creative in modifying the physical characteristics of the classroom. For example, in classrooms where desks are bolted down, students could sit on the tops of the desks to be able to face others in the group.

Student Responses to Active Learning

Beck (1995) conducted a study using a cooperative learning model based on feminist pedagogy that resulted in positive teacher–student and student–student interactions and satisfactory learning. Hezekiah (1993) cites the five basic feminist goals for the classroom ("atmosphere of mutual respect, trust and community, shared leadership, cooperative structure, integration of cognitive and affective learning, and action oriented field work" [pp. 55-56]) that would establish an environment for the development of critical thinking skills as the learner transforms information to knowledge. Wake et al. (1992) discuss shared governance in the classroom. They note that shared governance in nursing education produces professional nurses who will be prepared to practice in an ever-changing health care environment.

Price (1991) found that "interaction between the student and teacher ranked high as a positive contributor to learning" (p. 170). Price cited student responses to an interactive classroom:

> What's good is your understanding of conflicts we may be facing as new students, your continual encouragement, and the fact that you're always available to answer questions. . . . I don't function well, never have, when the question is memorizing. . . . I tend to learn very abstractly and not sequentially; my learning is not textbook learning. . . . I really find that I learn the most when I can apply it to myself and to someone else; that's the thing I can underline and say, "Yes, I learned that very well." . . . It's practical application, where it's applied to life, where your pattern of behavior is changed, something you can apply in your relationship with another human being. (pp. 170-171)

Summary

Nurses must possess a high level of critical thinking skills and a critical thinking disposition. Faculty must create opportunities for students to develop critical thinking as students progress through the curriculum. Faculty must become facilitators of learning and students must become active learners.

Critical thinking should be at the forefront of planning learning experiences for nursing students. If educators believe that "students can and should think their way through the content of their courses, . . . gain some grasp of the logic of what they study, . . . develop explicit intellectual standards, then they can find many ways to move instruction in this direction" (Barnes, 1992, p. 22). Faculty must create an environment that develops the traits of an ideal critical thinker and plan learning experiences that include strategies to develop the cognitive skills and subskills of critical thinking.

PLANNING LEARNING EXPERIENCES

Planning challenging encounters that will entice students to learn and develop critical thinking skills is a major task for any faculty member. Effective planning of any kind requires much time and effort; planning learning experiences is no exception. Careful planning of each learning experience gives teachers more self-confidence and aids in formative and summative evaluation of teaching. At least six steps are used in designing learning experiences:

1. Determine the learning outcomes for the specific class period
2. Create an anticipatory set
3. Select teaching and learning strategies
4. Consider implementation issues
5. Design closure to the learning experience
6. Design formative and summative evaluation strategies

Each of the stages is discussed in detail. All steps can be planned by both students and faculty. Novice faculty may find it helpful to design learning experiences in great detail (see Table 13-1), whereas more experienced faculty may use only a more general outline form.

Determining the Learning Outcomes

The first step is to determine the learning outcomes of the class. Several activities must be carried out before specific outcomes for any class period are developed. The first activity is assessment of the overall curriculum outcomes and the placement of the specific course in meeting the outcomes. Typically, general curriculum outcomes are stated in very broad terms and will likely not give the teacher any information about what to include in a specific class period. However, a thorough understanding of the broad curriculum goals is necessary so teachers can "connect" the specifics for the day to the broad curriculum outcomes. Course objectives and outcomes need to be reviewed to ascertain how the particular course "fits" within the curriculum (Ayer, 1986; Torres & Stanton, 1982). See Chapters 8 to 11 for additional information.

Teachers tend to design learning experiences within their own belief and value systems. Their own philosophies about teaching, learning, the curriculum, the ability of students, and how and what a nurse educator "should" do all influence the development of activities for a specific class period. Teachers need to be aware of these value systems and recognize the influence of them on their teaching and selection of teaching strategies (Creedy et al., 1992).

With these activities in mind, outcomes for a given experience can be established. There are several ways to identify outcomes. One way is to use behavioral objectives (see Chapters 9 and 10). For many, however, behavioral objectives imply rigid lists of specific content, faculty-dominated classrooms, and only one right answer to each examination question. Some believe that specific behavioral objectives need to be abandoned, given the important issue of development of critical thinking abilities in students (Bevis, 1993). In another approach, general outcomes or competencies are identified, and the path to achieving them is left open. How they are written depends on individual school requirements, the overall curriculum design, the content of the course, and the beliefs or values of the individual faculty member.

Creating an Anticipatory Set

The second major step in planning a learning experience is to create an environment that invites all students to become interested in the content and to participate in the learning process. This activity is referred to as *creating an anticipatory set* (Ayer, 1986; deTornyay & Thompson, 1982; Maas, 1990). The activity typically takes little in-class time and merely sets the stage for active involvement in the learning process. Maas (1990) includes three elements in an anticipatory set: active participation, relevance to the students, and relevance to the class period. Preclass readings; active, thought-provoking questions; and a class exercise that emphasizes students' prior knowledge are examples of activities that can be used as an anticipatory set. The anticipatory set prepares students for the main activity or content of the class period.

Selecting a Teaching Strategy

Selecting the particular teaching strategy is the third step in lesson planning. Faculty must consider multiple factors as they select a particular strategy. The first is the content itself. For example, teaching abstract concepts is probably better accomplished through mind mapping (Rooda, 1994), whereas psychomotor skills are better taught through demonstration (Kelly, 1992). The philosophy underlying the broad curriculum outcomes also influences the selection of teaching strategies. In a school that has adopted the principles of critical thinking, the traditional lecture would seldom be used as a strategy. Last, faculty must consider teaching strategies that are feasible. Questions to consider may include the amount of time available, room size, distance learning delivery system being used, the availability of equipment, the number of students, time and money costs for both the teacher and the student, and learning styles of the students.

With these factors in mind, many different teaching strategies would be appropriate for any student group and class content. Throughout the course, it is important to vary the strategies. Using the same type of anticipatory set followed by lecture and then the same closure can be very boring for students. For example, faculty may create interest for the students by using lecture some of the time and role play, demonstration, and reflection at other times.

Varying the strategies also has the advantage of appealing to all types of learners (see Chapter 2). Few of the teaching strategies are equally stimulating to all types of learners. It is not particularly important that teachers use strategies that appeal to all learners in every class, but it is important for them to use strategies that appeal to all types of learners throughout the course. Questioning is a teaching strategy that should be used consistently; it can even be used in every class (Paul, 1995). "Helping students to ask their own questions should perfect their ability to think critically about information and how to process it" (Hunkins, 1985, p. 296). Strategies that appeal to one type of learner can also be used for the preclass assignments or activities, and strategies for other types of learners can be used for the classroom experience.

Teaching Strategies and Critical Thinking

The actual steps in designing learning experiences do not change when critical thinking concepts are applied to the curriculum. Teaching strategies should be selected for the development of critical thinking skills. Development of these skills in students should be a planned activity throughout all stages of the curriculum. Any strategy selected should be selected for a particular reason, and all strategies should lead to the development of advancing levels of critical thinking.

Cognitive Levels

Cognitive levels must be considered during lesson planning. Several theorists have written about the various cognitive levels of students. Perry (1970) identifies four levels including nine stages of intellectual development. Belenky et al. (1986) have demonstrated that women and men differ in intellectual development in several major areas. One example is that women typically have a silent stage of cognitive development, which is the first level. This stage is characterized by a powerless, dependent fear of authority figures. Men typically do not go through the silent stage.

Hickman (1993) examined the theories of Perry (1970), Belenky et al. (1986), and others and integrated their thinking on cognitive levels with Benner's (1984) levels of skill acquisition. Hickman's (1993) thoughts are related directly to the licensed nurse, but her ideas can also be applied to the undergraduate nursing student. The beginning nursing student is a *novice* in critical thinking. Thinking is characterized as dualistic (everything is black or white). Little or no critical thinking is used. The novice depends on authority for knowledge and is usually silent. The next cognitive level is the *advanced beginner*. In this stage, thinking at the multiplicity level occurs. Students use subjective knowledge to begin seeing recurring themes, but they fail to differentiate important cues. Students at this level require assistance in establishing priorities. The next stage is the *competent student nurse*. At this stage students continue to use subjective knowledge, but they do so consciously and they use the subjective knowledge in deliberate planning activities. The last cognitive level is the *proficient student nurse*, who is at the relativistic level of intellectual development. Relativism is the recognition that opinions differ in quality and require supporting evidence to be valid. Relativism is equated with procedural knowledge, connected knowledge, or both. Students no longer see information as only black and white; they begin to see how things "fit" together and notice where information is missing. They begin to think critically.

It would be hoped that students completing a basic nursing education program would have attained the relativism level of cognitive development. Most undergraduate students will not have attained the final level, which is commitment in relativism. Commitment in relativism describes the expert nurse who integrates knowledge with experience and uses personal reflection to derive constructed knowledge (Hickman, 1993). Many graduate students will have already moved to this level. Undergraduate nursing students will likely move to the final level of cognitive development after they are licensed and have many more real-life nursing experiences and the time to reflect on and integrate those experiences.

The cognitive level of students must be addressed when learning experiences are designed. Moving students from the cognitive level of dualism to the level of relativism should be a major goal of nursing education. The level of cognitive development also influences the selection of teaching strategies. Bowers and McCarthy (1993) suggest that students who exhibit thinking at the informed commitment (relativistic) level would probably feel frustrated if they were expected to think at a dualistic level. For example, proficient student nurses would rather discuss implications of abnormal blood gas values (relativistic thinking) than respond to questions about normal findings (dualistic thinking).

Implementation Issues

The fourth stage of lesson planning is implementation of the learning experience. In this stage, two major activities are considered. The first is the *timing*. How much time will be spent on the strategies selected to develop the anticipatory set? What backup plans are made to account for a lesson that takes much less or more time than anticipated? What can be cut or what can be added? What are the most crucial concepts to be covered if time is short? The sample plan (Table 13-1) contains estimated times, with more detail included in a more extensive version of the plan.

The second activity in this stage is to plan for the *tools* needed to implement the class. In this case, tools can refer to many things. Tools can be instructional media and equipment such as an overhead projector, slide projector, computer, or video information system (Table 13-1). Tools can also refer to the information technology tools used to establish the learning community, such as computer conferencing or videoconferencing. Plan to check the equipment for correct working order. Nothing can ruin a well-planned learning experience quite so effectively as instructional media that do not work! Tools could also be the classroom itself. How should the chairs be arranged? Do you want to use a podium? Does the screen for the overhead projector work? The last set of tools is the paper products. What handouts does the faculty member need? How much lead time is needed for typing and copying the handouts? Are the computer slides or transparencies ready? Are there items that need to have copyrights cleared? Who does that and how much time does it take? Assessing and planning for the amount of time and the tools necessary for implementation of the teaching strategy are activities that should not be left to the last minute.

Designing Closure

The last step in designing the learning experience is planning for closure. Closure may be as simple as a few sentences that summarize the major concepts. In this case, the time allowed for closure would be very short. However, closure can take a large amount of class time, especially when dealing with sensitive or emotional content. Applying major concepts to similar or new areas of interest is another example of a closure technique (deTornyay & Thompson, 1987). This time may also be used to create the anticipatory set for the next class period by discussing how the content of the class relates to the content of the next class period.

Designing Formative and Summative Evaluation Strategies

During the lesson planning phase, both formative and summative evaluation need to be considered (Ayer, 1986). Chapter 14 contains information about

> **TABLE 13-1   Sample Plan for a Learning Experience: Ethics in Leadership**

1. Outcomes: Identify ethical theory used for own decision making Discuss implications of use of ethical theories in the workplace

ACTIVITY	CONTENT	TIME	STRATEGIES

2. Anticipatory set
  a. Preclass
     assignment
 	
  b. In-class exercise
	a. Ethical theories
	   Ethical case
	   examples
	b. Ethical situations
		a. 2 hr
		
		b. 10 min
			a. Text reading
			   Ethical survey
			b. Individual
			   reflection to
			   identify the most
			   difficult question
			   on the survey and
			   write how/why
			   answered

3. Implementation
   Tools:
    Overhead projector
    Overhead slides
	a. Three ethical
	   theories from text
		40 min	a. Large group discussion
			  (1) Overheads of
			     the theories'
			     main points
			  (2) At each main
			     point, ask "What
			     does this mean to
			     you?" and "Give
			     an example of how
			     the point would
			     be seen in
			     practice."

	b. Application
	  (1) Identify own
	     theory used
	  (2) Apply to fami-
	     liar situation
	  (3) Apply to new
	     situation
	  (4) Apply to
	     workplace
	     decision making
		30 min	b. Small group discussion
			  (1) "Which theory do
			     you use?"
			  (2) "Give example
			     of how you used
			     the theory."
			  (3) "How would
			     a nurse
			     administrator
			     use the theory to
			     make ethical
			     decisions?"
			  (4) "How could use of
			     the theories lead to
			     conflict in the
			     workplace?"

4. Closure	Emphasize class outcomes	20 min	Small group reports Overall summary

classroom assessment, and Chapters 21 to 23 contain information about assessment of learning outcomes. These chapters should assist in this stage of planning.

Evaluation activities should occur throughout the learning experience. Many formative evaluation techniques are available (see Chapter 14). Frequent formative evaluation is important for assessment of students' understanding of content. Varying the types of formative evaluation used is important. For example, some of the time, the objectives can be evaluated, and at other times, the teaching strategy used can be evaluated. Frequent self-evaluation is critical. Faculty should ask whether the time, tools, strategy, and content were organized and planned effectively and what could have been done differently to enhance student learning.

Summary

Designing effective learning experiences involves at least six distinct stages. A well-designed experience that enhances student learning cannot be done in a haphazard manner or at the last minute. Enhanced student learning and the development of critical thinking skills are the outcomes of well-planned learning experiences.

TEACHING STRATEGIES

There are many different teaching strategies. Those with the most application to nursing education are presented throughout the rest of the chapter. Each strategy is described with its advantages and disadvantages. Teaching tips are also included. Last, additional references are provided in which the reader may find a more detailed description of the strategy. Any discussion about teaching strategies would be incomplete without a review of learning resources, including instructional media or distance education delivery systems. These are discussed in Chapters 17, 18, and 19.

The lecture is presented first, because this teaching strategy is frequently used by many teachers. Many other strategies can be used in nursing education. These strategies are alphabetized for ease of location. Each strategy discussed may have its place in a course, but its use depends on the content, the teacher, and the learners.

Most of the strategies described after the lecture involve active learner participation in the learning process and emphasize adult learning and critical thinking concepts. Both teachers and students may resist this type of learning because the strategies are more flexible and less teacher centered than those typically used in the traditional college classroom. However, if one accepts that the learner must actively engage with the content or information to transform it into knowledge, the classroom should become student centered. Thus the traditional lecture may not always be the most appropriate strategy.

Lecture

Definition. Teacher presentation of content to students, usually accompanied by some type of visual aid or handout.

Use. Clarify complex, confusing, or conflicting concepts; provide background information not available to students; change of pace from more experiential learning strategies; cover background information from scattered sources.

Teaching tips
1. Increased student participation can be achieved if the format of the feedback lecture is used (Fuszard, 1995). For example, in a feedback lecture of 1 hour, a 6- to 10-minute group discussion period is inserted between two 20-minute lecture times.
2. Use visual aids, handouts, study guides so students can follow the sequence of the lecture.
3. Read the article "What Is the Most Difficult Step We Must Take to Become Great Teachers?" by Nelson (2001) for some ideas on how to decrease the amount of class time devoted to lecture.

Advantages. Time efficient for covering complex material; should raise further student questions that lend themselves to other teaching strategies.

Disadvantages. Decreases student involvement in learning when content is readily available and easy to understand in a text or other reading assignment; lengthy preparation time for faculty; little involvement in the topic for students other than sitting through the lecture; may have a high cost in preparation and development of handouts and visual aids.

Additional reading. deTornyay & Thompson, 1982; Fuszard, 1995; Hoover, 1980; McKeachie, 1986; Nelson, 2001.

Algorithms

Definition. Step-by-step procedure for solving a complex procedure; breaks tasks into yes/no steps.

Use. Any course in which frequent practice is required for student mastery of content, in which rules aid in problem solving, or in which the content can be broken into yes/no stages.

Teaching tips
1. Assess content for appropriate use of algorithm as a teaching strategy.
2. Develop algorithm and accompanying student explanations of how to use.
3. Allow 6 to 8 hours for the development of the first algorithms.
4. Additional algorithms on similar content typically take less time to develop.

Advantages. Shows students how to "spot" the most relevant information for problem solving; develops reliable, complex problem-solving abilities even in novice students; decreases the amount of one-on-one instruction often required when teaching problem-solving techniques; effective in teaching complex procedures that involve many steps; when used with case studies, may enhance learning; saves faculty teaching time over lecture type of presentations; saves student time in trying to remember and understand complex phenomena.

Disadvantages. Teacher must clearly define the steps or students will not be able to accurately complete the task; students may need to be taught how to use algorithms in problem solving; development of algorithms can be time consuming for faculty.

Additional reading. Connor & Tillman, 1990.

Argumentation/Debate/Structured Controversy/Dilemmas

Definition. The process of inquiry or reasoned judgment on a proposition aimed at demonstrating the truth or falsehood of something; involves the construction of logical arguments and oral defense of a proposition; requires the recognition of assumptions and evidence and use of inductive/deductive reasoning skills; allows identification of relationships.

Teaching tips
1. Strategy works best in an issues or topics course for students at a higher level of cognitive thinking.
2. For the purpose of forming productive debate teams, it is helpful for students to know each other.
3. Faculty should introduce the basic topics and structure the debate format early in the course to allow students adequate preparation time.
4. Debate teams usually consist of five students: two students debate for the topic, two debate against the topic, and the fifth student acts as the moderator.
5. Debates follow a specified format, including opening comments, presentation of affirmative and negative viewpoints, rebuttal, and summary (Fuszard, 1995).

Advantages. Develops analytical skills; develops ability to recognize complexities in many health care issues; broadens views of controversial topics; develops communication skills.

Disadvantages. Requires a fairly high level of knowledge about subject on the parts of both those presenting the debate and the audience; may require teaching students the art of debate; requires increased student preparation time; can create anxiety and conflict for students because of the confrontational nature of debate; students without adequate public speaking skills may also have increased anxiety.

Additional reading. Brookfield, 1992; Candela et al., 2003; Fuszard, 1995; Garrett et al., 1996; Metcalf & Yankou, 2003; Mottola & Murphy, 2001; Pederson, 1993; White et al., 1990.

Case Study/Case Problem/Case Report/Research Case/Case Scenario

Definition. In-depth analysis of a real-life situation as a way to illustrate class content; applies didactic content and theory to real life, simulated life, or both.

Teaching tips
1. A well-designed case that illustrates the most important class concepts is critical to the success of learning with this method.

2. Before the class period, analyze the case with the intent of determining the potential ways students could analyze the case but be prepared for student questions and comments that previously have not been considered (be able to say, "I don't know" or "I haven't considered that before" if necessary).

3. A safe, open, nonthreatening classroom environment is crucial for active student participation.

4. During the class period, ask pertinent questions, draw out quieter students, correct misconceptions, and support students in their efforts.

5. At the conclusion of the class, provide a summary of the most important points and sources for more in-depth study.

6. Assist in students' comprehension of critical concepts with the use of tools such as concept maps, chalkboards, and overheads.

Advantages. Stimulates critical thinking, retention, and recall; associating the practical with the theoretical helps many students to recall important information; typical lecture material can be presented in more practical context; problem solving can be practiced in a safe environment without the threat of endangering a patient; especially good for adult learners who desire peer interaction, support for prior experience, and validation of thinking; an experienced nurse can readily devise a case study example from actual patient encounters.

Disadvantages. More effective when used with complex situations that require problem solving; not appropriate when concrete facts are the only content; developing cases is a difficult and time-consuming skill for many and the option of published cases should be considered; requires the use of good questioning skills by the faculty; poor student preparation for class may result in less learning; may frustrate students who desire content to be presented through more traditional strategies such as lecture.

Additional reading. Cascio et al., 1995; Casebeer, 1991; Fuszard, 1995; Pond et al., 1991; Taylor et al., 1994; Tomey, 2003.

Cooperative Learning/Collaborative Learning

Definition. Teams of learners work on assignments and assume responsibility for group learning outcomes.

Teaching tips

1. Design meaningful assignments that can be accomplished by small groups (a group of three to five heterogeneous [in ability, gender, ethnic status, experience, and so on] students is ideal).

2. Teach or verify groups' understanding of team roles and group process; assign or ask group to designate "leader," "recorder," "reflector," "reporter," and other roles as necessary.

3. Allow adequate time for reporting and processing of group work.

Advantages. Promotes active and reflective learning; encourages teamwork; provides opportunity for students to become accountable for own and others' work; group dynamics skills can be used; large learning assignments/projects can be accomplished efficiently; can be implemented in discussion groups/forums by using the Internet and group conferencing software.

Disadvantages. Students may resist frequent use of group assignments; possibility that not all students will participate equally.

Additional reading. Dansereau, 1983; Glendon & Ulrich, 1992; Matthews et al., 1995; McAlister & Osborne, 1997; *The Team Memory Jogger*, 1995.

Demonstration

Definition. Show how to do something.

Use. Complex mental or psychomotor skill acquisition.

Teaching tips
1. Show the steps of the process clearly, from start to finish.
2. Go through the process a second time, showing the rationale and allowing time for questions.
3. May help to demonstrate the process again.
4. Provide for immediate, individual, supervised practice sessions.

Advantages. Visibly showing a process often aids in retention; complex skills become more understandable as a result of the demonstration; demonstration allows an expert to model the skill.

Disadvantages. Students have differing levels in skill acquisition abilities; students who quickly master skills may become bored while the others are practicing; mastering psychomotor skills is usually very stressful for students; requires adequate faculty supervision, space, supplies, and equipment to provide realistic practice sessions; high faculty workload involved in supervision of student practice times; high cost of supplies and equipment may limit amount of practice time available to students.

Additional reading. Jeffries et al., 2003; Kelly, 1992.

Dialogue/Peer Sharing/Story Telling/Narrative Pedagogy

Definition. Dialogue involves a conversation between two or more people.

Teaching tips
1. A clear connection must be made between the objectives and the strategy or students will think the activity is a waste of time.
2. Create a possible list of topics and allow students to choose what they are interested in to promote active student learning.
3. Creating relevance in the stories or peer sharing will also increase student learning.
4. Informal meetings between faculty and students may help clarify and structure questions used to promote in-class discussion.
5. These strategies probably work best with small groups.

Advantages. Provides a point of reference from which to explore concepts from multiple points of view, including theoretical and practical; promotes reflection and critical analysis; truth seeking is activated; enhances affective learning and caring; increases contextual learning.

Disadvantages. Requires that faculty continually focus on the realistic; faculty may need to assist learners to focus or refocus on concepts being discussed throughout class period.

Additional reading. Koenig & Zorn, 2002; MacLeod, 1995; Nehls, 1995; Porter, 1995; Symonds, 1995; Yoder-Wise & Kowalski, 2003.

Games

Definition

- *"Game:* An activity governed by precise rules that involves varying degrees of chance or luck and one or more players who compete (with self, the game, one another, or a computer) through the use of knowledge or skill in an attempt to reach a specified goal (gain an intrinsic or extrinsic reward)."
- *"Simulation Game:* An activity that incorporates the characteristics of *both* a simulation and a game; a contest that also replicates some real-life situation or process" (deTornyay & Thompson, 1987, p. 27).

Teaching tips

1. Use this method for reinforcement of knowledge rather than introduction of new knowledge.
2. An open learning environment is crucial to learning with gaming—faculty must back out—the learning is student to student in this method.
3. Several distinct steps are involved in development of a game. See Fuszard (1995).
4. Debriefing after the game is critical so students clearly connect the game with the important concepts.
5. If faculty do not value gaming as a teaching strategy, they may unconsciously sabotage the game.

Advantages. Increases cognitive and affective learning; improves retention; fun/exciting; increases learner involvement; motivates learner; can help connect practice experiences to theory; students can learn from each other through the experience of the game; good for adult learners who take more responsibility for their own learning; adult learners can receive immediate feedback in learning situation and can also see the immediate application of theory to practice; learning from gaming lasts longer when compared with learning from traditional lecture.

Disadvantages. May be threatening to some learners; may be time consuming; may be costly to purchase or develop; may be difficult to evaluate level of learning if several players are involved; may require greater amount of space; should have introductory and summary sessions; takes longer than traditional lecture; faculty must set guidelines so the game does not get out of control.

Additional reading. Batscha, 2002; deTornyay & Thompson, 1987; Fuszard, 1995; Kuhn, 1995; Metcalf & Yankou, 2003.

Humor

Definition. The ability to perceive, enjoy, or express what is comical or funny; the quality of being laughable or comical; funniness.

Use. Provides break in content students may perceive as boring; emphasizes important points.

Teaching tips
1. The use of cartoons with relevant content can provide a break in tense class sessions.
2. Content-related quotes work as well as cartoons in many instances.
3. Humor should be used sparingly to be most effective.
4. Develop your own sense of humor first before implementing humor in a classroom (Ulloth, 2003a).

Advantages. "Increased attention and interest, student/teacher rapport, comprehension and retention of material, motivation toward learning, satisfaction with learning, playfulness, positive attitudes and classroom environment, productivity, class discussions, creativity, generation of ideas, quality and quantity of student reading, and divergent thinking, decreased academic stress and anxiety, dogmatism, boredom and class monotony" (Parrott, 1994, p. 37).

Disadvantages. Can be seen as "ridicule, sarcasm, racist or ethnic jokes. . . . The wrong kind of humor can be demeaning and destroy self-esteem and confidence, interfere with communication and sever relationships" (Parrott, 1994, p. 37); faculty time spent finding appropriate cartoons, anecdotes, and so on can be extensive; some students may find humor distracting from the topic at hand.

Additional reading. Parrott, 1994; Robbins, 1994; Ulloth, 2002; Ulloth, 2003a; Ulloth, 2003b.

Imagery

Definition. Mental picturing, diagramming, or rehearsal before the actual use of the information in practice.

Use. Best use is in combination with other strategies (e.g., with physical practice in psychomotor skill acquisition).

Teaching tips
1. Create a scenario that would mimic a real-life situation.
2. Use the scenario to demonstrate effective use of imagery.
3. Relaxation techniques provide a good example of how to use imagery techniques.
4. A supportive classroom environment is needed for the effective use of this strategy.

Advantage. Superior learning of psychomotor skills when imagery is combined with physical practice.

Disadvantages. Individuals have varying levels of innate imagery skills, so some students may need to be taught how to do imagery; does not provide a substitute for physical practice of a skill; using imagery and physical practice of the skill will require more student study time than if only physical practice is used; stress and performance fears may interfere with the productive use of imagery; may require teacher education to implement imagery strategy.

Additional reading. Bucher, 1993; Doheny, 1993.

Learning Contracts

Definition. Individualized written contract between teacher and student.

Teaching tips
1. Specific elements need to be included in the learning contract. See deTornyay & Thompson (1982).
2. Learning contracts can be either teacher or student initiated.
3. A high level of trust must be established between the student and the teacher for the successful implementation of learning contracts.

Advantages. Maximizes adult students' needs to direct their own learning; may also provide the structure needed by some adult students; builds on prior knowledge and life experiences of adult students; allows students to work at their own pace (i.e., some may need remediation and others may need more advanced or complex learning objectives); teacher-initiated contracts may be very motivating for some students.

Disadvantages. Students may not be familiar with the process of developing a learning contract and may become frustrated when the "normal" educational classroom is absent; students must be independent thinkers to be able to construct productive learning contracts; students must be self-disciplined to complete the contract; faculty and administrators may need in-service programs in the development, management, and acceptance of learning contracts when they are used as the only form of student summative evaluation for a class; little preparation time but potentially a larger workload for faculty, especially if an entire class has individualized contracts; additional student time will be required for a self-assessment of learning needs and development of the learning contract.

Additional reading. deTornyay & Thompson, 1982, 1987; Swansburg, 1995.

Literature Analogies/Newspaper Analysis/Metaphor Examination

Definition. Conceptual clarification with the use of literature to identify similarities and differences of concepts in the literature with those in nursing practice.

Use. Relating unfamiliar to familiar; clarifying abstractions.

Teaching tips
1. Requires clear identification of the concepts that would be appropriate to clarify with this strategy.
2. Finding "just the right" piece of literature to use may be difficult. Probably the best way to locate a usable source is to come across it while reading the newspaper for pleasure rather than for work-related reasons.
3. It is important to clarify and summarize the exercise at the conclusion of the class.

Advantages. Allows students to relate foreign concepts to familiar concepts; establishes framework for introducing new materials; raises awareness of multiple meanings associated with human-related concepts.

Disadvantages. Time consuming for faculty to identify appropriate literature related to concepts being studied; learners may have difficulty seeing relationships; reading nonnursing-specific content may be costly in terms of time for students.

Additional reading. Kirkpatrick, 1994; Young-Mason, 1988, 1991.

Mind Mapping/Concept Mapping/Pattern Recognition/Chunking

Definition. Learning complex phenomenon by diagramming the concepts and subconcepts.

Teaching tips
1. Organizing the course in like subjects can provide an example of mind mapping for the students.
2. Grouping specific class content can also provide students with examples of mind mapping.

Advantages. Better understanding and recall of complex phenomena; especially effective in stimulating long-term recall of like concepts; active involvement by the students in designing the maps will enhance analytic thinking processes; helps students recognize similarities and differences among concepts; helps clarify relationships between concepts.

Disadvantages. May take longer initially until both faculty and students understand how to organize the concepts; may not appeal to concrete or auditory learners.

Additional reading. Antonacci, 1991; Beitz, 1998; Daley et al., 1999; Reynolds, 1994; Rooda, 1994; Tschikota, 1993.

Portfolio

Definition. "A portfolio is a collection of evidence, usually in written form, of both the products and processes of learning. It attests to achievement and personal and professional development, by providing critical analysis of its contents" (McMullan et al., 2003, p. 288).

Use. Documentation of student skills from prior courses or life experiences.

Teaching tips
1. A content outline should provide the framework for the portfolio but not limit student creativity.
2. Guidelines for the portfolio must be clear.

Advantages. Typically high student motivation because of control over learning; motivated students typically learn more; helps teachers understand individual student goals and aspirations; encourages student reflection of learning; independent, self-confident, and self-directed students will excel with this method.

Disadvantages. Must be combined with reflective strategies to encourage student ownership of learning; requires new ways of thinking about the learning process by both teachers and students; portfolios may become bulky unless specific inclusion guidelines are established; students with low self-confidence will need much faculty assistance; time involvement may be high for students in development of portfolios and for faculty in evaluation of portfolios; extra costs may be involved in duplication, construction, and storage of portfolios; unless students clearly see the objective of a portfolio, the work involved may be viewed as busywork.

Additional reading. Jones, 1994; Ramey & Hay, 2003.

Poster

Definition. Visual representation of class concepts.

Teaching tips
1. Students need instructions about how to construct a poster.
2. Clear guidelines of the expected poster contents, as well as evaluation techniques, need to be developed and presented to students.

Advantages. Students can convey complex ideas through posters; posters can facilitate student creativity; assessment of students' critical thinking abilities can be done through the use of posters; posters provide students with feedback from peers, as well as faculty; students can learn from each other; students get a sense of achievement from producing posters; skills developed in the production of a poster will be valuable for students after graduation; evaluation of posters can be done quickly.

Disadvantages. Involves faculty time to develop poster assignment and evaluation techniques; can be frustrating to students who are not visual learners; some students may not be able to financially afford supplies needed to produce a poster.

Additional reading. Conyers, 2003; Duchin & Sherwood, 1990; Moneyham et al., 1996; Moule et al., 1998; Russell et al., 1996.

Problem-Based Learning

Definition. Learning is that "which results from the process of working towards the understanding or resolution of a problem" (Barrows & Tamblyn, 1980). The problem is a clinical situation presented as a stimulus for students to acquire specific skills, knowledge, and abilities in the solution of the problem. Problem-based learning (PBL) is usually used as an approach to the entire curriculum, and rather than focusing on separate disciplines or nursing specialties, in PBL clinical problems and professional issues are used as the focus for integrating all the content necessary for clinical practice.

Teaching tips
1. Develop realistic, comprehensive clinical problems that will prompt and develop intended learning outcomes.
2. Faculty workload can increase significantly, particularly during the development stages; requires close collaboration between various disciplines if the case or curriculum is interdisciplinary.

3. Orient students to PBL approach; allow sufficient time for students to research the problem and discuss answers.
4. Groups of six to nine students are most effective for PBL.

Advantages. Fosters active and cooperative learning, the ability to think critically, and clinical reasoning; students use skills of inquiry and critical thinking, as well as peer teaching and peer evaluation; the problem can be developed in paper and pencil formats, videotape/interactive videodisc, computer-assisted instruction, CD-ROMs, or the Internet; students often work in teams or groups; can be used in interdisciplinary learning environments to develop roles and competencies of each discipline; contextual learning motivates students and increases ability to apply knowledge in clinical situations; increases student responsibility for self-directed and peer learning.

Disadvantages. Involves faculty time in developing the problem situation; requires shifts of roles of faculty and student; extensive time needed for faculty to learn to use PBL; students require orientation to role of learner in PBL setting and must work through potential discrepancies in expectations and goals for learning.

Additional reading. Alexander et al., 2002; Baker, 2000a; Baker, 2000b; Barrows & Tamblyn, 1980; Choi, 2003; Creedy & Hand, 1994; Creedy et al., 1992; Frost, 1996; McAlister & Osborne, 1997.

Questioning/Socratic Questioning

Definitions

- *Questioning:* An expression of inquiry that invites or calls for a reply; an interrogative sentence, phrase, or gesture.
- *Socratic questioning:* Probing questioning to analyze an individual's thinking.

Teaching tips

1. Allow sufficient time to construct thought-provoking questions.
2. Faculty need to be prepared to facilitate the discussion that should follow a good questioning period.
3. Student learning is enhanced if a preclass assignment that will lead to adequate student preparation is designed.
4. Questioning can be used spontaneously, as an exploratory strategy, or with issue-specific content.
5. An open, trusting classroom environment is needed.
6. Appropriate phrasing of questions is required so that students do not feel belittled by the questioning experience.

Advantages. Promotes active thinking about conclusions to be drawn; increases interaction between students and faculty; promotes discussion from multiple points of view; allows students to discuss concepts from their own experiences; discloses underlying assumptions; increases the articulation of evidence; stimulates students to ask higher-level questions; promotes higher level of problem-solving skills; learning is transferred from classroom to clinical environment; promotes thinking skills to enhance test taking abilities.

Disadvantages. Presumes a thorough knowledge of content; preclass preparation by student and faculty must be thorough; student cannot rely on simple recitation of facts; implies there may be no right answer.

Additional reading. Browne & Keeley, 1990; Hunkins, 1976, 1985; Meyers, 1986; Paul, 1995; Sellappah et al., 1998; Wilen, 1987, 1991; Wink, 1993.

Reflection/Clinical Logs/Journal

Definition. Students detail personal experiences and connect them to classroom concepts.

Teaching tips
1. Clear objectives and expectations for the journal may decrease student perception of the exercise as busywork.
2. Using different approaches to journal writing (e.g., writing learning objectives, summary of the experience, a diary, focused argument) may increase student interest in the assignment.
3. Thoughtful feedback (not necessarily lengthy feedback) from the teacher is very important to student learning.
4. Group discussions about the journals and what students are saying may increase learning for all students.
5. Most frequent use is connecting classroom theories and curriculum objectives to actual practice situations.
6. Oral and written reflections are equally effective.

Advantages. Promotes learning from experiences; helps students learn how to transfer facts from one context to another; links the realities of nursing practice to the more ideal classroom model of nursing; encourages students to think about clinical experiences in relation to classroom models; student-centered learning is especially valuable to adult learners; helpful in demonstrating how to become a lifelong learner; stimulates critical thinking; situation provides a feedback loop between teacher and student so teaching emphasis can be modified to enhance student learning; can be used for all levels of nursing education.

Disadvantages. Teachers may want to revert to the expert role rather than concentrating on the students' experiences; student-directed learning may frustrate some teachers; faculty need to direct student learning through questioning and discussion that may cover topics in which they are not prepared; students may see it as only a required exercise and not take the time to make appropriate use of the learning opportunity; high time cost for faculty to construct reflection guidelines, read student reflections, and help individual students process their reflections; high time cost for students to complete reflections.

Additional reading. Brown & Sorrell, 1993; Fuszard, 1995; Heinrich, 1992; McCaugherty, 1991; Powell, 1989; Rosenal, 1995.

Role Play

Definition. A dramatic approach in which individuals assume the roles of others; usually unscripted, spontaneous interactions (may be semistructured) that are observed by others for analysis and interpretation.

Teaching tips

1. Faculty need to plan thoroughly for the role play, but they also need to be prepared to monitor and modify student actions and reactions if necessary.
2. Situations that involve conflicting emotions provide good scenarios for role playing.
3. Typical organization of the role play involves three stages:

    a. Briefing—setting the stage and explaining the objectives, which is usually the shortest stage
    b. Running—acting out the role play, which may take from 5 to 20 minutes
    c. Debriefing—discussion, analysis, and evaluation of the role-playing experience, which may last 30 to 40 minutes or more

4. The debriefing is probably the most important stage of the role play so students can clarify actions and so that decisions and alternative decisions can be explained, observation skills can be enhanced, and other interpersonal reactions can be anticipated.
5. Videotaping or audiotaping of the role play may aid in the debriefing stage.
6. The technique works best with small groups of students so all those not involved in the role play can become active observers.
7. Students should be encouraged to respond naturally to the role play and avoid phony acting.
8. Criticism should be directed to the behaviors exhibited in the role play and not to specific students.

Advantages. Increases observational skills; improves decision-making skills; increases comprehension of complex human behaviors; provides immediate feedback about the interpersonal and problem-solving skills used in the role play; provides a nonthreatening environment in which to try out unfamiliar communication and decision-making techniques; good for adult learners because of the connection to real-life situations and active participation; does not generate extra costs because props, handouts, and so on are typically not used.

Disadvantages. Students may be reluctant to participate; high time cost for faculty to develop scenarios; faculty who like control of the learning environment may be frustrated by this method; stereotypical behavior can be reinforced; role play can be a costly use of class time if it is not planned appropriately.

Additional reading. deTornyay & Thompson, 1982; Fuszard, 1995; Shearer & Davidhizar, 2003.

Self-learning Packets/Individualized Learning Packet/ Minicourse/Self-learning Module

Definition. Information on one concept presented according to a few specific objectives in a format that allows skipping of a section if the student has previously mastered the content; typically includes self-checks (pretests, posttests) of student learning throughout the self-contained packet.

Teaching tips
1. A self-learning packet has many distinct sections (deTornyay & Thompson, 1987).
2. Can be used for a single class period, an entire course, enrichment, or remedial learning.

Advantages. Good for adult learners who have busy lives and limited traditional study times; gives students control of when and where learning will occur; learning can occur without presence of the teacher; flexible, according to learner needs; good for teaching psychomotor skills; has been found to enhance learning over combined lecture and discussion methods.

Disadvantages. Students may procrastinate and not complete work in a timely manner; costly in time and money to prepare and update; printing costs may be high; students used to in-class learning may feel abandoned.

Additional reading. deTornyay & Thompson, 1982, 1987; Kelly, 1992; Schmidt & Fisher, 1992; Swansburg, 1995.

Seminar/Small or Large Group Discussions

Definition. A meeting for an exchange of ideas in some area; guided discussion of concepts.

Teaching tips
1. Student preparation time may be reduced by having students rotate as discussion facilitators so the individual student is responsible for in-depth preparation of only a few topics.
2. The teacher is a part of the group, sometimes acting as a participant or a consultant or the leader.
3. Energy, creativity, and planning by the teacher and the students are required for effective use of this strategy.
4. A clear connection of the seminar discussions to the course objectives is necessary or students will be bored and perceive the seminar as a waste of time.
5. Some control is needed so a vocal person (either student or teacher) does not dominate the discussion.

Advantages. Active student engagement with content; collaborative, cooperative learning, peer sharing, and dialogue facilitate comprehension and practical application of concepts; allows teachers to act as role models for concept clarification and expert problem solving; improves articulation in discussion; improves thinking skills; limited development time for teachers, but planning is still necessary to ensure effectiveness; does not typically require additional supplies such as handouts or audiovisuals; students can learn group problem-solving techniques.

Disadvantages. Requires that students possess adequate knowledge for active discussion and comprehension; may require great amount of student preparation time; may allow a student to "slip through" without sufficient knowledge or thinking skills; students may require instruction in how to participate in seminars.

Additional reading. Alters & Nelson, 2002; Callahan, 1992; Cohen, 1994; Dansereau, 1983; Davidson, 1994; deTornyay & Thompson, 1987; Glendon & Ulrich, 1992; Johnson & Johnson, 1991, 1993; Johnson et al., 1991; Johnson et al, 1981; Kramer, 1993; Nelson, 2000; Rather, 1994; Udvari-Solner, 1994; White et al., 1990; Wilen, 1990.

Simulation

Definition. A near representation of an actual life event; may be presented by using computer software, role play, case studies, or games that represent reality and actively involve learners in applying the content of the lesson.

Teaching tips
1. A sound lesson plan must be developed so that the content is addressed adequately.
2. Learning through simulation is best when combined with other strategies appropriate to the content.
3. Relevance of the simulation to real-life situations enhances retention.
4. Teacher preparation for simulations involves several steps.
5. In simulations, previously learned content is applied, so appropriate presimulation activities, assignments, etc. are required.
6. Student expectations should be stated at the beginning and end of the simulation.
7. Discussion about what happened during the simulation (debriefing) and a summary of the major points are critical components of learning through simulation.
8. Emphasizing the process rather than the details in the simulation will enhance student learning.
9. Simulations can also be used as an evaluation tool, especially in evaluation of psychomotor skills and decision making.

Advantages. May be developed to require the learner to resolve problems in a linear or nonlinear fashion; requires the application of knowledge and critical thinking skills; may be used in the classroom or in the laboratory as a structured activity or as an independent study assignment; can provide immediate feedback, corrective actions, or both; enhances decision-making skills and content retention; provides foundation for future discussions; involves the affective domain; promotes student–student, teacher–student, student–teacher interactions; serves as foundation for small or large group discussion; students can experience "real" situations without risk to patients; students can repeat experiences many times or the simulation can be stopped for discussion; all students can receive approximately the same experience without having to depend on the availability of the experience in the clinical agency; students increase their feelings of self-confidence and competence.

Disadvantages. Must be structured so that all learners will become involved in the situation and problem-solving process; must be realistic enough for transfer of learning to real situations; requires teacher–student summarization of the content to be learned; teachers may feel they have lost control of the learning environment; simulations can be time consuming to develop and costly to purchase.

Additional reading. Jeffries et al., 2003; deTornyay & Thompson, 1982, 1987; Rauen, 2001; Van Hoozer et al., 1987.

Writing

Definition. Learning through documentation of ideas in, for example, scholarly papers, informal journals, poems, and letters.

Teaching tips
1. Structure the writing assignment with final grading in mind.
2. Assess the paper in its entirety rather than concentrating on grammar and style issues.
3. Peer review of drafts may decrease time in grading and stimulate thinking and critiquing skills.
4. Specific grading criteria decrease the amount of subjective grading.
5. Increasing complexity in writing experiences through the curriculum increases the effect on stimulating critical thinking abilities.
6. Providing flexibility in topic selection for written assignments recognizes individual student learning needs and empowers students.
7. Teacher review of student drafts allows early assessment of student thinking/processing of the material and allows for early intervention if problems are detected.
8. Many forms of writing can be used such as journals, formal papers, creative writing assignments (e.g., poems or book reports), summaries of class content, letters to legislators and nurse administrators, and research critiques.

Advantages. Stimulates critical thinking through active involvement with the literature, learning to judge the quality of the literature, organizing interpretation of the literature into logical sequences, and learning to make judgments based on what was learned; students can discover their own beliefs and values when writing, nurses write in many formats, and writing projects in an educational setting allows for learning different mediums and styles; knowledge gained from the writing assignments can give confidence and helps to empower students in their own ideas; improves communication skills.

Disadvantages. Grading writing assignments can be subjective; many students may feel unprepared to complete writing assignments, which may lead to increased frustration and stress; students must understand the importance of learning through writing, or writing assignments will be viewed as just another thing to get completed; may be high time cost for students to complete the writing assignments depending on how the assignment is structured; typically high time cost for teachers to grade; may be almost impossible to implement in large classes; writing to learn concepts may be new to some teachers, and faculty development may be needed before all can fully participate in this type of teaching strategy.

Additional reading. Bowers & McCarthy, 1993; Bradley-Springer, 1993; Gehrke, 1994; Lashley & Wittstadt, 1993; Pinch, 1995; White et al., 1990.

SUMMARY

A large part of any faculty member's time is spent in planning learning experiences. Over the past several years, critical thinking and the shift from teaching to learning have assumed greater emphasis in the design of learning experiences in nursing education. Licensed nurses need to be able to think critically in the ever-changing health care environment, and faculty must integrate opportunities to think critically into learning activities so that students will attain appropriate outcomes for critical thinking.

Planning learning experiences involves at least six distinct steps. The steps are determining the outcomes for the specific class period, creating an anticipatory set, selecting a teaching strategy, considering implementation issues, designing closure to the class period, and designing formative and summative evaluation strategies. Careful planning is crucial to the enhancement of student learning.

Many teaching strategies are described in this chapter. Each has been defined along with its advantages, disadvantages, and related teaching tips. It is important to use different teaching strategies throughout the course because different strategies will engage students with varying learning styles, create interest for the students, assist in the development of critical thinking abilities, and enhance retention of the critical body of knowledge needed by licensed nurses.

REFERENCES

Alexander, J. G., McDaniel, G. S., Baldwin, M. S., & Money, B. J. (2002). Promoting, applying, and evaluating problem-based learning in the undergraduate nursing curriculum. *Nursing Education Perspectives, 23*(5), 248-253.

Alters, B. J., & Nelson, C. E. (2002). Perspective: Teaching evolution in higher education. *Evolution: International Journal of Organic Evolution, 56*(10), 1891-1901.

Antonacci, P. A. (1991). Students search for meaning in the text through semantic mapping. *Social Education, 55,* 174-181.

Ayer, S. J. (1986). Teaching practice experience: Linking theory to practice. *Journal of Advanced Nursing, 11,* 513-519.

Baker, C. M. (2000a). Problem-based learning for nursing: Integrating lessons from other disciplines with nursing experiences. *Journal of Professional Nursing, 16*(5), 258-266.

Baker, C. M. (2000b). Using problem-based learning to redesign nursing administration masters programs. *Journal of Nursing Administration, 30*(1), 41-47.

Bandman, E. L., & Bandman, B. (1995). *Critical thinking in nursing* (2nd ed.). Norwalk, CT: Appleton & Lange.

Barnes, C. A. (1992). *Critical thinking: Educational imperatives.* San Francisco: Jossey-Bass.

Baron, J. B., & Sternberg, R. J. (1986). *Teaching thinking skills: Theory and practice.* New York: W. H. Freeman.

Barrows, H., & Tamblyn, R. (1980). *Problem-based learning: An approach to medical education.* New York: Springer.

Batscha, C. (2002). The pharmacology game. *CIN Plus, 5*(3), 1, 3-6.

Beck, S. E. (1995). Cooperative learning and feminist pedagogy: A model for classroom instruction in nursing education. *Journal of Nursing Education, 34,* 222-227.

Beitz, J. M. (1998). Concept mapping: Navigating the learning process. *Nurse Educator, 23*(5), 35-41.

Belenky, M. F., Clinchy, B.M., Goldberger, N. R., & Tarule, J. M. (1986). *Women's ways of knowing: The development of self, voice and mind.* New York: Basic Books.

Benner, P. (1984). *From novice to expert: Excellence and power in clinical nursing practice.* Menlo Park, CA: Addison-Wesley.

Bevis, E. O. (1993). All in all it was a pretty good funeral. *Journal of Nursing Education, 32,* 101-105.

Bowers, B., & McCarthy, D. (1993). Developing analytic thinking skills in early undergraduate education. *Journal of Nursing Education, 32,* 107-114.

Bradley-Springer, L. (1993). Discovery of meaning through imagined experience, writing, and evaluation. *Nurse Educator, 18*(5), 5-10.

Brigham, C. (1993). Nursing education and critical thinking: Interplay of content and thinking. *Holistic Nursing Practice, 7,* 48-54.

Brookfield, S. (1992). Uncovering assumptions: The key to reflective practice. *Adult Learning, 3,* 13-14.

Brookfield, S. D. (1987). *Developing critical thinkers: Challenging adults to explore alternative ways of thinking and acting.* San Francisco: Jossey-Bass.

Brookfield, S. D. (1995). *Becoming a critically reflective teacher.* San Francisco: Jossey-Bass.

 Brown, H. N., & Sorrell, J. M. (1993). Use of clinical journals to enhance critical thinking. *Nurse Educator, 18*(5), 16-19.

Browne, M. N., & Keeley, S. M. (1990). *Asking the right questions: A guide to critical thinking* (3rd ed.). Saddle River, NJ: Prentice-Hall.

Bucher, L. (1993). The effects of imagery abilities and mental rehearsal on learning a nursing skill. *Journal of Nursing Education, 32,* 318-328.

Burns, K. R., & Egan, E. C. (1994). Description of a stressful encounter: Appraisal, threat and challenge. *Journal of Nursing Education, 33,* 21-28.

Callahan, M. (1992). Thinking skills: An assessment model for ADN in the '90s. *Journal of Nursing Education, 31,* 85-87.

Candella, L., Michael, S. R., & Mitchell, S. (2003). Ethical debates: Enhancing critical thinking in nursing students. *Nurse Educator, 28*(1), 37-39.

Carlson-Catalano, J. (1992). Empowering nurses for professional practice. *Nursing Outlook, 40,* 139-142.

Cascio, R. S., Campbell, D., Sandor, M. K., Rains, A. P., & Clark, M. C. (1995). Enhancing critical-thinking skills: Faculty-student partnerships in community health nursing. *Nurse Educator, 20*(2), 38-43.

Case, B. (1994). Walking around the elephant: A critical-thinking strategy for decision making. *The Journal of Continuing Education in Nursing, 25,* 101-109.

Casebeer, L. (1991). Fostering decision making in nursing. *Journal of Nursing Staff Development, 7,* 271-274.

Choi, H. (2003). A problem-based learning trial on the Internet involving undergraduate nursing students. *Journal of Nursing Education, 42,* 359-363.

Cohen, E. G. (1994). *Designing groupwork: Strategies for the heterogeneous classroom* (2nd ed.). New York: Teachers College Press.

Connor, S. E., & Tillman, M. H. (1990). A comparison of algorithmic and teacher-directed instruction in dosage calculation presented via whole and part methods for associate degree nursing students. *Journal of Nursing Education, 29,* 31-36.

Conyers, V. (2003). Posters: An assessment strategy to foster learning in nursing education. *Journal of Nursing Education, 42,* 38-40.

Creedy, D., & Hand, B. (1994). The implementation of problem-based learning: Changing pedagogy in nurse education. *Journal of Advanced Nursing, 20*(4), 696-702.

Creedy, D., Horsfall, J., & Hand, B. (1992). Problem-based learning in nurse education: An Australian view. *Journal of Advanced Nursing, 17,* 727-733.

Daley, B. J., Shaw, C. R., Balistrieri, T., Glasenapp, K., & Piacentine, L. (1999). Concept maps: A strategy to teach and evaluate critical thinking. *Journal of Nursing Education, 38*(1), 42-47.

Dansereau, D. F. (1983). *Cooperative learning: Impact on acquisition of knowledge and skills* (Report No. 341). Abilene, TX: U. S. Army Research for the Behavioral and Social Sciences.

Davidson, N. (1994). Cooperative and collaborative learning: An integrative perspective. In J. S. Thousand, R. A. Villa, & A. I. Nevin (Eds.), *Creativity and collaborative learning: A practical guide to empowering students and teachers.* Baltimore: Paul H. Brookes.

deTornyay, R., & Thompson, M. A. (1982). *Strategies for teaching nursing* (3rd ed.). New York: John Wiley.

deTornyay, R., & Thompson, M. A. (1987). *Strategies for teaching nursing* (4th ed.). New York: John Wiley.

Dewey, J. (1933). *How we think: A restatement of the relation of reflective thinking to the educative process.* Boston: Heath.

Doheny, M. O. (1993). Mental practice: An alternative approach to teaching motor skills. *Journal of Nursing Education, 32,* 260-264.

Duchin, S., & Sherwood, G. (1990). Posters as an educational strategy. *Journal of Continuing Education in Nursing, 2,* 205-208.

Facione, N. C., Facione, P. A., & Sanchez, C. A. (1994). Critical thinking disposition as a measure of competent clinical judgment: The development of the California critical thinking disposition inventory. *Journal of Nursing Education, 33,* 345-350.

Facione, P. A. (1990). *Critical thinking: A statement of expert consensus for purposes of educational assessment and instruction. The Delphi Report: Research findings and recommendations prepared for the committee on pre-college philosophy.* Newark, DE: American Philosophical Association. (ERIC Document Reproduction Service No. ED 315-423).

Ford, J. S., & Profetto-McGrath, J. (1994). A model for critical thinking within the context of curriculum as praxis. *Journal of Nursing Education, 33,* 341-344.

Frost, M. (1996). An analysis of the scope and value of problem-based learning in the education of health care professionals. *Journal of Advanced Nursing, 24*(5), 1047-1053.

Fuszard, B. (1995). *Innovative teaching strategies in nursing* (2nd ed.). Gaithersburg, MD: Aspen.

Garrett, M., Schoener, L., & Hood, L. (1996). Debate: A teaching strategy to improve verbal communications and critical thinking skills. *Nurse Educator, 21*(4), 37-40.

Gehrke, P. (1994). Finding voices through writing. *Nurse Educator, 19*(2), 28-30.

Glendon, K., & Ulrich, D. (1992). Using cooperative learning strategies. *Nurse Educator, 17*(4), 37-40.

Halpern, D. F., and Associates. (1994). *Changing college classrooms: New teaching and learning strategies for an increasingly complex world.* San Francisco: Jossey-Bass.

Heinrich, K. T. (1992). The intimate dialogue: Journal writing by students. *Nurse Educator, 17*(6), 17-21.

Hezekiah, J. (1993). Feminist pedagogy: A framework for nursing education? *Journal of Nursing Education, 32,* 53-58.

Hickman, J. S. (1993). A critical assessment of critical thinking in nursing education. *Holistic Nurse Practice, 7*(3), 36-47.

Hoover, K. H. (1980). *College teaching today: A handbook for postsecondary instruction.* Boston: Allyn & Bacon.

Hunkins, F. P. (1976). *Involving students in questioning.* Boston: Allyn & Bacon.

Hunkins, F. P. (1985). Helping students ask their own questions. *Social Education, 49,* 293-296.

Jackson, B. S. (1995). Critical thinking. *Capsules & Comments in Critical Care Nursing, 3,* 183-187.

Jeffries, P. R., Rew, S., & Cramer, J. M. (2003). A comparison of student-centered versus traditional methods of teaching basic nursing skills in a learning laboratory. *Nursing Education Perspectives, 23*(1), 14-19.

Johnson, D. W., & Johnson, R. T. (1991). Cooperative learning and classroom school climate. In B. Fraser & H. Walberg (Eds.), *Educational environments: Evaluation and antecedents and consequences* (pp. 90-104). Oxford: Pergamon Press.

Johnson, D. W., & Johnson, R. T. (1993). Creative and critical thinking through academic controversy. *American Behavioral Scientist, 37,* 40-53.

Johnson, D. W., Johnson, R. T., & Smith, K. (1991). *Active learning: Cooperation in the college classroom.* Edina, MN: Interaction Books.

Johnson, D. W., Maruyama, G., Johnson, R. T., Nelson, D., & Skon, L. (1981). Effects of cooperative, competitive, and individualistic goal structures on achievement: A meta-analysis. *Psychological Bulletin, 89,* 47-62.

Jones, J. E. (1994). Portfolio assessment as a strategy for self-direction in learning. In R. G. Brockett & A. B. Knox (Series Eds.) & R. Hiemstra & R. G. Brockett (Vol. Eds.), *New directions for adult and continuing education: No. 64. Overcoming resistance to self-direction in adult learning* (pp. 23-29). San Francisco: Jossey-Bass.

Jones, S. A., & Brown, L. N. (1991). Critical thinking: Impact on nursing education. *Journal of Advanced Nursing, 16,* 529-533.

Jones, S. A., & Brown, L. N. (1993). Alternative views on defining critical thinking through the nursing process. *Holistic Nursing Practice, 7*, 71-76.

Kataoka-Yahiro, M., & Saylor, C. (1994). A critical thinking model for nursing judgment. *Journal of Nursing Education, 33*, 351-356.

Kelly, K. J. (1992). *Nursing staff development: Current competence, future focus.* Philadelphia: J. B. Lippincott.

Kirkpatrick, M. K. (1994). NINE: Newspaper in nursing education. *Nurse Educator, 19*(6), 21-23.

Koenig, J. M., & Zorn, C. R. (2002). Using storytelling as an approach to teaching and learning with diverse students. *Journal of Nursing Education, 41*(9), 393-399.

Kramer, M. K. (1993). Concept clarification and critical thinking: Integrated processes. *Journal of Nursing Education, 32*, 406-414.

Kuhn, M. A. (1995). Gaming: A technique that adds spice to learning? *The Journal of Continuing Education, 26*, 35-39.

Kurfiss, J. G. (1988). *Critical thinking: Theory, research, practice and possibilities* (Report No. 2). Washington, DC: Association for the Study of Higher Education.

Lashley, M., & Wittstadt, R. (1993). Writing across the curriculum: An integrated curricular approach to developing critical thinking through writing. *Journal of Nursing Education, 32*, 422-424.

Maas, D. (1990). *Maintaining teacher effectiveness* [Videotapes]. (Available from Phi Delta Kappa International, P.O. Box 789, Bloomington, IN 47402-0789).

MacIntosh, J. (1995). Fashioning facilitators: Nursing education for primary healthcare. *Nurse Educator, 20*(3), 25-27.

MacLeod, M. L. P. (1995). What does it mean to be well taught? A hermeneutic course evaluation. *Journal of Nursing Education, 34*, 197-203.

Matthews, R. S., Copper, J. L., Davidson, N., & Hawkes, P. (1995). Building bridges between cooperative and collaborative learning. *Change, 27*(4), 35-40.

McAlister, M., & Osborne, Y. (1997). Peer review: A strategy to enhance cooperative student learning. *Nurse Educator, 22*(1), 40-44.

McCabe, P. P. (1992). Getting past learner apprehension: Enhancing learning for the beginning reader. *Adult Learning, 3*(1), 19-20.

McCaugherty, D. (1991). The use of a teaching model to promote reflection and the experiential integration of theory and practice in first-year student nurses: An action research study. *Journal of Advanced Nursing, 16*, 534-543.

McKeachie, W. J. (1986). *Teaching tips: A guidebook for the beginning teacher.* Lexington, MA: D. C. Heath.

McMullan, M., Endacott, R., Gray, M. A., Jasper, M., Miller, C., Scholes, J., et al. (2003). Portfolios and assessment of competence: A review of the literature. *Journal of Advanced Nursing, 41*(3), 283-294.

McPeck, J. (1981). *Critical thinking and education.* New York: St. Martin's Press.

Metcalf, B. L., & Yankou, D. (2003). Educational innovations. Using gaming to help nursing students understand ethics. *Journal of Nursing Education, 42*(5), 212-215.

Meyers, C. (1986). *Teaching students to think critically.* San Francisco: Jossey-Bass.

Miller, M. A. (1992). Outcomes evaluation: Measuring critical thinking. *Journal of Advanced Nursing, 17*, 1401-1407.

Moneyham, L, Ura, D., Ellwood S., & Bruno, B. (1996). The poster presentation as an educational tool. *Nurse Educator, 21*(4), 45-47.

Mottola, C. A., & Murphy, P. (2001). Antidote dilemma: An activity to promote critical thinking. *Journal of Continuing Education in Nursing, 32*, 161-164.

Moule, P., Judd, M., & Girot, E. (1998). The poster presentation: What value to teaching and assessment of research in pre- and post-registration nursing courses? *Nurse Education Today, 18*, 237-242.

Nehls, N. (1995). Narrative pedagogy: Rethinking nursing education. *Journal of Nursing Education, 34*, 204-210.

Nelson, C. (2000). What is the first step we should take to become great teachers? *The National Teaching & Learning Forum, 10*(1), 7-8.

Nelson, C. (2001). What is the most difficult step we must take to become great teachers? *The National Teaching & Learning Forum, 10*, 10.

Norris, S. P., & Ennis, R. H. (1989). *Evaluating critical thinking.* Pacific Grove, CA: Midwest Publications.

Parrott, T. E. (1994). Humor as a teaching strategy. *Nurse Educator, 19*(3), 36-38.

Paul, R. W. (1995). *Critical thinking: How to prepare students for a rapidly changing world.* Rohner Park, CA: Sonoma State University Center for Critical Thinking and Moral Critique.

Pederson, C. (1993). Structured controversy versus lecture on nursing students' beliefs about and attitude toward providing care for persons with AIDS. *Journal of Continuing Education in Nursing, 24,* 74-81.

Perry, W. G. (1970). *Forms of intellectual and ethical development in the college years: A scheme.* New York: Rinehart.

Pinch, W. J. (1995). Synthesis: Implementing a complex process. *Nurse Educator, 20*(1), 34-40.

Pless, B. S., & Clayton, G. M. (1993). Clarifying the concept of critical thinking in nursing. *Journal of Nursing Education, 32,* 425-428.

Pond, E. F., Bradshaw, M. J., & Turner, S. L. (1991). Teaching strategies for critical thinking. *Nurse Educator, 16*(6), 18-22.

Porter, E. J. (1995). Fostering dialogical community through a learning experience. *Journal of Nursing Education, 34,* 228-234.

Powell, J. H. (1989). The reflective practitioner in nursing. *Journal of Advanced Nursing, 14,* 824-828.

Price, J. G. (1991). Great expectations: Hallmark of the midlife woman learner. *Educational Gerontology, 17,* 167-174.

Ramey, S. L., & Hay, M. L. (2003). Using electronic portfolios to measure student achievement and assess curricular integrity. *Nurse Educator, 28*(1), 31-36.

Rather, M. L. (1994). Schooling for oppression: A critical hermeneutical analysis of the lived experience of the returning RN student. *Journal of Nursing Education, 33,* 263-271.

Rauen, C. A. (2001). Using simulation to teach critical thinking skills. You can't just throw the book at them. *Critical Care Nursing Clinics of North America, 13*(1), 93-103.

Reynolds, A. (1994). Patho-flow diagramming: A strategy for critical thinking and clinical decision making. *Journal of Nursing Education, 33,* 333-336.

Robbins, J. (1994). Using humor to enhance learning in the skills laboratory. *Nurse Educator, 19*(3), 39-41.

Rooda, L. A. (1994). Effects of mind mapping on student achievement in a nursing research course. *Nurse Educator, 19,* 25-27.

Rosenal, L. (1995). Exploring the learner's world: Critical incident methodology. *Journal of Continuing Education in Nursing, 26,* 115-118.

Russell, C. K., Gregory, D. M., & Gates, M. F. (1996). Aesthetics and substance in qualitative research posters. *Qualitative Health Research, 6,* 542-552.

Scheffer, B. K., & Rubenfeld, M. G. (2000). A consensus statement on critical thinking in nursing. *Journal of Nursing Education, 39*(8), 352-359.

Schmidt, K. L., & Fisher, J. C. (1992). Effective development and utilization of self-learning modules. *Journal of Continuing Education in Nursing, 23*(2), 54-59.

Sellappah, S., Hussey, T., Blackmore, A. M., & McMurray, A. (1998). The use of questioning strategies by clinical teachers. *Journal of Advanced Nursing, 28*(1), 142-148.

Shearer, R., & Davidhizar, R. (2003). Using role play to develop cultural competence. *Journal of Nursing Education, 42,* 273-276.

Siegel, H. (1980). Critical thinking as an educational ideal. *The Educational Forum, 45,* 7-23.

Swansburg, R. C. (1995). *Nursing staff development: A component of human resource development.* Boston: Jones and Bartlett.

Symonds, J. M. (1995). *RN students finding their voices: Narrative in nursing.* Paper presented at the First Annual RN-BSN meeting, Baltimore, MD.

Taylor, D. E., Barrick, C. B., & Harrell, F. H. (1994). Preparing students for health care reform: An innovative approach for teaching leadership/management. *Journal of Nursing Education, 33,* 230-232.

The Team Memory Jogger. Methuen, MA: GOAL/QPC.

Tomey, A. M. (2003). Learning with cases. *Journal of Continuing Education in Nursing, 34*(1), 34-38.

Torres, G., & Stanton, M. (1982). *Curriculum process in nursing: A guide to curriculum development.* Englewood Cliffs, NJ: Prentice-Hall.

Tschikota, S. (1993). The clinical decision-making processes of student nurses. *Journal of Nursing Education, 32,* 389-398.

Udvari-Solner, A. (1994). A decision-making model for curricular adaptations in cooperative groups. In J. S. Thousand, R. A. Villa, & A. I. Nevin (Eds.), *Creativity and collaborative learning: A practical guide to empowering students and teachers*. Baltimore: Paul H. Brookes.

Ulloth, J. K. (2002). The benefits of humor in nursing education. *Journal of Nursing Education, 41*(11), 476-481.

Ulloth, J. K. (2003a). Guidelines for developing and implementing humor in nursing classrooms. *Journal of Nursing Education, 42*, 35-37.

Ulloth, J. K. (2003b). A qualitative view of humor in nursing classrooms. *Journal of Nursing Education, 42*, 125-130.

Valiga, T. M. (1983). Cognitive development: A critical component of baccalaureate nursing education. *Image: The Journal of Nursing Scholarship, 15*, 115-119.

Van Hoozer, H. L., Bratton, B. D., Ostmoe, P. M., Weinholtz, D., Craft, M. J., Gjerde, C. L., et al. (1987). *The teaching process: Theory and practice in nursing*. Norwalk, CT: Appleton-Century-Crofts.

Wake, M. M., Coleman, R. S., & Kneeland, T. (1992). Classroom shared governance. *Nurse Educator, 17*(4), 19-22.

Watson, G., & Glaser, E. M. (1984). *Watson-Glaser critical thinking appraisal manual*. New York: Harcourt Brace & Jovanovich.

White, N. E., Beardslee, N. Q., Peters, D., & Supples, J. M. (1990). Promoting critical thinking skills. *Nurse Educator, 15*(5), 16-19.

Wilen, W. W. (Ed.). (1987). *Questions, questioning techniques, and effective teaching*. Washington, DC: National Education Association.

Wilen, W. W. (1990). *Teaching and learning through discussion: The theory, research and practice of the discussion method*. Springfield, IL: Charles C. Thomas.

Wilen, W. W. (1991). *Questioning skills for teachers: What research says to the teacher* (3rd ed.). Washington, DC: National Education Association.

Wink, D. M. (1993). Effect of a program to increase the cognitive level of questions asked in clinical postconferences. *Journal of Nursing Education, 32*, 357-363.

Yoder-Wise, P. S., & Kowalski, K. (2003). The power of storytelling. *Nursing Outlook, 51*, 37-42.

Young-Mason, J. (1988). Tolstoi's *The Death of Ivan Ilych:* A source for understanding compassion. *Clinical Nurse Specialist, 2*, 180-183.

Young-Mason, J. (1991). *The Secret Sharer* as a guide to compassion. *Nursing Outlook, 39*, 62-63.

14

IMPROVING TEACHING AND LEARNING

CLASSROOM ASSESSMENT TECHNIQUES

Connie J. Rowles, DSN, RN, CNAA, Pamela J. Cole, MA, RN, CS

Since the early 1980s, postsecondary education has been carefully scrutinized by political, economic, consumer, and educational forces to ensure appropriate student performance. As a result, institutions of higher education—faculty and students—are being held more accountable for student learning in the classroom (Angelo & Cross, 1993; Curtis, 1985; Halpern, 1994). To improve learning, educators are attempting to reform classroom instruction. One way is to use classroom techniques that allow assessment of learning (Cross, 1990). These techniques help the teacher gather data that will help to improve teaching and learning (McKeachie, 1994). The purpose of this chapter is to explain these techniques and how nursing faculty can use them to improve teaching and learning.

CLASSROOM ASSESSMENT

Formative evaluation is the foundation of classroom assessment. Bloom et al. (1981) describe formative evaluation as a tool useful in the process of evaluation to guide revisions and facilitate improvement of classroom instruction and student learning. By the late 1980s, Cross (1990) was advocating the use of teaching activities—classroom research—to ascertain whether students are learning and to discover the best methods for teaching. At present, these activities are called *classroom assessment techniques* (CATs) (Angelo & Cross, 1993; Halpern, 1994).

Classroom assessment "consists of **small scale** assessments conducted **continuously** in the college classroom by discipline-based **teachers** to determine what students **are** learning **in that class**" (Angelo, 1994, p. 5). Classroom assessment is (Angelo, 1994; Angelo & Cross, 1993):

1. *Learner-centered:* Students actively learn, become responsible for their own learning, and critically evaluate their own learning.
2. *Teacher-directed:* Teachers decide why, when, and how to include CATs in their classes.

3. *Mutually beneficial:* Teachers improve their teaching and students improve their learning with the use of CATs.
4. *Formative:* CATs help with learning, not with the evaluation or grading of student efforts.
5. *Context-specific:* Classes within different disciplines, courses, and even sections of a course develop their own personalities; and the techniques of classroom assessment may need to vary to "fit" the situation.
6. *Ongoing:* Frequent, current feedback to both the student and the teacher is an important feature in improving student learning.
7. *Rooted in good teaching practice:* Classroom assessment puts already established good teaching practices into a more systematic framework.

Thus classroom assessment provides for an assessment of learning in progress for both teachers and students in a nonthreatening environment. In addition, classroom assessment incorporates active learning strategies that facilitate learning (Astin, 1985; Halpern, 1994; McKeachie, 1994).

The term *classroom assessment* represents conceptual thinking. Techniques used for classroom assessment are called *CATs*. Many sources provide examples of CATs. The most comprehensive is the collection of 50 different techniques presented by Angelo and Cross (1993).

CAT Outcomes

There is an emerging body of evidence about the impact CATs have on both faculty and students. The evidence seems to support the thinking of Angelo and Cross (Angelo, 1994; Angelo & Cross, 1993). CATs can be a valuable tool for improving student learning. However, the evidence that CATs improve student learning outcomes is mixed. Boles (1999) found that using an e-mail–designed CAT improved student learning in a data communications class. However, Cottell and Harwood (1998) did not find the same results in an accounting class. Their conclusion was that many variables affect student learning outcomes and more study of CATs is needed.

Advantages of CATs

CATs can give immediate feedback to faculty about the learning that is happening in their classroom. As a result, midcourse classroom improvements can be made. CATs also give students feedback about their own learning. Students have a chance to make midcourse changes in their study habits.

Steadman (1998) studied the effects of using CATs in a community college setting. When using CATS, faculty found the following advantages: "ability to tune into students' voices, opportunity to engage in reflection on and systematic change of their teaching, student improvement and involvement in learning and the opportunity to join a community of other faculty committed to teaching" (Steadman, 1998, pp. 26-27). Student advantages include "increased control and voice in the classroom, students are more involved in their own learning and students benefit from improved teaching because faculty use feedback from CATS to improve instruction" (Steadman, 1998, p. 30).

Disadvantages of CATs

There are also disadvantages for students and faculty. CATs take up classroom time that is typically used for other activities, but the major disadvantage for faculty is the difficulty "in dealing with negative feedback" (Steadman, 1998, p. 27). Students also reported the use of class time as a disadvantage associated with CATs. CATs mean that students must be active participants in the classroom. Students who prefer to be passive participants in the classroom do not like the experience of CATs (Steadman, 1998).

Classroom Assessment Techniques

CATs are informal, formative evaluation tools and procedures used to monitor student learning. CATs involve immediate, continuous interaction between the student and teacher to validate, clarify, and facilitate learning. CATs can be used to assess students' attitudes, knowledge about course concepts, study habits, or even reactions to the teaching strategies used in a particular course. The three phases of developing and using CATs are planning, implementing, and responding (Angelo & Cross, 1993).

Planning CATs

During the planning phase, the teacher chooses a particular class in which to implement the CAT. The decision that formative evaluation could improve teaching and learning is based on information the instructor may have about the students' progress such as examination scores, student inability to verbalize or implement major course concepts, or frequent questions during class time.

During the second activity of the planning phase, the teacher clearly identifies the desired information to be gained by using a CAT. Most teachers have multiple goals for any one class period. These goals may come from a variety of sources, such as the overall curriculum plan, level objectives, course objectives, unit objectives, and so on. Because all these goals cannot possibly be measured with any one CAT in a single session, the teacher should focus on one specific goal. The activity in this part of the planning phase forces the teacher to reflect on and prioritize what specifically should be assessed (Fox, 2002).

The last activity in the planning phase is identification of the specific CAT to be used. Obviously, the most important feature in the selection of a CAT is a close match between what the CAT will measure and what the teacher has previously identified as the priority goal for use of the CAT. The selected CAT should be adjusted to fit the purpose of administration or the personality of the class. For example, Angelo and Cross (1993) describe an exercise called "everyday ethical dilemmas" (p. 271). They present the exercise as a brief ethical dilemma from which the students respond to two questions. The teacher then analyzes the student answers and presents the responses to the class, which generates further discussion about the ethical situation.

In one application of this CAT, the teacher modified the exercise and used it to frame an entire class period for a graduate class in nursing administration. The reading assignment for the class period described three different theories about ethical decision making. The goal for the class period was for the students to develop a better understanding of the ethical decision-making theories. Several typical situations involving ethical decision making by nurse administrators set the stage for the analysis of the ethical decision-making theories. The situations were discussed from the perspective of each of the theories. At the conclusion of the class, students reported a better understanding of the theories and a better understanding of how they as individuals made their own ethical decisions.

Implementing CATs

The second phase is the actual implementation of the CAT. A CAT can be used before, during, or after a class period. The class content could be taught, with administration of the CAT following, or the CAT could be administered first to set the stage for the rest of the class period. The timing of the administration of the CAT depends on the purpose of the classroom assessment and the particular content of the class session. Examining and organizing the results of the CAT into some sort of meaningful framework is the last activity in this phase.

Responding to the CAT

Reporting the results of the CAT to the students represents the final phase of CAT administration. First, the results of the CAT that have been organized in the prior phase need to be interpreted and arranged for presentation to the students. The feedback is presented in a manner to enhance student learning. The teacher should present results of the CAT to the students during the next scheduled class period. Some CATs involve very time-intensive interpretation and analysis. In such cases, the results of the CAT should be presented as soon as they are available. The less time it takes students to receive results, the greater will be the impact on improvement of student learning as a result of using the CAT.

The last activity in the responding phase is reflection (Angelo & Cross, 1993). The teacher evaluates use of the CAT. Did use of the CAT accomplish the goal established during the first phase? Did implementation of the CAT occur as it was planned? Was the outcome of use of the CAT enhanced student learning? What did the students think about use of the CAT? What did the teacher think about use of the CAT? Technically, answering these questions and others posed by the teacher completes the three phases of implementing a CAT. However, this phase usually stimulates further action. Use of another CAT, repeated use of the same CAT at a later date, and even course revision are some of the future actions that may be the result of the evaluation.

Examples of CATs

In examples 1 and 2, formal descriptions of two CATs are given (Angelo & Cross, 1993), and implementation is described. A teacher implemented these

CATs in a nursing classroom. Both of the CATs were adjusted by the teacher to best fit the personality of the class.

Example 1: Implementation of the One-Minute Paper

Implemented when. Before, during, or at the end of class.

Purpose/goal. To assess comprehension of major course concepts.

Activities. On a maximum of ½ page, the students answer one question such as

- What was the most important thing learned in class today?
  or
- What point was most confusing for you today?

Time involved

- 5 minutes for administration.
- 30 to 45 minutes to evaluate answers.
- Variable time in the next class to clarify problem areas.

Advantages

- Little class time is used.
- Minimal time to analyze results.
- Students will think about the class and evaluate what they did or did not learn.

Disadvantage. The desired results depend heavily on asking questions in the correct way.

A variation of this one-minute paper was used in a first-year associate degree nursing course. The goal for use of the CAT was to help students prioritize which aspects of nursing care were the most important for a variety of case scenarios.

Midsemester, at the end of a class, student groups were given scenarios to complete. Each group presented its scenario in class the following week. Immediately after each of the presentations, 2 to 3 minutes were allowed for students to write the most important point made by the presenters. Because there were 11 scenarios, there were 11 most important points selected by each student. At the conclusion of class, the sheets of most important points were collected. Students stated that they were satisfied with the class format for the day and asked to see how their most important points compared with the responses from the teacher.

During a later class session, each student was given a tally sheet that listed the most important points selected by the students and the most important points identified by the teacher. When students selected different most important points, frequencies were given. Students reported that the results sheet proved to be a good study tool.

Students performed well on the part of the examination regarding the unit taught that day. A drawback of the CAT was the time required to tally 11 most important points for 30 students. The task took approximately 6 hours to complete! Another disadvantage was that students sometimes had difficulty identifying just one most important point. Overall, however, the teacher thought the established goal was met.

Example 2: Implementation of the Self-Confidence Survey
Implemented when. Before, during, or at the end of class.
Purpose/goal. To identify areas of high and low self-confidence.
Activity. Answer survey items.
Time involved

- 1 to 10 minutes for administration.
- 5 to 30 minutes to evaluate answers.
- Variable time in the next class to discuss low and high confidence areas.

Advantages

- Little time used to administer and analyze results.
- Helps identify low and high confidence items.
- Helps teacher prioritize what to emphasize.
- Acknowledging low self-confidence may facilitate remedy of the problem.

Disadvantage. When many areas of low self-confidence are found, both students and faculty may feel depressed.

This self-confidence survey was implemented in a beginning nursing skills classroom course. The survey given to the students is provided in the box. The purpose of administering this CAT was to identify areas in which students did not feel confident and to guide the need for further instruction. Additionally, the teacher hoped students would be able to identify areas they should pursue for learning and boost their self-esteem by noting areas in which they felt confident.

This CAT was quickly prepared, students completed the form in approximately 3 minutes, and student responses were tallied in approximately 30 minutes. Results were shared with the students by using an overhead projector. Discussion ensued regarding areas of low self-confidence. For example, a clear pattern of low self-confidence was noted in the student responses to the following items: knowledge of medication action, side effects/adverse effects, and nursing considerations regarding medications. Through the resulting discussion, both the teacher and the students discovered ways to improve teaching and learning.

SUMMARY

This chapter has described classroom assessment and discussed implementation of the techniques associated with classroom assessment. Classroom assessment involves frequent, ongoing assessment learning. The major purpose of classroom assessment is to enhance the processes of teaching and learning. The three phases of classroom assessment are planning, implementing, and responding.

Although the term *classroom assessment* provides the conceptual background, the term *CATs* describes the "how to" of implementing classroom assessment. A description of the actual implementation of two CATs has been provided. CATs can be an important aid in helping both students and teachers improve student learning in the classroom.

NURSING SKILL SELF-CONFIDENCE SURVEY

This survey is to help both of us understand your level of confidence in your nursing skills. Please indicate how confident you feel about your ability to do the various items listed below. (Circle the most accurate response for each.)

Items	Self-Confidence in Your Ability			
Subcutaneous injections	None	Low	Medium	High
Intramuscular injections	None	Low	Medium	High
Hanging intravenous solutions	None	Low	Medium	High
Spiking an intravenous tubing	None	Low	Medium	High
Teaching a client breast self-examination	None	Low	Medium	High
Teaching a client testicular self-examination	None	Low	Medium	High
Administering oral medications	None	Low	Medium	High
Knowledge of medication actions	None	Low	Medium	High
Knowledge of medication side/adverse effects	None	Low	Medium	High
Knowledge of medical and nursing considerations	None	Low	Medium	High
Caring for a client postoperatively	None	Low	Medium	High
Caring for an orthopedic client	None	Low	Medium	High
Caring for a pediatric client	None	Low	Medium	High
Performing a dressing change	None	Low	Medium	High
Discharge planning/teaching	None	Low	Medium	High
Communicating with clients	None	Low	Medium	High
Communicating with staff	None	Low	Medium	High
Communicating with faculty	None	Low	Medium	High

Courtesy P. Cole, RN, MA, Ball State University College of Applied Sciences and Technology, Associate School of Nursing.

REFERENCES

Angelo, T. A. (1994). Classroom assessment: Involving faculty and students where it matters most. *Assessment Update: Progress, Trends, and Practices in Higher Education, 6*(4), 1-2, 5, 10.

Angelo, T. A., & Cross, K. A. (1993). *Classroom assessment techniques: A handbook for college teachers.* San Francisco: Jossey-Bass.

Astin, A. W. (1985). Student involvement: The key to effective education. In A. W. Astin, *Achieving educational excellence* (pp. 133-157). San Francisco: Jossey-Bass.

Boles, W. (1999). Classroom assessment for improved learning: A case study in using e-mail and involving students in preparing assignments. *Higher Education Research & Development, 18*(1), 145-159.

Bloom, B. S., Madaus, G. F., & Hastings, J. T. (1981). Formative evaluation. In B. S. Bloom, G. F. Madaus, & J. T. Hastings, *Evaluation to improve learning* (pp. 154-178). New York: McGraw-Hill.

Cottell, P., & Harwood, E. (1998). Do classroom assessment techniques (CATs) improve student learning? *New Directions for Teaching and Learning, 75*, 37-46.

Cross, K. P. (1990). Teaching to improve learning. *Journal on Excellence in College Teaching, 17*, 9-22.

Curtis, M. H. (Ed.). (1985). *Integrity in the college curriculum: A report to the academic community* (Project on redefining the meaning and purpose of baccalaureate degrees). Washington, DC: Association of American Colleges.

Fox, D. (2000). Classroom assessment data: Asking the right questions. *Leadership, 30*(2), 22-23.

Halpern, D. F. (1994). Rethinking college instruction for a changing world. In D. F. Halpern (Ed.), *Changing college classrooms: New teaching and learning strategies for an increasingly complex world* (pp. 1-12). San Francisco: Jossey-Bass.

McKeachie, W. J. (1994). Learning and cognition in the college classroom. In W. J. McKeachie (Ed.), *Teaching tips: Strategies, research, and theory for college and university teachers* (pp. 279-295). Lexington, MA: DC Heath.

Steadman, M. (1998). Using classroom assessment to change both teaching and learning. *New Directions for Teaching and Learning, 75,* 23-35.

15

TEACHING IN THE CLINICAL SETTING

Lillian Stokes, PhD, RN, Gail Kost, MSN, RN

The health care system is ever changing. Health care reform challenges faculty to prepare students for future roles and to practice in a health care system that is increasingly patient centered, wellness oriented, community based, population based, and technologically advanced. The clinical setting, where students can use newly acquired knowledge and skills, think critically, make clinical decisions, and acquire professional values necessary to work in this environment, has become increasingly more complex. The purpose of this chapter is to describe the environments for clinical teaching and learning, describe characteristics of effective clinical teachers, and describe teaching methods and models that facilitate learning in clinical settings.

THE CLINICAL LEARNING ENVIRONMENT

Practice Setting

The practice setting for clinical experiences may be any place where students interact with patients and families for purposes such as acquiring critical thinking, clinical decision making, psychomotor, and affective skills. The practice setting also provides an opportunity for students to learn to apply theory to practice, and according to Reilly and Oermann (1992), "learn how to learn, develop skill in handling ambiguity, and become socialized into the profession" (p. 77). This requires a variety of experiences in a variety of settings to facilitate skill acquisition in these areas. These settings range from acute care to community-based care settings. It is essential for the environment to be supportive and conducive to learning so that students will have opportunities to develop qualities and abilities needed by competent professionals (Williams, 2001).

Acute Care and Transitional Care Settings

Acute care and transitional settings provide clinical experiences for undergraduate students and for graduate students preparing for advanced practice roles.

These settings have become increasingly more complex. The reasons for some of the complexity include factors such as extensive technology, rapid patient turnover (declining length of stay), high rates of severe illness, and complex needs. Experiences in these settings enable students to practice skills and interact with patients with acute and chronic illnesses and their families. Students must be prepared to take care of patients within these complex settings.

Because of the complexity of the environment, safety risks for students, patients, and staff are increased. Faculty must use creative teaching and learning strategies to ensure safe practice while meeting curriculum objectives. Samples of strategies may include multiple assignments and nursing rounds. Additional strategies may include those that relate to developing students' critical thinking abilities including simulated clinical scenarios or labs, case studies, computer-assisted instruction, and interactive videos. It is important for faculty to become facilitators of learning, designers of clinical experiences, and developers of flexible skill sets that can be used across settings. Faculty must provide experiences to help students think, care, and act like nurses—and finally to *be* nurses (Tanner, 2002). For this to occur, the outcomes for specific learning experiences must be clearly identified and articulated. Shadow experiences, virtual simulations, guided and focused small group sessions, and selective and capstone experiences have a high potential for clinical education.

Community-based Settings

The focus of health care delivery is being switched from acute care inpatient hospital settings to the community. Several factors have facilitated this movement. These include social and technological changes and the economics and politics of health care reform (Sullivan, 1995). Thus clinical experiences may take place in institutions and community agencies such as ambulatory, care settings, nurse-managed clinics, homeless shelters, homes for battered women, physicians' offices, health maintenance organizations, daycare centers, and schools (Buttriss et al., 1995; Faller et al., 1995; Gaines, 1996; Oesterle & O'Callaghan, 1996; Peters, 1995; Simandl, 1996; Smith et al., 1996; Williams & Wold, 1996). Summer camps are also being used for special experiences (Totten & Fonnesbeck, 2002). The use of technology such as videoconferencing, wireless remote communication, information systems (Elfrink, 1996), and Web-based courses (DeBourgh, 2001) have made it possible for clinical experience to occur at a distance.

Establishing learning experiences in community-based settings may be challenging. Finding appropriate and sufficient experiences may be difficult because of the nursing shortage, economic constraints, the time required for students, and the fact that many agencies are not accustomed to having students and fear not being able to provide sufficient role models. Furthermore, nurses who are potential role models often cannot give the additional time required for students because of economic constraints.

The transition to community-based clinical teaching may require faculty to develop new clinical skills, modify teaching methods, and adapt to methods of clinical supervision such as being accessible by pager. Support may be given to faculty through faculty development programs and orientation by faculty who work in the community.

Clinical experiences are selected and planned to provide students with opportunities to work across settings and manage care for varied populations with an emphasis on prevention and primary care. It is important for nursing students to learn to work collaboratively with a variety of health disciplines (American Association of Colleges of Nursing [AACN], 1996). Therefore nursing students should be provided with opportunities to work as members of interdisciplinary teams and in practice settings when interdisciplinary practice models are used for joint planning, implementing, and evaluating outcomes of care.

The goal of interdisciplinary education is to foster interprofessional relationships while enhancing the contributions of each discipline (AACN, 1996). An expected outcome of interdisciplinary education is increased future collaboration among professionals. The assumption is that students who are taught together will learn to collaborate more effectively when they later assume professional roles in an integrated health care system (AACN, 1996; Bellack, 1995; Cook & Drusin, 1995; Larson, 1995; Lough et al., 1996).

Nursing faculty are increasingly participating in teams and designing interdisciplinary clinical courses and learning experiences (Erkel et al., 1995; McDaniel & Robertson, 1997; Watson, 1996). Successful course development and implementation depend on faculty's commitment to the goal of interdisciplinary practice; professional respect and role clarity; ability to secure clinical facilities and develop schedules for clinical experiences compatible with the concurrent coursework and curriculum progression in each discipline; identification of content and experiences with similarities, differences, and overlaps; and clarification of autonomy and role interdependency. Success also depends on the ability to identify philosophical similarities and differences in clinical practice and to establish clear communication through avenues such as frequent interdisciplinary clinical conferences (Cook & Drusin, 1995; Larson, 1995; Lough et al., 1996).

Rewards and benefits of interdisciplinary practice and education include clearer understanding of roles and better employment opportunities for graduates. The long-term outcome is improved access to care, quality care, and increased patient satisfaction (AACN, 1996) and safety.

Ongoing evaluation is imperative and contributes to revisions and course development. Staff at clinical practice sites, students, and faculty should be involved in evaluation activities.

Selecting Health Care Agencies for Student Experiences

Regardless of the setting or practice model in which clinical experiences occur, faculty have the responsibility for selecting appropriate health care agencies and negotiating a contract that specifies the rights and responsibilities of both the school of nursing and the health care agency. When considering a health care agency as a practice setting, faculty should determine that the philosophy of the agency is consistent with that of the school of nursing, the patient population is adequate to meet curriculum and course objectives, the agency is accredited and has sufficient staff, and the practice model is compatible with curriculum needs. The adequacy and availability of physical resources (e.g., conference space and library resources) for students and faculty should also be determined. Finding a practice setting that meets all of these criteria has become a challenge because of changes in the delivery of health care. For example, rapid patient turnover often means that faculty have to select what is available, rather than what best meets students' needs. The limitation in patient selection in turn creates a challenge for faculty to be creative in how to use "what's available" to ensure that curriculum needs are met. The role of the faculty is to help students make the connections and "make them fit."

Relationships with Health Care Agency Staff

The ability of the clinical faculty to facilitate students' learning can be enhanced when an effective working relationship is established with the clinical agency. This requires having an understanding of the roles of the individuals within the setting and communicating effectively with them. Roles do not exist in isolation but are patterned to dovetail with or complement the other roles. According to Piscopo (1994), "roles identify relationships, are interactional, and are reciprocal" (p. 113). Faculty must facilitate the development of relationships to maximize opportunities for learning.

According to Frieburger (1996), collaboration between students and nursing staff can be facilitated by sharing information about the nature of student experiences, including goals and objectives for experiences; the level of the students and what they can be expected to do; the clinical schedule; roles and responsibilities of students and faculty; and expectations of the staff. Having a manager orient the students to the clinical setting and having students work with staff early in the clinical experience promote positive student–staff interaction and provide an opportunity for role clarification and the development of collegial relationships (Frieburger, 1996).

Although clinical faculty have the primary responsibility for teaching and guiding students in the clinical area, others can facilitate the process. Therefore communication about the nature of experiences and roles and responsibilities should be ongoing, clear, and consistent. Such communication enables the staff to be in a better position to assist faculty in identification of appropriate experiences for students. Follow-up communication permits all within the practice setting to keep abreast of ongoing changes.

Selecting Clinical Experiences

Clinical experiences refer to all the activities in which students engage in the practice of nursing. Such experiences are essential for knowledge application, skill development, and professional socialization. Selection of clinical learning experiences requires that all faculty be knowledgeable about clinical education and have a sound understanding of the curriculum, the learner, and the learning environment (Fothergill-Bourbonnais & Higuchi, 1995).

Faculty have the responsibility of acquiring as much information about the affiliating agency as possible. The information can be obtained through agency websites, formal meetings with agency administrators, special orientation and information sessions, and meetings with and shadowing of personnel in the immediate care area. These meetings should be reciprocal so that faculty can learn about the agency and staff at the agency can learn about faculty and students.

Understanding the Curriculum

The curriculum is composed of a series of well-organized and logical entities. It is designed to build on prior knowledge and to reinforce learning. The manner in which the curriculum is organized facilitates the planning of learning experiences in a logical, rational sequence. As students make progress and engage in varied clinical experiences, it is the responsibility of the faculty to interpret the curriculum and to describe the relationships among different components of the curriculum.

The selection of experiences should be consistent with the desired curriculum outcomes. The outcomes are multiple and specific to the nursing program. For example, the expected outcomes for students in an undergraduate degree nursing program are different from those for students in a graduate degree program. Therefore the learning experiences that are selected and the practice opportunities provided for students should be congruent with the program objectives.

The clinical experiences should also help students prepare for outcomes in a progressive, developmental manner. Experiences with patients of different ages and with different levels of wellness and interactions with diverse populations should be provided. Faculty should have opportunities to use creative talents and their own clinical skills and expertise.

Understanding the Student

Clinical experiences provide opportunities for students to practice the art and science of nursing and enhance the ability to learn. To maximize these opportunities faculty must have full knowledge and understanding of each student and the student population. The nursing student population is culturally diverse and includes members of many ethnic and racial minority groups and an increasing number of men. In addition to traditional students, the population includes persons of all ages with prior degrees from a variety of disciplines who have many different health care experiences and technological skill levels (Karuhije, 1997). In addition, students differ in their level of knowledge and preferences for learning opportunities; therefore faculty must make a concerted effort to balance the learning needs, interests, and abilities of students when selecting clinical experiences (Goldenberg & Iwasiw, 1988). Such action can be facilitated by making an assessment of the knowledge, culture, and skills of the learner. The assessment helps the faculty determine whether students possess the psychomotor and decision-making skills needed for the experiences. The curriculum guides the selection of learning experiences and clinical assignments, organizes teacher learning activities, and facilitates the measurement of student performance (Carpenito & Duespohl, 1985).

Students are required to demonstrate multiple behaviors in cognitive, psychomotor, and affective domains. Consequently, clinical faculty must evaluate students in each of these areas. The evaluation must be ongoing (formative evaluation) to assist students in learning and terminal (summative evaluation) to determine learning outcomes. Constructive and timely feedback, which promotes achievement and growth, is an essential element of evaluation (Pugh, 1988). For a discussion of clinical performance evaluation, refer to Chapter 23.

Understanding the Clinical Environment

The clinical environment has been described as a place where students synthesize the knowledge gained in the classroom and apply it to practical situations. The environment may be an acute care or community-based setting. As a result of the difficulty in finding placements for students in inpatient settings because of shortened hospital stays and an increased focus on health promotion, community sites are increasingly being used. Community-based environments may include worksite venues such as health maintenance organizations (Schim & Scher, 2002), community settings (e.g., ambulatory care, home health care), long-term care facilities, schools, and art galleries (Chan, 2002).

Chan (2002) describes the clinical learning environment as "the interaction network of forces within the clinical setting that influence student learning outcomes"(p. 70). A number of forces affect expected outcomes, including the increased complexity of care required by patients with more severe illness, the nursing shortage, the rapid pace, and multiple health care professionals and activities. These forces coupled with the need to adjust to an environment that requires a merging of thinking skills and performance skills often result in increased anxiety among students. Regardless of the location of the practice setting, faculty and staff should provide an environment where caring relationships are evident (Hodge, 1988). The clinical practice setting should be a place where students feel that they are accepted and that their contributions are appreciated by individuals within the environment (Chan, 2002). Specific attributes of staff that are considered helpful include warmth, support in obtaining access to learning experiences, and willingness to engage in a teaching relationship (Dunn & Burnett, 1995). Clinical strategies can be developed to reduce anxiety in clinical environments, especially in acute care settings. Some strategies focus on the level of students. Two such strategies are peer coaching in which senior students coach beginning students (Broscious & Sanders, 2001) and placement of students in long-term care settings.

Scheduling Clinical Assignments

Although faculty schedule clinical experiences to promote learning, there is ongoing dialogue about the best way to schedule experiences, the length of the experience (hours per day, number of days per week, number of weeks per semester), the timing of the experience in relation to didactic course assignments, and student needs. Porter and Feller (1979) examined the achievement of baccalaureate nursing students who either had clinical experience in two alternating clinical sites over a 16-week period or experiences in one site for 8 weeks, followed by experiences in a second site for the last 8 weeks. No differences in scores on National League for Nursing achievement tests were found. Similarly, Dunn et al. (1995) reported no differences in clinical learning outcomes when clinical assignments occur either 1 or 2 days per week or in alternating 2-week blocks of time. Students reported being frustrated by nonsequential clinical experiences because of the inability to form relationships with nursing staff. Additionally, students described the impact of the organization, clinical experiences, and timing of assignments on work and family responsibilities (Dunn et al., 1995).

Although results of research about outcomes and student satisfaction with timing and scheduling of clinical experiences offer some guidance, faculty must deal with multiple variables. These include variables such as availability of patients and clinical facilities, course schedules, and student needs. Scheduling can also be influenced by the desire to have concurrent classroom and clinical experiences so that knowledge can be transferred and applied immediately. Clinical scheduling can be further complicated by the need to mesh schedules of students from more than one school of nursing. Thus ideal scheduling may not be a reality.

EFFECTIVE CLINICAL TEACHING

Clinical teaching involves the careful design of an environment in which students have opportunities to foster mutual respect and support for each other while they are achieving identified learning outcomes. Faculty who teach in the clinical setting are the crucial link to successful experiences for students. Research in nursing education indicates that effective clinical teachers are clinically competent; know how to teach; have collegial relationships with students and agency staff; and are friendly, supportive, and patient (Halstead, 1996; Nehring, 1990; Oermann, 1996; Reilly & Oermann, 1992; Sieh & Bell, 1994; Stuebbe, 1990).

Being knowledgeable and being able to share the knowledge with students in clinical settings are essential. Such knowledge includes an understanding of the theories and concepts related to the practice of nursing. Equally important is an ability to convey the knowledge in an understandable manner. Attention to three discrete teaching domains—instructional, evaluative, and interpersonal (Karuhije, 1997)—will facilitate acquisition of the teaching skills needed to foster success in clinical settings. *Instructional* refers to approaches or strategies used to facilitate a transfer of knowledge from didactic to practicum. *Evaluative* relates to making determinations about performance and achievement of goals. *Interpersonal* refers to relationships and interactions.

Competence in the clinical practice of nursing has been documented as being necessary for effective clinical teaching. Morgan and Knox (1987) and Nehring (1990) found that the best clinical teachers exhibit expert clinical skills and judgment. Skills such as these have been described by students as being particularly important. Students tend to describe effective clinical teachers as those who demonstrate nursing competence in a real situation (Horst, 1988; Pugh, 1988).

Knowledge of how to teach is also essential for effective clinical teaching. Wong and Wong (1987) contend that effective clinical teachers are expected to have expertise in the "art" of teaching. Equally important are teacher behaviors that facilitate learning and support students in their acquisition of nursing skills (McCabe, 1985). There is empirical evidence that correlates specific teaching methods with enhanced student learning; examples of such methods are use of objectives, effective questioning, and responding to questions (Brophy & Good, 1986; Meleca et al., 1981; Rosenshine & Stevens, 1986).

Krichbaum (1994) reported student learning to be significantly related to teacher behaviors, the use of objectives and provision of opportunities for practice. A study conducted by Pugh (1988) revealed that preparation and the ability to explain concepts clearly and stimulate learning are also important. Other effective behaviors include sharing anecdotal notes, being fair in evaluation (Pugh, 1988), communicating expectations clearly (Nehring, 1990), and providing positively timed and specific feedback (Nehring, 1990; Pugh, 1988).

Massarweh (1999) contends that teachers can use motivational and critical thinking strategies in clinical settings to promote learning. Motivational strategies "foster increased productivity, vision, direction and excitement for the profession" (p. 45). Included among motivational strategies are discussing semester goals and relating them to the clinical arena, exhibiting enthusiasm about the profession, discerning student expectations, establishing reward systems, and trying new and different teaching strategies. A strategy that facilitates critical thinking could be the use of nursing process maps, which are reported to be effective.

Teacher behaviors relating to interpersonal skills are reported to affect student outcomes. Behaviors such as showing respect for students and treating them with respect (Pardo, 1991), correcting mistakes without belittling (Nehring, 1990; O'Shea & Parsons, 1979; Sieh & Bell, 1994), and being supportive and understanding (O'Shea & Parsons, 1979) are reported to be effective.

Nursing students experience stress and anxiety in clinical learning situations (Elliott, 2002; Lo, 2002; Timmins & Kaliszer, 2002). Negative relationships with faculty can contribute to anxiety (Kleehammer et al., 1990). The effective clinical teacher recognizes students' need for supportive and collegial relationships and develops an interpersonal style that promotes a collegial learning environment (Halstead, 1996). A safe learning environment has been created when students feel comfortable in speaking openly (Massarweh, 1999). Positive relationships are nurturing and can enhance learning. Caring behaviors and a caring environment are essential. Knowing how to give feedback about clinical performance and written clinical assignments is an important element of teaching. One way to do this is to point out positive aspects of performance, as well as areas that require improvement (Knox & Morgan, 1985). Senior clinical faculty should serve as role models and mentor junior clinical faculty members to create a legacy of effective clinical teaching. Additional characteristics of effective teachers can be found in Box 15-1.

Often, expert clinicians have the desire to teach in the clinical area. Some have been preceptors and believe that to make the transition to a new role as clinical teachers they need further instruction and guidance. Because clinical teaching is an acclaimed role, the desire can become a reality. Universities are challenged to meet the learning needs of new clinical faculty, especially those who maintain full-time clinical practices. These individuals should be encouraged and provided with information about where and how they can engage in activities that will facilitate their acquisition of the knowledge and skills required for the roles. Some schools have developed modules for that

Box 15-1
CHARACTERISTICS OF EFFECTIVE CLINICAL TEACHERS

Effective clinical teachers
1. Create an environment that is conducive to learning that requires:
   - Knowledge of the practice area
   - Clinical competence
   - Knowledge of how to teach
   - A desire to teach
2. Are supportive of learners; such support requires:
   - Knowledge of the learners
   - Knowledge of the practice area
   - Mutual respect
3. Possess teaching skills that maximize student learning; this requires an ability to:
   - Diagnose student needs
   - Learn about students as individuals, including their needs, personalities, capabilities
4. Foster independence so that students learn how to learn
5. Encourage exploration and questions without penalty
6. Accept differences among students
7. Relate how clinical experiences facilitate the development of clinical competence
8. Possess effective communication and questioning skills
9. Serve as a role model
10. Enjoy nursing and teaching
11. Are friendly, approachable, understanding, enthusiastic about teaching, and confident with teaching
12. Are knowledgeable about the subject matter and are able to convey that knowledge to students in their practice areas
13. Exhibit fairness in evaluation
14. Provide frequent feedback

purpose. One method for meeting the challenge of educating clinical teachers is to use an online course to orient clinicians who are making the transition from the role of expert clinician to that of clinical teacher (Vinten et al., 2003).

In summary, effective clinical teachers are knowledgeable about nursing, know how to convey the knowledge to students in a meaningful way, are clinically competent, exhibit interpersonal skills that positively influence students' learning, and establish collegial relationships that often last well beyond a specific course or program.

CLINICAL TEACHING METHODS

Teaching methods refer to the orderly, logical course of action taken to accomplish a particular educational goal. The actual selection and use of a particular method or strategy should be based on expected outcomes, principles of learning, and learner needs. This section focuses on several strategies commonly used in clinical teaching: patient care assignments, clinical conferences, nursing rounds, and written assignments.

Patient Care Assignment

Patient care provides students with opportunities to integrate, synthesize, and use previously learned knowledge and skills. Some nursing courses require students to prepare in advance for their clinical experience. Advance preparation commences with making patient care assignments. Making clinical assignments may be the responsibility of the teacher, the teacher and student together (especially useful for beginning students), the student alone, the student with guidance from the teacher, or the nursing and health care staff or preceptors (McCoin & Jenkins, 1988). When students are permitted some input into selecting clinical assignments, this encourages students to be self-directed, as well as to choose experiences on the basis of their personal learning needs (Pond, 1995).

The selection of clinical assignments by students in collaboration with others has several benefits. It provides opportunities for students to (1) select experiences that are based on personal learning needs, (2) experience a degree of control over their education, and (3) interact with practicing professionals during the process of selecting experiences (Pond, 1995). The extent to which students are permitted to self-select experiences depends on the goals or expected outcomes of the program, the philosophy of the specific clinical instructor, and the availability of resources in the clinical setting to assist students (i.e., answer questions and provide guidance in selecting patients).

Involvement of the clinical faculty is important when students select their experiences. Faculty (1) serve as resource advisors and sources of emotional support (Weinholtz & Ostmoe, 1987), (2) communicate goals and intended outcomes, (3) assist students in assessing the congruency between personal learning needs and course objectives, (4) facilitate planning the experiences, (5) collaborate with students as they strive to meet goals, and (6) evaluate accomplishments.

Strategies for Making Clinical Assignments

Clinical assignments are an integral part of nursing practicum experiences. Several strategies for making clinical assignments have been adopted for clinical teaching. The strategy used in clinical instruction is often determined by factors such as the skill level of the student, the patients' severity of illness, the number of assigned students, and availability of patients and resources. Traditional or alternative strategies—dual and multiple assignments—are discussed.

The traditional strategy is one in which nursing students are taught in a clinical setting with a varying faculty–student ratio. Ratios ranging from 1:8 to 1:10 are recommended (Schuster et al., 1997). From a student perspective, this strategy involves the assignment of one student to one or two patients. The student assumes responsibility for the nursing intervention needed in the care of the patient and also works alone in planning, implementing, and evaluating nursing activities. Unlike the multiple assignments, emphasis is on two students caring for one patient. The clinical faculty member acts as a resource for discussing problems and concerns related to patient care.

There are two alternatives to the traditional method of clinical instruction: dual assignments and multiple assignments. The dual assignment strategy

(Fugate & Rebeschi, 1991; Gotschall & Thompson, 1990) involves assigning two students to one patient. This alternative is useful when the level or complexity of care is beyond the capabilities of one student (deTornyay & Thompson, 1987). Because students must work closely together to implement care, collaboration and communication between the students are requisites for effective use of this strategy. The following benefits can be derived from the use of the dual assignment strategy (Meisenhelder, 1987):

- An opportunity to further develop communication and time management skills
- Opportunities to evaluate and improve skills in organization
- Increased opportunities for faculty to assess the capabilities of each student and provide feedback
- Opportunities for collaboration
- Decreased number of patients for which the faculty member is responsible
- Decreased level of anxiety among students

When dual assignments are made, the faculty member has the responsibility of being certain that each student understands his or her specific responsibility. For 2-day clinical rotations, roles may be reversed on the second day of care (Gotschall & Thompson, 1990). Such reversal makes it possible for both students to provide direct care to the patient.

The strategy of multiple assignments is useful for beginning students and in cases when a limited number of patients are available. This strategy involves the assignment of three students per patient. Three roles are assumed: the doer, who provides the care; the information gatherer or researcher, who is responsible for obtaining information needed for the safe care of the patient; and the observer, who observes the student, the researcher, student–patient interactions, the responses of the patient to his or her care, and family members (VanDenBerg, 1976). This person also makes suggestions for improving care. As with dual assignment, the roles for each student must be clearly defined. Adequate time must be made available for collaboration and discussion among students.

The multiple assignment approach must meet learning objectives. Glanville's (1971) study to determine the effectiveness of this method as an approach to clinical teaching revealed similarity in the extent to which objectives were met and in the levels of achievement for students assigned to the multiple assignment approach and those assigned to the traditional method. VanDenBerg (1976) randomly assigned 22 first-year associate degree students to two groups, traditional and multiple assignments. Results showed that students assigned to the multiple assignment group demonstrated a significant increase in nursing knowledge compared with those assigned to the traditional group.

In light of the increasing complexity of learning environments and the instability of the patient census, consistent clinical assignments and multiple placement assignments were compared to determine learning outcomes (Adams, 2002). *Consistent* means students were assigned to a unit for a specific time frame or used more than one unit during the period. Quantitative measures revealed no difference in the two methods of clinical rotation. However, the perceptions of the benefit of consistent clinical assignments were positive.

In summary, faculty, staff, and students play a significant role in determining assignments. Assignments are made according to a number of factors, including course objectives, learner needs, skill level, complexity of the clinical environment, and patients' severity of illness. The assignments may be implemented as solo or multistudent experiences. Each has been considered beneficial in enhancing learning.

Clinical Conferences

Clinical conferences are group learning experiences that are an integral part of the clinical experience. The use of clinical conferences in nursing is common. Conferences can provide meaningful learning experiences and excellent opportunities for students to bridge the gap between theory and practice. Through conferences, students can develop critical thinking and clinical decision-making skills (Wink, 1995) and acquire confidence in their ability to express themselves with clarity and logic.

Types of Conferences

Two types of conferences, preclinical and postclinical, by nature are small group discussion periods that immediately precede or follow a clinical experience. Both provide opportunities for discussion. In preclinical conferences, students share information about upcoming experiences, ask questions, express concerns, and seek clarification about plans for care. Preclinical conferences also provide opportunities for faculty to correct student misconceptions, identify problem areas, assess student thinking, and identify students' readiness to implement care.

Postclinical conferences provide a forum in which students and faculty can discuss the clinical experiences, share information, analyze clinical situations, clarify relationships, identify problems, ventilate feelings, and develop support systems. As early as 1969, Matheney supported the use of clinical conferences for these purposes. The purposes of clinical conferences were later refined by others (Mitchell & Krainovich, 1982; Wolfe & O'Driscoll, 1979). A perusal of these purposes suggests that there is interaction between the teacher and the students, student to student, which both offers medium for learning and exchange and provides meaningful experience.

Student and Faculty Roles

Both students and faculty have specific roles in conferences. Students should be made aware of their role as active participants. As such, they should defend choices of care, clarify points of view, explore alternatives, and practice decision making (Carpenito & Duespohl, 1985). A student may also assume the role of group leader. Faculty serve as conference facilitators by doing the following:

- Being supportive and sharing information
- Being flexible yet keeping the discussion focused and moving in a meaningful way

- Encouraging participation and active involvement of all students by posing ideas and questions
- Providing feedback in a nonthreatening way
- Creating an environment that is conducive to discussion
- Assisting students in identifying relationships, patterns, and trends
- Facilitating group process

As conferences are facilitated, efforts should be made to ask higher-level questions. Higher-level questions assist students in applying knowledge to clinical situations (Wink, 1993). Conferences also provide opportunities for students to apply group process and develop team-building skills.

Planning for Clinical Conferences

Successful clinical conferences are planned. Matheney (1969) asserts that conferences should not be free-wheeling, spur-of-the-moment, and ad-libbing sessions. Plans for conferences should take into consideration the curriculum and the learner. An identification of the purpose, topic, process, strategies, and methods of evaluation are essential if the teacher is to be instrumental in bridging the gap between theory and clinical practice. As a result of advancing technology, conferences may take place through electronic media (DeBourgh, 2001).

Evaluating the Conference

The conference should be evaluated in light of its effectiveness. The teacher should obtain and provide feedback regarding the extent to which goals were accomplished, the effectiveness of the method(s) or strategies, and the degree of learning achieved. The data from the evaluation can be used for planning future conferences.

In summary, both preclinical and postclinical conferences play a significant role in facilitating the learning of students. Conferences afford opportunities for enhancing critical thinking and decision-making skills, as well as group process and team skills. Successful conferences are planned. Inherent in planning is identifying the purpose, selecting topics, selecting teaching methods, and conducting and evaluating the conference.

Nursing Rounds

The practice of nursing rounds is a teaching strategy that uses the patient's bedside for direct, purposeful experiences. These experiences may involve demonstration, interview, or discussion of patient problems and nursing care. Rounds also afford an excellent opportunity for the exchange of ideas about patient care situations. Rounds may involve clinical faculty, students, and staff. Often, they are directed by the faculty. However, the responsibility for the rounds may rest with either students or staff.

The use of rounds as a teaching strategy requires planning. Planning includes obtaining permission from the patient and providing information about the nature of the round and the role the patient is to play. After the session, patient participation should be acknowledged.

Written Assignments

Written assignments generally complement clinical experiences. Written assignments are considered to be useful in that they facilitate development of critical thinking, organize thinking, and promote understanding of content (Allen et al., 1989). Such assignments may include short papers, nursing care plans, clinical logs, journals (Williams & Wold, 1996), and concept maps. Findings from research on the use of clinical logs indicate that their use provides opportunities for students to reflect on clinical experiences, communicate with the teacher, identify mistakes and negative experiences, and learn from these experiences (Sedlak, 1992).

Electronic technology is increasingly being used to support clinical teaching. For example, Web-based clinical courses have been designed to assist faculty with facilitating the development of clinical knowledge among students (DeBourgh, 2001). Technology has been used to integrate content such as communication, collaboration, coaching, and cognitive apprenticeship strategies. Several advantages have been identified. Online discussions promote peer support, idea sharing, and clarification of concepts. E-journals and e-boards support reflection in that students have opportunities to make inquiries about performance, thoughts, feelings, and experiences. Faculty can identify learning needs, misconceptions, and faulty patterns.

MODELS OF CLINICAL TEACHING

Several models of clinical teaching are being used to educate nursing students. These models, alternatives to the traditional model, include preceptorship, the clinical teaching associate model, the paired model, clinical teaching partnership, and adjunct faculty joint appointments. Given the diversity of health care settings, faculty shortage, and the need for reduced faculty/student ratios, these models serve to enhance effective student learning, facilitate development of clinical skills, and promote role development.

Preceptorship

Preceptorship is a teaching model in which the student is assigned a preceptor. Preceptors, as described by Armitage and Burnard (1991), are experienced nurses who facilitate and evaluate student learning in the clinical area over a specified amount of time. Their role is implemented in conjunction with other responsibilities. The preceptor model is based on the assumption that a consistent one-on-one relationship provides opportunities for socialization into practice and bridges the gap between theory and practice (Kersbergen & Hrobsky, 1996). Preceptors are useful for students-at all levels. However, they are considered to be particularly useful for senior-level students (Kersbergen & Hrobsky, 1996; O'Mara & Welton, 1995) and graduate students in advanced practice roles.

Theoretically, the preceptor provides one-on-one teaching, guidance, and support and serves as a role model. In one model (Billings et al., 2002), the preceptor, faculty, and student form a triad to facilitate the student's acquisition of clinical competencies. The preceptor is selected jointly by the student and the faculty, on the basis of the student's self-identified learning needs. The preceptor and student meet before the clinical experience and discuss learning styles, the student's current competency attainment, and the desired outcome of the clinical experience. Although the faculty member has ultimate responsibility for the course and student learning outcomes, the student and preceptor are empowered to conduct formative and summative evaluation of the student's clinical performance.

Preceptors are expected to be clinical experts, be willing to teach, and be able to teach effectively (Wright, 2002). Benefits that have been derived from preceptorships include enhanced ability to apply theory to practice, improvement in psychomotor skills, increased self-confidence (Letizia & Jennrick, 1998), and improved socialization (Collins et al., 1993; Myrick & Awrey, 1988). Attributes of an effective preceptor are shown in Box 15-2.

In a preceptorship, the role of the nursing faculty is not lost. Preceptors and faculty work in a close relationship (Hsieh & Knowles, 1990). The faculty provide the link between practice and education. In providing this link, faculty monitor how well the students complete assignments and accomplish outcomes. Evaluation is a joint responsibility of faculty and preceptors.

The use of preceptors requires planning to ensure that they understand their role. This is facilitated through strategically planned orientation sessions. These sessions provide a forum for sharing information about the philosophy and theoretical base of preceptorship, expected outcomes, teaching strategies, and methods of evaluation. Formative and summative evaluations are made.

The literature documents projects that have been developed to prepare students and preceptors for the preceptorship experience (Trevitt et al., 2001). One reported project is a package that contains two self-paced learning modules, one for students and one for preceptors, and an accompanying video. The reported outcome was feeling more prepared for the experience.

Although preceptorships are widely used in nursing education, to date, empirical data to substantiate the effectiveness of the strategy are limited. Studies conducted by Olson et al. (1984) and Myrick (1988) included control and experimental groups to determine whether clinical preceptorships would enhance students' perception of competence. The results of both studies indicated no differences in the performance of students assigned to a preceptor

---

Box 15-2
ATTRIBUTES OF AN EFFECTIVE PRECEPTOR

1. Knowledge of the patient care area
2. Effective communication skills (verbal and nonverbal)
3. Experience in a particular clinical area
4. Ability to relate to health care personnel and client
5. Honesty
6. Effective decision-making skills
7. Genuine caring behaviors
8. Leadership skills
9. Interest in professional development

Used with permission from Lewis, K. E. (1986). What it takes to be a preceptor. *The Canadian Nurse/L'infirmière canadienne, 82*(11), December 1986, 18-19.

and those who did not have a preceptor. The findings are congruent with findings of others (Marchette, 1984). These findings are in contrast to results of studies conducted by Scheetz (1989) and Myrick and Awrey (1988), who reported students', faculty, and preceptors' testimonial documentation of how preceptorships enhance student performance. Student evaluations describe preceptorships as being valuable. The value is generally related to providing a sense of independence for patient care and promotion of a sense of satisfaction. Satisfaction from the perspective of clinical faculty has been reported as positive (Zerbe & Lachat, 1991).

Clinical Teaching Associate

The clinical teaching associate (CTA) model involves a staff nurse who collaborates with a designated faculty member and instructs a specified number of students in the clinical area (Baird et al., 1994; Phillips & Kaempfer, 1987; DeVoogd & Salbenblatt, 1989). Teaching responsibilities are assumed by the CTA, who also serves as a resource person and role model. A faculty member serves as lead teacher and has responsibilities for supervision and evaluation of clinical learning experiences, including assignment of grades and collaboration with the CTA about assignments and experiences.

Results from a survey of nurse managers, CTAs, faculty, and students, conducted to determine the effectiveness of this model, were positive (Baird et al., 1994). Positive comments were presented in terms of student learning, patient satisfaction, and benefits to teaching associates and faculty. The quality of patient care and patients' satisfaction with care were reported to be greater than with the traditional model. Nurses in the CTA role reported an increase in confidence. Faculty reported that students were more relaxed and more self-confident. Students related effectiveness to being able to assume increased responsibility compared with the traditional model. Overall scores for CTAs were higher in several areas. Reports from Phillips and Kaempfer (1987) were also positive.

Paired Model

The paired model is designed to pair a student and a staff nurse for a clinical day. It is an alternative to the one-patient, one-student model and is a variation of the preceptor model (Gross et al., 1992). During the course, each student has a specified number of days in a paired relationship. The remainder of the time is spent acquiring experiences by using the traditional model. The staff nurse plans the learning assignments. The faculty member oversees the clinical experiences and creates a learning environment for students. However, most of the faculty member's time is spent in the traditional role with other students who have not been paired. A nurse manager evaluates the staffing pattern and determines the number of students that can be paired during a clinical day.

The paired model has been viewed positively by students, faculty, and staff nurses in the service area. Earlier interaction, a sense of belonging in the clinical environment, feelings of being less anxious, and enhanced learning were mentioned by students as positive aspects of the model. The reasons for these positive outcomes were related to students being more comfortable in the clinical setting (Gross et al., 1992). Faculty were more effective as teachers. Staff nurses reported being challenged to think. Overall, the relationship between education and service was reported to be strengthened.

Clinical Teaching Partnership

The clinical teaching partnership is a collaborative model shared by the service setting and academic setting. Both institutions share a clinical nurse specialist (CNS) and a university faculty member (Shah & Pennypacker, 1992). The CNS serves as an adjunct faculty member who provides client assignments. The academic faculty member provides scheduling as determined by a given course. The faculty member and CNS collaborate in grading written assignments and in evaluating students, and both provide input into grade assignment.

Communication is reciprocal and essential to the success of this model. The faculty member shares information about problems that may influence the performance of students. The CNS keeps the faculty abreast of current student performance. The faculty member and CNS schedule conferences to discuss anecdotal records of students.

Shah and Pennypacker (1992) have identified benefits of the model to the faculty and to the CNS. Benefits for the academic faculty are (1) increased time to pursue scholarly activities and (2) a direct link with clinical staff for purposes of communication about policy procedural changes and new equipment. Benefits for the CNS include (1) joint involvement with academic and clinical settings, (2) direct avenues for collaborative projects such as writing and publication, (3) increased involvement in staff development, and (4) satisfaction in observing student development.

Informal feedback from students about this model was positive. Reports indicate that students learned several roles assumed by nurses and different ways of performing clinical skills and that students' ability to transfer theory learned in the classroom to clinical practice was enhanced. A study conducted by Jackson (1986) showed that students who were taught by faculty involved in clinical practice scored higher in three areas: (1) integration of theory into practice, (2) realistic perception of the work environment, and (3) use of nursing research. In addition, a higher degree of autonomy, greater self-concept and self-esteem, and enhanced professional and bicultural role behavior were reported.

Adjunct Faculty

Adjunct faculty are health care professionals who are employed in the service setting and also have a part-time academic appointment. Adjunct faculty may assume various roles, including those of preceptor, mentor, guest lecturer, and supervisor. These individuals may also collaborate on research projects. Faculty who are appointed in an adjunct capacity are RNs or professionals who are experts in areas such as clinical practice, research leadership, management, legislation, and law.

In summary, several models for clinical education of student nurses exist. Alternative models, collaborative in nature, have evolved because of changes in the complexity of health care. Among these models are preceptorships, the teaching associate model, the paired model, clinical teaching partnerships, and adjunct faculty. The nature of each model dictates the level of student that would benefit most. The paired and the clinical associate models have been used for beginning students, whereas the preceptorship model is widely used for students in the upper level of their program and graduate students. Empirical research on the effectiveness of these models has been sparse. There is a dire need for increased research on these models in terms of their effectiveness on student learning.

SUMMARY

Clinical teaching involves student–teacher interaction in experiential clinical situations that take place in diverse and often interdisciplinary practice settings. These settings may include acute care settings; transitional settings; and community sites including homeless shelters, clinics, schools, camps, and social service agencies. Faculty must have in-depth knowledge of behaviors that facilitate students' learning and development and have complete knowledge of the practice area and the health care providers. Effective clinical teachers are able to plan, facilitate, and evaluate experiences using instructive, evaluative, and interpersonal strategies. These strategies facilitate students' acquisition of the skills they need to become nurses.

A variety of teaching methods can be used to enable students to achieve desired outcomes. Patient assignments, clinical conferences, nursing rounds, and written assignments are among these. The skill level of students, patients' severity of illness, number of students, and patient care resource availability will affect the method used. Among the models suggested for educating nursing students are the traditional model and alternatives to this model, including preceptorships, the clinical teaching associate model, teaching partnerships, and adjunct faculty. Planning and ongoing contact with preceptors and agency personnel in the clinical setting are crucial to the success of any clinical experience. Clinical experiences prepare students for working in a health care system that is patient centered. Teaching in the clinical setting blends faculty's clinical expertise with teaching skills to prepare nurses for current and future roles in an ever-changing health care system.

REFERENCES

Adams, V. (2002). Consistent clinical assignment for nursing students compared to multiple placements. *Journal of Nursing Education, 41*(2), 80-85.

Allen, D., Bowers, B., & Dickelmann, N. (1989). Writing to learn: A reconceptualization of thinking and writing in the nursing curriculum. *Journal of Nursing Education, 28*, 6-11.

American Association of Colleges of Nursing. (1996). *Position statement: Interdisciplinary education and practice.* Washington, DC: Author.

Baird, S., Bopp, A., Schofer, K., Langenberg, A., & Matheis-Kraft, C. (1994). An innovative model for clinical teaching. *Nurse Educator, 19*(3), 23-25.

Bellack, J. (1995). Educating for the community. *Journal of Nursing Education, 34*(8), 342-343.

Billings, D. M., Jeffries, P., Rowles, C. J., Stone, C., & Urden, L. (2002). A partnership model of nursing education to prepare critical care nurses. *Excellence in Clinical Practice, 3*, 3.

Brophy, J., & Good, T. L. (1986). Teacher behavior and student achievement. In M. C. Wittrock (Ed.), *Handbook of research on teaching* (3rd ed). New York: Macmillan.

Broscious, S., & Sanders, H. (2001). Peer coaching. *Nurse Educator, 26*(5), 212-214.

Buttriss, C., Kuper, R., & Newbold, B. (1995). The use of a homeless shelter as a clinical rotation for nursing students. *Journal of Nursing Education, 34*(8), 375-377.

Carpenito, L., & Duespohl, T. (1985). *A guide for effective clinical instruction.* Gaithersburg, MD: Aspen.

Chan, D. (2002). Development of the clinical learning environment inventory: Using theoretical framework of learning environment studies to access nursing students perceptions of the hospital as a learning environment. *Journal of Nursing Education, 41*(2), 69-75.

Collins, P., Hilde, E., & Shriver, C. (1993). A five-year evaluation of BSN students in a nursing management preceptorship. *Journal of Nursing Education, 32*, 330-332.

Cook, S. S., & Drusin, R. E. (1995). Revisiting interdisciplinary education: One way to build an ark. *Nursing & Health Care: Perspectives on Community, 16*(5), 200-265.

DeBourgh, G. A. (2001). Using Web technology in a clinical nursing course. *Nurse Educator, 26*(5), 227-233.

deTornyay, R., & Thompson, M. (1987). *Strategies for teaching nursing.* New York: John Wiley.

DeVoogd, R., & Salbenblatt, C. (1989). The clinical teaching associate model: Advantages and disadvantages in practice. *Journal of Nursing Education, 28*(6), 276-277.

Dunn, S., Burnett, P. (1995). The development of a clinical learning environment scale. *Journal of Advanced Nursing, 22*, 1116-1173.

Dunn, S. V., Stockhausen, L., Thornton, R., & Barnard, A. (1995). The relationship between clinical education format and selected student learning outcomes. *Journal of Nursing Education, 34*(1), 16-24.

Elfrink, V. (1996). The nightingale tracker. *Computers in Nursing, 14*(2), 82-83, 88.

Elliott, M. (2002). The clinical environment: A source of stress for undergraduate nurses. *Australian Journal of Advanced Nursing, 20*(1), 34-38.

Erkel, E. A., Nivens, A. S., & Kennedy, D. E. (1995). Intensive immersion of nursing students in rural interdisciplinary care. *Journal of Nursing Education, 34*(8), 359-365.

Faller, H. S., McDowell, M. A., & Jackson, M. A. (1995). Bridge to the future: Nontraditional settings and concepts. *Journal of Nursing Education, 34*(8), 344-349.

Fothergill-Bourbonnais, F., & Higuchi, K. S. (1995). Selecting clinical experiences: An analysis of the factors involved. *Journal of Nursing Education, 34*(1), 37-41.

Frieburger, O. A. (1996). A collaborative approach to team building between staff and students in long-term care. *Nurse Educator, 21*(6), 7-12.

Fugate, T., & Rebeschi, L. (1991). Dual assignment: An alternative clinical teaching strategy. *Nurse Educator, 15*(6), 14-16.

Gaines, S. K. (1996). Clinical experiences in day care settings. *Nurse Educator, 21*(4), 23-27.

Glanville, C. (1971). Multiple student assignment as an approach to clinical teaching in pediatric nursing. *Nursing Research, 20*(3), 237-244.

Goldenberg, D., & Iwasiw, C. (1988). Criteria used for patient selection for student nurses' hospital clinical experience. *Journal of Nursing Education, 27*(6), 258-265.

Gotschall, L., & Thompson, C. (1990). Dual assignments: An effective clinical teaching strategy. *Nurse Educator, 15*(6), 6.

Gross, J., Aysee, P., & Tracey, P. (1992). A creative clinical education model. *Three Views, 41*(4), 156-159.

Halstead, J. A. (1996). The significance of student-faculty interactions. In K. R. Stevens (Ed.), *Review of research in nursing education* (Vol. VII). New York: National League for Nursing Press.

Horst, M. (1988). Students rank characteristics of the clinical teacher. *Nurse Educator, 13*(6), 3.

Hsieh, N., & Knowles, D. (1990). Instructor facilitation of the preceptorship relationship in nursing education. *Journal of Nursing Education, 29*(6), 262-268.

Jackson, N. (1986). Part-time faculty suggestions for policy. *Nursing Education, 13*(1), 36-40.

Karuhije, HF. (1997). Classroom and clinical teaching in nursing: Delineating differences. *Nursing Forum, 32*(2), 5-12.

Kersbergen, A. L., & Hrobsky, P. E. (1996). Use of clinical maps in precepted clinical experiences. *Nurse Educator, 21*(6), 19-22.

Kleehammer, K., Hart, A. L., & Keck, J. F. (1990). Nursing students' perception of anxiety-producing situations in the clinical setting. *Journal of Nursing Education, 29*(4), 183-187.

Knox, J., & Morgan, J. (1985). Important clinical teacher behaviors as perceived by university nursing faculty, students, and graduates. *Journal of Advanced Nursing, 10*, 25-30.

Krichbaum, K. (1994). Clinical teaching effectiveness described in relation to learning outcomes of baccalaureate nursing students. *Journal of Nursing Education, 33*(7), 306-315.

Larson, E. L. (1995). New rules for the game: Interdisciplinary education for health professionals. *Nursing Outlook, 43*, 180-185.

Letizia, M., & Jennrich, J. (1998). A review of preceptorship in undergraduate nursing education: Implication for staff development. *Journal of Continuing Education in Nursing, 29*(5), 211-216.

Lewis, K. (1986). What it takes to be a preceptor. *The Canadian Nurse, 82*(11), 18-19.

Lo, R. (2002). A longitudinal study of perceived level of stress, coping and self-esteem of undergraduate nursing students: An Australian case study. *Journal of Advanced Nursing, 39*(2), 119-126.

Lough, M. A., Schmidt, K., Swain, G. R., Naughton, T. M., Leshan, L. A., Blackburn, J.A., et al. (1996). An interdisciplinary model for health professions students in a family practice center. *Nurse Educator, 21*(1), 27-31.

Marchette, L. (1984). The effect of a nurse internship program on novice nurses' self-evaluation of clinical performance. *Journal of Nursing Administration, 15*(5), 6-7.

Massarweh, L. (1999). Promoting a positive clinical experience. *Nursing Educator, 24*(3), 44-47.

McCabe, B. (1985). The improvement of instruction in the clinical area: A challenge waiting to be met. *Journal of Nursing Education, 24*, 255-257.

McCoin, D., & Jenkins, P. (1988). Methods of assignment for preplanning activities (advance student preparation) for clinical experience. *Journal of Nursing Education, 27*, 85-87.

McDaniel, A. M., & Robertson, K. E. (1997). Teaching collaboration skills to baccalaureate nursing students: An interdisciplinary teaching project. *Journal of Nursing Education, 36*(6), 271-273.

Meisenhelder, J. B. (1987). Anxiety: A block to clinical teaching. *Nurse Educator, 12*(6), 27-30.

Meleca, C., Schimpfhauser, F., Witteman, J., & Sachs, L. (1981). Clinical instruction in a national survey. *Journal of Nursing Education, 20*, 32-40.

Matheney, R. (1969). Pre- and post-conferences for students. *American Journal of Nursing, 69*(2), 286-289.

Mitchell, C., & Krainovich, B. (1982). Conducting pre- and post-clinical conferences. *American Journal of Nursing, 82*, 823-825.

Morgan, J., & Knox, J. (1987). Characteristics of "best" and "worst" clinical teachers as perceived by university nursing faculty and students. *Journal of Advanced Nursing, 12*, 331-337.

Myrick, F. (1988). Preceptorship: A viable alternative clinical teaching strategy? *Journal of Advanced Nursing, 13*, 588-591.

Myrick, F., & Awrey, J. (1988). The effect of preceptorship on the clinical competency of baccalaureate student nurses. *Canadian Journal of Nursing Research, 20*(3), 29-33.

Nehring, V. (1990). Nursing and clinical teacher effectiveness inventory: A replication study of the characteristics of the best and worst clinical teachers as perceived by nursing faculty and students. *Journal of Advanced Nursing, 15*, 934-940.

Oermann, M. H. (1996). Research on teaching in the clinical setting. In K. R. Stevens (Ed.), *Review of research in nursing education* (Vol. VII, pp. 91-126). New York: National League for Nursing.

Oesterle, M., & O'Callaghan, D. (1996). The changing health care environment. *Nursing & Health Care: Perspectives on Community, 17*(2), 78-81.

Olson, R., Gresley, R., & Healer, B. (1984). The effect of an undergraduate clinical internship on the self-concept and role mastery of baccalaureate nursing students. *Journal of Nursing Education, 23*(3), 105-108.

O'Mara, A., & Welton, R. (1995). Rewarding staff nurse preceptors. *Journal of Nursing Administration, 25*, 64-67.

O'Shea, H., & Parsons, M. (1979). Clinical instructions: Effective and ineffective teacher behaviors. *Nursing Outlook, 27*, 411-415.

Pardo, D. (1991). *The culture of clinical teaching.* Michigan, UMI Dissertation Abstracts International, Vol. No. (B52 4), page No. (UMI No. AAT 9125450).

Peters, R. (1995). Teaching population-focused practice to baccalaureate nursing students. *Journal of Nursing Education, 34*(8), 378-383.

Phillips, S., & Kaempfer, S. (1987). Clinical teaching associate model: Implementation in a community hospital setting. *Journal of Professional Nursing, 3*(3), 165-175.

Piscopo, B. (1994). Organizational climate, communication, and role strain in clinical nursing faculty. *Journal of Professional Nursing, 10*(2), 113-119.

Pond, E. (1995). Student-selected clinical experiences. In B. Fuzard (Ed.), *Innovative teaching strategies in nursing.* Gaithersburg, MD: Aspen.

Porter, K., & Feller, C. (1979). The relationship between patterns of massed and distributed clinical practicum and student achievement. *Journal of Nursing Education, 18*, 27-34.

Pugh, E. (1988). Soliciting student input to improve clinical teaching. *Nurse Educator, 13*(5), 28-33.

Reilly, D., & Oermann, M. (1992). *Clinical teaching education* (2nd ed.). New York: National League for Nursing.

Rosenshine, B., & Stevens, R. (1986). Teaching functions. In M. C. Wittrock (Ed.), *Handbook of research in teaching* (3rd ed., pp. 376-391). New York: Macmillan.

Scheetz, L. (1989). Baccalaureate nursing student preceptorship programs and the development of clinical competence. *Journal of Nursing Education, 28*, 30-35.

Schim, S., & Scher, K. (2002). Worksite "lunch and learn": A collaborative teaching project. *Journal of Nursing Education, 41*(12), 541-543.

Schuster, P., Fitzgerald, D. A., McCarthy, P., & McDougal, D. (1997). Work load issues in clinical nursing education. *Journal of Professional Nursing, 13*, 154-159.

Sedlak, C. (1992). Use of beginning logs by beginning students and faculty to identify student learning needs. *Journal of Nursing Education, 31*, 24-27.

Shah, H., & Pennypacker, D. (1992). The clinical teaching partnership. *Nurse Educator, 17*(2), 10-12.

Sieh, J., & Bell, S. (1994). Perceptions of effective clinical teachers in associate degree programs. *Journal of Nursing Education, 33*(9), 389-394.

Simandl, G. (1996). Nursing students working with the homeless. *Nurse Educator, 21*(2), 18-22.

Smith, M., Barton, J., & Baxter, J. (1996). An innovative interdisciplinary educational experience in field research. *Nurse Educator, 21*(2), 27-30.

Stuebbe, B. (1990). Student and faculty perspectives in the role of a nursing instructor. *Journal of Nursing Education, 19*, 4-9.

Sullivan, E. (1995). A revolution in the making. *Journal of Professional Nursing, 11*(3), 137.

Tanner, C. (2002). Clinical education, circa 2010. *Journal of Nursing Education, 41*, 51-52

Timmins, F., Kaliszer, M. (2002). Aspects of education programmes that frequently cause stress to nursing students—Fact-finding sample survey. *Nursing Education Today, 22*, 203-211.

Totten, J. K., Fonnesbeck, B. (2002). Camp communities: Valuable clinical options for BSN students. *Journal of Nursing Education, 41*(2), 83-85.

Trevitt, C., Graslish, L., & Reaby, L. (2001). Students in transit: Using a self-directed preceptorship pack to smooth the journey. *Journal of Nursing Education, 40*(5), 25-28.

VanDenBerg, E. (1976). The multiple assignment: An effective alternative for laboratory experiences. *Journal of Nursing Education, 15*(3), 3-12.

Vinten, S., Kost, G., & Chalko, B. (2003, September). *Orienting the clinical educator: Developing faculty competencies.* Paper presented at the conference of the National League for Nursing, San Antonio, TX.

Watson, J. (1996). From discipline specific to "infer" to "multi" to "transdisciplinary" health care education and practice. *Nursing & Health Care: Perspectives on Community, 17*(2), 90-91.

Weinholtz, D., & Ostmoe, P. (1987). Selecting clinical teaching strategies. In H. Van Hoozer et al. (Eds.), *The teaching process theory and practice in nursing* (pp. 173-210). Norwalk, CT: Appleton-Century-Crofts.

Williams, A., & Wold, J. L. (1996). Healthcare for the future: Caring for populations in alternative settings. *Nurse Educator, 21*(2), 23-26.

Williams, J. (2001). The clinical notebook: Using student portfolios to enhance clinical teaching learning. *Journal of Nursing Education, 40*, 135-137.

Wink, D. (1993). Using questioning as a teaching strategy. *Nurse Educator, 18*, 11-15.

Wink, D. (1995). The effective clinical conference. *Nursing Outlook, 43*, 29-32.

Wolfe, Z., & O'Driscoll, R. (1979). How useful is the pre-clinical conference? *Nursing Outlook, 27*, 455-457.

Wong, J., & Wong, S. (1987). Towards effective clinical teaching in nursing. *Journal of Advanced Nursing, 12,* 505-513.

Wright, A. (2002). Preceptoring in 2002. *Journal of Continuing Education in Nursing, 33*(3), 138-141.

Zerbe, M., & Lachat, M. (1991). A three-tiered team model for undergraduate preceptor programs. *Nurse Educator, 16*(2), 18-21.

UNIT IV

TEACHING, LEARNING, AND INFORMATION RESOURCES

16

THE LEARNING RESOURCE CENTER

Kay E. Hodson-Carlton, EdD, RN, FAAN,
Pamela J. Worrell-Carlisle, PhD, RN

The Learning Resource Center (LRC) of today is a central hub of instructional activity for students, faculty, and professionals. The historic use of the LRC as a practice center for the knowledge acquisition and practice of nursing skills before performance of procedures in the health care setting is still a primary focus, but the contemporary LRC now serves as an exemplary multifunctional teaching and learning center. The intent of this chapter is to describe the LRC functions, instructional issues research, expanded LRC functions, and introduce management and operational issues for the administration of an LRC.

THE LEARNING RESOURCES CENTER: FUNCTIONS

Functions of the LRC, as well as its designation, vary widely from institution to institution. *Learning Resource Center* or *Learning Resources Center* is frequently used as the broad term for this teaching/learning support facility. Other examples of terms used to designate either the multifunctional facility or the associated clinical practice environment include *Center for Teaching and Lifelong Learning, Educational Resources, Office of Learning Technologies, Patient Safety Simulation Laboratory, Clinical Resource Center* or *Lab, Clinical Simulation Lab, Nursing Lab,* and *Nursing Skills Laboratory* (Childs, 2002; Nelson, 2003; Redford & Klein, 2003). Regardless of the specific name of this instructional facility, a multitude of teaching and learning activities remain the primary goals of the LRC.

The LRC facility is typically conceptualized as a multimedia environment where learners use visual, auditory, kinesthetic, and tactile abilities for the acquisition of cognitive, affective, and psychomotor skills for lifelong and multidisciplinary collaborative learning. The LRC can be a place for low-stress learning, role modeling, decision making and critical thinking, independent and group study, and all levels of multimedia instruction and evaluation. Students in fundamental clinical courses, as well as students preparing for advanced practice roles, are served by the LRC. In addition, enhanced functions of some LRCs around the country may include some or all of the following:

- Operation of multimedia and computer laboratories
- Technology support for nursing and/or associated health care discipline users of the facility
- Multimedia design, development, and production
- Faculty development and consultation support for teaching and learning activities
- Coordination of distance learning for nursing and/or associated programs
- Nursing clinical practice
- Continuing and lifelong education

Teaching and Learning in the Learning Resource Center

Nursing Skill Instruction

It is not by chance that nursing skill development and medication administration are essential teaching and learning foci of almost all LRC units. The Joint Commission on Accreditation of Healthcare Organizations (cited in Koerner, 2003) claims that inadequate training or orientation is the cause of threats to patient safety in 87% of cases. Medication administration and equipment use errors top the list of safety violations. Thousands of cases of injury or death occur annually, and one half of the errors are related to medication administration, with 62% of the medication errors involving intravenous (IV) pumps. Preparation of competent caregivers is a critical role of nursing education.

Changes in the health care environment affect faculty capacity to prepare students adequately. First, as the severity of illness of hospitalized and home health care patients increases, students in clinical practice are confronted with providing more complex nursing care earlier in and throughout their undergraduate program experience. The traditional debate over whether it is ethical to teach students psychomotor skills in the practice setting or in the simulation laboratory is complicated by increased severity of illness. Second, increased dependence on technology (e.g., medical equipment) requires that students and staff be trained to use a greater variety of equipment. Manufacturers' updates of the equipment dictate the need for frequent retraining. Also, the increasing use of computerized systems for care and medication documentation adds to the complexity of clinical experiences. Third, turnover in staff, use of registry personnel, floating among assigned units, and a shortage of RNs with extensive clinical experience can decrease the availability of competent preceptors for student nurses. The academic institution's role in teaching nursing skills has never been more salient than in today's dynamic health care milieu.

The debate on how to best teach psychomotor skills to undergraduates has been a part of nursing education for many decades (Corcoran, 1977; Olsen, 1999; Stern, 1988). Implementation of the nursing process requires competency in a complex set of cognitive, social-emotional, and psychomotor skills. Psychomotor skill acquisition is now understood as a multidimensional learning event, yet evidence-based practice in this area is rudimentary.

The role of the LRC in nursing skill instruction has traditionally been to provide a setting in which students can observe and practice in a simulated environment. The goals of instruction are to decrease anxiety and increase knowledge and skill through use of a simulated patient encounter before students have contact with patients in clinical practice. Teaching nursing skills in the LRC encompasses several issues, which are summarized in Box 16-1.

Defining and Identifying Essential Nursing Skills

Defining psychomotor skills and identifying the essential skills to be taught in the undergraduate curriculum have been examined by several authors. Oermann (1990) delineates three types of psychomotor skills: fine, manual, and gross. Fine motor skills are used for tasks that require precision. Manual skills are used in tasks requiring manipulation and possible repetition. Gross motor skills involve the large muscle groups and require more movement. Alavi et al. (1991) categorize skills as fundamental, general therapeutic and diagnostic, and specialized therapeutic and diagnostic (Table 16-1). Fifty-nine faculty members generated the categories according to frequency of use of the skill and availability of opportunities to practice the skill. This suggests that psychomotor skills are hierarchical and that task analysis and leveling of skills may be beneficial instructional strategies. In addition, incorporating this hierarchical analysis and leveling into research when teaching strategies are compared would strengthen the design. For example, the best instructional strategy for teaching a task that requires fine and manual motor skills, such as tracheostomy care, might differ from the preferred teaching strategy for wheelchair to bed transfer.

Many psychomotor skills are involved in delivering nursing care (Alavi et al., 1991; Sweeney et al., 1982; Sweeney et al., 1980), and the identification of "essential" skills has proven to be controversial. It is common to consult with staff in the practice setting to determine current skill sets in high demand, yet Olsen's literature review (1999) indicates that academia and the service sector differ in perceptions of essential skills. In addition, Sweeney et al. (1982) report that faculty often do not agree with each other on which skills are a priority for teaching. One explanation for such a discrepancy may be curriculum differences among the diploma and associate and baccalaureate degree programs. Authors who looked at these differences during the 1980s found

---

Box 16-1
ISSUES IN NURSING SKILL INSTRUCTION

- Defining and Identifying Essential Nursing Skills
- Implementing Instructional Strategies and Evaluation
  Competency Levels
  Integrating Learning Domains
  Simulations
  Traditional Faculty Role or Self-Directed, Technology-Enhanced Model
  Student Preferences and Satisfaction
- Identifying Conceptual and Theoretical Frameworks for Instructional Design

TABLE 16-1	Psychomotor Skill Categorization Scheme	
FUNDAMENTAL	**GENERAL THERAPEUTIC & DIAGNOSTIC**	**SPECIALIZED THERAPEUTIC & DIAGNOSTIC**
Mobilization	Inspection	Oxygen therapy
Range of motion	Auscultation of bowel, breath, and	Oropharyngeal suction
Body mechanics	heart sounds	Tracheostomy suction
Lifting	Palpation	Stoma therapy
Showering	Percussion	Nasogastric tube
Bed-bathing	Ear/nose/throat assessment	Eye toilets
Mouth care	Neurological assessment	Eye irrigation and drops
Hair care	Integrated physical assessment	Nose drops
Positioning	Specimen collection	Orthopedic applications
Pressure area care	Medication administration	Baby bath
Handwashing	Bandage application	Assessment of neonatal
Bed making	Surgical asepsis	and child development
Feeding	Wound drainage	CVP measurement
Assisting with	Removal of sutures/staples	Intercostal catheter care
bedpan/urinal/commode	IV therapy	CPR
Assessment of	Isolation technique	
TPR & BP	Catheterization	
Height and weight	Urinalysis	
measurement	Cleansing enema	
	Suppositories	
	Hot and cold application	

Modified from Alavi, C., Loh, S. H., & Reilly D. (1991). Reality basis for teaching psychomotor skills in a tertiary nursing curriculum. *Journal of Advanced Nursing, 16*(8), 957-965.
BP, Blood pressure; *CPR,* cardiopulmonary resuscitation; *CVP,* central venous pressure; *TPR,* temperature, pulse, and respiration.

that baccalaureate programs incorporated critical thinking, technology, theory, communication, research, individualized care, and the liberal arts core but gave less priority to basic psychomotor skills (Olsen, 1999). Faculty assigned to teach psychomotor skills perceive that their colleagues do not value this skill instruction within the baccalaureate curriculum (Minnesota Baccalaureate Psychomotor Skills Faculty Group, 1998). The educational preparation of respondents should be considered in studies comparing differences between service and academia. An alternative explanation for the discrepancy is that with the dynamic infusion of technology into health care and increased levels of illness severity, the nursing program needs to more closely align skill instruction with the service setting.

Implementing Instructional Strategies and Student Evaluation

Competency Levels. Another consideration in teaching psychomotor skills is competency level (Benner, 1984; Hallal & Welsh, 1984; Olsen, 1999). A checklist is typically used by faculty to evaluate competency before the student's performance of the skill at a health care facility. Traditionally, checklists have also been used to increase interrater reliability of evaluators and to communicate expectations to students. The checklists can also be retained by students as personal performance critiques; examples might be placed in students' portfolios (Ryan & Hodson-Carlton, 1997).

Checklist items are generally derived from nursing textbooks and health care agency procedure manuals. When checklists are generated from various sources, the potential for discrepancy between service and educational settings is introduced. Variability in checklist design can compromise measurement of competency. In addition, the degree of detail of critical behaviors may vary from checklist to checklist. Mooney (1993) suggests that detailed checklists become overwhelming to students who are at the novice level of performance, but others may argue for a detailed task analysis.

Instead of expecting optimal mastery of a skill at the beginning of a nursing education program, skill checklists could be designed to measure levels of competency (Alavi et al., 1991). Leveling competencies might also reduce the effect of stress and anxiety on motor and cognitive performance because students would gain confidence and experience during their undergraduate program. One approach in the literature is Dave's taxonomy (1970), a system for categorizing behaviors that involve neuromuscular coordination. The five levels of skill are imitation, manipulation, precision, articulation, and naturalization. Alavi et al. (1991) have used this framework for leveling psychomotor skills. Students are expected to perform at the precision or articulation levels before performing the skill in the clinical setting.

Integrating Learning Domains. For the past few decades, many (Bolton, 1984; Doheny, 1993; Gomez & Gomez, 1984; Hodson et al., 1985; Smith, 1992) have advocated rethinking effective teaching strategies for psychomotor skills. Oermann (1990) suggests that a psychomotor skill initially be broken down and the conceptual aspects be taught separately from the motor processes. However, psychomotor skills are not performed apart from the affective and cognitive components in patient care, and at some point, students must have an integrated learning experience that simulates the clinical experience. For example, maintaining sterile technique while changing a dressing is a basic skill that requires demonstration of a minimal level of competence for the safety of the patient. However, the complexity of dressing changes varies. In addition, being able to communicate effectively to ease a patient's apprehension during a painful dressing change is an important skill. Changing dressings on a critically ill, ventilator-dependent patient with multiple trauma in an intensive care setting demands further competence. Eerden (2001) cites the National League for Nursing Accrediting Commission, Inc. (NLNAC) standard revisions and notes that the focus is on simulating the skills and critical thinking used in the clinical context. Eerden developed critical thinking vignettes for each of two to three skills courses in an associate degree program. For each vignette, students were graded on three to five psychomotor skills, communication, teaching, reading environmental cues, referral to community resources, collaboration, management concepts, and critical thinking. Students performed with faculty observing while they interacted with a standardized patient (SP) in the lab setting. This more comprehensive approach to integration and evaluation of psychomotor, cognitive, and affective domains is attainable in a simulated environment.

Simulations. Simulations are a common and increasingly important strategy used in the LRC to link multidimensional learning to practice and performance. Simulations can include the use of mannequins for the practice of psychomotor skills, entire sequence(s) of nursing clinical actions with computerized and virtual reality simulators, and human simulation with actors.

The use of mannequins and models in the LRC has a historical precedent, beginning in nursing education with "Mrs. Chase," the prototype mannequin first used in the 1950s (Herrmann, 1981). These "realia" and human actors role playing individuals with specific health conditions are used to simulate nursing procedures and health care situations and provide the learner with an opportunity to practice nursing skills in a controlled environment.

An entire range or continuum of simulations is available for nursing and health care education. Ziv et al.'s (2000) categories of simulation-based training provide a good framework for the discussion of integration of simulation in nursing skills and are described here. The categories include the following:

- Simple models or mannequins
- Simulated/standardized patients
- Computer screen–based clinical case simulators
- Realistic high-tech procedural simulators (task trainers)
- Virtual reality (VR)
- Realistic, high-tech interactive patient simulators (RPSs)

Simple models or mannequins are relatively low-tech, low-cost simulators used to teach basic cognitive knowledge or hands-on psychomotor skills. Examples of these models are the enema administration model, injection and IV arm(s), and abdominal suture models available from such companies as Armstrong Medical Industries, Inc. *(http://www.armstrongmedical.com)*, GAUMARD Scientific Company *(http://www.gaumard.com)*, Health Edco *(http://www.healthedco.com)*, Medical Plastics Laboratory, Inc. *(http://www.medicalplastics.com)*, and NASCO *(http://www.eNasco.com)*.

Simulated or standardized patients (SPs) are often used for training and assessment in history taking, physical examination, and communication skills. The use of SPs has been one of the most studied and frequently used simulation-based instructional tools in medical education since the 1960s (Barrows, 1993). Individuals are trained to play a scripted patient role for education and evaluation purposes (Ziv et al., 2000). Gibbons et al. (2002) describe one such successful use in nursing education. The use of SPs in a health assessment course for nurse practitioners and nurse anesthetists resulted in improved clinical evaluation and increased faculty and student satisfaction.

The use of computer screen–based clinical case simulators proliferated in the 1980s with the emergence of the personal computer in nursing programs. For example, Klaassens (1992) describes positive experiences with the use of computer-based simulations that allow students to practice problem solving in patient situations in a safe and nonthreatening environment. White (1995) reports that the use of computer-based patient simulations with the addition of interactive video enhanced the problem-based learning of students in a primary health care graduate nursing curriculum. The computer-based simulation with the interactive video component allows for the demonstration of nonverbal cues and allows the graduate nursing student to associate responses with the videotaped patient. Screen-based computer simulations continue to be available and are used for a wide variety of nursing clinical specialties. The media format has evolved from the computer disk of the early 1980s to CDs, DVDs, and the Internet.

Realistic high-tech procedural simulators (task trainers) are described by Ziv et al. (2000) as instructional tools that enhance static models with audio-visual, touch/feel interactive cues, and sophisticated computerized software. Examples used primarily for medical and advanced nursing education include the Harvey Cardiology Patient Simulator, which presents auscultatory and pulse findings of numerous cardiovascular conditions; an ultrasound system with a functional control panel, mock transducers, and a realistic patient-mannequin; and laparoscopic high-tech surgery task trainers.

VR is an evolving technology that uses "highly interactive computer simulations that sense the user's position and replace or augment the feedback of one or more senses—giving the feeling of being immersed, or being present in the simulation" (Sherman & Craig, 1995, p. 37). Simpson (2002) explains that there are two forms of VR: immersive and nonimmersive. In nonimmersive VR, a three-dimensional computer-generated image on a desktop computer system is used. Immersive VR systems usually require the user to "gear up" in a technology-linked helmet, hand-control device, data glove, and body suit within a multimedia-equipped, cave-like environment. VR has become a "reality" in the practice setting and in nursing, allied health, and medical education (Simpson, 2003). Several nurse authors have examined the use of VR for distraction during painful procedures with children and adolescents (Merril & Barker, 1996; Schneider & Workman, 2000; Wint et al., 2002; Worley et al., 2002).

The VR CathSim Intravenous Training system can provide students or staff with the opportunity to practice IV line insertion (Agazio et al., 2002; Chang et al., 2002). Jeffries et al. (2003) incorporated VR into a multimedia, interactive CD-ROM program to teach 12-lead electrocardiography (ECG). They report that the program produced cognitive gains, skill performance, student satisfaction, and student confidence in ability to perform the skill that were comparable to those associated with the traditional lecture and demonstration model of instruction. VR is an emergent technology holding significant potential for responding in areas where the nursing faculty shortage is critical and for training in underserved regions. However, the cost of producing VR, the dynamic nature of the emergent technology, and the limited number of users at any one time on a system will likely affect the utility of this exciting medium in health care education (Koerner, 2003).

According to a review by Ziv et al. (2000), RPSs were first used in the late 1960s for anesthesia training. Common features of an RPS include a full-length mannequin, a computer workstation, and interface devices that actuate mannequin signs and drive monitors. In a realistic lifelike patient simulator, computers are used to record drug levels, generate and display blood pressures and heart sounds, and control motion actuators. RPSs are now commercially available. An example is the UltraSim, an ultrasound training simulator available from MedSim Advanced Medical Simulations, Ltd. (*http://www.MEDSIM.com*).

The UltraSim is a complete system simulator with B-mode and color and spectral Doppler echocardiography capabilities and an intuitively designed, generic control panel. The simulator provides all of the necessary clinical data and a detailed, annotated analysis for each patient case. Another example is the PediaSim, which is available from Medical Education Technology at *http://www.meti.com/*. The SimMan, available through Laerdal at *http://www. laerdal.com/*, is yet another example of a high-tech patient simulator.

As Ziv et al. (2000) indicate, these devices represent a paradigm shift from the traditionally available instrumented mannequins with which health care educators and providers are acquainted. Implications for future exploration of this high-tech simulation in nursing education are vast. A 2003 $375,000 grant from the Laerdal Medical Corporation to the National League for Nursing (NLN) will support a 3-year, national, multi-site, multi-method study on the use of simulation in RN education programs. Eight project sites of diploma, associate, and baccalaureate degree nursing programs from across the country will participate in a research study exploring ways in which simulations can be used effectively to facilitate student learning and create learning communities (Corcoran, 2003).

A type of simulation not addressed in the model described by Ziv et al. (2000) is that of a day, a part of a day, or a specific care experience in a clinical agency. For example, Sullivan et al. (1977) designed a simulated hospital day in the college laboratory so the students would experience integrated care rather than separate nursing skill modules. McDonald (1987) describes an 18-hour on-campus simulated clinical experience used as a senior-level substitute for the emergency department experience. Experiences include guided imagery, video role playing, telephone role playing, and evaluative feedback. Reichman and Weaver-Meyers (1984) have also used a role-playing simulation to provide the student with experience in working with a visually impaired patient who has glaucoma and cataracts, and Manderino et al. (1986) describe the results of senior-level students' performance of a cardiac arrest simulation.

Advantages of the simulation strategies include the addition of realism and decision making to patient like situations in the laboratory setting, teaching potential in cognitive and affective realms and psychomotor skill performance, the ability to control multiple extraneous variables present in the actual clinical environment, minimized ethical concerns, and evaluative possibilities. Positive outcomes for students when they use simulations include increased student organization and integration of separate skill modules, faculty identification of students' level of performance in clinical skills, increased student confidence, and smoother transition from laboratory to health care setting, improved performance assessment, error management, improved safety culture, and new research possibilities (McDonald, 1987; Sullivan et al., 1977; Ziv et al., 2000).

In terms of barriers to the adoption of simulations, Hanna (1991) reports that the most frequently cited *disadvantage* of simulations is the amount of time required for the design of the simulation. Other disadvantages include the time and staff needed to prepare, assemble, and maintain the supplies, space, and equipment required for the simulation; plans for and continual orientation of new and reassigned faculty to the simulation(s); and continual updating and revisions required for use of the simulation on a recurring basis (Sullivan et al., 1977). Nehring et al. (2002) point out the additional administrative consideration of maintenance expenses including the purchase of equipment and compensation of faculty for training and practice. Addition of the role-playing element can also add managerial time, especially if nonstudent volunteers or individuals from outside the institution need to be scheduled and compensated for participation. Visible costs, especially with the more complex simulation tools, are relatively high; whereas cost benefits may be indirect, unsubstantiated, and long term (Ziv et al., 2000).

Traditional Faculty Role or Self-Directed, Technology-Enhanced Model. Two competing instructional strategies for teaching psychomotor skills have been the focus of most research on psychomotor skill instruction. One is the traditional faculty-mediated model of lecture and demonstration, followed by student practice and return demonstration to establish competence. Demonstrations and return demonstrations have been, and continue to be, a strategy commonly used in the LRC to develop and refine psychomotor skills because of the ability to control the environment and simulate clinical practice. The effectiveness of teaching by using the demonstration and return demonstration strategy has been described by several authors. Davis and Fusner (1994) describe a 2-hour campus laboratory demonstration of the skills associated with intravenous (IV) therapy that was followed by an 8-hour IV skills day in an outpatient surgery unit. Brigham et al. (1991) describe a campus laboratory participatory learning module for acquisition of skills related to asepsis and universal precautions. Materials for a series of stations, including sterile gloving, opening of sterile materials, and simple dressing change, were assembled and maintained by the laboratory staff. During a scheduled laboratory session, faculty demonstrated the skills at each station and then evaluated return demonstration by the students.

In an attempt to enhance learning and reduce student anxiety in traditional skill demonstration and return demonstration settings, instructors have explored alternative approaches to supplement some of the commonly used teaching strategies. In a performance-centered skills fair, Byrum et al. (1996) incorporated games, music, posters, and a relaxed, flexible atmosphere to involve the learner in practice and review of required skills. Robbins (1994) integrated humor, media, and music with laboratory instruction in fundamental nursing skills. Doheny (1993) and Bucher (1993) used mental imaging practice as a student support for learning motor skills.

Others have examined the effects of faculty feedback during psychomotor skill acquisition. Baldwin et al. (1991) conducted a study to determine whether the use of mediated instruction without instructor input, and hence less instructor-student contact time, would adversely affect performance outcomes. Performance of a skill (blood pressure measurement) by two groups of students was evaluated and compared: one group prepared by reading the textbook, viewing a videotape, and practicing in the laboratory without faculty assistance and the other group had the additional assistance of faculty demonstration of skills and supervised laboratory practice. The study had methodological limitations. However, results indicated that faculty contact is an important element when students are learning to perform a psychomotor skill. Salyers (2001) modified the instructional approach with small samples of students. In the control group, the traditional approach was used; whereas in the experimental group, students learned content and observed demonstration from a technology format, then used class time to practice and received faculty feedback. Salyers reported greater cognitive gains in the experimental group but observed no significant difference in competence of skill performance. Students reported greater satisfaction with the traditional approach.

The alternative to the traditional faculty role is a self-directed approach, replacing the lecture and demonstration with technology and media. Instead of the traditional faculty role in lecture and demonstration, various forms of media including videotapes or DVDs; CD-ROM simulations; Internet learning objects, such as those found on MERLOT *(http://www.merlot.org)*; and VR are used—often in a modular format. Many institutions have designed and implemented modular learning approaches to the teaching and evaluation of nursing skills. In general, the "module" has a pretest and posttest (which may be computerized or offered on the World Wide Web), specific objectives and outcomes, a listing of structured activities with designated resources, and a multimedia integration plan. The advantages of technology-mediated instruction include learner control of pace, consistent content, repetition as needed, multiple examples, and sensory input to meet the needs of different learning styles.

In research designed to compare the traditional and technological approaches, three questions are typically included: (1) Are there differences in performance of the skill? (2) Are there differences in cognitive gains? and (3) Are there differences in student satisfaction? Several authors (Baldwin et al., 1991; Love et al., 1989; Oermann, 1990) have documented that self-directed technology-based instruction, rather than faculty lecture and demonstration, can produce comparable results in performance of psychomotor skills. Jeffries (2001) describes the use of an interactive, multimedia CD-ROM program to teach oral medication administration to baccalaureate nursing students in comparison with the traditional lecture with videotape. Jeffries' well-designed study produced findings consistent with earlier research and new insights. Students in the self-directed technology group demonstrated skill levels equal to those achieved with the traditional method, scored significantly higher on the cognitive assessment, expressed greater satisfaction, and used 31% less time preparing for return demonstration. Jeffries et al. (2003) compared the traditional lecture, self-study module, and demonstration with an interactive, multimedia CD-ROM with VR and a self-study module for teaching 12-lead electrocardiography (ECG) to baccalaureate nursing students. No differences were found in cognitive assessment, student satisfaction, self-efficacy regarding skill competence, or ability to perform the skill. No differences in computer proficiency were found between the groups, but the levels were based on self-report. Age was not reported as a variable in the research design, yet the participants ranged in age from 21 to 53 years. Actual computer skill proficiency may vary in this age range and could account for the lack of effects. In summary, the self-directed technology-mediated models of instruction produced skill performance comparable to that achieved with the traditional method, but cognitive gains were inconsistent.

Another variation of self-directed learning is the use of peers or videotape for obtaining feedback during practice of psychomotor skills. Videotape has a long history of use in the LRC for teaching and evaluating communication and psychomotor skills (Carpenter & Kroth, 1976; Graf, 1993; Iversen, 1978; Memmer, 1979; Quiring, 1972). Memmer describes videotape replay as a tool that nursing students can use to learn to evaluate their own proficiency in using sterile technique. After presentation of classroom content, faculty skill demonstration, and student practice, students were videotaped performing a simulated dressing change on a "patient." Students subsequently observed, critiqued, and evaluated the videotaped performance, as did the instructor, by using a predetermined skills checklist. Variations of this strategy of videotaping psychomotor skills have been examined by others (Bauman et al., 1981; Cowan & Wiens, 1986; Hill et al., 2000; Matthews & Viena, 1988; Graf, 1993). Having students videotape skills practice and then critique themselves or peers offers several potential advantages. Students must think about the skill to evaluate the taped performance and thus have another opportunity to create mental images and procedural knowledge. Self-critique provides more ownership in evaluation and less antagonism toward faculty, and perhaps, is less stressful. A methodological requirement for confirming that approach as effective or even preferable is the validity of the student evaluator's knowledge and accuracy in critiquing a peer's performance. Further study is needed to determine the effect of self or peer evaluation in nursing skill performance.

More recently, Miller et al. (2000) examined student satisfaction and performance levels in two groups of baccalaureate nursing students. One group was evaluated with competency checklists by faculty during the return demonstration, and the other students videotaped their performance, then submitted the tape to faculty for evaluation. Skills included administration of oral and IV medications and rectal suppositories; mixing medications; IV therapy; regulation of IV flow rates; nasal cannula and oxygen mask use; incentive spirometry; insertion of a urinary catheter; open gloving; application of a dry dressing; and insertion, maintenance, and removal of a nasogastric tube. Students with faculty present had a higher mean score on checklists for IV medication administration. Although the overall number of satisfactory ratings was higher for the videotaped students (93.1% versus 88.2% for the first skill set and 84.5% versus 79.2% for the second skill set), only differences in oral medication administration were significant between the two groups. Collectively, faculty spent less time evaluating students when the videotaped methods were used (235.46 minutes in videotaping versus 420.18 minutes in faculty-present evaluation). However, satisfaction ratings on a 5-point Likert scale indicated that both faculty and students preferred the faculty-present method. Although videotaping was perceived as more convenient by both students and faculty, both groups of students believed the experience was moderately stressful.

Student Preferences and Satisfaction. Student responses to the incorporation of media and technology into the curriculum have been examined and found to be dependent on the questions being asked and when the data are collected. Miller et al. (2000) report that students prefer to have faculty present to evaluate their psychomotor skills rather than to make a videotape and submit the tape to faculty. Perceived advantages include immediate feedback and greater learning. Elfrink et al. (2000) monitored students' acceptance scores for use of a handheld computer for managing data in community health nursing. Student frustration with using the system changed over time. Acceptance scores declined from week 1 to week 6, but then increased from week 6 to week 13. Designing evaluation that acknowledges a learning curve may be important when student attitudes are being measured. Jeffries (2001) reports higher student satisfaction scores for interactive CD-ROM instruction for oral medication administration ($\bar{x}=1.83$) compared with the traditional faculty lecture ($\bar{x}=1.31$). However, the restricted scale only ranged from -1 to $+2$. Jeffries et al. (2003) found no differences in student satisfaction between faculty-mediated and multimedia, self-directed instruction for performing 12-lead ECG. As with other aspects of nursing skills instruction, student preferences are complex and not clearly understood. Because students have a range of learning styles that include preferences for social interaction, responsiveness to criticism, and need for sensory input, the variability in student attitudes toward the type of instruction used and the degree of technology infusion should be anticipated. The addition of a measurement of learning style during comparison of instructional strategies would increase understanding of the variables influencing learner behavior and satisfaction.

Identifying Conceptual and Theoretical Frameworks for Instructional Design

Learning Theory. The foundation for nursing skill instruction can be grounded in social or observational learning theory (Bandura, 1986) and information-processing theories of learning, regardless of the instructional design. There are four types of observational learning effects that can shape behavior. Inhibition occurs when a learner refrains from behaving in a particular way because he or she has observed the consequences another experienced. Disinhibition occurs when a learner observes another behave in a socially unacceptable way and go unpunished. Facilitation is the result of seeing another be rewarded in some way that a learner values for behaving in a particular way. Potential exists for facilitation, inhibition, and disinhibition when students observe peers in skill practice and return demonstration with faculty critique. The fourth type is true observational learning in which a behavior is learned by observation of a model and subsequent imitation. Although all four effects may occur when students learn nursing skills, true observational learning can form a foundation for instruction. According to Bandura (1986), attention, retention, production, and motivation are critical factors in observational learning. Information processing theories of learning use the computer analogy to explain learning (Snowman & Biehler, 2003). Analysis of instructional input can inform the selection of strategies for teaching nursing skills.

Attention to a model must occur for observational learning to take place. Research with social learning theory and information-processing theory indicates that attention is more likely to occur when the following conditions are met:

- The model is perceived as competent
- The model is respected

- The consequences observed for executing the behavior are valued
- The sensory register is not bombarded by unlimited input
- Prior knowledge storage in long-term memory is adequate
- Novelty exists
- The teacher provides cues to important data
- Accommodations for individual differences in learning style are made

After observation, a behavior must be retained or remembered so that the student can imitate it. In addition to learning the process or steps involved in the behavior, a learner may have to remember other information such as why or when the behavior is to be performed. For the information to be encoded into long-term memory and retrieved for later use, the learner must have opportunities to rehearse or actively think about it (Snowman & Biehler, 2003). Rehearsal encompasses not only repetition but thinking about how new information is different from or similar to previous learning (Ausubel et al., 1978). Retention is also enhanced when the information is organized in a meaningful way for the learner according to cognitive style. For example, information may be stored as mental images or verbal propositions or both. Retrieval is facilitated when information is encoded in both images and language (Clark & Paivio, 1991). Cognitive style will influence retention and organization; some learners focus on the broad concepts and miss details, and others miss the conceptual meaning and more easily learn the steps of a process. Factual information such as the steps in a procedure, which have few meaningful links to prior knowledge, may be organized more efficiently by using memory strategies (mnemonics) such as rhymes, acrostics, acronyms, or loci methods (Snowman & Biehler, 2003). Retention can be facilitated by the following:

1. Actively rehearsing and organizing the information: note taking, summarizing, outlining, diagramming, telling, acting, teaching, performing, questioning, using mnemonic devices
2. Providing verbal, visual, and tactile or kinesthetic input and output
3. Offering rationales for why the behavior is important
4. Comparing and contrasting new information with previous learning

Production of a new behavior may be initially imitation; later, automatization or mastery occurs through practice with feedback on competence (Snowman & Biehler, 2003). Production is enhanced when there is limited time between observation and imitation. Learners are motivated to produce the behavior when they perceive the consequences to be rewarding. Feedback to reward accuracy or to correct errors is necessary and needs to be delivered within a limited amount of time after performance. The following are required to facilitate production of a new behavior:

1. Practice of skills
2. Immediate and accurate feedback
3. A valued consequence for completing the task

Bandura (1993) asserts that a learner's belief in his or her own ability to be successful, or self-efficacy, is an important motivational factor in observational learning. Self-efficacy is the result of previous learning attempts, persuasion by others that the learner is capable, emotional state, and seeing successful models whom the learner perceives as being like him or her. Learners with high self-efficacy have higher expectations of themselves, visualize themselves being successful, engage in more analytical and evaluative thought in problem solving, work longer at reaching their goals, and approach a new learning task with energy and curiosity. The implications for nursing skill instruction include the following:

1. Stress and anxiety will affect performance
2. Previous success and failure will affect feelings of confidence
3. Students with a history of difficulty in developing psychomotor skills may need more encouragement, instruction, and positive feedback

Faculty can design instruction with the use of these concepts to facilitate learning. These concepts would apply to both traditional faculty-directed instruction and media- or technology-mediated models and could be tested through research.

Expanded Functions of the Learning Resource Center

Depending on the particular institutional goals and financial support, the scope of the LRC functions may include more dimensions than the sole focus of nursing skill teaching and learning. The following discussion expands on the more common functions and covers technology support and/or development and production, distance education, clinical practice, links to clinical practice, and lifelong learning.

Technology Support

In many LRCs, technology support and/or development and production are expanded functions. Support for technology use in the nursing program can be a substantive responsibility of the LRC personnel. This often includes the operation and management of computer labs and the design, development, and production of multimedia and Internet-based products. Childs (2001) surveyed clinical resource centers in 349 American Association of Colleges of Nursing (AACN) schools of nursing and found that 40% of the units managed classroom media services, 38% coordinated the use of technology, and 23% produced multimedia resources.

A common practice is the partnering of the nursing LRC with other technology services within the institution to provide this technology support and/or the development and production of multimedia products. A case study example is the School of Nursing LRC at Ball State University *(http://www.bsu.edu/nursing)*. Staffed with technology support personnel at the nursing academic unit level, the LRC is the initial point of technology service for students, faculty, and staff in the nursing program. However, a wide variety of institutional support services work in partnership with the school to offer more comprehensive services. These partnerships include personnel consultation, design, development and production staff, and financial support for the purchase of hardware and software at the unit level. In this case, institutional technology support services partnering with the school of nursing LRC include University Computing Services *(http://www.bsu.edu/web/ucs)*, Teleplex *(http://www.bsu.edu/web/teleplex)*, University Libraries *(http://www.bsu.edu/libraries)*, the Office of Teaching and Learning Advancement *(http://www.bsu.edu/web/otla/)*, Extended Education *(http://www.bsu.edu/distance)*, and Office of Research and Sponsored Programs *(http://www.bsu.edu/web/research)*.

Distance Education

The coordination of distance education for the nursing program has been a natural evolution for some LRCs, especially those LRC units that have historically had technology support and/or the development and production of multimedia as one of their essential functions. Typically, the nursing unit LRC partners with other institutional services in the support of distance education. The LRC director and staff are generally key support personnel for the development, implementation, and evaluation of the distance learning offerings, courses, and programs. In almost all cases, this function is done in close partnership with other institutional technology and teaching and support entities (e.g., library, extended education, telecommunications, computer services, and marketing). Resources that provide a comprehensive overview of the current status, strategies, support, and evaluation of distance education overall and, specifically, in nursing education are available (Hodson-Carlton et al., 2003; Moore & Anderson, 2003).

Clinical Practice

The LRC is a vital link to the practice setting in various capacities. The LRC may serve as a center for clinical practice for faculty and students. For example, a physical assessment classroom or lab areas may be designed to serve as a clinic for providing health assessment services, or a simulated home health care room can serve as a place to teach families how to care for patients in the home. LRCs also can serve as resource centers for community groups (e.g., wellness programs or patient teaching). The LRC can therefore also offer an opportunity for providing services and teaching opportunities and generating income. The LRC may also be the point from which faculty and students provide health care services to patients at a distance. This might include telehealth applications, computer conferencing in which faculty and students provide health counseling (Billings & Phillips, 1991) or preventive health services, and data management services in underserved areas (Puskar et al., 1996).

Many LRCs are increasingly serving as a bridge, sometimes virtual, to clinical practice. In several instances the LRC of one institution is physically and technologically linked to one or more health care institutions. In the early 1990s, Simpson (1990) advised closing the rapidly expanding technological gap between the school and the automated environment of the health care workplace by integrating computer terminals at the bedside of each practice unit in the LRC and the functional networking of each of those terminals to a "real" hospital information system through a collaborative partnership with the vendor. The goal of this redesigned learning laboratory was to prepare the student to practice in the increasingly automated health care environment through use and practice with the "real" automated tools of the health care workplace. There are examples of LRCs that are serving as a bridge to clinical practice at the health care agency. Doorley et al. (1994) describe the internal institutional and external collaboration required to allow students to access the hospital information system from the LRC at the school of nursing site. Electronic connectivity with the clinical agency hospital information system allows nursing students to create patient care plans from computers in the LRC and enter the information into the patients' records after review of the care plans with the clinical instructor. Hilgenberg and Damery (1994) report on a similar collaborative project between a school of nursing and a major clinical site to introduce and orient baccalaureate nursing students to use of an automated hospital information system. The School of Nursing at Ball State University is another case study example of a collaborative partnership among the university, a regional health care center, and a health care information system vendor to provide student orientation to computerized documentation in the LRC before practice at the health care agency.

It is realistic to envision the need for ongoing partnerships to develop such bridges as technology applications in acute and home care clinical agencies expand at a phenomenal rate. For example, Vautier et al. (2003) provide an excellent summary of the application of technology within the Emory Hospital system in Atlanta. Applications include the following:

- Automated staffing/scheduling systems
- Long-distance cardiac/hemodynamic monitoring systems delivered via radiofrequency telemetry
- Handheld devices with resources (e.g., clinical algorithms, drug reference systems)
- Satellite broadcasts of surgical training, operating room techniques, and electronic tracking of surgical patients
- Web-based communication between the emergency department and emergency medical services
- Emergency department patient information systems for tracking and record retrieval
- Access to, monitoring, and record keeping for continuing education
- Computerized training on safety procedures, basic life support, and advanced life support
- Online access to policy and procedure manuals
- Electronic communication systems for clinical staff with links to protocols and Internet resources

The Nightingale Tracker (NT) project, developed and pilot tested by the Fuld Institute for Technology in Nursing Education (FITNE), is another example of the type of health care communication/instructional model that may be supported by the LRC (Elfrink, 1996; Elfrink et al., 2000). The NT is a computerized interactive communication system designed to assist with such interrelated functions of the community health student clinical assignment as assignment generation, preplanning, patient visit, postclinical documentation, and evaluation and follow-up (Elfrink, 1996). Students can use the NT in the field for patient data retrieval, recording clinical data, and Internet access. With the help of a computerized system such as the NT or another advanced telecommunications system, faculty present in the LRC may serve as a resource to students located at the health care setting.

Lifelong Learning

Rapidly expanding electronic networks create the potential for the LRC to play a key role in the delivery of continuing education or lifelong learning. Many health care and health care–related academic institutions now have World Wide Web home page sites, some with "virtual tour" and "virtual course" delivery, thus providing access to lifelong learning at the learner's time and place (Hodson-Carlton, 1996). Alumni and others may access continuing education programs and modules that provide just-in-time learning through the facilities of the LRC. With downsizing and outsourcing of education in health care facilities, the LRC may provide access to information and networking opportunities. Both computer technologies and interactive television may be used as delivery systems. There are also examples of partnerships with external organizations for the delivery of this continuing education. One example is the NLN sponsorship of continuing education developed with Indiana University School of Nursing.

Management and Operation of the Learning Resource Center

Physical Structure

The facility and physical layout of an LRC varies widely, depending on the scope of services and the particular institutional objectives for the unit. The central, organizational core of most LRCs is generally located within or near the nursing and health care program(s). In physical size dimensions, Childs (2001) reports that 75% of 349 AACN school of nursing respondents indicated that the LRC facility was less than 4000 square feet, 50% indicated a size of less than 2000 square feet, and the largest LRC size was reported as 15,000 feet. However, since the phenomenal growth of the Internet, the LRC increasingly has a virtual space, as well as a physical space dimension.

Billings (1996) created a checklist of considerations for physical space, as well as for virtual space. Considerations for physical space included use flexibility, conference room space, telecommunication infrastructure, storage and distribution space, current and future work space for staff and faculty, space for student and patient privacy, compliance with Occupational Safety and Health Administration (OSHA) and Americans with Disabilities (ADA) codes, custodial storage, carrels and space for a variety of changing work functions, viewing ability, maintenance and repair work space, and space for learning aids and display or bulletin boards. Dimensions cited as important to include in considerations for virtual space are computer-based technologies with Internet connections, access to patient database systems and institutional data sets, customer access from homes and work sites, access to a broadcast/receive site for technology-based conferences, capabilities for student-faculty contact from remote sites, connections to libraries and electronic information distribution systems, and local and wide area networks. Consideration of such design and operational issues remains current.

Because distance learning has increased and more education, agency, and/or foundation partnerships have been formed, the physical space of the LRC is sometimes located at remote or distant locations. In some cases, the LRC unit is actually administratively responsible for the supplies, equipment, and, sometimes staffing of the clinical practice environment at the remote location. This might take the form of a mobile, transportable community clinic, a community nursing center at various locations, and/or a satellite, branch LRC. Stone (2003) reports on one such remote, rural LRC development: Aunt Hattie's barn was converted into a modern LRC when the traditional facilities were unable to accommodate an increasing student population.

A visit to selected LRC home pages on the World Wide Web reveals the diversity in the physical design and size of nursing skill practice areas. For example, the Clinical Simulation Lab at the Shady Grove Center of the University of Maryland *(http://www.nursing.umaryland.edu/departments2.htm)* is designed to replicate multiple clinical settings in one lab (i.e., a basic hospital unit and critical care, pediatric, maternity, and neonatal units). Other examples are located at Northern Illinois University *(http://www.nursing.niu.edu/kuczek/310lab.htm)* and University of Kansas *(http://www2.kumc.edu/son/Building/skillslab.htm)*.

Learning Resource Center Administration and Personnel

Childs (2001) reports significant variations in administrative position titles and organizational structure, academic qualifications, and salaries of LRC directors from institution to institution A review of Childs' findings from the 349 respondents reveals the following typical profile of the LRC administrator: a full-time employee (40%) with faculty academic status (49%), typically titled "LRC Coordinator" (41%) with a master's degree (59%) and academic rank of assistant professor (33%) who reports to a department chair (42%) and earns a salary in the range of $35,000 to $50,000.

Responsibilities of the LRC administrator role can also vary widely depending on the institutional goals and support. Support for teaching and learning activities is usually a predominant role of the LRC administrator. This role generally includes assisting faculty and students with curriculum development and implementation and integration of technology; coordination of unit activity with other institutional and extra-agency technology support areas; and fiscal, personnel, hardware, and software management including grant writing and teaching functions. When respondents were asked to select responsibilities of their LRC management role in Childs' (2002) LRC survey, two of the top three responsibilities involved working with faculty in a consultative role: consulting with faculty on the use of the clinical resource center (n = 216, 78.8%) and consulting with faculty on teaching resources available in the clinical resource center (n = 211). Other responsibilities cited in the survey include administration, committee work, remedial sessions for students, consultation with other faculty or departments, evaluation of student performance, management of classroom media services, coordination of technology in the school or program, acting as a resource for the community and alumni, production of multimedia resources, research, community service, and "other" (including such duties as Web page management, course teaching, grant acquisition, coordination of distance learning, and acting as liaison to the library).

Student staffing is also a critical personnel component of many LRC units. Childs (2002) reports that more than 85% of the 276 AACN school of nursing respondents indicated the use of some sort of student help (e.g., work-study employees or undergraduate or graduate student employees) paid for by the academic unit. A wide range of student work responsibilities were cited, including serving as core staff during evening and weekend hours, setting up supplies and equipment for teaching and learning activities, cleaning equipment and the practice and evaluation area, teaching skills, serving as student mentors, and assisting the other LRC staff members in the operation and maintenance of the facility.

Professional staff positions may also be allocated as LRC support for technical, computer networking, secretarial, and skill practice laboratory supervision. Some institutions have successfully employed faculty or RN staff as preceptors in the LRC to provide assistance and feedback to students who are practicing skills. Often, these individuals will also evaluate the students' performance of the skills before performance of the skill in the health care setting.

The increasing focus on technology integration for the position is affecting the LRC personnel composition. Each institution is faced with personnel "retooling" and the addition of student and professional personnel having knowledge and experience with computer and multimedia technology, including the maintenance and operation of local and wide area networks. In the 2001 survey of LRCs, Childs (2002) found it rare for the director to be the only staff member of the LRC (13%). Seventeen percent reported that a media specialist was on the LRC staff.

There can be frequent turnover in LRC personnel because of the lack of standardization of LRC director position duties, qualifications, and benefits from institution to institution; wide variations in LRC unit staff composition; and the heavy dependence of the position's stability on the administrative prerogative of the chief executive officer of the institution. For example, Childs (2001) found most LRC managers had been in the position 0 to 2 years (38%). However, stability and the presence of high-quality personnel in this position are increasingly important as the pervasiveness of technology in the profession continues. The effective use of this position and the LRC staff composition can have far-reaching benefits for the institution in terms of effective and efficient technology integration and use at the unit level and successful internal and external resource collaborative efforts.

Fiscal Management: Budget and Operating Costs

Significant variations exist in budgetary allocations and the fiscal management policies of LRCs. Budgets for the LRC may range from very limited available funds for the nursing unit LRC, managed by the administrative officer of the entire unit, to budgets in excess of a million dollars, managed by the LRC director. According to Childs' (2002) descriptive study, overall budgets for the clinical resource centers ranged from less than $5000 per year to more than

$45,000, with 78% of the 276 units operating on budgets of $25,000 or less. The primary source for funding of the LRC is the supporting institution, often augmented by student clinical or technology fees.

Regardless of the individual variations, a key trend is the movement toward internal and external collaboration and partnerships for the most effective use of resources, and in some cases, revenue generation. Nassif et al. (2003) describe such experiences in sharing laboratory space between nursing and pharmacy technician students. Another example is the nursing unit that uses an institutional computer laboratory rather than obtaining support for the personnel, equipment, and supply expenditure for this laboratory from the unit budget. Revenue for the nursing unit LRC may also be generated by costing out services and equipment to other units through the collaborative sharing of skill practice laboratory or computer laboratory space and resources.

Some have also reported on the feasibility of an LRC in health care facilities, thus providing opportunities for sharing of LRC resources by two or more agencies. Often the cost-efficiency potential of the LRC as a clinical assessment center has been the incentive for the development of the LRC at the health care site. For example, in the late 1980s, del Bueno et al. (1987) described how clinical assessment centers could reduce orientation costs for new employees and increase the benefits, in terms of employee screening and training, to the health care institution of such assessment centers. Mackin (1996) and Baughman (1996) describe the challenges, the issues, and the potential of the LRC in the health care facility. Charron (1996) advocates maximizing the hospital and collegiate learning resources through the establishment and sharing of a hospital-based electronic nursing LRC by the hospital staff development department and five collegiate schools of nursing.

Additional Learning Resource Center Operational Issues: Safety, Evaluation, and Networking

Additional LRC issues are important to consider in the operation of the facility. The following discussion focuses on three dimensions: safety, evaluation, and professional networking opportunities.

The operation of a nursing skill practice area, typically the most common function of the majority of LRCs in the United States, must include consideration of safety issues typical of clinical experiences in health care institutions and community health experiences. In their discussion of ways educators can reduce the risk of injury to students and potential litigation charging educational negligence, Goudreau and Chasens (2002), Higginbotham (2000), and Redford and Klein (2003) provide dimensions that may be used to develop a proactive plan to ensure student safety in the skills laboratory. Some of the dimensions of such a proactive plan with suggestions to promote lab safety are summarized in Table 16-2.

Although evaluation is increasingly a critical component of success and continuing functionality of any entity, there are no specific standards for the evaluation of LRCs. Guides and recommendations related to evaluation of the nursing LRC from a cost/benefit analysis and/or program/instructional

TABLE 16-2 Proactive Plan: Promoting Safety in Skills Lab	
POTENTIAL RISKS	**SUGGESTIONS TO REDUCE INJURY RISK(S)**
Use of dangerous materials & equipment such as needles, crutches, etc. outside of faculty-supervised times	Student instruction on safe operation of equipment is part of new student orientation
	Lock areas where needles are stored
	Require students' yearly attendance at OSHA in-service
	Develop guidelines for using needles/syringes that students must sign
	Partner with institution's environment specialist for compliance with use & maintenance of hazardous materials, supplies, and equipment
Malfunctioning equipment such as electric beds, wheelchairs, and other electronic equipment	Contractual agreement with associated clinical facility and/or commercial vendor for annual maintenance checks and repairs as needed
Latex allergy	Partner with institution's Office of Disabled Student Development
	Obtain medical verification of physical impairment
	Provide accommodation compliance with Americans with Disabilities Act and the Rehabilitation Act of 1973
Back injuries	Provide supervised practice in transferring patients, emphasizing both student and patient safety
Bloodborne pathogens	Use same protective measures in skills lab as would be used in clinical setting (e.g., use of gloves)
	School maintains documentation of student training in standard precautions
Student live participation in procedures versus simulation	Student who volunteers to undergo/perform procedure is asked to sign consent/release from liability form that discloses risks and hazards

service perspective have also been scarce in the literature. Available reports usually focus on one aspect of LRC operation, such as budgetary analysis, rather than providing a comprehensive evaluation of the entire LRC operation (i.e., curriculum, faculty and student support, and fiscal accountability). For example, in the mid 1980s, Hodson et al. (1988) described the development and use of a computerized management program to automate much of the paperwork involved in the operation of a skills laboratory; however, there was no accompanying description of costs, nor did they indicate whether or how the system was used to measure the effectiveness of the LRC. Reimer (1992) describes the design and development of a computerized cost analysis system to more efficiently track the costs of the skills laboratory operation and plan budgetary allocations. However, again, there is no subsequent follow-up description of linking costs to lab effectiveness and productivity.

Some sources have suggested LRC evaluation criteria or benchmarking dimensions (Wilson, 1999). For example, Billings (1996) proposes that areas for benchmarking might include customer satisfaction, congruence of resource support with functions, cost-effectiveness of technology, and customer accomplishment of learning outcomes. duBoulay and Medway (1999) also emphasize the need for unit evaluation to substantiate the continuing value of the instructional unit. Areas deemed critical for inclusion in an evaluation plan are learning outcomes, benefits to students, and value for money.

In summary, it appears that the area of LRC evaluation needs more attention, especially in an era of soaring costs, budget reductions, and demand for measurable outcomes. Until LRC comprehensive performance and outcome standards are established, it is recommended that existing units, at a minimum, use evaluation questionnaires or surveys for their diverse on-site and virtual customers.

As diverse as LRCs are across the country, there have been increasing efforts toward developing professional networking among LRC directors during the last 2 decades. In the early 1980s a few LRC directors identified the need for a periodic LRC National Conference at which LRC directors from across the country could collaboratively explore the issues of teaching and learning in the LRC and network with each other about operational issues of the unit. In 1996 this national conference was broadened to include an international perspective and has become a biennial event held in different regions of the country. Although a planning committee of LRC directors from across the country develops the programs for these conferences, the conferences are typically hosted by the continuing education or LRC unit of the host educational institution. For example, the tenth biennial North American Learning Resources Center Conference takes place in 2004 and will be sponsored by the Intercollegiate College of Nursing/Washington State University College of Nursing. There has been enough interest in such professional networking that the National Conference on Nursing Skills Laboratories was initiated in the mid 1990s by the LRC/continuing education unit at the San Antonio, Texas, branch of the University of Texas. Focused on the areas of organization and management of nursing skills laboratories, teaching and learning processes for acquiring nursing skills, and strategies to enhance clinical evaluation and skills verification, the fifth biennial national conference on nursing skills laboratories is scheduled for 2005 in San Antonio, Texas *(http://www.nursing. uthscsa.edu/CE_Events/2005/June23.htm)*. Other professional networking opportunities for LRC directors and others include subscription and participation in the NurseLRC LISTSERV and membership in the 2002 established International Association for Clinical Nursing Simulation and Learning (INACSL). The LISTSERV address is majordomo@douglas.bc.ca with the message *Subscribe NurseLRC*. A great deal of information is exchanged in the LISTSERV communication, including tips on the use of simulations, comparative equipment pricing and recommendations, and ideas for teaching and learning in the skills laboratory. The mission of INACSL is to promote and provide the development and advancement of clinical simulation and LRCs, and INACSL is committed to and supports collaboration, application of resource management concepts, integration of teaching strategies, research, and scholarship and information dissemination.

In summary, the management and operational issues for the administration of an LRC are complex and often vary widely depending on institutional goals and budget allocation for the facility. LRC dimensions that vary widely across the country include physical and virtual space, personnel composition, qualifications, responsibilities, and funding allocations. One of the areas of management that requires further exploration is the development and implementation of comprehensive evaluation. A positive trend during the last 2 decades has been increasing professional networking.

SUMMARY

The LRC remains an integral part of nursing education programs for the purpose of nursing skills instruction and holds the potential for enhanced functions with the integration of technological supports and bridges to clinical practice. Several issues regarding the function of the LRC have been discussed. The range of uses for LRCs across nursing programs is due to variability in operational budgets and institutional and unit goals. Budget constraints affect media and technology infusion, faculty involvement and responsibilities, administration and staffing, and the design of the physical space and virtual presence. Budget allocations often reflect the institution's philosophy and goals regarding the importance of teaching psychomotor skills within the curriculum or the willingness to assume responsibility for technology management. Agreement on essential nursing skills and minimal levels of behavioral competencies has yet to be achieved in nursing. The intellectual skills and motor processes that allow a student to think critically about the how, why, and what while actually performing continue to be underestimated in both research and instructional design. A lack of national standardization in identifying and measuring essential nursing skill competencies has the potential effect of minimizing the importance of dedicating resources to the LRC. For example, if accrediting agencies were to stipulate nursing skill competencies or proficiencies for best practice, the instructional methods and evaluation practices would need to be organized and standardized under the management of an academic unit such as an LRC. Laboratory practice, the use of media and technology, skill demonstrations and return demonstrations, and simulations are common elements in nursing skill instruction. Infusion of technology into instruction adds another dimension for study. Initial research indicates that faculty-mediated instruction and media/technology instruction produce similar skill performance and self-directed, media/technology forms of instruction can yield higher cognitive gains. In the future the design and evaluation of instructional strategies for teaching nursing skills can be enhanced by using conceptual frameworks from observational learning theory and information processing. The functions of the LRC offer many opportunities for research and evaluation.

REFERENCES

Agazio, J. B., Pavlides, C. C., Lasome, C., Flaherty, N. J., & Torrance, R. J. (2002). Evaluation of a virtual reality simulator in sustainment training. *Military Medicine, 167*(11), 893-897.

Alavi, C., Loh, S. H., & Reilly, D. (1991). Reality basis for teaching psychomotor skills in a tertiary nursing curriculum. *Journal of Advanced Nursing, 16*(8), 957-965.

Ausubel, D. P., Novak, J. D., & Hanesian, H. (1978). *Educational psychology: A cognitive view* (2nd ed.). New York: Holt, Rinehart, & Winston.

Baldwin, D., Hill, P., & Hanson, G. (1991). Performance of psychomotor skills: A comparison of two teaching strategies. *Journal of Nursing Education, 30,* 367-370.

Bandura, A. (1986). *Social foundations of thought and action: A social cognitive theory.* Englewood Cliffs, NJ: Prentice-Hall.

Bandura, A. (1993). Perceived self-efficacy in cognitive development and functioning. *Educational Psychologist, 28*(2), 117-148.

Barrows, H. S. (1993). An overview of the uses of standardized patients for teaching and evaluating clinical skills. *Academic Medicine, 68,* 443-453.

Baughman, D. (1996, April). *Simulation laboratory in a hospital.* Paper presented at the Learning Resources for Life Long Learning Conference, Indianapolis, IN.

Bauman, K., Cook, J., & Larson, L. (1981). Using technology to humanize instruction: An approach to teaching nursing skills. *Journal of Nursing Education, 20*(3), 27-31.

Benner, P. (1984). *From novice to expert: Excellence and power in clinical nursing practice.* Menlo Park, CA: Addison-Wesley Publishing Co., Nursing Division.

Billings, D. (1996). Designing nursing learning centers of the future. *Computers in Nursing, 14*(2), 80-81.

Billings, D., & Phillips, A. (1991). Computer conferencing: "The school nurse" in the "electronic school district." *Computers in Nursing, 9*(6), 215-218.

Bolton, J. G. (1984). Educating professional nurses for clinical practice. *Nursing and Health Care, 5*(7), 385-389.

Brigham, C. J., Foster, S. L., & Hodson, K. E. (1991). A participatory learning module: Asepsis and universal precautions. *Nurse Educator, 16*(1), 22-25.

Bucher, L. (1993). The effects of imagery abilities and mental rehearsal on learning a nursing skill. *Journal of Nursing Education, 32*(7), 318-324.

Byrum, C. D., Rudisill, P. T., & Singletary, M. B. (1996). The traveling salvation show: A performance-centered skills fair. *Journal of Nursing Staff Development, 12*(4), 198-203.

Carpenter, K. F., & Kroth, J. A. (1976). Effects of videotaped role playing on nurses' therapeutic communication skills. *The Journal of Continuing Education in Nursing, 7*(2), 47-53.

Chang, K. K., Chung, J. W., & Wong, T. K. (2002). Learning intravenous cannulation: A comparison of the conventional method and the CathSim Intravenous Training System. *Journal of Clinical Nursing, 11*(1), 73-78.

Charron, H. S. (1996, April). Maximizing hospital and collegiate learning resources through partnerships. Paper presented at the Learning Resources for Life Long Learning Conference, Indianapolis, IN.

Childs, J. (2001). *CRC survey.* University of Southern Maine College of Nursing and Health Professions. Retrieved August 15, 2003, from http://www.usm.maine.edu/conhp/Survey%20results%20for%20web.pdf

Childs, J. C. (2002). Clinical resource centers in nursing programs. *Nurse Educator, 27*(5), 232-235.

Clark, J., & Paivio, A. (1991). Dual coding theory and education. *Educational Psychology Review 3*(3), 149-170.

Corcoran, R. D. (2003). Letter from *NLN CEO NLN UPDATE A Biweekly Publication of the National League for Nursing, 6*(11).

Corcoran, S. (1977). Should a service setting be used as a learning laboratory? *Nursing Outlook, 25,* 771-776.

Cowan, D., & Wiens, V. (1986). Mock hospital: A preclinical laboratory experience. *Nurse Educator, 11*(5), 30-32.

Dave, R. H. (1970). *Psychomotor levels in developing and writing behavioral objectives.* Tucson, AZ: Educational Innovators Press.

Davis, J. A., & Fusner, S. J. (1994). Teaching venipuncture in an outpatient surgery unit. *Nurse Educator, 19*(2), 40-42.

del Bueno, D., Weeks, L., & Brown-Stewart, P. (1987). Clinical assessment centers: A cost-effective alternative for competency development. *Nursing Economics, 5*(1), 21-26.

Doheny, M. O. (1993). Mental practice: An alternative approach to teaching motor skills. *Journal of Nursing Education, 32*(6), 260-264.

Doorley, J. E., Renner, A. L., & Corron, J. (1994). Creating care plans via modems: Using a hospital information system in nursing education. *Computers in Nursing, 12*(3), 160-163.

Eerden, K. (2001). Using critical thinking vignettes to evaluate student learning. *Nursing and Health Care Perspectives, 22*(5), 231-235.

Elfrink, V. (1996). The Nightingale tracker. *Computers in Nursing, 14*(2), 82-83, 88.

Elfrink, V., Davis, L., Fitzwater, E., Castleman, J., Burley, J., Gorney-Moreno, et al. (2000). A comparison of teaching strategies for integrating information technology into clinical nursing education. *Nurse Educator, 25*(3), 136-144.

Gibbons, S. W., Adamo, G., Padden, D., Ricciardi, R., Graziano, M., Levine, E., et al. (2002). Clinical evaluation in advanced practice nursing education: Using standardized patients in health assessment. *Journal of Nursing Education, 41*(5), 215-221.

Gomez, G. E., & Gomez, E. A. (1984). The teaching of psychomotor skills in nursing. *Nurse Educator, 9*, 35-39.

Goudreau, K. A., & Chasens, E. R. (2002). Negligence in nursing education. *Nurse Educator, 27*(10), 42-46.

Graf, M. A. (1993). Videotaping return demonstration. *Nurse Educator, 18*(4), 29.

Hallal, J., & Welsh, M. (1984). Using the computer laboratory to learn psychomotor skills. *Nurse Educator, 9*(4), 34-38.

Hanna, D. R. (1991). Using simulations to teach clinical nursing. *Nurse Educator, 16*(2), 28-31.

Herrmann, E. K. (1981). Mrs. Chase: A noble and enduring figure. *American Journal of Nursing, 81*, 1836.

Higginbotham, E. (2000). The liability risks when students practice nursing. *RN, 63*(9), 90.

Hilgenberg, C., & Damery, L. (1994). Introduction to an automated hospital information system in baccalaureate education: A pilot project. *Journal of Nursing Education, 33*(8), 378-380.

Hill, R., Hooper, C., & Wahl, S. (2000). Look, learn, and be satisfied: Video playback as a learning strategy to improve clinical skills performance. *Journal for Nurses in Staff Development, 16*(5), 232-239.

Hodson, K. E., Manis, J., Thayer, M., Webb, S., Hunnicutt, C., & Hoogenboom, A. (1988). Computerized management program for the skills laboratory of a school of nursing. *Computers in Nursing, 6*(5), 215-221.

Hodson, K. E., Worrell, P. J., & Alonzi, V. P. (1985). Design and development of cognitive mastery testing using an authoring system. *Computers in Nursing, 3*(4), 166-172.

Hodson-Carlton, K. E. (1996). Reengineering of the learning environment: Linking the nursing student with the healthcare community. *Computers in Nursing, 14*(1), 19-20.

Hodson-Carlton, K., Siktberg, L., Flowers, J., & Scheibel, P. (2003). Overview of distance education in nursing: Where are we now and where are we going? In M. Oermann & K. Heinrich (Eds.), *Annual review of nursing education: Volume I* (pp. 165-189). New York: Springer.

Iversen, S. M. (1978). Microcounseling: A model for teaching the skills of interviewing. *Journal of Nursing Education, 17*(7), 12-16.

Jeffries, P. R. (2001). Computer versus lecture: A comparison of two methods of teaching oral medication administration in a nursing skills laboratory. *Journal of Nursing Education, 40*(7), 323-330.

Jeffries, P. R., Woolfe, S., & Linde, B. (2003). Technology-based vs. traditional instruction: A comparison of two methods for teaching the skill of performing a 12-lead ECG. *Nursing Education Perspectives, 24*(2), 70-75.

Klaassens, E. (1992). Strategies to enhance problem solving. *Nurse Educator, 17*(3), 28-31.

Koerner, J. (2003). The virtues of the virtual world: Enhancing the technology/knowledge professional interface for life-long learning. *Nursing Administration Quarterly, 27*(1), 9-17.

Love, B., McAdams, C., Patton, D. M., Rankin, E. J., & Roberts, J. (1989). Teaching psychomotor skills in nursing: A randomized control trial. *Journal of Advanced Nursing, 14*(11), 970-975.

Mackin, J. (1996, April). The learning resource center in the health care facility. Paper presented at the Learning Resources for Life Long Learning Conference, Indianapolis, IN.

Manderino, M. A., Ganong, L. H., Yonkman, C. A., & Royal, A. (1986). Evaluation of a cardiac arrest simulation. *Journal of Nursing Education, 25*(3), 107-111.

Matthews, R., & Viena, D. C. (1988). Evaluating basic nursing skills through group video testing. *Journal of Nursing Education, 27*(1), 44-46.

McDonald, G. F. (1987). The simulated clinical laboratory. *Nursing Outlook, 35*(6), 290-292.

Memmer, M. K. (1979). Television replay: A tool for students to learn to evaluate their own proficiency in using sterile technique. *Journal of Nursing Education, 18*(8), 35-42.

Merril, G L., & Barker, V. L. (1996). Virtual reality debuts in the teaching laboratory in nursing. *Journal of Intravenous Nursing, 19*(4), 182-187.

Miller, H., Nichols, E., & Beeken, J. (2000). Comparing videotaped and faculty present return demonstrations of clinical skills. *Journal of Nursing Education, 39*(5), 237-240.

Minnesota Baccalaureate Psychomotor Skills Faculty Group. (1998). Conversations: An experience of psychomotor skills faculty. *Journal of Nursing Education, 37*(7), 324-325.

Mooney, N. E. (1993). Juggling performance checklist: Teaching psychomotor skills to nurses. *Journal of Continuing Education in Nursing, 24*(1), 43-44.

Moore, M. G., & Anderson, W. G. (2003). *Handbook of distance education.* Mahwah, NJ: Lawrence Erlbaum Associates.

Nassif, D., Herrington, K., Delaney, M., Carr, C., & Deshotels, D. (2003). Introducing interdisciplinary collaboration to nursing and pharmacy technician students. *American Journal of Health-System Pharmacy, 60*(9), 951.

Nehring, W. M., Lashley, F., & Ellis, W. E. (2002). Critical incident nursing management using human patient simulators. *Nursing Education Perspectives, 23*(3), 128-132.

Nelson, A. (2003). Using simulation to design and integrate technology for safer and more efficient practice environments. *Nursing Outlook, 51*(3), S27-S29.

Oermann, M. H. (1990). Psychomotor skill development. *Journal of Continuing Education in Nursing, 21*(5), 202-204.

Olsen, R. K. (1999). Teaching psychomotor nursing skills in simulated learning labs: A critical review of the literature. In K. R. Stevens & V. R. Cassidy (Eds.), *Evidence-based teaching: Current research in nursing education.* Sudbury, MA: Jones and Bartlett.

Puskar, K. R., Lamb, J., Boneysteele, G., Serecka, S., Rohay, J., & Tusore-Mumford, K. (1996). High touch meets high tech: Distance mental health screening for rural youth using teleform. *Computers in Nursing, 14*(6), 323-329.

Quiring, J. (1972). The autotutorial approach: Effect of timing of videotape feedback on sophomore nursing student's achievement of skill in giving S9 injections. *Nursing Research, 21*(4), 332-337.

Redford, D. S., & Klein, T. (2003). Informed consent in the nursing skills laboratory: An exploratory study. *Journal of Nursing Education, 42*(3), 131-133.

Reichman, S. L., & Weaver-Meyers, P. (1984). Glaucoma and cataracts: A nurse-patient simulation for nursing students. *Journal of Nursing Education, 23*(7), 314-315.

Reimer, M. S. (1992). Computerized cost analysis for the nursing skills laboratory. *Nurse Educator, 17*(4), 8-11.

Robbins, J. (1994). Using humor to enhance learning in the skills laboratory. *Nurse Educator, 19*(3), 39-42.

Ryan, M., & Hodson-Carlton, K. (1997). Portfolio applications in a school of nursing. *Nurse Educator, 22*(1), 35-39.

Salyers, V. L. (2001). The effect of alternative instructional methods on cognitive knowledge and psychomotor skill acquisition for beginning nursing students. *Dissertation Abstracts International, Part B, 62*(12), 5646. (UMI No. AA13035640).

Schneider, S. M., & Workman, M. L. (2000). Virtual reality as a distraction intervention for older children receiving chemotherapy. *Pediatric Nursing, 26*(6), 593-597.

Sherman, V. R., & Craig, A. B. (1995). Literacy in virtual reality: A new medium. *Computer Graphics, 29*, 37-44.

Simpson, R. L. (1990). Technology: Nursing the system: Closing the gap between school and service. *Nursing Management, 21*(11), 16-17.

Simpson, R. L. (2002). The virtual reality revolution: Technology changes nursing education. *Nursing Management, 33*(9), 14-15.

Simpson, R. L. (2003). Welcome to the virtual classroom: How technology is transforming nursing education in the 21st century. *Nursing Administration Quarterly, 27*(1), 83-86.

Smith, B. E. (1992). Linking theory and practice in teaching basic nursing skills. *Journal of Nursing Education, 31*(1), 16-23.

Snowman, J., & Biehler, R. (2003). *Psychology applied to teaching* (10th ed.). Boston: Houghton Mifflin Co.

Stern, S. B. (1988). Are we preparing baccalaureate students for practice? *Nurse Educator, 13*(4), 3-4.

Stone, S. (2003). Frontier School of Midwifery and family nursing news: Aunt Hattie's barn becomes the student learning resource center. *Frontier Nursing Service Quarterly Bulletin, 78*(3), 13-14.

Sullivan, K., Gruis, M., & Poole, C. (1977). From learning modules to clinical practice. *Nursing Outlook, 25*(5), 319-321.

Sweeney, M., Hedstrom, B., & O'Malley, M. (1982). Process evaluation: A second look at psychomotor skills. *Journal of Nursing Education, 21*(2), 4-17.

Sweeney, M. A., Regan, P., O'Malley, M., & Hedstrom, B. (1980). Essential skills for baccalaureate graduates: Perspectives of education and service. *Journal of Nursing Administration, 10*(10), 37-44.

Vautier, A., Connor, J., Fragala, P., Hart, M., Brown, K., Sverdlik, B., et al. (2003). The Emory Experience. *Nursing Administration Quarterly, 27*(1), 18-28.

Wilson, M. (1999). Using benchmarking practices for the learning resource center. *Nurse Educator, 24*(4), 16-20.

White, J. E. (1995). Using interactive video to add physical assessment data to computer-based patient simulations in nursing. *Computers in Nursing, 13*(5), 233-235.

Wint, S. S., Eshelman, D., Steele, J., & Guzetta, C. E. (2002). Effects of distraction using virtual reality (VR) glasses during lumbar punctures in adolescents with cancer. *Oncology Nursing Forum, 29*(1), 8-15.

Worley, B., Wint, S. S., Eshelman, D., Steele, J., & Guzetta, C. E. (2002). Level of sedation may influence effect of virtual reality glasses during distraction therapy. *Oncology Nursing Forum, 29*(7), 1029.

Ziv, A., Small, S. D., & Wolpe, P. R. (2000). Patient safety and simulation-based medical education. *Medical Teacher, 22*(5), 489-496.

17

Using Media, Multimedia, and Technology-Rich Learning Environments

Enid Errante Zwirn, PhD, MPH, RN

As institutions of higher education and their schools of nursing create learning communities that are convenient, accessible, and student focused, media, multimedia, and electronically mediated technologies are increasingly used to support and enhance the teaching and learning that occur in these communities. The purposes of this chapter are to define the various types of media, to present a systematic course of action to guide the selection and use of media and the environments in which they are used, and to describe how the roles of faculty and students change when they use media or multimedia and adopt technology-rich learning environments.

MEDIA

The term *media* refers to the models, images, and audio or video aids used to convey messages. Each type of media accomplishes specific purposes and has advantages and disadvantages (Table 17-1). Instructional media are typically categorized as follows: *realia and models*, providing visual, tactile, auditory, kinesthetic, and sometimes olfactory channels for learning; *still visuals* (non-projected and projected), providing information to be carried visually to a more concrete level than the level of verbal symbols alone; *moving visuals*, providing for motion and the manipulation of temporal and spatial perspectives for learning; and *audio media*, providing for the recording and transmission of information that can be accessed aurally. Each of these categories of instructional media is discussed along with consideration for use.

Realia and Models

Realia are actual objects that provide the learner with the most concrete learning experiences, whereas *models* "are three-dimensional representations of a real thing . . . and may be larger, smaller, or the same size as the objects [they represent]" (Heinich et al., 1996, p. 412). Models have some

TABLE 17–1   **Advantages and Disadvantages of Various Types of Media and Multimedia**

CATEGORY	ADVANTAGES	DISADVANTAGES
Realia and models (mannequins, models, patients)	Represent reality Can be manipulated Facilitate simulating psychomotor skills Models decrease risk to patients	Expense Difficult to use with a large audience
Nonprojected still visuals (photographs, diagrams, graphics, posters, cartoons, handouts)	Inexpensive to produce Can be developed by students Easy to transport or distribute	Difficult to display to a large group Graphic materials have high culturals specificity
Projected still visuals (overhead transparencies, slides, hard copy used with document cameras)	Easy to produce with presentation software Quick way to project enlarged materials	Requires use of projector and screen display Room must be darkened
Moving visuals (films, videotapes, videodiscs)	Effective way to show motion and sound Can be used independently by students	Requires projection equipment
Audio (audiotapes, compact discs)	Inexpensive Easy to use and store Facilitates self-paced and independent study Portable	Requires equipment (CD-player, tape deck) Tapes may be erased and reused
Multimedia (CAI, CD-ROM, interactive videodiscs, virtual reality, Internet, & WWW)	Engages all senses Facilitates interactive, collaborative, and independent learning Cost-effective when used with large numbers of students	Expensive to produce/ purchase Requires specific hardware to use

CAI, Computer-assisted instruction; *WWW,* World Wide Web.

advantages over realia in that they can be modified to accentuate certain details or disassembled to provide interior views. Realia and models are most often used in classroom demonstrations or in learning resource centers to provide students with an opportunity to practice nursing skills and simulate patient care.

Whether they are using realia or models, students should be encouraged to handle and manipulate each medium. To facilitate easy student access, the instructor may need to bring more than one of the same item to a group of students. Another suggestion is for the instructor to place a series of different objects, with their supportive texts and instructions, around the classroom and have learners visit each in turn. Learning resource centers provide students with opportunities for individual or group learning during scheduled class periods or at other times convenient for the students (for additional discussion see Chapter 16).

Nonprojected Still Visuals

Nonprojected visuals do not require projection for viewing. These graphic materials include still pictures, drawings, charts, graphs, posters, and cartoons designed specifically to communicate a message to the viewer. Some of these materials might be posted or distributed during class meetings; others might appear in prepared course handouts.

Graphic materials often include verbal and symbolic visual cues, and as forms of communication, are becoming more important within a global society in helping to overcome language and other barriers to communication. Faculty should be aware that visual symbols can mean different things to students from different cultural groups, and sometimes students misinterpret the intended meaning (Fleming & Levie, 1978; Heinich et al., 1996; Teague et al., 1994).

Still pictures are "photographic (or photograph-like) representations of people, places and things" (Heinich et al., 1996, p. 113). Still pictures are readily available, easy to use, and relatively inexpensive; but the size of a still picture may limit its use with a group, unless multiple copies of the same picture are obtained or the picture is enlarged. Still pictures also only provide a two-dimensional representation; pictures of the same objects, taken from different angles, offset this problem.

Drawings, sketches, and diagrams "employ the graphic arrangement of lines to represent persons, places, things, and concepts. Drawings are, in general, more finished and representational than sketches, which are likely to lack detail" (Heinich et al., 1996, p. 114). Drawings are more likely than photographs to be correctly interpreted because drawings are less detailed and pertinent images are more easily seen. During presentations, faculty and students can use drawings, sketches, and diagrams to enhance specific instructional content.

Graphs improve the ability to communicate numerical information efficiently and effectively. Graphs can also show "relationships between units of the data and trends in the data" (Heinich et al., 1996, p. 115). Types of graphs include circle graphs, which show percentages or portions of a whole; bar graphs, which show relative performance of one or more items against one or more factors; line graphs, which provide for an overview of continual trends; and picture graphs, which are variations of bar graphs in which symbols depicting the items represented in the data are used. Graphs can be made easily by faculty and students using presentation software.

Posters "incorporate visual combinations of images, lines, colors, and words. They are intended to catch and hold the viewer's attention at least long enough to communicate a brief message, usually a persuasive one" (Heinich et al., 1996, p. 117). Posters should communicate a single idea "and when kept on display, are a continuing reminder of information being used" within an instructional setting (Teague et al., 1994, p. 8).

The most effective posters convey a single, simple message. Posters can be designed by nursing students or faculty to stimulate interest in new topics, to increase motivation, to promote safety, or to promote good health practices. By designing their own posters, students can be encouraged to select and present key concepts (Moneyham et al., 1996; Sorenson & Boland, 1991). Posters that depict successful community partnerships or clinical research efforts are often designed for and displayed at nursing conferences.

Cartoons are simple line drawings. These rough caricatures of real or imagined persons or sentient animals are among the most widely available of the visual formats. Cartoons, through their wit and wisdom, appeal to all age groups. However, cartoons that fall outside the intellectual and experiential range of students or patients may not be understood or appreciated.

When editorial cartoons are used, it is important to remember that people tend to project their own feelings and prejudices onto cartoons. Thus cartoons that are easily interpreted and well received by one group of learners may not be meaningful, or might even be offensive, to another group. Students can be encouraged to draw their own cartoons relating to a wide variety of subjects—including student life, community health issues, and health promotion—to reinforce instruction.

Projected Still Visuals

"Projected visuals are . . . media formats in which still images are enlarged and displayed on a screen. Such projection is usually achieved by passing a strong light through transparent film (overhead transparencies, slides, and filmstrips) magnifying the image through a series of lenses, and casting this image onto a reflective surface" (Heinich et al., 1996, p. 140). Not only are new developments in the projection of computer-generated visuals onto a reflective surface becoming more common in nursing education, but the projection equipment itself is becoming smaller and even portable. ELMOs* (for *Electricity Light Machine Organizations*) attach to a laptop computer and allow faculty and students to "present images of virtually anything, to anyone, anywhere, at any time" (ELMO, 2003). As nurse educators develop greater expertise with integration of ELMOs, document cameras, digital cameras, and WhiteBoards, these technologies will join the ranks of overhead and slide projectors in ease of use.

Moving Visuals

Moving visuals include film and video-related technologies (including videocassettes), video on the World Wide Web, and digital versatile disks (DVDs) and compact discs (CDs) that incorporate stored motion pictures. Moving visuals add motion to the projected visual image and present a process more effectively than other media. Moving visuals permit safe observation of phenomena that might be hazardous to view directly. Faculty can also use moving visuals to dramatize events and situations, explore personal and social attitudes, enhance problem-solving instructional situations, and teach the subtleties of unfamiliar cultures. Finally, moving visuals serve as a method of gaining student attention to the topic and cue the learner to the most relevant components of instruction.

Film: Thomas A. Edison believed that film would revolutionize education and would give "new life to curricular content and provide students with new motivation for learning" (Heinich et al., 1996, p. 204). Although this dream

---

*ELMO Corporation, Plainview, NY.

was not realized, the applications of *film attributes* to changing space and time provide for unique and attractive learning options. Spatial perspectives are commonly modified by "zooming in" or "out." The compression of time can appear to have taken place through time-lapse photography. The expansion of time can be demonstrated by filming in slow motion. Animation can be achieved through use of a series of drawings or photographs evidencing small displacements in the space of objects or images or by the use of computers.

The limitations of film (size, weight, expense, and technical complexities) have been so modified by the adoption of video-related technologies (such as videocassettes, satellite television, DVDs, and CDs) that film as a medium is receiving less emphasis (Teague et al., 1994). The positive attributes of film, realized by newer video technologies, provide unique features for teaching, such as instant production and playback.

DVD technology: This technology can be categorized as either still or moving visual media. DVD technology offers the capacity to provide motion video, a combination of motion and still video, or still video alone. DVD is a "high density mass storage medium . . . capable of storing large amounts of information due to improvements in recording density and use of multiple layers per side" (Mehlinger & Powers, 2002, p. 311). DVD technology is now coupled with computer-managed instruction, providing the learner with ready access to textual, numerical, and graphic instructional material.

ScreenWatch Producer 5.0*: This is a "full-motion and full-screen recording software" that combines the instructor's voice (or video) with computer applications (such as spreadsheets, and PowerPoint[†] or interactive whiteboard content) in real time for Web streaming (Meonske, 2003).

Audio Media

Audio media include "the various means of recording and transmitting the human voice and other sounds for instructional purposes" (Heinich et al., 1982, p. 140). Audio media tend to be inexpensive, simple to use, easily adapted, and portable. Audio media can be used in nursing education for self-paced instruction, mastery learning, drill and practice, interview skills, or performance evaluation. Audiotape recordings can be used to record patient data to be communicated between teams of nurses ("shift reports") or to record nursing students' responses to a field experience before returning to the health care agency.

Cassette tapes are inexpensive, virtually immune to shock and abrasion, and easy to store. However, because cassette tapes use magnetic storage, data can be lost when tapes are exposed to elevated levels of electromagnetic radiation as might be found near some diagnostic medical equipment. Accidental erasure of cassette tapes, by rerecording, can be prevented by fracturing and removing the small plastic tabs on the back of the cassette. Many commercial cassettes are already packaged in this fashion. An efficient addition to use of cassette tape-recorded speech is the audio feature known as *rate-controlled audio playback*. This feature allows for the tape to be played back at a rate faster or slower than the rate at which it was recorded without altering either the pitch

---

[*]OPTX International, Magalia, CA,
[†]Microsoft Corporation, Mountain View, CA.

or the intelligibility of the original. Learners wishing to revisit a recorded lecture can listen at their own pace without distortion. Books on tape can be heard at rates as much as 50% faster than originally spoken.

CDs provide for high-quality digital recording and random access capabilities (the learner can move quickly between recorded tracks for individual selection). CDs, unlike cassette tapes, do not degrade under normal use and can be accessed without distortion for many years. Audio material that is already in digital form can be copied (or "burned") on to new CDs at relatively little cost.

Real Audio is a computer application that captures sound and stores it as files that can be transmitted over the Internet, opened, and used at a later date. Real Audio can also be used to support multimedia presentations to provide sound or narration to accompany the presentation.

Faculty may wish to reconsider the use of audio media. Media go in and out of favor, and audio media have been supplanted, in the popular view, by more sophisticated technologies that integrate audio media with other channels of learning. However, audio media may easily serve many instructional and learning needs because of their ease of use, portability, and low cost.

MULTIMEDIA

The term *multimedia* refers to any combination of video, audio, text, and graphics. A *multimedia computer* is a "computer configured with the necessary hardware to be able to use multimedia software that combines text, sound, video, and animation" (Mehlinger & Powers, 2002, p. 313). The strengths of several media can be combined to appeal to a variety of learning styles and facilitate learning. The benefits of using multimedia include reduction in the cost of teaching and learning and improved learning effectiveness as a result of increased learner motivation, improved retention of learning, interactivity, satisfaction, and opportunities for peer and faculty collaboration (Gleydura et al., 1995).

ELECTRONICALLY MEDIATED LEARNING

Computer-based Instruction

Computer-based instruction, computer-assisted instruction, computer-assisted learning, and *computer-based training* refer to the use of the computer to guide learning and create learning communities (Gleydura et al., 1995). The computer programs (software) can be used as tutorials, simulations, and tests or to enrich or remediate learning. In a distributed computing environment in which students work on a network that provides access to software, files, and electronic mail, computer-mediated learning promotes dialogue, inquiry, collaboration, and shared interactive learning experiences. These networks create virtual classrooms and knowledge communities that can be accessed at any time and any place (Brown & Duguid, 1996).

Tutorials teach new concepts to students. A tutorial program assumes that the student has little or no prior knowledge of the particular subject matter.

Generally, tutorials present facts and principles, ask the student to interact with the content by answering questions, and then on the basis of the student's response, provide feedback and move on to the next component of the lesson.

Simulations, in the context of computer-based instruction, fulfill the same goals of simulations in general; but computer simulations have additional multimedia capabilities. Programs that teach learners about a wide variety of subjects are being used in nursing schools to allow learners to individualize decision making, develop critical thinking skills, and create plans for patient care. Most of these programs use text, audio, video, graphic, and motion capabilities (Bolwell, 1995).

Testing by computers gives the faculty member the opportunity to develop, grade, administer, and perform statistical measurements of an examination (item analysis, standard deviation, mean, median, mode) with ease. A wide variety of computerized test development software programs are available to facilitate the development and administration of tests (Kirkpatrick et al., 1996).

Computer-based testing can also be used to assess learning needs and learning styles (Billings, 1991), administer pretests or posttests to determine mastery, or simply to provide the student with an opportunity to practice taking tests related to specific content areas for self-evaluation of learning. Another example of the use of the computer to facilitate testing is the use of software for preparing students for licensing or certification examinations (Billings et al., 1996; Ross et al., 1996).

Virtual Reality

In virtual reality, learners vicariously interact within "virtual worlds" through "the display and control of synthetic scenes by means of a computer and peripherals which sense a user's movements, such as data gloves, helmets, or joysticks" (Gayeski, 1993, p. 6). Although the potential of virtual reality in nursing education has yet to be fully explored, it is believed that virtual reality will bring about two major changes in education. First, education by textbook abstractions will be supplanted by experiential learning in naturalistic settings; second, the focus in education will move from written texts to a reliance on imagery and symbols (Helsel, 1993).

The World Wide Web

The World Wide Web is an intuitive, multimedia platform for accessing information. Information contained on the Web is not in alphabetical or hierarchical order but is organized in relationship to other information, referred to as *hyperlinks.* The same information can be accessed through multiple paths. Databases from around the world can be easily, quickly, and almost effortlessly reviewed; needed information can be downloaded onto one's own computer and printed out (Levine & Baroudi, 1993). As our society moves from an industrial to a knowledge economy, nurse educators will increasingly find themselves working in what has been called "integrated learning environments" that "[combine] in-class teaching and learning modalities with robust electronically mediated experiences" (Skill & Young, 2002, p. 25).

SELECTING MEDIA

Regardless of type and attributes, media should be selected to facilitate teaching and learning. Several principles can be used to guide selection.

Media should be selected for the learner's level of readiness. As instructional technologies become more complex, students must be trained in their appropriate use. Instruction in the use of the computer, DVDs, and CDs is necessary before a student can independently access a computer-based instructional package. Until that time, other media need to be used to present that content.

Media should be selected for use in an environment that is conducive to learning. The environment for learning should be physically comfortable, should be emotionally supportive, and should encourage students to participate. Students should have convenient access to this environment, and support staff should be available to assist with technical problems (Khoiny, 1995; North, 2002).

Media should contain information relevant to the learner's interest and use. Relevance and motivation are closely linked. Carl Rogers (1902-1987), the renowned clinical psychologist, emphasizes this principle when he notes that "the time for learning . . . would be cut to a fraction of the time currently allotted if the material were perceived by the learner as related to his own purposes" (Spradley, 1990, p. 311).

Media should be appropriate for the audience. It is known that more effective communication occurs when the source and the receiver are similar. To enhance communication, faculty might choose pictorial examples that reflect the composition of the intended audience (Fleming & Levie, 1978). Males and females, young and older adults, persons of many ethnic backgrounds, and persons wearing or not wearing identifiable uniforms may all be depicted as nursing students. A visual with outdated styles of uniforms or equipment will quickly cause students to question the competence of the content being presented.

Media should provide learners with opportunities to apply knowledge. Application—whether by answering questions, manipulating models, or identifying application in patient care—helps students integrate the content presented. Media should never stand alone.

Media should be selected to support the learning experience. Edgar Dale (1969) has arranged various teaching methods into a hierarchy of lesser to greater abstraction—from the most concrete experiences to the most abstract experiences—in the form of a cone (Figure 17-1). As the teaching methods move away from the cone's base, they become more and more abstract. According to Dale (1969), the learner is able to more profitably apply the more abstract instructional activities *only* after having experienced that content on a more concrete level that would give meaning to the abstract representation of reality. Faculty, cognizant that instructional media provide different degrees of experimental concreteness, can choose media that match the level of abstraction desired within a teaching-learning experience. For example, learning in a real situation might include field study or internships in clinical agencies.

Learning through interpretation of a real situation might include demonstration, simulations, role playing, or dramatizations in conferences held after an incident has taken place. Learning through vicarious representations of the real situation might include listening to audio recordings, interacting with computer programs, or watching videotapes or DVDs in learning laboratories. Learning through verbal descriptions of the real recorded situation might occur through listening to live lectures, participating in discussion sessions, or reading about the situation.

Media carry messages from the sender or transmitter (a human being or an inanimate object) to the receiver. Faculty should first identify the content of the lesson and the information the learner should receive, then match media choice to the particular lesson content or the objectives of the lesson. Several media alternatives for presenting the instruction, providing for practice, or evaluating student performance could be made available.

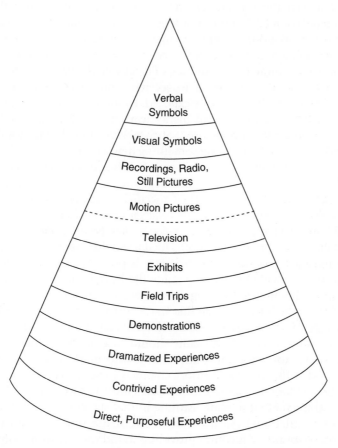

FIGURE 17-1   Dale's cone of experience. (From Audio-Visual Methods in Teaching, Third Edition, by Edgar Dale, Copyright 1969 by Holt, Rinehart and Winston, Inc., reprinted by permission of the publisher.)

Cost, preferred learning styles, and preferred teaching styles play important roles in media selection. Media must be eliminated from consideration if their costs cannot be justified. *Cost-effective media* achieve objectives at lower cost when capital and running costs (costs incurred during use) between alternative media are compared. Fortunately, even with all the considerations noted previously, nurse faculty members have many media choices that can be used to satisfy the demands of the messages that need to be transmitted.

If the messages are to be informational only (the receiver of the information is not held responsible for measurable, specific actions or performance), a medium providing *one-way or unidirectional communication* is sufficient. These applications may be viewed primarily as presentation media and technology and lend themselves well to formal presentations. Examples of one-way communication media include printed handouts, traditional textbooks, audiotapes or videotapes, materials available in reference centers, and dial-access retrieval systems.

If the messages are to be instructional (the receiver of the instruction is to give demonstrable proof that he or she has learned), *two-way communication* is required between the transmitter and the receiver. These applications can include interactive media and technology and are designed for individual use but may be used in group learning settings as well. Examples of two-way communication include a lecture followed by exercises, computer-mediated instruction, programmed texts, and tests (Teague et al., 1994).

Learners become accustomed to receiving messages from the types of media to which they are frequently exposed. By looking at the typical forms of instruction used at institutions of higher learning, faculty can rapidly determine those media traditionally used. Such observation should not deter the nurse faculty member from trying something new, because the novelty of a different instructional medium often receives much learner attention.

Romiszowski (1981) suggests that faculty follow two rules when attempting to match media with the level of specificity required by the established objectives. First, *"If you expect a certain behavior from the learner after instruction, you should give him opportunities to practice that behavior during instruction"* (p. 348, italics in original). Instructional media should be provided to the learner in locations where practice of the behavior is possible. Although auditory or visual instruction may initially help guide the learner, materials to which the learner can apply the new learning directly must be made available. Learning laboratories in which learners can first watch instructional videos or films and then go to the materials to practice the skills depicted follow this rule.

The second rule states that faculty should "use the most appropriate sensory channels for communicating the information to be learned" (Romiszowski, 1981, p. 349). Sensory channels include vision, sound, touch, smell, taste, and kinesthetics. If the objectives include psychomotor behaviors, instructional media that provide learning in that sensory channel (i.e., realia, models, or simulations) are most desirable. If the objectives include only recognition of sounds, a medium providing sound transmission only, such as an audiotape or a CD, should suffice.

In summary, media selection is based on three important considerations: What are the learner's objectives? What are the learner's special needs? What are instructional strategies selected by the faculty? The selection of appropriate media may be initially challenging and time consuming. However, learner acceptance and dependence on technological applications are high. Nursing faculty who familiarize themselves with and select (often with student input) appropriate media will find that presentation of information, provision for student practice, and evaluation of student performance are not only facilitated but enriched.

USING MEDIA

Once faculty and students have selected appropriate media, they are ready to integrate it into the course or assignments. Using media involves planning and preparation and becoming a showperson.

Planning for Using Media

Heinich et al. (1996) constructed a procedural model with the acronym *ASSURE*, "because it is intended to ASSURE effective use of media in instruction" (p. 34). The *six steps of the ASSURE model* ask that the educator do the following:

1. *A*nalyze learners for general characteristics, specific entry competencies (knowledge, skills, and attitudes about the topic), and learning styles.
2. *S*tate objectives or learning outcomes as specifically as possible. Objectives should be stated behaviorally (what the student will be able to do, the conditions under which the student's performance is to take place, and the criteria established for success).
3. *S*elect, modify, or design instructional materials.
4. *U*se those materials and follow them up with class discussion, small group activities, or individual projects and reports.
5. *R*equire learner response to help process the knowledge or skills and obtain feedback before formal assessment takes place.
6. *E*valuate the media used for their impact and effectiveness.

The ASSURE model provides a systematic plan for incorporation of media into learning experiences. It is especially useful to attend to those three areas of media application most often overlooked: the initial analysis of learner characteristics, the reinforcement of correct learning by requiring learner response, and the final evaluation of chosen media in aiding the learner's attainment of stated objectives.

Preparing and Using Media

It is also necessary to prepare carefully for using media. Teague et al. (1994) suggest the following five-step utilization procedure for faculty and students when they are preparing to use instructional media:

1. Preparing yourself: Carefully review the instructional materials to be used for content appropriate to the established objectives. If a study

guide is provided with the medium, the instructor should identify which related audience preparation or suggested follow-up activities might be explored. Sometimes only a portion of the instructional materials should be used, and that portion should be identified.

2. Preparing the environment: The environment must often be adjusted for use of the media. Tasks might include rearrangement of seating for optimum viewing, hearing, and accommodation of individuals with mobility challenges; setting up and testing of the necessary equipment; and controlling ventilation and available room light.

3. Preparing the audience: Preparing the audience for instruction is the most crucial step in the entire process of using media. Bring the audience to the point at which they are ready to learn. This may be accomplished by presenting a broad overview of the content of the presentation, by pointing out specific content to which the learner is to pay special attention, or by defining unfamiliar vocabulary or visual cues. Learners can also be provided with a guide or set of questions to be answered during or after use of the materials. When learners are well prepared, they are more active participants and are more likely to see relevance of the media to the topic being presented.

4. Using the media: Faculty and students who have prepared themselves well are confident that their learners will experience the planned outcomes when the media are used. They will demonstrate technical ease with the equipment and be able to "troubleshoot" technical breakdowns. Last, they understand that they, too, "are an instructional medium" and apply effective media use practices.

5. Combining the media with other learning: Instructional media are components of planned sequences of learning activities and must be integrated with the entire instructional design process to be maximally effective. It is important that content presented within instructional media be connected to content provided by other sources, namely, reading materials, other students, and faculty (Teague et al., 1994). As noted earlier, media should never stand alone.

Faculty can maintain an appraisal checklist on which they can record pertinent data about each medium or instructional material reviewed. Data in one generalized checklist include title, producer and distributor, length, brief description, entry capabilities required (what the learner must be able to do before the medium can be applied successfully), rating, requirements, and strong and weak points. Another evaluation guide includes many of these considerations and adds, among other considerations, evaluative areas about the material's consistency with the local curriculum and freedom from bias, prejudiced attitudes, and concepts (Teague et al., 1994).

Presentation Skills

Media are often a component of courses and presentations; thus faculty should consider presentation factors that must be performed effectively if a presentation is to be successful. Behavior, such as dominance, and physicality, such as movement and body position, should be considered, as well as projection principles.

Body Position and Movement

If the front of the classroom is thought of as a stage, the position directly centered and closest to the audience is the most dominant. Thus if the audience is to attend to a model or screen, the model or screen should be placed "front and center," with the presenter off to the side. When moved away from the learners and toward the right (as seen by the audience), a person or medium that occupies that position becomes less strong.

Many speakers, for emphasis or to signal the beginning of a new topic, successfully use movement. If the presenter moves from a less to a more dominant position in front of the learners, the point being made at that time is likely to be underscored. Movement toward a centered visual adds dramatic emphasis to that visual and increases learner interest.

Movement may be excessive, however, if it distracts the learner from the points being made. The presenter should also avoid distracting mannerisms. Such mannerisms may remain unknown to the presenter unless he or she has had an opportunity to be videotaped during a presentation. Videotaping and other similar forms of feedback allow the presenter to become aware of nervous movements or oft-repeated and unnecessary phrases, such as "you know."

Body positions assumed by the presenter have been rated for strength. The full-front body position is the strongest. The three-quarter full-front position is the second strongest. The one-quarter view, with the back nearly turned toward the audience, is the weakest position. Thus, for the strongest presentation, when pointing to an aspect of a projected image, a faculty member should point with the arm closest to the screen, while facing front, rather than making a one-quarter turn away from the learners.

Projecting Media

Projection principles are applied to a wide variety of projected media (including overheads, slides, computer graphics, and videotapes) to increase legibility and visibility. The "two by six rule" suggests that the closest a viewer should be placed to a projected image is two times the width of the screen. Conversely, the farthest a viewer should be placed from a projected image is a distance no greater than six times the width of the viewing screen (Heinich et al., 1996; Teague et al., 1994).

The projected image should fill the screen, and the bottom of the projected image should be at the viewer's eye level. The projection equipment or the presenter should not block the view of learners, if possible.

The projection equipment should be placed parallel to the screen to prevent "keystoning" (a projected image that is trapezoidal rather than rectangular). Correction of keystoning, to maintain a parallel relationship between the projection equipment and the screen, may require moving the projection equipment or moving or tying back the bottom of the screen.

One last consideration for projected images is the placement of the screen. A screen placed in the corner of a classroom allows for simultaneous use of a projected image and a chalkboard. To lessen the amount of ambient light that reaches the screen and reduces image brightness, the presenter should place the screen in front of the windows that have the greatest light leakage.

Heinich et al. (1982) include four general tips for an individual involved in presenting audio or visual material. They suggest that the presenter do the following:

1. Promote a relaxed environment through the wise use of humor and by being natural and enthusiastic.
2. Keep a surprise in store by using unexpected conclusions or surprising visuals.
3. Control attention by maintaining eye contact and keeping the light source on the area to which attention is to be drawn. Turning off the visual's light source will again make the presenter the focus of the presentation.
4. Keep sight and sound synchronized. This requires careful scripting and watching the screen to be sure text and visuals match.

Presentation skills are not difficult to learn. The presenter (faculty member or student) who follows effective presentation guidelines provides for a more enjoyable, smoother, and stronger learning experience.

DESIGNING MEDIA

With the advent of low-cost, easy-to-use computer presentation systems, desktop publishing, and authoring software, more instructional material and courses are being developed by nursing faculty for their own and their colleagues' use (Goodman & Blake, 1996; Miller & Brigham, 1996). Nursing students can also develop and use instructional materials for patient instruction or class presentations.

In addition to decisions about the design of projected materials, slides, or visuals to be used alone or with other media (multimedia), the effectiveness of the visuals must be considered. "The effectiveness of visuals is measured by the degree of learner recall of its content" (Teague et al., 1994, p. 257); thus whatever visuals are used should attract attention and hold the interest of the learner. Visual messages should adhere to the following basic design principles:

- *Balance,* which is "a form of equilibrium within a composition that is used to provide coherence for all the other elements" (Teague et al., 1994, p. 258).
- *Emphasis,* which helps the student identify the main theme. Note that English-speaking Americans are accustomed to reading from left to right and from top to bottom, but that order is not universally followed. Pointers, used to direct the student, would be placed to the right if the materials were developed for the use of Israelis or to the top if they were to be used for a Chinese audience (Teague et al., 1994). In a classroom of diverse students, the significance of linguistic and cultural variance cannot be overlooked; assuming that every audience is com-

posed only of English-speaking Americans places other groups at a disadvantage.

- *Simplicity,* which makes it easier for the student to identify key elements. Faculty are admonished to "limit text messages to 20 words for projected visuals. . . . Use a single line, rather than multiple lines for titles, place captions for a graphic inside the image area when possible, and . . . avoid placing words close to the edges of a visual page" (Teague et al., 1994, p. 259).
- *Unity,* which provides for "continuity of thought and ideas" through overlapped images, using a border around common objects or repeating shapes and colors (Teague et al., 1994, p. 259).

Other considerations for development of graphic materials include the following visual elements of design:

- *Lines,* which "attract attention by directing the eye to a specific object or area," or can "create a variety of effects such as motion, instability, or calmness" (Teague et al., 1994, p. 260).
- *Shapes,* which can be used to "attract attention or represent universal images recognized across cultures so as to provide clearer visual communications. Shapes might be geometric, symbolic, or abstract representations of familiar objects" (Teague et al., 1994).
- *Color and contrast,* which can serve to either unify or differentiate elements of a design. "Harmonious colors in a design unify its appearance" (Teague et al., 1994, p. 260), whereas "contrasting colors can be used to highlight or emphasize a portion of the design" (Teague et al., 1994, p. 260). Although the use of black and white can sometimes be preferable for reasons of visual simplicity, "research indicates that the appropriate use of color makes a visual more attractive to the viewer" (Teague et al., 1994, p. 260). Attractive visual sources are deemed more influential in instruction designed to produce attitudinal change (Fleming & Levie, 1978).
- *Texture,* which is usually represented in visuals through the use of "repetitious patterns created in variations of lines and dots." (Teague et al., 1994, p. 261). These patterns may take on a characteristic of cloth or other material forms. "Texture can provide emphasis to certain parts of a visual as well as contribute to the overall unity." (Teague et al., 1994, p. 261). Texture can be created in a visual presentation through a variety of means, ranging from pencil strokes to complex computer graphical software (Teague et al., 1994, p. 261).
- *Space,* which can be used to create a visually pleasing presentation. "Space can be either negative or positive. The unused or open portions of a design are referred to as negative [or 'white'] space," (Teague et al., 1994, p. 262) and can help prevent the visual from becoming unnecessarily complicated and crowded. Positive space, the portion of the design that is filled with text or images, should be the focal point of the design.
- *Size,* which can "attract attention to certain elements of a visual. Larger images usually gain greater attention from the viewer, if all other visual

elements are equal [in size]" (Teague et al., 1994, p. 261). For creating projected visuals, use of a font size of 18 points or larger is recommended (Pacific Lutheran University, 1999), and the images should be prepared by using the landscape, or horizontal, plane.

Collins (1991) suggests that technology-mediated instruction will influence teaching and learning in eight "shifts" that will dramatically change the teaching-learning environment. These shifts will move the student from a passive learner to one who is independent and self-directed. The faculty role will change from that of content provider to that of mentor and facilitator. (This shift in faculty roles has been referred to as "moving from the 'sage-on-the-stage' to the 'guide on the side.'")

Collins expects the following:

1. A shift *from lecture and recitation to coaching*. If the direction for the content is provided by means of interactive technologies, faculty will be able to spend more of their time facilitating student learning.
2. A shift *from whole-class instruction to small-group instruction*. Students need no longer move in lockstep through material. Faculty, interacting more with individual students and small groups of students, can address student misunderstandings and assess learning.
3. A shift *from working with better students to working with weaker students*. The faculty member is freed to identify and target student populations at risk and devote more time to those students who need more help.
4. A shift from every student learning the same thing to *different students* being recognized, and perhaps being rewarded for *learning different things*.
5. A shift toward *more engaged students*. With interactive technology, attention is ensured because instruction comes to a halt when there are no responses from learners.
6. A shift toward *assessment on the basis of products and progress* rather than on test performance. Nursing students will be assessed on projects that include realistic tasks that incorporate what is being learned and show how these concepts and principles are applied to new areas.
7. A shift *from a competitive to a cooperative goal structure*. Students will share their own work, developed from extensive databases, through networked communication systems. Faculty will generate new methods of assessment according to the collaborative nature of student products.
8. A shift *from the primacy of verbal thinking to the integration of visual and verbal thinking*. Multimedia has the capacity to engage a variety of senses. The visual support for learning will supplement the auditory (listening) mode, and learners will integrate and use both channels.

HIGH-TECH CLASSROOMS

If located on campus, the shifts that Collins mentions often occur within spaces variously referred to as *high-tech, mediated, technology-rich,* or *technology-*

enabled classrooms. A convergence of technologies has produced teaching-learning environments in which actively engaged students, using high-tech communications equipment, can participate in desktop experiments, collaborative learning activities, and student-faculty dialogue.

Technologies may differ in classrooms considered "high-tech." The usual technologies that might be found in high-tech classrooms include ceiling-mounted video projector(s), an instructor workstation with videoconferencing and World Wide Web (WWW) interactivity, multiple interactive student workstations, multiple student microphones, a document camera, an electronic WhiteBoard, and networked printers.

The seating arrangements in high-tech classrooms may also differ. All, however, have innovative seating arrangements to encourage students to take more active and collaborative roles in the learning process (Graetz & Goliver, 2002; Skill & Young, 2002). For example, the Massachusetts Institute of Technology (2001) has transformed some traditional classrooms with chairs on one level, into amphitheater-style rooms with fixed tables and loose chairs to encourage group work. Arizona State University has some classrooms with team-based seating where the instructor has the ability to project student work on to main screens. The Rose-Hulman Institute of Technology, with its completely networked campus environment, requires that every student purchase a specified laptop computer at the time of enrollment. Also, at Rose-Hulman, many classrooms are equipped with network and power connections with which students can access software and applications for individual or group work. At Texas A&M University, in large classes of approximately 100 students, one computer is provided for every two students. Students at Texas A&M sit in teams (for collaborative work), at rectangular tables, perpendicular to the placement of the faculty workstation (for ease of faculty observation) and may observe projected materials on screens on both sides of the classroom (so students do not have to turn from side to side) (Cordes & Froyd, 2002).

Furniture should "facilitate learning, not just be a place to sit" (Cornell, 2002, p. 37) In high-tech classrooms one no longer sees rows of single chairs with armrests. Furniture is selected that "[helps] the instructor and student achieve their goals using the methods and tools of their choice" (Cornell, 2002, p. 37). Cornell, in the chapter, "The Impact of Changes in Teaching and Learning on Furniture and the Learning Environment," speaks to five aspects of furniture functionality that support the emerging paradigm of teaching and learning. Rooms must be able to be *readily reconfigured* from lecture to small group setups and unused equipment must be able to be easily stored ("fold-n-go"). Ubiquitous *access to technology* should be available to students and faculty ("plug-n-play"). *Presentation, modification, recording, and retrieval of information* for both faculty and students must be supported ("say-n-see"). The environment must *provide for both individual student concentration and student collaboration* ("relate-n-reflect"). Last, Cornell emphasizes that the teaching-learning environment should be *"fun, energetic, and enjoyable"* ("inspire-n-invite").

In "Improving the Environment for Learning: An Expanded Agenda," Chism and Bickford (2002) contrast new assumptions about learning space design with the old and share implications for current educational design practices. These implications include designs that (1) consider the whole campus as a potential learning space, (2) facilitate social interaction, (3) expand per-student space allocation, (4) amplify both faculty and student input, and (5) foster broad participation and collaboration among "multiple actors" in the design process.

MEDIA AND NEW ROLES FOR FACULTY AND STUDENTS

Goldberg (1999), in *Overcoming High-Tech Anxiety*, states "Historically people have always flourished when offered the opportunity for exploration and settlement of new frontiers. The electronic frontier offers such a world of opportunities and possibilities" (p. xv). Higher education is experiencing a paradigm shift from teaching to learning; the previous paradigm is no longer seen as having the "capacity to solve problems and generate a positive vision of the future" (Barr & Tagg, 1998, p. 708). Media have the potential to support and enhance learning experiences, and the use of media, by both nursing faculty and students, will help them find ways both to "produce information that can be used to build knowledge, and a way of communicating that information" (Goldberg, 1999, p. 155).

The shift from content-centered presentations to shared quests between students and faculty to use existing information to answer questions and solve problems will facilitate modeling, foster creativity, and enhance active and collaborative learning. Recognition of, and respect for, individual competencies, needs, and interests will make it possible for each student to travel a unique route to successful education in nursing. Faculty who remain open to change and administrators who anticipate and support what forms education might take in an age rich in instructional media (especially electronic information) will find themselves sometimes anxious, many times challenged, and always growing.

SUMMARY

This chapter explored the use of media, multimedia, and technology-rich learning environments in educational settings for nurses. By gaining an understanding of the basic precepts of media and modifications supportive of a new teaching learning paradigm, learning experiences for nursing students and faculty will become more fruitful, effective, and fulfilling.

REFERENCES

Billings, D. (1991). Assessing learning styles using a computerized learning style inventory. *Computers in Nursing, 9*(3), 121-125.

Billings, D., Hodson-Carlton, K. E., Kirkpatrick, J. M., et al. (1996). Computerized NCLEX-RN preparation programs: A comparative review. *Computers in Nursing, 14*(5), 272-286.

Bolwell, C. (1995). *Directory of educational software for nursing.* Alexandria, VA: Stewart Publishing, Inc.

Brown, J. S., & Duguid, P. (1996). Universities in the digital age. *Change, 28*(4), 11-19.

Chism, N. V. N., & Bickford, D. J. (2002) Improving the environment for learning: An expanded agenda. In N. V. N. Chism & D. J. Bickford (Eds.), *The importance of physical space in creating supportive learning environments: New directions for teaching and learning* (92) (pp. 91-97). San Francisco: Jossey-Bass.

Collins, A. (1991). The role of computer technology in restructuring schools. *Phi Delta Kappan, 73*(1), 28-36.

Cordes, D., & Froyd, J. (2002) Engineering classrooms before and after innovation. Paper presented at Pedagogical Network for Engineering Education, Copenhagen, Denmark. Retrieved March 12, 2004, from cordes@cs.ua.edu

Cornell, P. (2002). The impact of changes in teaching and learning on furniture and the learning environment. In N. V. N. Chism & D. J. Bickford (Eds.), *The importance of physical space in creating supportive learning environments: New directions for teaching and learning* (pp. 33-42). San Francisco: Jossey-Bass.

Dale, E. (1969). *Audio-visual methods in teaching* (3rd ed.). Austin, TX: Holt, Rinehart, & Winston.

ELMO. (2003). Retrieved March 22, 2004, from http://www.elmo-corp.com/presentation/menu.htm

Fleming, M., & Levie, W. H. (1978). *Instructional message design: Principles from the behavioral sciences.* Englewood Cliffs, NJ: Educational Technology Publications.

Gayeski, D. M. (Ed.). (1993). *Multimedia for learning.* Englewood Cliffs, NJ: Educational Technology Publications.

Gleydura, A. J., Michelman, J. E., & Wilson, C. N. (1995). Multimedia training in nursing education. *Computers in Nursing, 13*(4), 169-175.

Goldberg, B. (1999) *Overcoming high-tech anxiety.* San Francisco: Jossey-Bass.

Goodman, J., & Blake, J. (1996). Multimedia courseware, transforming the classroom. *Computers in Nursing, 14*(5), 287-296.

Graetz, K. A., & Goliber, M. J. (2002). Designing collaborative learning spaces: Psychological foundations and new frontiers. In N. V. N. Chism & D. J. Bickford (Eds.), *The importance of physical space in creating supportive learning environments: New directions for teaching and learning* (pp. 13-22). San Francisco: Jossey-Bass.

Heinich, R., Molenda, M., & Russell, J. D. (1982). *Instructional media and the new technologies of instruction.* New York: John Wiley.

Heinich, R., Molenda, M., Russell, J. D., & Smaldino, S. E. (1996). *Instructional media and technologies for learning* (5th ed.). Englewood Cliffs, NJ: Merrill.

Helsel, S. K. (1993). Virtual reality and education. In D. M. Gayeski (Ed.), *Multimedia for learning.* Englewood Cliffs, NJ: Educational Technology.

Khoiny, F. E. (1995). Factors that contribute to computer-assisted instruction effectiveness. *Computers in Nursing, 13*(4), 165-168.

Kirkpatrick, J. M., Billings, D. M., Carlton, K. H., Cummings, R. B., Hanson, A. C., Malone, J., et al. (1996). Computerized test development software: A comparative review. *Computers in Nursing, 14*(2), 113-125.

Levine, J. R., & Baroudi, C. (1993). *The Internet for dummies.* Indianapolis, IN: IDG Books Worldwide.

Massachusetts Institute of Technology. (2001, December 12). New classrooms offer high-tech education in physics, mechanical engineering. *TechTalk,* 1-3. Retrieved June 16, 2003, from http://web.mit.edu/newsoffice/tt/2001/dec12/classroom.html

Mehlinger, H.D., & Powers, S.M. (2002) *Technology and teacher education: A guide for educators and policymakers.* Boston: Houghton-Mifflin Company.

Meonske, N. (2003, February). ScreenWatch Producer 5.0 multimedia lectures direct to the Web. *Syllabus, 16*(2), 38-39.

Miller, A. M., & Brigham, C. (1996). Creating your own computer-assisted instruction and interactive videodisc programs. *Perspectives on Community, 17*(4), 198-202.

Moneyham, L., Ura, D., Ellwood, S., & Bruno, B. (1996). The poster presentation as an educational tool. *Nurse Educator, 21*(4), 45-47.

North, J. D. G. (2002). Put your money where your mouth is: A case study. In N. V. N. Chism & D. J. Bickford (Eds.), *The importance of physical space in creating supportive learning environments: New directions for teaching and learning* (pp. 73-80). San Francisco: Jossey-Bass.

Pacific Lutheran University. (1999). *Designing presentation visuals.* Retrieved March 23, 2004, from http://www.plu.edu/libr/media/designing_visuals.html

Romiszowski, A. J. (1981). Media selection. In A. J. Romiszowski (Ed.), *Designing instructional systems* (pp. 339-359). New York: Nichols.

Ross, B., May, F., Nice, A., & Billings, D. (1996). Using computer NCLEX-RN review software to identify and assist students at risk for failing the computerized NCLEX-RN. *Nurse Educator, 21*(2), 39-43.

Skill, T. D., & Young, B. A. (2002). Embracing the hybrid model: Working at the intersections of virtual and physical learning spaces. In N. V. N. Chism & D. J. Bickford (Eds.), *The importance of physical space in creating supportive learning environments: New directions for teaching and learning* (pp. 23-32). San Francisco: Jossey-Bass.

Spradley, B. W. (1990). *Community health education. Community health nursing: Concepts and practice* (3rd ed.) (pp. 296-323). Glenview, IL: Scott, Foresman/Little, Brown Higher Education.

Sorenson, E. S., & Boland, D. (1991). Use of the poster session in teaching research critique to undergraduate nursing students. *Journal of Nursing Education, 30,* 334-340.

Teague, F. A., Rogers, D. W., & Tipling, R. N. (1994). *Technology and media.* Dubuque, IA: Kendall/ Hunt.

18

TEACHING AND LEARNING
AT A DISTANCE

Charlene E. Clark, MEd, RN, FAAN,
Roy W. Ramsey, EdD, MEd, BA

As colleges and universities struggle to become more competitive in the educational marketplace, administrators and faculty are striving to create attractive and cost-effective learning options that will improve teaching and learning. Distance education delivery systems that encourage innovation and flexibility have the potential for maximizing use of institutional infrastructure, improving access to credit courses, and providing consistency for learning at multiple locations. In nearly every educational setting, there has been a shift in organizational structure and pedagogy to accommodate distance teaching and learning.

Distance education is broadly defined as students receiving instruction in a location other than that of the faculty. This separation of teacher and student could be as close as within the same community or campus or as far away as across states or continents. The options of available delivery systems to implement distant academic courses or continuing education opportunities have become increasingly competitive and are frequently defined by cost; administrator; and faculty knowledge, acceptance, and readiness. Additionally, the computer and computer-based communication systems continue to have a positive and dramatic effect on teaching and learning, thus becoming invaluable tools for distance instruction. Because many different instructional delivery systems are available, faculty should find the discriminatory material presented in this chapter useful.

Distance education delivery systems are undergoing rapid change. In many cases technologies are merging with others to form a blend of delivery or are being replaced by new and innovative delivery options. Obsolescence of existing media within the next decade will be commonplace. However, the concepts related to leading, planning, using, supporting, administering, and evaluating student learning will remain applicable. The virtual classroom, defined for this purpose as the learning environment occurring wherever the student can access information, has become more common as colleges and universities endeavor to offer efficient and effective higher education opportunities to students anyplace and anytime.

In recent years, academic institutions have adopted the practice of extending curricular access to an audience that is more diverse and geographically separated by embracing the use of innovative educational technologies (Armstrong & Frueh, 2003; Billings et al., 1994a, 1994b; Clarke & Cohen, 1992; Dirksen et al., 1993; Fulmer et al., 1992; Heinich et al, 1999; Moore & Anderson, 2003; Novotny, 2000). A multitude of media comparison studies specific to distance education continue to maintain that there does not appear to be a negatively significant difference in learning between on-site and distance education students (Armstrong & Frueh, 2003; Billings & Bachmeier, 1994; Keck, 1992; Nichols et al., 1994; Simonson et al., 2000; Souder, 1993). The topic of "no significant difference" has become such a popular area of research that the International Distance Education Certification Center (IDECC) has published a summary of 355 reports and papers by Thomas L. Russell (1999). In addition, TeleEducation NB (2004) a nonprofit organization devoted to technology and training, created a website that identifies a historical chronology of research findings from this compilation with quotes from various publications about no significant difference. In nearly all comparison research, the findings are similar: distant learners perform as well or better than learners in the face-to-face environment.

Distance learning tends to capitalize on a constructivist, or problem-solving, approach to learning. This approach is in direct contrast to Gagne's (1979) distinct learning groups, which are based on a hierarchy of complexity and the need for mentoring and role modeling. However, distance learning seems to support Piaget's (2001) position that learning is not just inherent or experiential in nature, but a combination of both. Driscoll (2000) identifies constructivism as " . . . gaining popularity and momentum at the same time interactive, user-friendly computers are becoming widely available" (p. 394). Although other instructional media are not excluded from this consideration, the computer has had a huge impact on the learner's ability to construct and manage his or her own learning environment. Distance learning and computer-based instruction have created a newfound independence.

Although learning outcomes are similar for on-site and distance students, there is a continued need for development of a cohesive and engaging community environment within the delivery option. Moore and Kearsley (1996) consider distance education from a systems point of view by defining the social and structural framework for the virtual dynamics of this type of teaching and learning. Nursing faculties must consider this as they move forward with designing instructional approaches that incorporate distance delivery technologies.

The variety of options available to support distance instruction continues to increase as technologies improve and the transformation from a teacher focus to a learner focus becomes more prominent. "Sole reliance on the use of lecture is no longer an accepted teaching method. Instead, faculty are integrating the use of technology into their teaching and promoting the active involvement of students in the learning process" (Finke, 1998, p. 4). Online course management software has had an impact on this transformation by providing a learning environment that incorporates a support system for management including course information, announcements, communication for synchronous and asynchronous collaboration, and assessment. The shift to computer-based instruction has become so dramatic that selected offerings to distance students are designed entirely for online teaching and learning. "Three-fifths (62.5%) of the colleges and universities that participated in the 2002 Campus Computing Survey offer at least one complete online/Web-based college course" (Green, 2003, p. 14).

With this shift to computer-based instruction, the number of courses offered exclusively in the form of face-to-face instruction is substantially decreasing. However, many courses offer a blended, or hybrid, approach with other technologies such as interactive television, which can be accomplished by satellite, broadcast, microwave, or optical fibers and other electronic methods including audioconferencing, videoconferencing, videostreaming, and specialized computer applications. This chapter covers selected strategies used in educating students who are geographically dispersed and separated from a main campus of instruction. An overview of delivery systems, their advantages and disadvantages, and other pertinent information specific to each medium are also presented in Table 18-1.

SELF-DIRECTED LEARNING

For learning to occur, there must be a change in performance, or a potential for change, as a result of instruction (Driscoll, 2000). Not all students enter nursing education with the same background or understanding. Nor do all students learn in the same way or at the same pace. Instruction that is designed to meet a specific level of student development, which may have already been obtained through other means, does not necessarily meet the criteria set forth in Driscoll's definition. Through self-direction, the student learns by discovery in a constructivist approach, a method frequently used in nursing education. Nursing faculties have used autotutorial, individualized, or self-directed study to enhance curricula in a variety of pedagogically innovative and effective ways (Goldrick et al., 1990; Novotny, 2000). A wide range of design, development, and implementation of curricula has resulted in alternative strategies for use of the broadened terms of *independent, individualized,* and *guided study.* Regardless of the terminology chosen to describe the independent learning process, it should be clearly understood that the teacher is involved, at least somewhat, in leading, advising, planning, and evaluating student learning.

Independent study can be viewed from three quite different perspectives: (1) the course for which academic credit(s) is assigned at the time of enrollment; (2) the guiding materials to support the concept of learning most often referred to as *self-directed, individualized, autotutorial,* or *self-study;* and (3) the interaction built into the learning environment in support of the emotional, psychological, and educational needs. Components of motivation, critical thinking, and decision making should be included in the design and development of these materials as a stimulant for learning and the discovery process (Dick et al., 2000; Keller, 1999; Smith & Ragan, 1999; Ramsey, 2002).

Students at both undergraduate and graduate levels frequently have an opportunity to negotiate for an independent study course that will carry academic credit. Such work may be arranged to fulfill a credit deficit or to allow

TABLE 18–1   Instructional Delivery Systems

TYPE	ADVANTAGES	MAJOR DISADVANTAGES	COSTS RELATED TO TECHNOLOGY
I. Self-directed and independent study	Learner-centered Students can work at own convenience within a defined period Individual responsibility and accountability are encouraged Various strategies can be included A variety of media can be incorporated into the learning process	Requires a balance of curricular structure and flexibility Requires student self-discipline Entails possibility of limited feedback about performance	Initial labor-intensive costs to development of materials (self-directed) Time and involvement related to maintenance of materials Media enhancements are labor intensive and costly for initial development
II. Web-based instruction	Learner-centered Access anyplace and anytime Accommodates communication between many students Encourages collaborative educational endeavors Learner is exposed to multiple points of view in collaborative learning environment.	Other students are not seen; therefore nonverbal cues are missing Requires computer literacy and proficiency Requires self-motivation Technology and hardware-related problems 24/7 technical assistance	Modem Computer Charges for computer access Conferencing software Electronic access to full-text library resources Technology support Instructional design of courses
III. Satellite	Real-time video Requires minimum technical assistance at receive sites once downlink is positioned to satellite	One-way video; return audio is by telephone or instant message Requires technical staff at origination site	Satellite uplink and downlink equipment Rental fees for satellite access Technical staff salaries
IV. Broadcast television/ cable	Organized, well-planned presentations Scenarios can be produced to augment lectures Can be recorded off-air by home videocassette recorder for later viewing Convenient and easy to use	Real-time interaction with faculty member or other students is limited Programs are usually preproduced Requires technician, producers, and production facilities	Air time Support staff salaries Production studio

V. Interactive videoconferencing	Learner-centered Provides live visual interaction Equipment can usually be operated by students and faculty	A local coordinator within each classroom is available to handle needs and concerns at each site Sometimes presentation and media enhancements are limited	ISDN and proprietary networks require line fees High demand on network bandwidth Salaries to provide scheduling and technical support
VI. Videostream	Learner-centered Access anywhere Real-time/anytime delivery Archives available for on-demand use	Quality is directly related to connection speed and available bandwidth Limited two-way interaction Requires computer literacy Technical problems are common	High-speed line access High-quality computer Production staff salaries Support staff salaries
VII. Audioconferencing	Learner-centered Lowest cost of real-time distance learning strategies' Can be taught from or received at any location that has telephone access	Because live visual contact is missing, students may feel isolated A local coordinator handles needs and concerns at each site Styles of class presentation may need to be altered Visual learners and students with hearing limitations may be at a disadvantage	Long-distance telephone toll charges Audioconferencing equipment at receive sites, if more than one student is enrolled Salaries for site coordinators

ISDN, Integrated Services Digital Network.

the student to pursue a specialized theory or clinical interest not otherwise available within the nursing curricula. In such cases, the student usually works with the teacher to establish learning outcomes, and the process of meeting expectations for successful completion of the course is negotiated between learner and teacher. As the title implies, although there may be occasional meetings with the supervising faculty member, ultimate responsibility rests with the student to plan and execute the course.

The cost to implement an independent study course for academic credit is minimal and mostly related to the faculty member's time commitment. Tuition is paid by the student, as would be the case for any credit course.

Many nursing programs have designed portions of curricula to provide student independence as an accommodation for a personal learning pace for selected educational activities. The computer, supplemented with online courseware and access to the Internet, is commonly used to facilitate this individualized learning process. The pathways for meeting the educational objectives are clearly defined in materials presented to the students; however, the learners make choices as to the speed at which they will attain the objectives. Such guided study frequently includes learning modules or packets and regularly incorporates required activities that include a hands-on practice component. Computer-assisted instruction is another popular category of individualized discovery in which the instructional program controls the sequencing of events according to individual response. Simulation training has also become a popular computer-based option. Learning assessment is typically integrated for immediate and formative feedback (Goldrick et al., 1990; Heinich et al., 1999; Simonson & Thompson, 1997).

Modules, learning packets, Web-based instruction, computer-assisted instruction, and simulation training have an initial high cost because the design and development of these resources is labor intensive. However, once the materials have been developed and appropriately revised, incorporating piloted documentation, the ongoing expense is quite minimal. Learning modules used for this teaching strategy should be evaluated and updated frequently to ensure currency with literature, research, and practice.

Full-course correspondence instruction, one of the oldest versions of individualized distance instruction, is quickly yielding to computer-based instruction. For many years, correspondence instruction provided economical and efficient access to courses for many learners when special circumstances prevented them from following the more traditional approach (Pittman, 2003; Tallman, 1994). It is also used for special certification courses when student time and availability are limited. Although correspondence instruction remains a viable means for some course delivery when computer and Internet access are not available, it is rapidly losing popularity as a learning option. Most courses previously developed as correspondence text-based programs have been, or are being considered for redevelopment as Web-based options.

The primary advantages of Web-based instruction are the immediacy of access to content and the ability to correspond with the instructor and other students in real time (synchronous) or at any time (asynchronous). Students who enroll in these college or university courses are provided online access and all the features of the course management software. Videocassettes, audio-tapes, CD-ROMs, digital versatile disks (DVDs), videostreams, or other embedded media may supplement online materials. Learning assessment is commonly conducted online and is characterized by the ability of the faculty member to monitor student progress and provide feedback by e-mail or online discussion.

Web-based courses can be successful learning options for the independent and highly motivated student. Because the onus is on the learner to complete course work, students may find they lack the motivation to complete an online offering. Principles of systematic motivational design are needed for Web-based instruction (Bonk & Dennen, 2003; Clark, 1998; Dick et al., 2000; Keller, 1999; Ramsey, 2002; Smith & Ragan, 1999). Design features that allow for learner choice and control lead to a sense of duty and increased responsibility. These features coupled with interactive communication give the student a sense of community and social connectivity.

The number of credits that can be obtained through Web-based courses is a policy usually established by the institution conferring the degree. However, it is not uncommon to find that most colleges and universities allow a substantial percentage of course work leading to an undergraduate or graduate degree to be earned through an online format. Some degree programs are available totally online. Chapter 19 provides further discussion of online teaching and learning.

DISTANCE DELIVERY SYSTEMS

Distance delivery systems selected for inclusion in this chapter represent those strategies and technologies most commonly used at this time and those projected for use in the near future.

Classroom Instruction and Educational Television

Classrooms initially designed for on-campus seat-time instruction are common to nearly every college or university in the world. As demand for interactive distance education with the same instructional context grew, classrooms were designed or converted to incorporate video-based technology. Delivery was accomplished by using a variety of networked systems. Although they are expensive, these networks have done an excellent job of transmitting two-way interaction and linking multiple classrooms as an initiative to replicate the original classroom environment. Over time, computer-based technology has had an enormous impact on these networks by providing a means to more efficiently compress the video and audio components in a digital format that is then sent over fiberoptic networks. These dedicated fiberoptic networks have nearly eliminated the more expensive and labor-intensive delivery options, such as microwave, instructional television fixed systems, closed-circuit television, and satellite. The tremendous advantage of this type of delivery system is the ability to reach a vast number of students. The biggest disadvantages are cost and a highly structured learning environment that sometimes limits interaction, learner focus, and the sense of the social learning community.

Blended Delivery Options

Multiple delivery modalities can provide enrichment to the distance education experience. This is frequently referred to as a *blended,* or *hybrid, approach* to distance learning. For example, online courseware may be used as a supplement to a traditional classroom course by providing synchronous components, asynchronous components, or both to the instructional process (Salzer, 2002). Online courseware frequently becomes a clearinghouse for course materials, assignments, and electronic transfer. The use of multiple technologies has become very popular and more directly associates learning with the student's educational objectives (Shearer, 2003).

Data Networks

Data networks have become the backbone for transmission of digital information directly, indirectly, and by wireless means. Applications are independently accessed from personal computers or devices or provided from any multitude of servers through routers, switches, and gateways; thus a true virtual relationship of information and interaction has become possible. Education has accepted the challenge of incorporating data infrastructure into the design and development of effective instruction, making global teaching and learning possible. Because data networks have influenced almost every aspect of distance education in nursing, the challenge for nurse educators is to continue to look for innovative ways to design learning environments that optimize the use of these networks. The ability to access a vast amount of information in a short period is changing the way resources are delivered and the way students and educators participate in the instructional process. Steeples et al. (2002) suggest that network learning design should include access to resources, communication and social interaction, learning assistance, feedback for performance and opportunities for reflection, and synchronous and asynchronous support (pp. 326-329). Data networks are also providing a bridge for practitioners to reach populations in remote and underserved areas, although there are many locations where telecommunication services are not yet available. In the future, wireless networks may have a significant impact on the ability to reach these populations (McCaughan, 2003; Puskin, 2003).

Bandwidth

Bandwidth is a word heard frequently in reference to data networks and their capabilities for transmitting data. Heinich et al. (1999) define bandwidth as "the range of frequencies an electronic communications channel can support without excessive deterioration" (p. 401). In other words, when the amount of electronic communication exceeds the channel's capability, quality of transmission deteriorates dramatically. Interactive videoconferencing, multimedia, and video applications typically demand large amounts of bandwidth and must be evaluated carefully for use on some data networks. A process of compressing a rich medium to make it more compatible with available bandwidth is common practice.

Wireless networks are also subject to bandwidth limitations. Although wireless technology is popular with students at educational institutions throughout the world, instructors are sometimes reluctant to rely on it in the classroom because of limited bandwidth caused by heavy student use. However, faculty are optimistic that bandwidth limitations will be reduced in the near future, allowing for reliable integration of wireless technology throughout a campus.

There is also a trend in nursing for use of wireless personal devices. Use of such devices allows information to be accessible from the Internet and downloadable to a personal digital assistant (PDA). These devices have tremendous implications for clinical instruction, research, and practice.

Interactive Delivery Types

Each medium has identifiable differences specific to the technology and is briefly described in this section. However, the similarities of required support, planning, and implementing use of technology in the classroom and online represent the major focus. Faculty must consider intricacies of the total responsibilities of designing and melding the variety of distance education strategies for effective use in the telecommunications classroom. Within this overall process, students must be oriented to the technology and the expectations of the learner receiving instruction through distance education. Gibson (1996) indicates that student outcomes are influenced by both process and content of learning in what is referred to as *academic self-concept*. Clear and concise orientation is an important step toward improved academic self-concept. A summary of adapting strategies specifically for teaching on television can be found in Table 18-2.

Interactive Videoconferencing

Interactive videoconferencing is live face-to-face conferencing between two or more participants at various locations with digitally transmitted audio and video components over data networks. Interactive videoconferencing is used in a variety of educational applications for both large- and small-group discussions. It also is used for conducting meetings and collaborative ventures. Interactive educational videoconferencing provides synchronous communication and an opportunity for teachers and students to conduct live interactions in a face-to-face environment. Continuous two-way communication with learners located at distant sites is possible, as well as one-on-one mentoring for nursing clinical practice. Likewise, meetings are conducted by using this technology as a means to augment conversations, collaborate on special issues, and share information without a travel burden. Interactive videoconferencing also allows the sharing of documents, instructional media, and computer-based presentations.

Videoconferencing transmissions involve data networks and may use dedicated fiberoptics for connection, telephone lines, or the Internet. Elaborate instructional videoconferencing systems with satellite, broadcast, or microwave are used throughout the world, although many of these systems are decreasing in popularity because of cost and the convenience of other videoconferencing systems (Clark, 1993; Cowell et al., 1992; Heinich, 1999; Walsh & Reese, 1995). More common instructional videoconferencing systems are self-contained units that are relatively easy to use once data configurations have been established.

Integrated Services Digital Network

Integrated Services Digital Network (ISDN) is a digital dial-up means of telephone access to networking. ISDN is touted to have greater transmission reliability and provides much faster communication than some other options, such as fraction T-1 networks, frame relay (FR), and asynchronous transfer mode (ATM). T-1, FR, and ATM are typically very expensive and out of reach for many small-scale users. ISDN typically uses leased telephone lines; can carry data, voice, and video; and is a widely used option for providing distance education. For distance teaching, one ISDN videoconferencing unit is connected to another by dialing one unit to the other, much like a telephone call. Multiple connections can be accomplished with the addition of controlling hardware and software. ISDN accommodates interactive communications for both small and large classroom systems.

Internet Protocol Videoconferencing

Internet Protocol Videoconferencing (IPVC), sometimes called *videoconferencing over IP*, uses the Internet and a proprietary protocol, H.323, to connect one videoconferencing unit to another. Because IPVC uses the Internet, bandwidth is greatly affected. The amount of bandwidth used is directly proportional to data rate and quality selected for an IPVC conference. Much like ISDN, multiple connections can be accomplished with the addition of controlling hardware and software. Most IPVC systems are designed for small-group interaction, although connections are possible for most video-based classroom systems. As bandwidth increases and compression protocols become more efficient, the use of IPVC for meetings and distance education will increase. IPVC technology has excellent potential for fulfilling nursing education's need for an active learning process.

Satellite Videoconferencing

Satellite videoconferencing is expensive and requires an "uplink" from the origination site to communicate with the orbiting satellite and a "downlink" at each of the selected receive sites. The visual component is only from the origination site; however, students in the receiving location(s) may participate with audio interaction through telephone connections or by means of computer instant messaging.

Equipment to establish satellite access is too expensive for many institutions because the cost of uplinks commonly exceeds $250,000 and the cost of downlinks ranges from $3000 to $5000. Fees for use of this technology can be as high as $700 per hour. This technology is often used in training and academia when the audience is large and spread over a diverse geographic area. The Centers for Disease Control and Prevention in Atlanta, Georgia, has extensively used satellite broadcasts to reach large populations of health care workers with clinical updates and health care forums. Likewise, kindergarten through grade 12 education has used satellite to broadcast course content to rural area schools that cannot afford teachers for every subject.

Satellite origination in education typically involves a simulated classroom in a television production studio located at the uplink site. The production is professionally designed; and special lighting and audio and other production equipment are used. Costs for this service and technology are high. Technical staff are necessary to support the studio classroom, and classes move along in a rigid time frame, much the same as broadcast programming.

Use of satellite requires that students cluster at each downlink location for classes. Because neither the teacher nor the students have the opportunity to see learners from other sites as they participate in course discussion, it is helpful to have a photograph of each student enrolled at the multiple sites. These pictures can be superimposed on the uplink by a technician at the origination site while the student is speaking from his or her location, thus increasing the feeling of belonging to a single community within all classroom settings.

The economics of scale continue to make this delivery mechanism a good option for distance education. However, this technology has lost much of its popularity because of improved access to computer-based systems and availability of the Internet. Videostreaming technology has also become a competitive strategy for reaching these same populations.

Broadcast and Closed-Circuit Television

Many viewers can simultaneously receive presentations transmitted via electromagnetic waves, broadcast, microwave, and fixed systems (instructional television fixed systems). Such programming may be distributed widely through commercial and noncommercial narrow and broadband broadcasting. Cable channels, which are considered a closed-circuit application, also carry broadcast programs.

Courses offered through broadcast or cable medium are usually one-way video and audio transmissions. If the presentation is a live broadcast, telephones or computer instant messaging may be used to communicate with the instructor. Typically, broadcast and cable offerings "fit" within an allotted airtime and are sometimes rebroadcast from tape, so interaction is not possible. Telephone "office hours" can be arranged to provide a link between student and faculty member, or a computer-based forum may be established for synchronous or asynchronous interaction to help prevent feelings of isolation.

Television signals transmitted in the microwave spectrum (above 2000 MHz) require that courses offered through this medium be limited to viewing by those students who gather at a designated electronic classroom. Instructional television fixed systems is a one-way video, two-way audio system in which both video and audio components are carried on the microwave band.

When planning for use of broadcast, the instructor should remember that most courses taught through this medium do not have viewing restricted to only those who enroll; anyone who has a working television and is located within the broadcast range or cable access area can view this programming. However, audio and instant messaging from the viewer would only be accepted from registered course participants who are connected through telephone or the Internet to the origination site.

Open broadcast is infrequently used as a medium for delivery of academic university courses; however, many educational programs are delivered to homes and kindergarten through grade 12 classrooms through local cable services under a community-franchised access agreement. This technology is also losing popularity because of improved access to computer-based systems and availability of the Internet. Videostreaming technology has also become a competitive strategy for reaching these same populations.

Fiberoptic transmission is similar to microwave in accomplishing educational delivery. However, rather than signals being carried above the ground by microwaves between towers, fiberoptic cabling is buried between all sites. This has been most economically used in geographic areas that have a generally flat terrain and would pose few environmental barriers to laying cable. An additional advantage of fiberoptic cabling is that it can transmit more signals with higher quality than other types of cabling. Though the cost of installing an optical fiber network is higher than that of a microwave system, maintenance expenses are significantly lower because the fiber is protected from weather and vandalism. Additionally, digital transmission on fiberoptic data networks is usually accomplished by compressing the video and audio components to conserve bandwidth. This allows for sharing of bandwidth, thus reducing cost. However, quality of the transmission is directly proportional to the data rate used.

Audioconferencing

Instruction transmitted over phone lines is a delivery strategy commonly referred to as *audioconferencing*. A teacher located at the origination site, not necessarily a classroom, interacts with students in one or more receiving sites (Hardy & Olcott, 1995; Henry, 1993; Moore, 1994). Some distance teaching universities and colleges incorporate audioconferencing in a blended manner with other technology as a required component of curricula. Contracts for this service are commonly developed with third-party providers. Courses to be offered through this medium must be selected and designed carefully to ensure that they are developed in a pedagogically correct manner. Seminars, forums, discussion, and some lecture classes with activities that encourage critical thinking lend themselves well to this economical technology (Hardy & Olcott, 1995; MacIntosh, 1993; Simonson & Thompson, 1997). As an adjunct to audio communication, use of computers between class sessions for collaborative assignments and correspondence with peers at other sites should be encouraged. Use of electronic whiteboards and document-sharing software provides an added level of interaction to the audioconference; however, this requires supplemental equipment, thus raising the cost of delivery.

If the blend of instruction does not include a visual component, photographs of the instructor and students may be shared by electronic or other means at the beginning of the course. In addition, students should be encouraged to identify themselves and their location when they speak during the audio class sessions to facilitate a feeling of classroom community. Activities that provide opportunity for some student socialization should also be incorporated into early class sessions at the same time students are provided orientation to use of the technology. Because the teacher is unable to identify nonverbal cues, teaching strategies should include more questioning to determine class understanding of content being addressed. Methods of drawing students into discussion should be planned and appropriately incorporated into classes throughout the course.

As with other instructional delivery strategies, it is imperative that marketing, site selection, effective communication, and ongoing course coordination be managed efficiently. The teacher and administrators must work together closely to ensure that these components of the total educational plan are in place.

Videostreaming

Videostreaming is an emerging technology that allows users to receive real-time video and audio transmissions at a computer via an Internet connection. Videostreaming involves the digital encoding of a television signal into a compressed video format so it can be served on networks for viewing at a place other than the site of origination. This is a one-way audio and video delivery modality that is gaining popularity in higher education for enriched distance education delivery. When a student is connected to the network at a high rate of data transmission, the videostream will play through the appropriate software plug-in on a personal computer. Because the video transmission is compressed for use on limited bandwidth data networks, video quality is much poorer than that of transmissions typically viewed on television. The picture size is normally reduced, and interruption of signal is common as the computer buffers content and tries to optimize the delivery.

Live videostreaming is a synchronous (real-time) distance learning technology. It is one-way audio and video transmission but can be supplemented with various forms of instant messaging or online chat for interaction. The instructor reads messages as they arrive and normally responds to these questions as he or she would any other questions from the origination site. Because of transmission delays, telephone conferencing is not a good option for interaction. Because quality is poorer than that of television, special consideration must be given to teaching methods and the use of supplemental materials.

A primary disadvantage of videostreaming is that it places a high demand on bandwidth; therefore network management personnel must monitor use carefully. Videostreaming continues to be problematic for low network connection speeds.

Videostreaming can also be an asynchronous (anytime) distance learning technology. Streaming media can be stored on a video server, or compact disc (CD) or DVD, for on-demand access. This means the learner can access archived lectures or videostreams as needed within the context of instruction. "Today, with archived streaming video available on the Web, no one must be in a classroom to hear a lecture. Students can hear it live anywhere or hear it later as many times as they'd like" (Strauss, 2002, p. 13).

Courses and Curricula on the Internet and World Wide Web

Computers and the development of Web-based instruction have had a tremendous impact on education. Armstrong and Frueh (2003) contend that the computer has become a major influence in distance education by providing an interactive technology that allows learners to participate at any time or from any place. Web-based instruction provides an innovative and interactive way to bridge time and distance. Through use of the computer, students at multiple sites can collaborate with others and ask questions without synchronous connection (Cragg, 1994). Instruction is a medium that supports multiple student interactions without requiring participants to be gathered in a central place at a specified time (Moore & Anderson, 2003; Tuckey, 1993). Students have the opportunity to participate in synchronous and asynchronous discussion. They may participate in live chat sessions, during which conversation occurs in text, or threaded discussions, in which they read others' materials asynchronously, respond, and return to the computer dialogue later to provide additional input. Although all students read the conference correspondence provided by classmates or faculty members, personally directed e-mail messages can also be sent to only selected individuals. Online interaction can be facilitative in encouraging students to work on collaborative projects. Having adapted to this medium, students may be encouraged to apply its usefulness in their professional careers.

Computers are used in almost every aspect of the nursing profession including storage and retrieval of data; collaborating, advising, and promoting consensus-building skills; and health teaching (Armstrong & Frueh; 2003; Doorley et al., 1994; Hekelman et al., 1993; Novotny, 2000). Web-based instruction, however, does have disadvantages. The lack of a visual and audible interface with the teacher and other students is a potential problem. Online interaction and sharing of photographs can help, but there is little to compensate for the lack of visual cues. Some special forms of character messaging and emphasis placed on words can be used to illustrate emotion and add expression to writing. Practical skills are difficult to demonstrate in the online environment. The use of compressed media-rich delivery and simulations can help, but these are sometimes costly to produce and require additional time to prepare. Poor access to the Internet can also be a disadvantage, although the number of households with computers and access to the Internet is increasing.

Faculty who have taught courses by computer reflect that self-discipline is as crucial for the faculty member as it is for students (Boston, 1992; Novotny, 2000). Depending on the design of the course, the teacher must regularly check threaded discussions to respond to questions and post additional questions or assignments. However, faculty who become enamored with this strategy and the technology should be cautioned to regulate their time to avoid becoming overcommitted and overdirective to the course.

Web-based courses and computer conferencing are becoming ubiquitous as universities and schools of nursing seek to provide access to education for new and continuing learners. As courses and even schools of nursing become "virtual," nursing faculty and administrators must define guidelines, develop mechanisms to accept credits obtained through this medium from another institution, establish workload policies, and institute new systems of faculty rewards.

ADAPTING TEACHING FOR DISTANCE EDUCATION

Although there are differences in the technology and intricacies of various distance education delivery systems, there are commonalities that should be considered regardless of the medium to be used. See Table 18-2 for a summary of specific strategies for teaching with television. Primary to teaching through a distance delivery system is the understanding that there must be modifications to the style of teaching and to the materials used (Dirksen et al., 1993; Hegge, 1993; Novotny, 2000; Purdy & Wright, 1992; Shomaker, 1993; Tingen & Ellis, 2000). In a qualitative research study by Wolcott (1993), faculty respondents indicated that planning as a team rather than individually, emphasizing content rather than process, and using a syllabus to cohesively link content were important elements of the distance education planning process. Despite the time involved in making these adjustments, overall faculty perceptions of distance education delivery systems are reported as positive (Armstrong & Frueh, 2003; Billings et al., 1994b; Dillon & Walsh, 1992; Dirksen et al., 1993). However, also worthy of note are faculty-described concerns related to fear of technology, resistance to change, and fear of being replaced by technology (Charp, 1995). Personal bias can also be an obstacle to change (Ridenour et al., 2003). Consistently reported throughout the literature as being imperative to faculty satisfaction is an adequate operational and administrative infrastructure to support teaching endeavors.

Needs Assessment

Before a distance education program is initiated, the need for its introduction into the proposed geographic area should be determined to ensure adequate student participation. Nursing education administrators have embraced distance learning because there is perceived need and demand. A move forward with the curriculum implies a commitment from the university that students will be able to complete a significant portion, if not all, of the academic or continuing education program through distance instruction. Strategic marketing of a course or program in a new geographic area is usually effective in ensuring adequate registration. Once the program has been initiated, student satisfaction serves as the best method of promoting the program.

As more courses are offered at a distance through Web-based instruction, statistics indicate that the number of requests for this type of instruction from resident on-campus students is increasing (Palloff & Pratt, 2003). This fact is changing how nurse educators and administrators are thinking about the traditional face-to-face modality for meeting learning needs. "Attracting students is an outcome of Web presence" (Ridenour et al., 2003, p. 50). Turning attention to the learner will allow the individual to determine how technology can best serve his or her learning style and needs. Assessment for computer

TABLE 18-2 **Teaching with Television, Interactive Videoconference, and Videostream: Adapting Teaching Strategies**

STRATEGY OR USE IN TV COURSES	TEACHING STRATEGIES
Lecture Provides an efficient method of presenting much factual information in a short period	Lectures "come alive" through presentation of bits or chunks of material (10- to 15-minute segments) interspersed with some type of feedback, such as live or Web-based question-and-answer forum Provide a variety of material by using interactive communication with other strategies Strive to get audience to interact mentally with the material being presented; give them pretests to motivate; use organizers to focus on central ideas Enhance lecture with Web- and computer-based materials, graphs, charts, and other media such as slides, overheads, videotapes, and computer graphics Be certain guest speakers are aware that this is an interactive TV class. Instruct them to adapt their presentation for this medium of instruction
Discussion Generates feeling that all learners are important Facilitates collaborative process Provides a change of pace and a chance for all to participate Includes stimulating questions and develops critical thinking skills	Can bring in multiple points of view, experiences; students enjoy the variety of perspectives of others Preassign individuals to give specific reports that enhance discussion Call on students frequently; establish a dialogue between reception sites Allow sufficient time for students at all sites to respond to questions and enter the discussion Ask open-ended questions Repeat/rephrase question while waiting for students to prepare a response. Encourage all reception sites to participate Encourage participation from reception sites by looking into the camera or focusing camera with a close-up on the site (two-way video)
Interview Experts or clients bring additional information or viewpoints to the class in an interview format	Segments can be prerecorded with guest "live" for questions or available by telephone Moderator should make frequent summaries and clarifications and keep interview moving and to the point
Panel Discussion Helps bring in a wide range of informed opinions	Students should be prepared by previous assigned reading Four panel members is optimum. Be sure wide-angle camera can show the entire panel Panel members can be at different locations—live and online—but be sure to guide discussion to all panel members Moderator's summaries are crucial to bring out important points, because presentation is not as orderly and systematic as it is in the on-campus classroom Encourage panel to develop visual aids

> **TABLE 18-2 Teaching with Television, Interactive Videoconference, and Videostream: Adapting Teaching Strategies—cont'd**

STRATEGY OR USE IN TV COURSES	TEACHING STRATEGIES
Role Playing Adds variety to teaching strategies Encourages collaboration and student involvement	Role playing can be recorded ahead and shown during class Prepare learners ahead of time, because there is less spontaneous activity than in a classroom Encourage response from students at all reception sites Use role playing in groups at local sites or as a prerecorded "vignette" Keep role playing segments short so that other students can react Follow up role playing with discussion to bring out important learning, feelings, etc. Role playing can be used to follow up a previous assignment such as "What would you do in this situation?"
Reactor Panel Stimulates audience participation by "getting the ball rolling" through the use of an audience reaction team, made up of a few members of a large audience who act as representatives of the group to react to a speaker	Preassign a number of individuals to fill this role; they can be at the same or different locations Can be used to encourage others at reception sites to participate Conversely, can be used with large groups when the network time won't allow much participation by students; allows for some "audience interaction" with the speaker
Buzz Groups When group is too large at an individual site for discussion or when topic to be discussed is facilitated by off-the-air discussion groups	Sites with large enrollment should divide into groups of 5 to 10 for discussion purposes Give buzz groups explicit instructions as to the task to be accomplished: e.g., "develop one question" or "agree on one disadvantage"; keep instructions clear and simple Have groups report back on the air
Question and Answer Question-and-answer periods can be built into classes to provide feedback to both speaker and participant Stimulates discussion Keeps student attention	Participants should be encouraged to make note of questions or comments as the program goes along so they are ready to respond Respect for individuals' questions is necessary; provide opportunity through computer, fax, or 800 number to answer questions from individuals who did not have a chance to participate during the class session
Case Study Simulation Helps individuals to weigh and test values, separate fact from opinion, and develop critical thinking skills	Case studies should be sent as part of advance materials so the learners can identify the facts and issues and prepare responses If oral case studies are presented, they can add a change of pace; keep these short (5 to 10 minutes) so that others in the group can assimilate the details Use slides, videotapes, or computer-assisted instruction to enhance the case study

Continued

TABLE 18-2 Teaching with Television, Interactive Videoconference, and Videostream: Adapting Teaching Strategies—cont'd

STRATEGY OR USE IN TV COURSES	TEACHING STRATEGIES
Group Work Sessions	
Provides opportunity for practical work sessions in a collegial/collaborative environment	Give clear directions for group work activities; teach and develop collaborative learning skills before use with activity; monitor effectiveness of work groups at all sites
	Use team-building skills to develop collaborative learning
Encourages participation and builds group rapport at local sites	Activities can be organized or guided by local group leaders or site coordinators
	Variety increases interactivity and critical thinking
Demonstration	
Shows steps of procedure efficiently, in shorter time, with visual reinforcement	Plan ahead so camera positions are appropriate
	Use text to highlight or focus attention on key points
	Speak and demonstrate slowly and repeat as needed
Debate	
Clarify points/positions	Plan ahead and give clear directions
Helpful for values clarification and developing critical thinking and communication skills	Have groups develop criteria for judging
	Be sure students at all sites can hear points; repeat as needed
	Can preassign positions to be debated to specific groups
Supports learning in the affective domain	
Multimedia/Graphics/Slides	
Provides visual clarity and close-up view of selected material	Keep graphics simple
	Use "horizontal" or "landscape" aspect
	Use large letters
	Use contrasting background/foreground (blue, gray, and pastel are best as background colors)

Adapted for use with permission from Billings, D. (1995). *Guide to teaching on television*. Indiana University School of Nursing, Indianapolis. Unpublished manuscript.

literacy is critical for faculty and students to prevent frustration created by lack of understanding of technology and its use.

Origination Site

The classroom remains an essential component of distance education delivery. However, the increasing number of Web-based courses and online supplements is changing how the classroom is used for distance instruction. When electronic classrooms are needed to support all or portions of a course, the commitment to technology and the site must be considered as a long-term investment because the cost of equipping the facility will be substantial. A newly designed classroom may comprise complete multimedia systems including computerized presentation systems and wired and wireless high-speed data networks. Visual presentation can be at the touch of a button from a single control module. Camera control, videocassette recorder (VCR), DVD, CD, electronic whiteboard, and audiocassette technology are typically integrated into the classroom design for quick and easy access (Suvajian, 2003).

When the opportunity to select a totally new site within a geographic area exists, its location should be considered with respect to its centrality to population, access to public transportation, and relationship to library and computing resources. However, universities generally opt to have the origination site located on an existing campus, although the selection of the building in which a traditional classroom will be converted to an "electronic origination classroom" can become a political quagmire within the institution.

When there is a commitment to online delivery, there must also be a financial commitment to infrastructure including data networks and computing resources for hardware, software, and instructional media. Personnel for technical support must also be included in this plan.

Reception Site Development

When distance education technologies that include off-site learning facilities are used, a site coordinator, carefully selected to provide support to faculty and students, is essential to having the program run smoothly. Moore (1995, pp. 1-5) suggests the following "five C's" of this resource person's role:

1. A willingness and ability to *communicate* effectively
2. *Competence* in handling technical needs and serving as an instructional assistant
3. *Control* of events that helps instill student confidence in the system
4. *Caring* demonstrated for student achievement and success
5. *Continuity* of role from one semester to the next

It is apparent, from the multiple tasks that must be accomplished at each distant site to ensure a smoothly delivered program, that a site coordinator, not necessarily a nurse, is an invaluable resource who serves as the extended arm of the teacher (Clark, 1993; Hampton et al., 1994; Moore, 1995, Shomaker, 1995).

For Web-based instruction, personnel who manage the online courseware are needed to provide support to faculty and students to ensure that each online component runs smoothly. A faculty support team that focuses on content and not technology is also needed to mentor the online instruction process (Judson & Hook, 2003).

Logistics of ensuring availability of library, computer, and audiovisual resources must be handled by administrative and support staff. Such resources are essential to successful course delivery; however, teaching faculty, although responsible for planning and implementing the presentation of the course content, should not be expected to coordinate the plethora of other relevant activities. Support efforts to ensure efficient registration; advising; locating physical resources; hiring of technicians, site coordinators, or proctors; handling of syllabus and other course materials; obtaining copyright permissions;

arranging travel (if a part of the instruction design); and providing other similar services are essential to the success of any distance education delivery program. Support needs will vary depending on the medium being used.

Clinical Site Development

Creating collateral clinical experience for distance learners can be a challenge for health care educators. It may be necessary to replicate all aspects of clinical practice to meet curriculum mandates for successful skill development and competence. This requires coordination with health care agencies for creation of consistent, high-quality clinical experiences. Site visits may be required to ensure accuracy and calibration with instruction at the main campus. Preceptors and clinical coordinators may need to be hired to act as mentors to distant students, to ensure adequate skill development, and to support the alliance between programs and agencies.

Distance videoconferencing technologies can also be implemented to provide for interactive consultation. These technologies, along with other telecommunication systems, make it possible for faculty to work with students remotely, when it has been traditionally done in person. Electronic document transfer, online evaluation instruments, and collaboration over interactive networks have made it feasible to assess student performance at a distance and to guide the student's clinical experience.

Preparing Faculty

Orientation to technology and ongoing development are needed for faculty teaching distance education courses. This is a way to create new understanding and to advance existing expertise to new levels of pedagogical effectiveness. Faculty must intricately understand the delivery mechanism to give full attention to the learners instead of the technology. Formative development is a desired approach because it improves specific instructional strategies and ensures strong learning focus.

If they are given an orientation early in their commitment to teaching the course, faculty will have time and opportunity to incorporate innovative tactics into their design and presentation style and to modify teaching materials appropriate to the technology. For example, presentation software, slides, and printed copy used for television delivery should be altered for better accommodation to a horizontal 3 × 4 format. Likewise, graphics, interactive activities, and multimedia need to be carefully developed and evaluated for Web-based courses.

Continuous and formative updates during the course of instruction ensure that strategies are being implemented appropriately and that learning focus is maintained. The formative nature of these updates allows for adjustments and modifications to both teaching and learning so faculty and students can maintain good social presence in the learning environment for the duration of the course.

COURSE ENHANCEMENTS AND RESOURCES

Courses that are enhanced with the use of media may have instructional advantages over traditional or fully online courses. "Segmented models show media-enhanced courses having higher success and lower withdrawal rates than traditional or fully online courses. When media-enhanced and fully online classes are matched with traditional sections, media-enhanced versions are superior in having greater numbers of students succeeding with an A, B or C grade, and fewer withdrawals" (Hartman et al., 2000, p. 158). This position indicates that supplemental enhancement to a course leads to greater student satisfaction and success.

In a blended approach to distance education, the learning value of the course is increased through supplemental media and several adjunct resources that support instructional delivery. Electronic document exchanges, fax machines, mail and courier services, e-mail, and voice mail are necessary enhancements. Through use of these tools, faculty and students have increased opportunities for communication throughout the term of instruction. Some universities have made available toll-free telephone numbers for enrolled students' use to facilitate their communication with faculty, registrar, financial aid advisors, and other home campus support services. Additionally, many universities are moving forward with a "portal" that will provide a personalized online interface to all university and educational activities.

EVALUATION

Ongoing evaluation of student learning will provide the best measure of learning success and will provide faculty with information to improve teaching strategies and the use of technology for distance learning. "Evaluation of learning is defined as *the systematic process of collecting and interpreting information as a basis for decisions about the learner*" (Nugent, 2003, p. 349). In order for institutions to make informed and reasonable decisions about the worth of current and future distance learning programs, this type of evaluation data is essential (Thompson & Modupe, 2003).

Evaluation of distance education delivery systems should also occur both formatively and summatively (Clark, 1993). Student and faculty perceptions of the technology and delivery efficacy should be explored, as well as the rate of student success within the course. Reasons for student attrition should be researched, and constructs should be designed to reverse negative trends (Gibson, 1996).

Evaluation data should also include the cost of the course to the university. Factors considered will include salaries or wages for faculty, technicians, site coordinators, and other support staff; equipment; potential lease fees for facilities and communication systems; travel costs for faculty; mailing or courier charges; and other resources needed for course implementation. All expenditures must be evaluated against the income generated through tuition and provided by other financial support sources.

SUMMARY

Increased opportunities for access to higher education are becoming more readily available for students who live and work in areas remote from a central campus, as well as within a wired or wireless central community. Informational and educational technologies are regularly used to reach undergraduate and graduate nursing students, as well as RNs seeking nonacademic continuing education. As technology improves and increased research provides greater direction for use of selected paradigms, nursing faculty will find additional challenges to propel curricula and curricular applications far into the future.

Leaders must carefully assess data collected about distance education to set new parameters for future learning. For nursing education, it will be necessary to determine the extent to which distance delivery will be a part of the educational process. Will it become the single most important process? Will it be used to support other more traditional processes? Will it provide additional opportunities to extend learning in a more collaborative way with other organizations and institutions of higher education? Without a doubt, the advancement of computer-based data networks, innovative design of instruction, and creative leadership will provide a solid platform for distance learning environments in the future.

REFERENCES

Armstrong, M., & Frueh, S. (Eds.). (2003). *Telecommunications for nurses: Providing successful distance education and telehealth* (2nd ed.). New York: Springer.

Billings, D., & Bachmeier, B. (1994). Teaching and learning at a distance: A review of the nursing literature. In L. R. Allen (Ed.), *Review of research in nursing education* (pp. 1-32). New York: National League for Nursing.

Billings, D., Durham, J. D., Finke, L., Boland, D., Manz, B., & Smith, S. (1994a). Collaboration in distance education between nursing schools and hospitals. *Holistic Nursing Practice, 8*(3), 64-70.

Billings, D., Durham, J., Finke, L., Boland, D., Smith, S., & Manz, B. (1994b). Faculty perceptions of teaching on television: One school's experience. *Journal of Professional Nursing, 10,* 307-312.

Bonk, C. J., & Dennen, V. (2003). Frameworks for research, design, benchmarks, training, and pedagogy in Web-based distance education. In M. G. Grapham & W. G. Anderson, (Eds.), *Handbook of distance education* (pp. 21-35). Mahwah, NJ: Lawrence Erlbaum Associates.

Boston, R. L. (1992). Remote delivery of instruction via the PC and modem: What have we learned? *American Journal of Distance Education, 6*(3), 45-57.

Charp, S. (Ed.). (1995). Editorial. *T.H.E. Journal, 22*(11), 6.

Clark, C. E. (1993). Beam me up, nurse! Educational technology supports distance education. *Nurse Educator, 18*(2), 18-22.

Clark, R. E. (1998). Motivating performance: Part 1—diagnosing and solving motivation problems. *Performance Improvement, 37*(8), 39-46.

Clarke, L., & Cohen, J. A. (1992). Distance learning: New partnerships for nursing in rural areas. In P. Winstead-Fry, J. C. Tiffany, & R. V. Shippee-Rice (Eds.), *Rural health nursing: Stories of creativity, commitment, and connectedness* (pp. 359-388). New York: National League for Nursing.

Cowell, J. M., Kahn, E. H., & Bahrawy, A. A. (1992). The school nurse development program: An experiment in off-site delivery. *Journal of Continuing Education in Nursing, 23,* 127-133.

Cragg, C. E. (1994). Nurses' experiences of a post-RN course by computer mediated conferencing: Friendly users. *Computers in Nursing, 12,* 221-226.

Dick, W., Carey, L., & Carey, J. O. (2000). *The systematic design of instruction* (5th ed.). New York: Addison-Wesley.

Dillon, C., & Walsh, S. (1992). Faculty: The neglected resource in distance education. *The American Journal of Distance Education, 6*(3), 5-21.

Dirksen, S. R., Hoeksel, R., & Holloway, J. (1993). RN/BSN distance learning through microwave. *Nurse Educator, 18(2)*, 13-17.

Doorley, J., Reener, A., & Corron, J. (1994). Creating care plans via modems: Using a hospital information system in nursing education. *Computers in Nursing, 12*, 160-163.

Driscoll, M. (2000). *Psychology of learning for instruction* (2nd ed.). Needham Heights, MA: Allyn & Bacon.

Finke, L. (1998). Teaching in nursing: The faculty role. In D. Billings & J. Halstead (Eds.), *Teaching in nursing: A guide for faculty* (p. 4). Philadelphia: W. B. Saunders.

Fulmer, J., Hazzard, M., Jones, S., & Keene, K. (1992). Distance learning: An innovative approach to nursing education. *Journal of Professional Nursing, 8*, 289-294.

Gagne, R., & Briggs, L. (1979). *Principles of instructional design* (2nd ed.). New York: Holt, Rinehart and Winston.

Gibson, C. (1996). Toward an understanding of academic self-concept in distance education. *The American Journal of Distance Education, 10(1)*, 23-36.

Goldrick, B., Appling-Stevens, S., & Larson, E. (1990). Infection control programmed instruction: An alternative to classroom instruction in baccalaureate nursing education. *Journal of Nursing Education, 29*, 20-25.

Green, K. C. (2003). Digital tweed, chapter two: New beginnings. *Syllabus, 16(10)*, 14 & 41.

Halstead, J., Hayes, R., Reising, D., & Billings, D. (1995). Nursing student information network: Fostering collegial communications using a computer conference. *Computers in Nursing, 13*, 55-59.

Hampton, C. L., Mazmanian, P. E., & Smith, T. J. (1994). The interactive videoconference: An effective CME delivery system. *The Journal of Continuing Education in the Health Professions, 14*, 83-89.

Hardy, D. W., & Olcott, D., Jr. (1995). Audio teleconferencing and the adult learner: Strategies for effective practice. *The American Journal of Distance Education, 9(1)*, 44-60.

Hartman, J., Dziuban C., & Moskal, P. (2000). Faculty satisfaction in ALNs: A dependent or independent variable? In J. Bourne (Ed.), *Proceedings of the 1999 Sloan Summer Workshop on Asynchronous Learning Networks* (pp. 151-172). Nashville, TN: Center for Asynchronous Learning Networks at Vanderbilt University.

Hegge, M. (1993). Interactive television presentation style and teaching materials. *Journal of Continuing Education in Nursing, 24*, 39-42.

Heinich, R., Molenda, M., Russell, J. D., & Smaldino, S. E. (1999). *Instructional media and the new technologies for learning* (6th ed.). Upper Saddle River, NJ: Prentice-Hall.

Hekelman, F., Niles, S., & Brennan, P. F. (1994). Gerontologic home care: A prescription for distance continuing education. *Computers in Nursing, 12*, 106-109.

Henry, P. R. (1993). Distance learning through audioconferencing. *Nurse Educator, 18*(2), 23-26.

Judson, L. H., & Hook, J. (2003). Designing a course on the Web using WebCT. In M. Armstrong & S. Frueh (Eds.), *Telecommunications for nurses: Providing successful distance education and telehealth* (2nd ed., pp. 85-108). New York: Springer.

Keck, J. F. (1992). Comparison of learning outcomes between graduate students in telecourses and those in traditional classrooms. *Journal of Nursing Education, 31*, 229-234.

Keller, J. (1999). Motivational systems. In H. Stolovitch & E. Keeps (Eds.), *Handbook of human performance technology: Improving individual and organizational performance worldwide* (2nd ed.). San Francisco: Jossey-Bass.

MacIntosh, J. A. (1993). Focus groups in distance nursing education. *Journal of Advanced Nursing, 18*, 1981-1985.

McCaughan, T. W. (2003). Opportunities and challenges of telecommunications for nurses. In M. Armstrong & S. Frueh (Eds.), *Telecommunications for nurses: Providing successful distance education and telehealth* (2nd ed., pp. 1-18). New York: Springer.

Moore, M. G. (1994). Audioconferencing in distance education [Editorial]. *The American Journal of Distance Education, 8*(1), 1-4.

Moore, M. G. (1995). The five Cs of the local coordinator [Editorial]. *The American Journal of Distance Education, 9*(1), 1-5.

Moore, M. G., & Anderson, W. G. (Eds.). (2003). *Handbook of distance education.* Mahwah, NJ: Lawrence Erlbaum Associates.

Moore, M. G., & Kearsley, G. (1996). *Distance education: A systems view.* Belmont, CA: Wadsworth.

Nichols, E., Beeken, J., & Wilkerson, N. (1994). Distance delivery through compressed video. *Journal of Nursing Education, 33,* 184-186.

Novotny, J. (Ed.). (2000). *Distance education in nursing.* New York: Springer.

Nugent, K. E. (2003). Evaluation of learning outcomes. In A. Lowenstein & M. Bradshaw (Eds.), *Fuszard's innovative teaching strategies in nursing* (3rd ed., pp. 349-365). Gaithersburg, MD: Aspen.

Palloff, R. M., & Pratt, K. (2003). *The virtual student: A profile and guide to working with online learners.* San Francisco: Jossey-Bass.

Piaget, J. (2001). *The psychology of intelligence* (2nd ed.). (M. Piercy & D. E. Berlyne, Trans.) New York: Routledge.

Pittman, V. V. (2003). Correspondence study in the American university: A second historiographic perspective. In M. G. Grapham & W. G. Anderson (Eds.), *Handbook of distance education* (pp. 21-35). Mahwah, NJ: Lawrence Erlbaum Associates.

Purdy, L. N., & Wright, S. J. (1992). Teaching in distance education: A faculty perspective. *The American Journal of Distance Education, 6*(3), 2-4.

Puskin, D. S. (2003). An overview of telemedicine: Through the looking glass. In M. Armstrong & S. Frueh (Eds.), *Telecommunications for nurses: Providing successful distance education and telehealth* (2nd ed., pp. 135-165). New York: Springer.

Ramsey, R. W. (2002). *Improving nursing student motivation to learn.* Ft. Lauderdale, FL: Nova Southeastern University.

Ridenour, N., Kossman, S., & Mock, D. (2003). In M. Armstrong & S. Frueh (Eds.), *Telecommunications for nurses: Providing successful distance education and telehealth* (2nd ed.). New York: Springer.

Russell, T. L. (1999). *The no significant difference phenomenon.* Retrieved February 23, 2004, from http://www.idecc.org

Salzer, J. S. (2002). Web-based instruction. In A. Lowenstein, & M. Bradshaw (Eds.), *Fuszard's innovative teaching strategies in nursing* (3rd ed., pp. 210-226). Gaithersburg, MD: Aspen.

Shearer, R. (2003). Instructional design in distance education: An overview. In M. G. Grapham & W. G. Anderson (Eds.), *Handbook of distance education* (pp. 275-286). Mahwah, NJ: Lawrence Erlbaum Associates.

Shomaker, D. (1993). A statewide instructional television program via satellite for RN-to-BSN students. *Journal of Professional Nursing, 9,* 153-158.

Shomaker, D. (1995). The culture broker in post-RN education: A view from a distance. *Nursing Outlook, 43,* 129-133.

Simonson, M., Smaldino, S., Albright, M., & Zvacek, S. (2000). *Teaching and learning at a distance: Foundations of distance education.* Upper Saddle River, NJ: Prentice-Hall.

Simonson, M. R., & Thompson, A. (1997). *Educational computing foundations.* Upper Saddle River, NJ: Prentice-Hall.

Smith, P., & Ragan, T. (1999). *Instructional design* (2nd ed.). New York: Wiley.

Souder, W. E. (1993). The effectiveness of traditional vs. satellite delivery in three management of technology master's degree programs. *The American Journal of Distance Education, 7,* 37-53.

Steeples, C., Jones, C., & Goodyear, P. (2002). Beyond e-learning: A future for networked learning. In C. Steeples & C. Jones (Eds.), *Networked learning: Perspectives and issues* (pp. 323-341). London: Springer.

Strauss, H. (2002). New learning spaces, smart learners, not smart classrooms. *Syllabus, 16*(2), 12-17.

Suvajian, J. (2003). It's all in the presentation at URI. *Syllabus, 16*(11), 33-35.

Tallman, F. D. (1994). Satisfaction and completion in correspondence study: The influence of instructional and student-support services. *The American Journal of Distance Education, 8*(2), 43-57.

Teleeducation NB (2004). *Teleeducation NB Teleeducation.* Retrieved February 23, 2004, from http://www.teleeducation.nb.ca/English/index.cfm

Thompson, M. M., & Modupe, E. I. (2003). Evaluating distance education programs. In M. G. Grapham, & W. G. Anderson (Eds.), *Handbook of distance education* (pp. 567-584). Mahwah, NJ: Lawrence Erlbaum Associates.

Tingen, M., Ellis, L. (2000). Teaching by distance education. In A. Lowenstein & M. Bradshaw (Eds.), *Fuszard's innovative teaching strategies in nursing* (3rd ed., pp. 183-195). Gaithersburg, MD: Aspen.

Tuckey, C. (1993). Computer conferencing and electronic white board in the United Kingdom: A comparative analysis. *The American Journal of Distance Education, 7*(2), 58-72.

Walsh, J., & Reese, B. (1995). Distance learning's growing reach. *T.H.E. Journal, 22*(11), 58-62.

Wolcott, L. L. (1993). Faculty planning for distance teaching. *The American Journal of Distance Education, 7*(1), 26-36.

19

TEACHING AND LEARNING IN ONLINE LEARNING COMMUNITIES

Judith A. Halstead, DNS, RN,
Diane M. Billings, EdD, RN, FAAN

The proliferation of online courses in higher education over the last 10 years has been phenomenal. Initially used primarily to provide education to students who lived geographically distant from campus, the online courses offered on today's college campuses are just as likely to attract students who are living on campus as those who live at a distance. The current generation of new students, many of whom were accustomed to using technology throughout their elementary and secondary education, are seldom intimidated by the computer and fully expect faculty to incorporate technology into their classroom learning activities.

Online learning in nursing education is not limited to single course offerings. Entire nursing degree programs are available online, especially for those students who are seeking BSN completion degrees and graduate degrees. Providers of continuing education programs are also using online technology to reach out to larger audiences of health care professionals who appreciate the flexibility and convenience of having their educational needs met in their own homes. Online learning has revolutionized higher education and continuing education, erasing place and time boundaries for institutions, students, and faculty.

Despite the increasing presence of technology and online education in higher education, teaching in online learning communities (OLCs) remains a new experience for many nurse educators. Faculty who teach online courses and students who take online courses must reconceptualize their roles as teachers and learners to be successful in these courses. In addition, multiple administrative issues must be considered when the choice is made to implement online education. This chapter defines online learning, identifies factors that must be considered in the planning and implementation of online learning, and describes online course design issues. In addition, this chapter discusses the implications of online learning for the teaching and learning process, as well as the development needs for faculty and students. The chapter concludes with evidence of the effectiveness of online teaching and learning.

DEFINING ONLINE LEARNING

A variety of terms are associated with online learning. *Computer-mediated instruction* is defined as instruction that incorporates the use of technology to facilitate the achievement of identified learning outcomes. Computer-mediated instruction may include the use of multimedia, the Internet, e-mail, computer discussion boards, and audiostreaming or videostreaming. Online learning is an example of computer-mediated instruction. *Online learning* uses the World Wide Web (WWW) of the Internet to provide course materials to students. Faculty and student interactions are conducted through the Web with the use of computer discussion boards and e-mail communication. Learning activities are accomplished online, and student evaluation is also facilitated through online activities.

There is considerable variation in how the WWW is used to provide online course materials to students. Some courses are described as *Web-enhanced or Web-supported*, meaning that they are not conducted entirely online; rather, the class typically continues to meet face to face, but aspects of the course are available to students online. For example, faculty may choose to post syllabi, course handouts, and answers to study questions online for students to access. In Web-enhanced or Web-supported courses, the majority of student-faculty interactions are conducted in the traditional sense in the classroom setting.

Another variation of the online course is the *hybrid course*, which is a combination of online discussion with only occasional (three to four times per semester) class meetings. In a hybrid course a combination of technologies may be used to meet the needs of students. For example, for those students who are enrolled in hybrid courses but live far away from the campus, one-way or two-way videoconferencing may be used to "connect" them to the class during the times of on-campus class meetings. Finally, a course may be a *fully Web-based* course, in which all student-faculty interactions are conducted online and there are no scheduled class meetings.

Student–student and student–faculty interactions in online learning may occur asynchronously or synchronously, depending on the desired nature of the interaction. *Asynchronous* interactions are those that are not time and place dependent. E-mail, threaded discussions on discussion boards, and archived videostreams are examples of interactions that are asynchronous. Participants involved in an asynchronous interaction can choose to access or respond to the communication at a time that is convenient for them. *Synchronous* interactions are those that occur in "real time" and require participants to be present at a specific time to participate in the discussions. Class meetings, teleconferencing, live videostreams, chat rooms, and videoconferencing are examples of synchronous interactions. It is also possible to use e-mail in a synchronous fashion, if those involved in the e-mail messaging prearrange the time for sending and responding to the messages. Electronic "office hours" during which the faculty member is available to promptly answer any student e-mails sent during that period is an example of using e-mail in a synchronous fashion.

Regardless of the type of online course the faculty member is teaching, it is important to remember that it is the nature and quality of student–faculty interactions within the course that will ultimately determine students' satisfaction with the learning experience. When designing a course for online learning, faculty must consider how interactions between students and faculty will be fostered to promote the development of an *OLC*. A learning community is one in which there is a free exchange of information in a supportive environment with the intent that the participant's learning needs will be met. Careful planning by faculty helps to ensure that an OLC will develop and that students will not feel isolated from the other members of the class. The remainder of this chapter provides information that will help faculty to successfully plan and implement online learning experiences that will promote the development of learning communities.

PLANNING ONLINE LEARNING EXPERIENCES

Many institution and program issues must be considered when the decision is made to engage in online education. To successfully plan and implement online education, institutions and individual programs must identify how the needed infrastructure for online education will be sustained and how faculty and student development and support needs will be met. It is common for planning committees consisting of administrators, technology staff, student support personnel, and faculty to be charged with addressing and monitoring these issues. Specific issues that should be addressed include institutional planning, technology support, marketing, faculty development, learner support services, and assessment of the online learning courses (Bonnell & Halstead, 1999).

Institutional Planning

One of the first issues to be considered in the implementation of online education is the institutional organizational structure that will be necessary to support the delivery of the programs. For example, should the technology support services be centralized within the institutional structure or decentralized in the individual schools and programs? Who within the institution will provide administrative oversight for the development of online education? Does the institution already employ the technical and instructional design personnel needed to provide course design and delivery support or will additional positions need to be created and funded? How will the development of online courses be funded? Technology fees or distance education fees may need to be assessed of students in addition to tuition fees. Some institutions offer in-state tuition to those students who live out of state but enroll in online courses. Will faculty receive additional compensation for designing and teaching online courses? Many institutions provide either overload pay or release time to faculty during the semester in which they initially develop a course for online delivery or teach the course.

Technology Support

Another issue that needs to be addressed before implementation of online education is the issue of technology support. As previously mentioned, it is important to determine whether the institution already employs personnel with the required expertise to work with faculty to design and deliver online education or whether additional personnel need to be hired. Will this support be centralized or decentralized within the institution, or will a combination of centralized and decentralized support be more effective? What level of technology support will be provided to faculty and students (Halstead & Coudret, 2000)? Other important considerations include acquisition and maintenance of the hardware and software necessary to support online education. Is the institution's current computer network system capable of providing online access to students and faculty with speed and reliability, or are upgrades required? Do faculty have access to the level of hardware and software needed? Is there a plan to replace computer hardware and software on a regular schedule to maintain sufficient resources?

It is also important for the institution to make a decision about what software will be used to support the delivery and management of online courses. Course management systems are comprehensive software programs specifically designed for this purpose. A course management system "hosts" the course and allows faculty and students to access the course online by simply accessing the Web and logging in to the system with an individualized login and password. A course management system provides all of the tools required to effectively manage an online course—course materials management, student tracking options, communication tools (e-mail, threaded discussion boards, chat, group discussion), online testing, and grade recording and reporting (Dell, 2002). There are a variety of commercial vendors and course management systems from which to choose. Some of the larger university systems have chosen to design and support their own course management systems. Using a course management system to deliver online courses provides faculty with a relatively easy-to-use, consistent template on which to build their courses. It also provides students with a consistent learning environment with which they can become comfortable. There are advantages and disadvantages associated with each of the various commercial programs available; each institution needs to evaluate the programs to determine which will best meet the needs of the university.

Marketing

Some consideration must also be given to how the online courses or programs will be marketed to the target audience. It is also important to be clear about the forces that are driving the desire to offer online education. Is the institution or nursing program interested in offering online education to primarily serve and retain the current student population or to extend course or program offerings to a wider market? An understanding of the reasons for engaging in online education will help guide marketing decisions. Before an online course or program is developed, it can be helpful to conduct an environmental scan to gauge the market and identify which other universities are offering online education and the nature of the courses offered online. What niche does the proposed course or program fill that is not being met by another institution? A needs assessment can also be conducted among prospective students to identify the level of interest in enrollment in an online course or program and the reasons for their interest in online education, as well as the level of computer skills and availability of Internet access present within the targeted population. Having this information before an online offering is planned can help ensure that the learners' educational needs will be met.

It is also important to acknowledge that some of the most strategic marketing of online education may need to occur "internally" within the institution (Billings, 2002). Online education is still new to many faculty, students, and administrators. Faculty who are "early adopters" of technology and online education will need to communicate the potential advantages of online learning to faculty who are more skeptical.

Faculty Development

When implementation of online learning is initiated, faculty development needs will likely be focused on the following five areas: instructional design, technology management, time management, student–faculty interactions, and student evaluation (Halstead & Coudret, 2000). Before any online course development is begun, it is important to assess the knowledge and comfort level of faculty regarding conversion of traditional classroom courses into online courses and to determine what level of instructional design support will be needed. Orientation of faculty and support staff to the chosen course management system will also be important. Development of expertise in online teaching typically involves a gradual learning process. Scheduling a series of educational sessions focused on such topics as technology and time management, developing online courses that promote student–faculty interaction, and student evaluation, for faculty and support staff throughout the academic year can help faculty acquire the knowledge and skills necessary to successfully design and teach online courses. These topics are covered in more depth later in this chapter.

Learner Support

Introducing online education into a program will have a major impact on the delivery of learner support services, especially if the introduction of online education affects more than just a few individual courses. All aspects of the institution's student support services will ultimately be affected and need to be reconsidered to best serve the needs of students who are geographically distant from the campus, as well as those who are on campus (Mills et al., 2001). Students who enroll in distance education courses, including online programs, must have access to the same type of learner support services as those students who are enrolled in traditional courses on campus. The admission and registration processes may need to be restructured so that distant students will be able to accomplish these tasks without being physically present on campus. Financial aid services may also be affected and will need to be structured to provide support to students who live far away from campus. Faculty will need to consider how student advisement will be managed to accommodate distant learners. Are library resources and services such as catalog searches, access to databases, and interlibrary loan requests available online in sufficient quality and quantity to provide the learner with adequate resources to support learning? Are bookstore services available online to students?

Students who are unfamiliar with online learning will also require an orientation to the course management system and any other technology that they may be required to use in their course work. The institution needs to consider how it can provide orientation to technology for distant learners, as well as technology support when students encounter problems. Students who are new to online learning frequently need some initial guidance in how to manage their time when they are taking online courses. It is easy for students to underestimate the amount of self-direction that is required to be successful in online learning.

The decision to deliver online education will also result in the need for the institution to make financial decisions regarding tuition costs and additional student fees. Will students who reside out of state, but enroll in online programs, be eligible for in-state tuition? Will additional technology or distance education fees need to be assessed of students who enroll in online courses to support the delivery of student services? Many universities or colleges automatically charge students on-campus usage fees, such as activity fees and parking fees. Will these fees be waived for students who never come to campus? These decisions and others related to the delivery of student support services will require the consideration and collaboration of numerous departments in the institution so that students will have a quality learning experience.

Assessment and Evaluation of Online Courses

Faculty and administrators also need to give consideration to how online courses and programs will be assessed and evaluated to determine whether curriculum and program outcomes are being met, as well as for the purpose of continuous quality improvement. Most states have established guidelines for the delivery of distance education through the government bodies that regulate higher education. Accrediting agencies have also identified standards, principles of good practice, or guidelines for providing quality distance education. Faculty should familiarize themselves with the guidelines that apply to their particular state, institution, and program as they undertake the planning of online learning.

FACULTY ROLE IN ONLINE LEARNING

The faculty member's role as an educator does undergo a change when he or she is teaching online courses (Halstead, 2002). First of all, real-time, face-to-face interaction with students becomes limited, with most interactions confined to threaded discussion "conversations," e-mail messages, and the occasional phone call. Most importantly, in online courses the educator is less likely to be the primary source of information for the students. Instead, the educator's primary role becomes one of facilitating the student's learning experiences. The students assume more responsibility for identifying their own learning needs and being self-directed in how they choose to meet the identified learning outcomes for the course. For some faculty, this results in feeling a loss of control over the learning process.

Becoming a "facilitator" of learning, however, does not lessen the need for the educator or the importance of the educator's role in the learning process. The educator retains responsibility for identifying the expected outcomes of the course, designing learning activities that will promote active student involvement in the learning process, and evaluating student performance.

Facilitating online discussion is another important role for faculty who are teaching online. It is also important for the educator to provide frequent feedback to students, so that students will know whether they are achieving the desired outcomes. Use of formative evaluation techniques throughout the course to assess student learning will help assure the educator that the students are learning what they need, even though faculty and students are not meeting together in a classroom on a weekly basis.

Two of the most common concerns of faculty who are engaged in online teaching for the first time are related to how to facilitate and manage asynchronous online discussion and how to manage time most effectively. The amount of communication that can be generated by students in online courses can be overwhelming if the educator has not given some prior thought to how to manage it.

Successful management of asynchronous discussion requires the educator to initially identify the purpose of the discussion and to be sure that all students are contributing to the discussion (Halstead, 2002). As the online discussion continues to unfold, the educator may find it necessary at times to change the direction of the discussion or to correct any factual errors students may have made in their postings. However, most of the time, it is only necessary for the faculty to comment periodically to help guide the discussion. It is not desirable to respond to every comment made by students in online discussion; faculty should strive to avoid dominating the conversation, reserving their comments for emphasizing key concepts, praising students and providing feedback as appropriate, and other similar contributions.

Time management frequently becomes an issue for faculty teaching online courses because of the amount of student communication typically generated within the course through threaded discussion postings, e-mail, and phone calls. Because online courses promote student flexibility and convenience in learning, students tend to access the course, post comments, and send e-mails to faculty at all hours of the day, 7 days a week. The faculty member who is on the receiving end of all of this communication can quickly become overwhelmed. That is why it is essential to implement time management strategies before the course begins. By having a plan in place, faculty can respond to student comments in a timely manner while still retaining a sense of control.

Some strategies for managing online communication that have proven helpful include (1) deciding how quickly to respond to student inquiries (e.g., within 48 hours) and informing students of this time frame so that they will know when to anticipate an answer; (2) establishing individual student electronic file folders in which to retain a record of course communication; (3) using a separate e-mail account for student communications, so that student e-mail is automatically separated from other professional or personal correspondence; (4) establishing "electronic" office hours to interact with students; and (5) creating and saving standardized responses to the most commonly asked questions that can be quickly accessed and individualized for students. Faculty may also find it helpful to "block" out scheduled amounts of time each week to devote to the online course.

There are other aspects to time management that faculty who are teaching online courses need to consider. Because of the increased student interaction typically experienced in online courses, faculty can anticipate spending more time teaching the course online than they would if the course were offered in the traditional classroom setting. The class size of the online course will also affect the time needed to teach the course. Some institutions have established a maximum enrollment for online courses because of the increased time commitment for the faculty. Policies regarding class size vary among institutions.

Despite the potential increase in time demands for faculty who teach online, faculty do experience the same convenience and flexibility in teaching online courses as students enrolled in online courses do. With careful time management, faculty can incorporate their responsibilities for online teaching into their schedules at a time that is most convenient for them. Faculty can remain in contact with their students even when they are traveling and attending professional conferences. Online teaching helps to promote maximum flexibility in balancing the demands of the various aspects of the faculty role: teaching, scholarship, and service.

DESIGNING COURSES AND LEARNING ACTIVITIES FOR THE ONLINE LEARNING COMMUNITY

At some point in their careers, most educators will use all or part of an OLC to enhance or deliver a course. Evidence for best practices indicates that course design influences how students learn and the productive use of their learning time (Boettcher & Conrad, 1999; Bonk & King, 1998; Palloff & Pratt, 1999). Although working with a team of instructional design specialists is essential, course management software provided by most colleges, universities, and health care agencies is becoming easier to use; and preset templates simplify course authoring. Ultimately, however, faculty are responsible for the design and integrity of courses that are moved to the OLC and must be aware of course design basics.

Nurse educators can guide their Web course design according to theories of teaching and learning and instructional design (Bolan, 2003; Bonk & Cunningham, 1998; Jeffries, 2000; Sternberger, 2002). These theories suggest that course design should integrate teaching and evaluation strategies adapted for online environments that are appropriate for the course content and assist students in acquiring the requisite knowledge, skills, and values. Basic principles of course design are discussed here with references to the nursing literature.

1. *Start with the learner*. The student is the focal point for designing online courses. Educators must assess student learning styles, learning needs, current knowledge, motivation, and adaptive needs (see Chapter 10). Understanding the learner's technology skills is also important, and

learner support resources are essential to the success of any online course.

2. *Define learning outcomes/objectives/competencies.* Specifying the learning outcomes is a curricular process and should be completed within the context of course and curriculum development (see Chapter 9). Outcomes in all domains of learning can be facilitated within online courses, and the course design can accommodate a variety of learning domains and levels within the domains.

3. *Organize content into short, logical units* such as lessons or modules. Courses designed for the classroom are typically planned for the semester and class hour schedule of the institution. With Web-based courses, however, there is more flexibility in scheduling, and thus the content can be organized with additional attention to pedagogical principles.

4. *Create learning activities.* Learning activities provide students with opportunities to practice and apply course principles and to receive feedback about their learning. Learning activities should require active participation—interaction with the content, course, classmates, and the teacher. Additionally, learning activities should be designed for the higher levels of the cognitive domain and assist the students in moving from comprehension to synthesis and evaluation (Malloy & DeNatale, 2001; Peterson et al., 2001).

5. *Create evaluation and grading plans.* The evaluation and grading criteria should be clearly stated. A variety of strategies for evaluation can be adapted for use in online learning environments (see Teaching in the Online Learning Community).

6. *Use graphic design principles.* Although course design is improved by working with a graphics designer, the use of colors, fonts, and visuals must support the teaching and learning and not serve as the primary feature of the course. The course designer should integrate media such as videostreaming, audiostreaming, and visuals thoughtfully (see Chapter 17).

TEACHING IN THE ONLINE LEARNING COMMUNITY

In repeated studies of teaching in courses conducted fully or partially online, findings demonstrate the importance of effective teaching strategies and well-designed learning experiences (Billings et al., 2001; Billings et al., 2002). In general, teaching practices used in the classroom are also effective in the online environment. These educational practices have been derived from work by Chickering and Gamson (1987) and adapted for use in the online classroom (Chickering & Ehrmann, 1996; Edwards et al., 1999; Kirkpatrick, 2002; Malloy & DiNatale, 2001; Mastrian & McGonigle, 1999). See Table 19-1.

The educational practices listed in Table 19-1 can be activated by a variety of teaching strategies. Strategies should engage all learners, be varied, allow for diversity, and require creativity. Strategies that work particularly well in online classrooms include round robin, debate, questions that require analysis, synthesis, evaluation, and reflection, short written work, and collaborative

TABLE 19-1 Educational Practices in Online Courses

EDUCATIONAL PRACTICE	EXAMPLES IN ONLINE COURSES
High expectations	Communicate learning outcomes and expectations in several places in the course; expect success; online learning is not easier than or less than classroom expectations
Active learning	Use case studies; problem-based learning; discussion; round robin; critical thinking vignettes
Rich, prompt feedback	Create self-graded activities; structure learning activities that require students to produce work for review by self, students, and faculty
Interaction with faculty	Use online office hours; use course e-mail for individual communications; be available to answer noncourse-related questions; share examples of faculty work; participate in socialization activities
Interaction with classmates	Use group projects to promote collaborative work; structure communication tools for small-group work, learning circles, chats; create opportunities for students to share reflections and experiences; ensure places for public and private communication for class members
Time on task	Time spent on learning activities should be reasonable; allow sufficient time between assignments; structure online classroom so students are not reading voluminous and nonessential postings and online time is productive and related to course outcomes; create separate "social spaces" as options for participation
Respect for diverse ways of learning	Create options for learning and evaluation; present choices for content and learning activities; encourage diverse opinions while creating norms of respect; use reflective journals to assist students to assess their own needs, styles, and values

group work. See Box 19-1 for a discussion forum from a fully online Web course showing the use of a variety of teaching–learning strategies. Each module in the discussion forum identifies the learning activity for the students to engage in and discuss among themselves.

Just-in-Time Teaching and Learning

Most nursing courses now use some form of online course support to create community, to administer tests and surveys, or simply to post course resources. Just-in-time teaching (Novak et al., 1999) is a strategy that combines active learning in the classroom with the use of online course resources. The educator uses online assignments to facilitate learning course concepts before students participate in classroom activities. For example, an assignment might require students to read lesson content and complete an online assignment that tests their ability to apply the content in a variety of ways. Students receive feedback about their learning before they come to the classroom. Faculty and students are then better prepared to use classroom time to clarify misunderstood concepts or solve more complex problems.

Box 19-1
DISCUSSION FORUMS

Introductions Introduce yourself: tell us where you work, why you are taking this course, and anything else you want us to know about you!

Module 1: Focus on the Learner Post a description of your learners, how you will assess their needs, and what support they need in your Web course.

Module 2: Debate Question: Should ALL nursing courses be designed to be offered only on the Internet? Participants with last names A-M will argue the affirmative; participants with last names N-Z will argue the negative. Participant with first last name with A, summarize the affirmative; person with first last name with Z (or last of alphabet) summarize the negative.

Module 2: Treasure Hunt In this course, find the various strategies used to inform learners about the course expectations and learning outcomes to be attained. Post your findings and comment on the value of each strategy.

Module 2: Round Robin Post a response to the question, "How can we assist learners in Web courses to obtain feedback?"

Module 3: Chat Summary Summarize the work of your chat room discussion.

Module 4: One-Minute Paper "Online Learning Communities" Write a "one-minute paper" describing what helped you become a member of the online learning community in this course.

Module 5: Muddiest Point What is still not clear to you at this point in the course? Post your questions and all (faculty and participants) will try to clear up your muddiness.

Student Lounge This is the place to kick back and relax.

Question Office Post your questions about the course content, process, or technical aspects here. Answers will be provided within 24 hours.

Facilitating Discussion in the Online Learning Community

Facilitating discussion in the OLC is one of the most important roles of the educator who is engaged in online teaching. Effective facilitation of online discussion promotes critical thinking, active learning, collaborative learning, and reflective thinking.

To facilitate online discussion, the educator must first establish a learning community through activities that promote personal student interaction and allow the class to get acquainted with each other as individuals. Sharing pictures, using "ice breaker" activities, and posting brief introductory messages during the first week of the course are just a few examples of some activities that can promote interaction among the students before discussion of course content begins. Establishing a discussion forum that can be used by students to ask course questions and promote student dialogue without faculty presence can also be helpful in promoting a learning community. Some faculty elect to schedule periodic face-to-face interactions to promote a sense of community, but this is not always possible or even necessary. A learning community can be successfully built online without the participants ever meeting each other.

Palloff and Pratt (1999) identify six elements that are key to building OLCs and promoting interaction: honesty, responsiveness, relevance, respect, openness, and empowerment. For meaningful online discussion to occur, students must be able to expect that they will receive honest, respectful, constructive feedback and prompt responses from faculty and students. The subject matter and discussion need to be relevant to real life. Respect for students as equal participants in the learning process and empowering them to be self-directed, responsible learners is also important. Finally, students need to feel free to share their thoughts and feelings without fear of retribution in the form of lower grades. By creating an OLC that adheres to these principles, faculty will more likely be successful in getting the level of discussion they desire in their online courses.

Faculty can also promote online discussion among all students by clearly establishing expectations for participation within the course. If weekly online discussion is expected, this should be stated in the course syllabus. During the first 2 to 3 weeks of the course, those students who are not participating in the online discussion should be actively sought out. The lack of participation early in the course is likely due to technology issues or the inability to be self-directive in learning (Halstead & Coudret, 2000). Reaching out to the student at this critical point in the course may make a difference in whether the student will be successful in completing the course.

Learning assignments that foster higher-level discussion are those that promote analysis or critique of a concept. Some examples of higher-level learning assignments that promote student interaction with content include concept clarification, case studies, and debates. Identifying a challenging clinical problem and having students brainstorm solutions or debate the pros and cons of a given solution to the problem are other examples of higher-level discussion techniques that promote discussion and interaction. It is relatively easy for students to identify real-life issues in nursing practice that can be used to generate online discussion. The classroom assessment techniques of Angelo and Cross (1993) such as "muddiest point," "minute paper," "pro and con," and "analytic memo" can also be used to stimulate interaction and higher-level thinking in online discussion.

Varying the students' roles in discussion can also help promote interaction and ensure participation by all students. Students can take turns being assigned the role of discussion leader or summarizer of the week's discussion. Teams of students can be formed for small-group discussion of a topic, with the team summarizing its discussion at a later point for the whole class to consider. By carefully selecting discussion topics that foster higher-level thinking, periodically altering the roles that students have in the discussion, and allowing students to identify areas of content that they would like to discuss in depth, faculty will likely be successful in facilitating meaningful online discussion.

Clinical Teaching and the Online Learning Community

Although the clinical practice experiences required in nursing cannot be taught online, the tools and strategies that are the strengths of the OLC can be used to support clinical experiences for students (DeBourgh, 2001; Vinten & Partridge, 2002;). E-mail and chat and discussion forums link students to instructors and preceptors, expert nurses, health care professionals, and clients in the broader community of professional practice. In the clinical teaching environment the knowledge learned in the didactic course is applied. Here apprenticeship strategies, use of preceptors, and interaction with colleagues facilitate knowledge transfer. For example, Nesler et al. (2001) found that precepted clinical experiences for students in Web courses were important components for professional role socialization, and Billings et al. (2001) found that effective teaching practices within the Web course correlated highly with socialization and preparation for real-world work.

EVALUATING AND GRADING LEARNING OUTCOMES

Evaluation is as important in online courses as it is in the classroom or clinical practice environment. Best practices indicate that evaluation begins with clearly stated and communicated learning outcomes or competencies; provides students with an opportunity to learn and practice the expected behaviors and receive feedback during the learning process; and concludes with judgment or "grading," indicating the degree to which learning has occurred. Special considerations for these evaluation practices as they pertain to the online environment are discussed here.

Timing of Evaluation

Evaluation in online courses, particularly those courses that are fully online, assumes greater significance because of the asynchronous nature of the course and the lack of face-to-face communication. Faculty must therefore be deliberate about the timing of the evaluation and thoughtful in choosing evaluation strategies and providing feedback throughout the course.

Formative evaluation is essential to learning in online courses. Case studies, critical thinking vignettes, and self-tests provide students with opportunities to practice and receive formative evaluation when teaching feedback is included in the test or scenarios. Adapting classroom assessment techniques (CAT) (see Chapter 14) to the online learning environment is another way to help both students and faculty gauge students' understanding of course concepts. For example, a CAT such as an online "muddiest point" or electronic survey early in the course can help faculty to modify the course or teaching strategies as the course progresses. Taking advantage of the features of an online grade book will help students keep track of their own progress.

Summative evaluation occurs after students have had the opportunity to learn and apply course content. Evaluation strategies that work well in the classroom usually work well in online courses (see Chapter 21). Strategies that are particularly effective include written work, games, debates, discussion, portfolios, electronic poster presentations, and tests (Bloom & Trice, 1997; Reising, 2002; Rossignol & Scollin, 2001).

Evaluation in online courses should take advantage of the course management tools such as discussion forum, e-mail, testing, and portfolio management. Online grade books assist students in tracking their own progress, and to the extent possible, in determining when they are ready for summative or final evaluation such as taking a final exam.

Academic Integrity in Online Courses

Academic integrity must be observed and protected in the online community, as well as in the classroom. Policies may need to be written to include online courses or may need to be adapted to be more inclusive of the online course. In addition, norms of respect for individuals and their ideas must also be observed. All expectations must be communicated to the student.

Plagiarism involves using the work of another without attributing credit to the original author. The electronic environment provides students with easy access to papers and projects from students throughout the world, as well as from students in similar or previous courses within the same school. Faculty have a responsibility to assist students in learning the conventions of citing published work and to be proactive in offsetting the potential for plagiarism. Simple measures include developing an honor code statement, requiring students to submit copies of all cited references, selectively altering assignments each semester, and choosing assignments that can be completed only by using original work such as a care plan for a specific patient. More complicated and expensive measures include purchasing plagiarism detection software.

Exam Security

Online testing poses risks for exam security, and it is the responsibility of faculty to take reasonable measures to ensure test security and confront instances of cheating. As in the classroom, methods for ensuring test security can be simple and low cost, or they may be complicated and involve additional human and fiscal resources (Reising, 2002). Easy-to-manage security in online tests includes having students log in with a user name and password, using timed tests, and using test software features to scramble test answers or generate alternative versions of exams. More complex measures to prevent or track cheating include tracking Internet protocol (IP) addresses for the computers on which students are taking a test and hiring proctors.

EFFECTIVENESS OF ONLINE LEARNING

Because the use of online learning has increased, educators have been concerned about assessing the effectiveness of their own online courses and programs. Findings from several studies are being used to guide the process of assessing effectiveness and to set the stage for continuous quality improvement in these courses and programs.

Studies of the effectiveness of online courses reveal that online learning is as effective as it is in the classroom (Leasure et al., 2000) and that the findings of "no significant differences" are consistently true when one media format is compared with another (see Chapter 17). Students also tend to be satisfied with online learning (Billings et al., 2001) and favor the online format (Wills & Stommel, 2002). DeBourgh (2003) notes that student satisfaction with computer-mediated distance education was most associated with the perceived quality of the instruction and the effectiveness of the instructor. Buckley (2003) notes that although there were no differences in learning outcomes between a classroom, a Web-enhanced, and a Web-based nutrition course for undergraduate nursing students, students expressed the greatest satisfaction with the Web-enhanced version of the course.

Other researchers examined the effectiveness of the educational practices within Web courses. For example, Billings et al. (2001) found that the use of active learning strategies and ample opportunity for interaction within the course were correlated with outcomes such as student satisfaction, socialization, and preparation for real-world work. VandeVusee and Hanson (2000) found that faculty could facilitate active learning by carefully structuring the discussion forums that were used to promote outcomes of critical thinking.

Nurse educators will continue to monitor the effectiveness of the use of technology, the educational practices within the OLC, and the outcomes of the courses and educational programs in which online teaching and learning occur. Using the opportunities of new learning environments will continue to challenge assumptions about teaching and learning, and in the long run, result in improvement of pedagogical practices.

SUMMARY

Online learning is a dynamic process that has been proven in many instances to be as effective as traditional classroom learning. The rapid development and adoption of online education is having a significant impact on higher education. Nurse educators are leaders on university and college campuses in implementing online education and will continue to be in the forefront of identifying the best practices for designing, implementing, and evaluating online programs of education.

REFERENCES

Angelo, T., & Cross, P. (1993). *Classroom assessment techniques.* San Francisco: Jossey-Bass.
Billings, D. (2000) A framework for assessing outcomes and practices in Web-based courses in nursing. *Journal of Nursing Education, 39,* 60-67.
Billings, D. (2002). Internal marketing. In D. Billings (Ed.), *Conversations in e-learning.* Pensacola, FL: Pohl Publishing.
Billings, D., Connors, H., Skiba, D. (2001). Benchmarking best practices in Web-based nursing courses. *Advances in Nursing Science, 23*(3), 41-52.
Bloom, K. C., & Trice. L.B. (1997). The efficacy of individualized computerized testing in nursing education. *Computers in Nursing, 15*(2), 82-88.
Boettcher, J., & Conrad, R. (1999). *Faculty guide for moving teaching and learning to the Web.* Retrieved February 22, 2004, from League for Innovation in the Community College Web site: http://www.league.org
Bolan, C. (2003). Incorporating experiential learning theory into the instructional design of online courses. *Nurse Educator, 28*(1), 10-14.

Bonk, C., & Cunningham, D. (1998). Searching for learner-centered, constructivist, and sociocultural components of collaborative educational learning tools. In C. Bonk & K. King (Eds.), *Electronic collaborators* (pp. 25-50). Mahwah, NJ: Lawrence Erlbaum Associates.

Bonk, C., & King, K. (Eds.). (1998). *Electronic collaborators*. Mahwah, NJ: Lawrence Erlbaum Associates.

Bonnell, K., & Halstead, J. A. (1999, February 23). *Are you ready to deliver a distance education program?* Paper presented at Proceedings from Stop Surfing-Start Teaching 1999 National Conference, University of South Carolina, Myrtle Beach, SC.

Buckley, K. M. (2003). Evaluation of classroom-based, Web-enhanced, and Web-based distance learning nutrition courses for undergraduate nursing. *Journal of Nursing Education, 42*(8), 367-369.

Chickering, A., & Ehrmann, S. (1996). *Implementing the seven principles: technology as a lever.* Retrieved March 3, 2004, from http//www.tltgroup.org/programs/seven.html

Chickering, A., & Gamson, Z. (1987). *Seven principles of good practice in undergraduate education.* Racine, WI: Johnson Foundation.

Clark, R. C., & Mayer, R. E. (2003). *e-Learning and the science of instruction: Proven guidelines for consumers and designers of multimedia learning.* San Francisco: Jossey-Bass Pfeiffer.

DeBourgh, G. A. (2001). Using Web technology in a clinical nursing course. *Nurse Educator, 26*(5), 227-233.

DeBourgh, G. A. (2003). Predictors of student satisfaction in distance-delivered graduate nursing courses: What matters most? *Journal of Professional Nursing, 19,* 149-163.

Dell, D. (2002). Learning management systems. In D. Billings (Ed.), *Conversations in e-learning.* Pensacola, FL: Pohl Publishing.

Edwards, N., Hugo, K., Cragg, B., Peterson, J. (1999). The integration of problem-based learning strategies in distance education. *Nurse Educator, 24*(1), 36-41.

Halstead, J. A. (2002). How will my role change when I teach on the Web? In D. Billings (Ed.), *Conversations in e-learning.* Pensacola, FL: Pohl Publishing.

Halstead, J. A., & Coudret, N. A. (2000). Implementing Web-based instruction in a school of nursing: Implications for faculty and students. *Journal of Professional Nursing, 16*(5), 273-281.

Jeffries, P. (2000). Development and test of a model for designing interactive CD-ROMs for teaching nursing skills. *Computers in Nursing, 18*(3), 118-124.

Leasure, A. R., Davis, L., & Thievon, S. (2000). Comparison of student outcomes and preferences in a traditional vs. World Wide Web-based baccalaureate nursing research course. *Journal of Nursing Education, 39,* 149-154.

Malloy, S., & DeNatale, M. (2001). Online critical thinking. *Nurse Educator, 26,* 101-197.

Mastrian, G., & McGonigle, D. (1999). Using technology-based assignments to promote critical thinking. *Nurse Educator, 24*(1), 45-47.

Mills, M., Fisher, C., & Stair, N. (2001). Web-based courses: More than curriculum. *Nursing and Health Care Perspectives, 22*(5), 235-239.

Nesler, M., Hanner, M. B., Melburg, V., & McGowan, S. (2001). Professional socialization of baccalaureate nursing students: Can students in distance nursing programs become socialized? *Journal of Nursing Education, 40*(7), 293-302.

Novak, G., Patterson, E., Gavrin, A., & Christian, W. (1999). *Just-in-time teaching: Blending active learning with Web technology.* Upper Saddle River, NJ: Prentice Hall.

Palloff, R., & Pratt, K. (1999). Building learning communities in cyberspace: Effective strategies for the on-line classroom. San Francisco: Jossey-Bass.

Peterson, J., Henning, L., Dow, K., Sole, M. (2001). Designing and facilitating class discussion in an Internet class. *Nurse Educator, 26*(1), 28-32.

Reising, D. (2002). Online testing. In D. Billings (Ed.), *Conversations in e-learning.* Pensacola, FL: Pohl Publishing.

Rossignol, M., & Scollin, P. (2001). Piloting use of computerized practice tests. *Computers in Nursing, 18*(2), 72-86.

Smith-Stoner, M. (2003). Videostreaming in nursing education. *Nurse Educator, 28*(2), 66-70.

Sternberger, C. (2002). Embedding a pedagogical model in the design of an online course. *Nurse Educator, 27*(4), 170-173.

Thurmond, V. (2002). Considering theory in assessing quality of Web-based courses. *Nurse Educator, 27*(1), 20-24.

VandeVusee, L., & Hanson, L. (2000). Evaluation of online course discussions. *Computers in Nursing, 18*(4), 181-188.

Vinten, S., Partridge, R. (2002). E-learning and the clinical practicum. In D. Billings (Ed.), *Conversations in e-learning* (pp. 187-196). Pensacola, FL: Pohl Publisher.

Wills, C., & Stommel, M. (2002). Graduate nursing students' precourse and postcourse perceptions and preferences concerning completely Web-based courses. *Journal of Nursing Education, 41*(5), 193-201.

EVALUATION

20

THE EVALUATION PROCESS
AN OVERVIEW

Mary P. Bourke, PhD(c), RN, Barbara A. Ihrke, PhD, RN

Nursing faculty are responsible for appraising student learning, course, curriculum, and program outcomes and their own teaching practices; they are accountable to students, peers, administrators, employers, and society for the effectiveness of the nursing program. The purpose of this chapter is to present an overview of the process by which nursing faculty can evaluate these outcomes and report results to stakeholders. This chapter is a link to subsequent and previous chapters that cover specific evaluation activities and strategies. The chapter delineates a step-by-step evaluation process including the use of models; selection of instruments; data collection procedures; and the means to interpret, report, and use findings that can be used to make decisions about improvement in student learning; faculty performance; and course, curriculum, and program quality.

DEFINITION OF TERMS

The many terms used to describe evaluation and evaluation activities are often used interchangeably. The following definitions are used throughout this chapter.

Evaluation

Evaluation is a means of appraising data or placing a value on data gathered through one or more measurements. Evaluation also involves rendering judgment by pointing out strengths and weaknesses of different features or dimensions. Evaluation is the "step in the assessment process in which measures of quality and productivity are examined against some standard of performance" (Gates et al., 2002, p. 6).

Grading

Grading, often confused with evaluation, involves quantifying data and assigning value. Grades serve two purposes. Grades notify students of their achievement and inform the public of student performance (Shoemaker & DeVos, 1999).

Assessment

Assessment, in the broadest view, refers to processes that provide information about students, faculty, curricula, programs, and institutions. More specifically, assessment refers to measures of student abilities and changes in knowledge, skills, and attitudes during and after participation in courses and programs (Angelo & Cross, 1993; Davis, 1993; Gates et al., 2002). Assessment data can be obtained to place students in courses, to provide information about learning needs (Chapter 2), and to determine achievement in individual courses and programs (Chapters 14 and 21 to 24). Findings are used to improve student learning and teaching (Chapter 14) and to improve courses and programs (Forker, 1996).

Curriculum Evaluation

Curriculum evaluation is the process of determining the outcomes of student learning as a result of participation in a program or plan of learning. Curriculum evaluation involves establishing outcomes and verifying the extent to which these have been achieved (see Chapter 24).

Program Evaluation

Educational program evaluation or program review encompasses a broader view of the educational program and examines component parts, including faculty, students, fiscal effectiveness, and curriculum and instructional outcomes. Program reviews are typically conducted by the faculty as a self-study and are undertaken to respond to accreditation reviews by state, education, and professional accrediting bodies (see Chapter 24).

Accreditation

Accreditation is a peer review process that serves as a mechanism of ensuring quality of educational programs. Accreditation signifies that an institution, school, or program has defined appropriate outcomes, maintains conditions in which they can be met, and is producing acceptable outcomes (Millard, 1994). Accreditation involves the following (Millard, 1994):

- Developing a statement of program mission, goals, and outcomes
- Conducting a self-study about the extent to which outcomes are being attained
- Undergoing on-site review by an external group of peers
- Being reviewed by an independent accrediting body that reads both the self-study and the site report of the peer reviewers and makes recommendations for accreditation

Schools of nursing may be accredited by state and regional agencies and national nursing organizations. Historically and currently, there are two organizations with interests in accrediting nursing education programs: the National League for Nursing Accrediting Commission and the Commission on Collegiate Nursing Education. Effective accreditation programs must be simple, relevant, and cost-effective. Regardless of the agency or organization providing accreditation services, nursing faculty must be aware of the standards and participate in the process of their development and review.

PHILOSOPHICAL APPROACHES TO EVALUATION

A philosophy of evaluation involves the evaluator's beliefs about evaluation. The philosophy will influence how evaluations are conducted, when evaluations are conducted, what methods are used, and how results are interpreted. A philosophy is reflected in attitudes and behavior.

In nursing education, evaluations or judgments are made about performance (students), program effectiveness (a nursing curriculum or program), instructional media (a textbook, a computer-assisted instruction program), or instruction (course, faculty). Evaluation activities in nursing education are conducted from various perspectives, and these perspectives influence outcomes. Therefore evaluators should be aware of the perspective or orientation they have toward evaluation.

Several philosophical perspectives tend to influence evaluation. Educators who rely on goals, objectives, and outcomes to guide program, course, or lesson development will likely have an *objectives* approach to evaluation. The merits of the activity or program are largely indicated by the success of students in meeting those objectives. A *service* orientation emphasizes the value evaluation can have in assisting educators to make decisions about learners and the teaching–learning process. Although all evaluation involves judgment, the evaluator with a *judgment* perspective will focus on establishing the worth or merit of the employee, student, product, or program. Others have a *research* orientation to evaluation and emphasize precision in measurement and statistical analysis to gain general understanding of why students and programs do or do not succeed. The focus in this perspective is on tools, methods, and designs and the validity and reliability of instruments. Yet another orientation is the *constructivist* view that emphasizes the values of the stakeholders and builds consensus about what needs to be changed. Although faculty, in their role as evaluators, use a combination of these perspectives, one is likely dominant, and faculty should be aware of the perspective they bring to evaluation activities because the philosophical orientation toward evaluation will guide the evaluation process and influence outcomes.

THE EVALUATION PROCESS

Evaluation is also a process that involves the following systematic series of actions:

1. Identifying the purpose of the evaluation

2. Identifying a time frame
3. Determining when to evaluate
4. Selecting the evaluator(s)
5. Choosing an evaluation design/framework or model
6. Selecting an evaluation instrument(s)
7. Collecting data
8. Interpreting data
9. Reporting the findings
10. Using the findings
11. Considering the costs of evaluation

The steps can be modified depending on the purpose of the evaluation, what is being evaluated (for example, students, instruction, program, or system), and the complexity of the units being evaluated.

Identifying the Purpose of the Evaluation

As in the research process, the first step in the evaluation process is to pose various questions that can be answered by evaluation. These questions may be broad and encompassing, as in program evaluation, or focused and specific, as in classroom assessment (Box 20-1). Regardless of the scope of the evaluation, the purpose or reason for conducting an evaluation should be clear to all involved.

Identifying a Time Frame

The next step in the evaluation process is to consider *when* evaluation should occur. Time frames for evaluation can be described as formative or summative.

Formative Evaluation

Formative evaluation (or assessment) refers to evaluation taking place during the program or learning activity (Kapborg & Fischbein, 2002; Whitman et al., 1992). Formative evaluation is conducted while the event to be evaluated is occurring and focuses on identifying progress toward purposes, objectives, or outcomes to improve the activities, course, curriculum, program, or teaching

---

Box 20-1
PURPOSES OF EVALUATION

1. To facilitate learning—or change behavior of an employee or student
2. To diagnose problems—to find learning deficits, ineffective teaching practices, curriculum defects, etc.
3. To make decisions—to assign grades, to determine merit raises, to offer promotion or tenure
4. To improve products—to revise a textbook, to add content to an independent study module
5. To judge effectiveness—to determine whether goals or standards are being met

and student learning. Formative evaluation emphasizes the parts instead of the entirety.

One *advantage* of formative evaluation is that the events are recent, thus guarding accuracy and preventing distortion by time. Another major advantage of formative evaluation is that the results can be used to improve student performance, program of instruction, or learning outcome before the program or course has concluded (Sims, 1992). *Disadvantages* of formative evaluation include making judgments before the activity (classroom or clinical performance, nursing program) is completed and not being able to see the results before judgments are made. Formative evaluation can also be intrusive or interrupt the flow of outcomes. There is also a chance for a false sense of security when formative evaluation is positive and the final results are not as positive as predicted earlier.

Summative Evaluation

Summative evaluation (or assessment), on the other hand, refers to data collected at the end of the activity, instruction, course, or program (Kapborg & Fischbein, 2002). The focus is on the whole event and emphasizes what is or was and the extent to which objectives and outcomes were met for the purposes of accountability, resource allocation, assignment of grades (students) or merit pay or promotion (faculty), and certification (Davis, 1994). Summative evaluation therefore is most useful at the end of a learning module or course and for program or course revision. Summative evaluation of learning outcomes in a course usually results in assignment of a final grade.

The *advantages* of performing an evaluation at the end of the activity are that all work has been completed and the findings of evaluation show results. The major *disadvantage* of summative evaluation is that nothing can be done to alter the results.

Determining When to Evaluate

The evaluator must also weigh each evaluation event and determine *when* evaluation is most appropriate. Typically, both formative and summative evaluations are appropriate and lend respective strengths to the evaluation plan.

In determining when to evaluate, the evaluator must also consider the frequency of evaluation. Evaluation can be time consuming, but frequent evaluation is necessary in many situations. Frequent evaluations are important when the learning process is complex and unfamiliar and when it is considered helpful to anticipate potential problems if the risk of failure is high. Finally, important decisions require frequent evaluations (Box 20-2).

Selecting the Evaluator(s)

An important element in the evaluation process is the evaluator. Selection of an evaluator involves deciding who should be involved in the evaluation process and whether the evaluator should be chosen from the "inside" (internal evaluator) or from the "outside" (external evaluator). Both have merits.

> **Box 20-2**
> **SITUATIONS IN WHICH FREQUENT EVALUATION IS USEFUL**
>
> - Learning is complex
> - Trends are emerging
> - Problems have been identified
> - Problems are anticipated
> - There is a high risk of failure
> - Serious consequences would result from poor performance

Internal Evaluators

Internal evaluators are those directly involved with the learning, course, or program to be evaluated, such as the students, faculty, or nursing staff. Many people have a vested interest in evaluation (stakeholders) and can be selected to participate in the evaluation process. There are advantages and disadvantages associated with internal evaluators, and often several evaluators are helpful to obtain the most accurate data.

Advantages of using internal evaluators include their familiarity with the context of the evaluation, experience with the standards, cost-effectiveness, and potential for less obtrusive evaluation. Additionally, the findings of evaluation can be easily used because the results are known immediately. *Disadvantages* of using internal evaluators include bias, control of evaluation, and reluctance to share controversial findings. When internal evaluators are chosen and employed, it is important to note their position in the organization and where responsibility and reporting lines exist.

External Evaluators

External evaluators are those not directly involved in the events being evaluated. They are often employed as consultants. State, regional, and national accrediting bodies are other examples of external evaluators.

The *advantage* of using external evaluators is that they do not have a bias, are not involved in organizational politics, may be very experienced in a particular type of evaluation, and do not have a stake in the results. *Disadvantages* of using external evaluators include expense, unfamiliarity with the context, barriers of time, and potential travel constraints.

Because evaluators are so critical to the evaluation process, faculty should select evaluators carefully. Box 20-3 lists questions to be asked in the selection of an evaluator.

Choosing an Evaluation Design/Framework or Model

This step of the evaluation process involves selecting or developing an evaluation model. An evaluation model represents the ways the variables, items, or events to be evaluated are arranged, observed, or manipulated to answer the evaluation question. A model serves to clarify the relationship of the variables to be evaluated and provides a systematic plan or framework for the evaluation.

Box 20-3
QUESTIONS TO ASK WHEN SELECTING AN EVALUATOR

1. What is the evaluator's philosophical orientation?
2. What is the evaluator's experience?
3. What methods or instruments does the evaluator use? Have experience with?
4. What is the evaluator's style?
5. Is the evaluator responsive to the client?
6. Does the evaluator work well with others?
7. Is the evaluator supportive versus critical?
8. What is the evaluator's orientation to evaluation?

Evaluation models for nursing education may be found in the nursing literature or may be developed by nurse educators for a specific use. Although evaluation models have been adapted from those used in education (Guba & Lincoln, 1981; Madaus et al., 1988; Scriven, 1972; Stake, 1967) and business, nursing education evaluation models may more closely reflect the aspects of nursing education and practice that are being evaluated (Billings et al., 2001; Germain et al., 1994; Kapborg & Fischbein, 2002).

Using an evaluation model has several advantages. A model makes variables explicit and often reflects a priority about which variables should be evaluated first or most often. A model also gives structure that is visible to all concerned; the relationships of parts are evident. Using an evaluation model also helps focus evaluation. It keeps the evaluation efforts on target: those elements that are to be evaluated are included; those not to be evaluated are excluded. Finally, a model can be tested and validated.

A model should be selected according to the demands of the evaluation question, the context, and the needs of the stakeholders. Several models are used in nursing evaluation activities, and they are described briefly here. For detailed information and an example of the use of one model, see Chapter 24, Educational Program Evaluation.

Decision-oriented Models: CIPP

The concepts of the CIPP model (context, input, process, and product) facilitate delineating, obtaining, and providing useful information for judging decision alternatives (Stufflebeam & Associates, 1971; Stufflebeam & Webster, 1994). *Context* evaluation identifies the target population and assesses its needs. *Input* evaluation identifies and assesses system capabilities, alternative program strategies, and procedural designs for implementing the strategies. *Process* evaluation detects defects in the design or implementation of the procedure. *Product* evaluation is a collection of descriptions and analysis of outcomes and correlates them to the objectives, context, input, and process information, resulting in the interpretation of results.

The CIPP model measures the weakness and strengths of a program, identifies the needs of the target population, identifies options, and provides evidence of beneficial results or lack thereof. In this model, evaluation is performed in the service of decision making; hence, it should provide information useful to decision makers. Evaluation is also a cyclic, continuing process, and therefore must be implemented through a systematic program.

Client-centered Models

Stake's (1967) Countenance model focuses on the goals and observed effects of the program being evaluated in terms of antecedents, transactions, and outcomes (Stufflebeam & Webster, 1994). *Antecedents* are conditions that exist that may affect the outcome; for example, students with prior college experience will affect the outcome of freshman scores. *Transactions* are all educational experiences and interactions; and *outcomes* are the abilities, achievements, attitudes, and aspirations of students that result from the educational experience. The purpose of this model is to promote an understanding of activities in a given setting. Case studies and responsive evaluations (Stake, 1967) elicit information about the program from those involved in this action-research approach to educational evaluation. In this model, evaluators must make judgments on the comparison of goals and the outcomes.

Assessment Models

Assessment models focus on the outcomes of general and professional education. Assessment models tend to be locally developed and locally implemented, and the results are used by the participants for course, curriculum, and program improvement. Assessment begins with educational values; works best when the program has clear purposes; and makes a difference when it illuminates questions of concern to the stakeholders, is ongoing, and meets responsibilities to students and the public (The American Association of Higher Education [AAHE] Assessment Forum, 1994).

Stern and Kramer (1992) describe the Kean College approach to outcome assessment. In this model, each department was given ownership of the evaluation process. The step-by-step process for each department consisted of "(a) establishing program and specific course objectives that were stated in measurable terms; (b) developing an instrument or other means of assessing students' achievement of those objectives; (c) conduction of the pilot study of the instrument of measure chosen; and (d) analyzing the data and implementing change as needed" (p. 621). The results were to be used to enhance and improve programs. Because the evaluation belonged to the department and findings were not to be used for teacher evaluation or tenure, the responsibility for change also rested there.

Another well-known example of the use of an assessment model is Alverno College (Loacker & Mentkowski, 1993; Voorhees, 2001). Assessment is an integral component of the curriculum because both the students and faculty monitor the direction of learning and the coherence of instruction. Portfolios are one of the key strategies used in the assessment process.

Naturalistic, Constructivist, or Fourth-generation Evaluation Models

Fourth-generation evaluation is a "sociopolitical process that is simultaneously diagnostic, change-oriented, and educative for all the parties involved" (Lincoln & Guba, 1985, p. 141). Fourth-generation evaluation takes into account the values, concerns, and issues of those involved in the evaluation (students, faculty, clients, and administrators). The result is a construction of and consensus about needed improvements and changes (Swenson, 1991). Both the evaluator and the stakeholders are responsible for change.

Fourth-generation evaluation incorporates techniques of evaluator observation, interviews, and participant evaluations to elicit views, meanings, and understanding of the stakeholders. Thus the evaluation becomes not the opinion or judgment of the evaluator but the working toward meaning, understanding, and consensus of all involved in the process. This responsive evaluation informs and empowers the stakeholders for reflection and change.

Quality Assurance Models: Total Quality Management, Continuous Quality Improvement

Adapted from business and nursing services, quality assurance models can be used to guide evaluation and improve educational programs and nursing programs. Total Quality Management (TQM) and Continuous Quality Improvement (CQI) are structured approaches that examine organizational processes as a way of understanding their contributions to outcomes. Organization-wide participation is focused on meeting the customer's needs and continuously improving the processes that contribute to an effective organization and organizational outcomes (Clark & Rice, 1994). The process involves all stakeholders and uses team knowledge to improve decision making. Benchmarking is used in the "pursuit of continuous quality improvement" (Murphy, 1995).

Benchmarking

Benchmarking has been widely used in the business arena, including health care, but has been used less often in educational settings. Benchmarking refers to the measurement and comparison of selected criteria with previously recognized ideal criteria. Licensing exam pass rates of nursing programs are compared, thus permitting evaluation of a program according to national standards. The number of students passing the licensing exam is an indication that an overall program has been successful in the teaching–learning process. Benchmarking or "best practices" is "a process improvement technique that provides factual data that allows institutions to compare performance on specific variables in order to achieve best-of performance" (Billings et al., 2001, p. 42). Palomba and Banta (1999) define benchmarking as "the process of identifying and learning from institutions that are recognized for their outstanding practices" (p. 333). Gates et al. (2002) refer to benchmarking as the "comparison to leading-edge peers" (p. 98), thus relying "on the comparison of performance with that of external peers" (p. 143). Others have interchanged goals and objectives with the term *benchmarks* (Lignuagaris-Kraft et al., 2001).

Welsh and Metcalf (2003) refer to performance benchmarking as a method of evaluating institutional effectiveness. Although most definitions indicate evaluation at an institutional level, benchmarking can also be used at the divisional or college level. Nursing programs evaluate themselves in comparison with nursing programs that are recognized for outstanding practices. Individual courses are judged against courses developed by "leading-edge peers" who are specialists in content and teaching–learning practices. Although, few researchers have used benchmarking as an approach to assessment of the teaching–learning process (Parry & Dunn, 2000), it is a valid assessment model.

Billings et al. (2001) measured performance indicators in Web-based nursing courses, and the mean of each indicator was "reported as the benchmark" (p. 46). According to Billings et al., one begins the process of assessment by defining the benchmarks to be used. Thus benchmarks depend on the evaluation purpose and can be defined for institutions, programs within institutions, or individual student performance.

Models for Evaluating Online Learning Environments

With increasing use of online courses and programs, educators must also use models for evaluating the unique aspects of these learning environments. Many online courses are compared with their classroom counterparts, and claims of increased critical thinking, comprehension, and academic success are made. However, when one examines the research closely, the evaluations are often incomplete or inadequate. Without a model or framework to be used as guide for the school, faculty, or administration, a one-dimensional evaluation may result.

Evaluation models for online learning must account for the use of the technology, student support, faculty development, and effective use of principles of teaching and learning, as well as program outcomes. Formative evaluation is particularly important in the initiation of online courses and programs and typically includes usability testing and peer review of the courses (see Chapters 17, 18, & 19).

Selecting an Evaluation Instrument

After a model has been selected and the variables to be evaluated and their relationship to each other have been identified, the evaluator then selects evaluation instruments that can be used most easily to obtain the necessary data. The selection of evaluation instruments is determined by the evaluation question and the evaluation model.

Types of Instruments

Many evaluation instruments can be used or adapted to elicit information about nursing education activities. Commonly used instruments are discussed briefly here. Actual examples of evaluation instruments are provided in related chapters.

Questionnaire. A questionnaire is a method in which a person answers questions in writing on a form. The questionnaire is usually self-administered. The person reads the question and then responds as instructed. Questionnaires are cost-effective but often lack substance. Questions must be clear, concise, and simple (Polit & Hungler, 1999). This type of instrument is often used to "measure qualitative variables, such as feelings, attitudes and other behavioral and health-related variables" (Svenson, 2001, p. 47). Questionnaires could be used to measure a student's level of confidence in the clinical setting or to determine students' satisfaction with the nursing program after graduation.

Interview. An interview involves direct contact with individuals participating in the evaluation. Exit interviews, for example, are often conducted as a faculty member leaves the school of nursing or as students graduate. Interviews can be used to elicit both qualitative and quantitative data. Interviews can be conducted with an individual or in focus groups. Students or external evaluators may be assigned to collect the data (Angelo & Cross, 1993). The interview should be scheduled at a time that is convenient for both the interviewer and the participant.

The interviewer should provide a quiet private room or office to allow the participant to speak in privacy. A participant may open up more if he or she feels that the conversation will be private and confidential. An objective outline should be created and followed during the interview, and notes should be kept in a file. Great care must be taken to avoid personalizing the information. One negative aspect of interviews is that they are time intensive (Polit & Hungler, 1999).

Observation. Observation is the direct visualization of performance of a task or behavior. Observation or performance appraisal is useful for evaluation of clinical performance, skill competence, and development of attitudes and values. Observation allows for immediate feedback and opportunity for remediation. Difficulties often arise in scheduling observation; and when there are no objective criteria for observation, observations are biased opinions that skew results. The student, knowing he or she is being observed, will often inadvertently distort accuracy of data collected because of anxiety. Also, distortion of one problem observed can affect results of future observed outcomes. To avoid obtaining inaccurate results, the observer must have an objective tool that can be used to collect information accurately and without bias.

If the student is aware of objective criteria before evaluation, he or she has a clear understanding of expected behavior. Prior preparation will decrease anxiety among students, enabling a fair assessment. Faculty may provide a list of skills to be observed and the criteria for competence to the student. The student has a responsibility to prepare for the observation according to the criteria specified. This will give the student a sense of control over his or her educational experience and evaluation, thus decreasing anxiety.

Rating Scale. A rating scale is used to measure an abstract concept on a descriptive continuum. The rating scale is designed to increase objectivity in the evaluation process. Rating scales work well with norm-referenced evaluation, although they are not the best tools to use for this type of evaluation. Grades can easily be assigned to the ratings.

Checklist. A checklist is two-dimensional in that the expected behavior or competence is listed on one side and the degree to which this behavior meets the level of expectation is listed on the other side. With a detailed checklist of items and well-defined criteria being measured, the evaluator can easily identify expected behavior or acceptable competence. This type of instrument is useful for formative and summative evaluations. A checklist can be used to evaluate a student's performance of clinical procedures. The steps to be followed can be placed in sequential order, and the observer can then check off each action that is taken or not taken.

Attitude Scale. An attitude scale measures how the participant (usually a student) feels about a subject at the moment when he or she answers the question. Several popular types of attitude scales are used in nursing education evaluation.

The most popular is the *Likert scale*. In a Likert scale, several items in the form of statements (10 to 15 recommended) are used to express an opinion on a particular issue. Each item represents a construct of that issue; for example, a particular item may express an opinion about Latino students in nursing when the theme of the survey is diversity. Participants are asked to indicate the degree to which they agree or disagree. Equal numbers of positively and negatively worded items should be used to prevent bias in the responses.

Semantic differential is another scale used to measure attitude. Bipolar scales are used to measure the reaction of the participant. Each item on the scale is followed by bipolar adjectives such as good-bad, active-passive, or positive-negative. The number of intervals between each adjective is usually odd so that the middle interval is neutral. A list of five to seven intervals is adequate. Analysis is performed by adding values for each item, which is similar to what is done with the Likert scale (Cox & West, 1986). Both the Likert scale and the semantic differential provide interval data for analysis.

Self-Report, Journal, Diary. A self-report, journal, or diary is a student's written narrative of his or her critical reflections, thoughts, fears, goals progress, improvements needed, and tasks completed. These reports can involve a one-time assignment or a continuous record over a semester of clinical experience or even a curriculum. A spiral notebook is a useful tool for keeping a progressive record together. The notebook can be evaluated on a daily, weekly, or semester basis. The more frequent the evaluation, the more effective this tool will be in the evaluation process.

The diary or journal is valuable in a long-term analysis of the student's progress. The value of this tool is directly correlated with the planning and construction of its intended purpose and how it is used. Diaries or journals require student compliance and may involve considerable time to grade.

Anecdotal Notes. Anecdotal notes are the instructor's notations or comments on student performance or behavior during clinical experience. The value of these notes will be directly related to the objectives to be measured. Planning and identification of what is to be noted will prevent negative bias or lack of constructive value. Anecdotal notes are a valuable tool when accumulated and then used for a summative evaluation of the student's performance. This continual assessment allows the student to be judged fairly, especially in cases in which the student may have performed unsatisfactorily during one clinical learning experience, thus preventing the possibility that one event will cloud the entire clinical experience.

Selection and Development of Evaluation Instruments

The evaluator should give careful consideration to selection (or development) of an evaluation instrument(s). Several guidelines can be used for selecting evaluation instruments. The instrument should have the following characteristics:

1. Appropriate for what is being evaluated
2. Appropriate for the domain being evaluated
3. Comprehensive: inclusive of all variables in the evaluation model
4. Easy to use: understandable to the evaluator and user
5. Cost-effective
6. Time efficient
7. Valid and reliable

When evaluation tools or instruments are not available, faculty can develop their own. However, the cost of development can be significant in terms of time. Schools of nursing tend to have instruments developed that can be used as a starting point for evaluation activities.

Although there are many advantages to use of existing instruments, Polit and Hungler (1999) point out that the potential for serious problems must be understood before any instrument is used. First, the selection of an inappropriate or technically inadequate instrument will lead to inadequate measurement of desired data. The instrument must meet minimum standards of validity, reliability, and interpretability. Second, the instrument or tool must be valid. Third, faculty must consider that the use of some existing instruments, such as examinations, increases the chance of material not being taught or learned according to the objectives but according to material being tested or observed. An evaluation of the instrument with these criteria will increase success in measuring accurately what is intended to be evaluated.

Reliability and Validity of Evaluation Instruments Used in Nursing Education

When any instrument is used, its validity and reliability for evaluation should be ensured. Special procedures can be used to determine reliability and validity of instruments used for clinical evaluation, program evaluation, and examinations given to measure classroom achievement. Specific procedures are discussed in appropriate chapters of this book. A general overview of the concepts of validity and reliability is provided here.

Validity. Measurement validity verifies that faculty are in fact collecting and analyzing results they intend to measure. Measurement validity, particularly in the area of educational assessment and evaluation, has attributes of relevance, accuracy, and utility (Prus & Johnson, 1994). *Relevance* of an instrument is achieved when the instrument measures the educational objective as directly as possible. The instrument is *accurate* if it is measuring the educational objective precisely. The instrument has *utility* if it provides formative and summative results that have implications for evaluation and improvement. Thus valid evaluation instruments have relevance for the local program or curriculum and can provide meaningful results that indicate directions for change (Prus & Johnson, 1994).

Although there are several types of validity, measurement validity is now viewed as a single concept (Goodwin, 1997). Content-related evidence, criterion-related evidence, and construct-related evidence are considered categories of validity. For interpretation, evidence from all categories is ideal. The validity of an instrument can best be determined when faculty understand the nature of the content and specifications in the evaluation design, the relationship of the instrument to the significant criterion, and the constructs or psychological characteristics being measured by the instrument (Gronlund, 1993).

Content-related evidence refers to the extent to which the instrument is representative of the larger domain of the behavior being measured. Content-related evidence is particularly important to establish for clinical evaluation instruments and classroom tests. For example, with classroom tests, the following question is raised: "Does the sample of test questions represent all content described in the course?" In clinical evaluation, the question posed is "Does the instrument measure attitudes, behaviors, and skills representative of the domain of being a nurse?"

Criterion-related evidence refers to the relationship of a score on one measure (test, clinical performance appraisal) to other external measures. There are two ways to establish criterion-related evidence, concurrent and predictive. *Concurrent evidence* is the correlation of one score with another measure that occurs at the same time. The most common example of concurrent validity is correlation of clinical course grades with didactic course grades. Concurrent validity of the instrument is said to occur, for example, when there is a high correlation between clinical evaluation and examination scores in a class of students. *Predictive study,* on the other hand, is a correlation with measures obtained after completion of an event or intervention, such as a course or lesson. For example, there may be predictive validity between course grades and licensing examination or certification examination scores.

Criterion-related evidence is used to relate the outcomes of one instrument to the outcomes of another. In this sense it is used to predict success or establish the predictability of one measure with another one. Criterion-related evidence is established by using correlation measures. One example is the correlation between grade point average and scores on licensing or credentialing examinations. When there is a high positive correlation between the grade point average and the examination score, there is said to be criterion-related evidence.

Construct-related evidence is a relationship of one measure (e.g., examination) to other learner variables such as learning style, IQ, clinical competence, or job experience. Construct-related evidence is used to infer the relationship of a test instrument and student traits or qualities to identify what factors might be influencing performance. Examples include the relationship of IQ scores, Student Achievement Test (SAT) scores, and other test scores or working for pay as a student nurse and clinical performance.

Reliability. Reliability is the extent to which an instrument (self-report examination, observation schedule, or checklist) is dependable, precise, predictable, and consistent. Pedhazur and Schmelkin (1991) refer to reliability as the "degree to which test scores are free from errors of measurement." Reliability answers the question, "Will the same instrument yield the same results with different groups of students or when used by different raters?" According to Newby (1992), "Reliability in testing refers to the idea that tests should be consistent in the way that they measure performance" (p. 253).

Several types of reliability—stability reliability, equivalence reliability, and internal consistency reliability—are relevant to evaluation instruments and achievement examinations. *Stability reliability* of an instrument is the perceived consistency of the instrument over time. An assumption of stability in results is assumed. *Equivalence reliability* entails the degree to which two different forms of an instrument can be used to obtain the same results. For example, when two forms of a test are used, both tests should have the same number of items and same level of difficulty. The test is given to the group at the same time as the equivalent test is given or the equivalent is administered at a later date. *Internal consistency reliability* is associated with the extent to which all items on an instrument measure the same variable and with the homogeneity of the items. This reliability is considered only when the instrument is being used to measure a single concept or construct at a time.

Because the validity of findings is threatened when an instrument is unreliable, faculty should use measures to ensure instrument reliability. Millman (1994) advises that the reliability of the instrument is related to the number of items on the instrument and therefore that increasing the number of items on an instrument whose reliability is in doubt will increase its reliability. Additionally, measures of individual students are less reliable than measures of groups, and faculty can also use groups as a way of increasing reliability of some instruments.

Collecting Data

The next step of the evaluation process is use of the evaluation instrument to gather data. Although the instrument will determine to some extent what data are collected and how, several other factors should be considered at this time. These include the data collector, the data sources, amount of data, timing of data collection, and informal versus formal data collection.

Data Collection

Consideration must be given to *who* is collecting the data. In some instances the data are gathered by the evaluator, as for example, the faculty member evaluating clinical performance of the students. In other situations, instruments may be administered by students or research assistants. If the data collectors are not familiar with the data-collecting procedures, they should be oriented to the task. Interrater reliability must be ensured when more than one person is collecting data.

Data Source

Before evaluation, the evaluator must identify sources from which the data will be collected. Will the data be observed (as in clinical evaluation), archival (as when grade point average is obtained from student records), or reported (as obtained from a longitudinal questionnaire of graduates)? At this time in the evaluation process, it is important to determine whether it is possible to have access to records, particularly if permission must be obtained from the participants.

Amount of Data

The amount of data to be collected must also be determined and specified. All data may be collected, or a sample may be sufficient, but a decision must be made. For example, in clinical evaluation, or classroom testing, it is impossible to collect data about each instance of clinical performance or knowledge gained from the classroom experience. In this instance, a sampling procedure is used and is guided by the clinical evaluation protocol or the blueprint or plan for the classroom test. It is important to note that the sampling plan must be established at this stage of the evaluation process.

Timing of Data Collection

When is the best time to collect the data? An understanding of the context of evaluation is helpful here. Should the data be collected at the beginning, middle, or end of the activity being evaluated? When gathering data from students, it is important to allow adequate time and to gather data when students are able to give unbiased responses. (For example, course evaluation data collected immediately after test results have been given may not yield the most reflective responses.)

Formal versus Informal Data Collection

Decisions about use of formal and informal data must also be made. Data can be obtained in a formal manner, such as by using a structured evaluation tool. Data can also be collected with informal methods, such as in the form of spontaneous comments made by students. The evaluator must decide whether both formal and informal data will be used in the plan.

Interpreting Data

This step of the evaluation process involves translating data to answer the evaluation questions established at the beginning of the evaluation process. This involves putting the data in usable form, organizing data for analysis, and interpreting the data against preestablished criteria. When data are interpreted, the context, frame of reference, objectivity, and legal and ethical issues must also be considered.

Frame of Reference

Frame of reference refers to the reference point used for interpretation of data. Two frames of reference are discussed here, norm-referenced interpretation and criterion-referenced interpretation.

Norm-referenced Interpretation. *Norm-referenced interpretation* refers to interpreting data in terms of the norms of a group of individuals who are being evaluated. The scores of the group form a basis for comparing each individual with the others. In norm-referenced evaluation, there will always be an individual who has achieved at the highest level, as well as one who has achieved at the lowest level.

Norm-referenced interpretation permits evaluators to compare achievement of students in several ways. Students in the same group can be compared and ranked. Students can be compared with students in another group or class section or with national group norms, as in the case of licensing examinations or nursing specialty certification examinations. Thus an *advantage* of norm-referenced interpretation is the ability to make comparisons within groups or with external groups and to use the data for predictive purposes, such as admission criteria. A *disadvantage* of using norm-referenced interpretation is the focus on comparison, which may foster a sense of competitiveness among students.

Criterion-referenced Interpretation. In criterion-referenced interpretation, on the other hand, results are judged against preestablished criteria and reflect the degree of criteria attainment. Criterion-referenced evaluation is typically used in competence-based learning models in which the goal is to assist the learner to achieve competence in or mastery of specified learning outcomes. Because students are compared with the outcome and not each other, all students can achieve competence.

The *advantages* of criterion-referenced interpretation include emphasis on mastery and the potential for all learners to achieve, increased learner motivation, sharing and collaboration among students, and ability to give clear progress reports to learners. *Disadvantages* of criterion-referenced interpretation include the inability to compare students with each other or with other groups.

Issues of Objectivity and Subjectivity

The issues of objectivity and subjectivity in evaluation always arise when data are interpreted. Different evaluators can look at the same data, yet render different judgments. The differences may be a result of evaluator bias or degrees of difference in objectivity. Studies of performance appraisals in work settings have shown the effects of recency—interpreting findings when other favorable findings have preceded the evaluation (Polit & Hungler, 1999). In some ways, faculty need to accept that there is a certain amount of subjectivity in evaluation: after all, this is "evaluation" and not "measurement." However, faculty should recognize subjectivity and the role it may play in interpretation of findings.

Legal Considerations

There may also be *legal aspects* involved in interpretation of findings. Legal consideration is particularly important in the area of student rights. How will results of evaluation be shared? What data about students can be collected? Does evaluation involve protection of human subjects? Will there be moral or ethical dilemmas in reporting the data? Who is affected by evaluation? How will they respond to the results? What impact will evaluation have on a student, a program, or a curriculum? Thus the evaluator and the audience must be aware of the context of evaluation because these elements can influence how the evaluation is conducted, how results are reported, what will change as a result of the evaluation, and how due process will be handled. See Chapter 3 for additional discussion of legal aspects of evaluating students' academic and clinical performance.

Reporting the Findings

In this step of the evaluation process, the results of evaluation are communicated to appropriate persons. Factors to consider when findings are reported include when, how, and to whom the findings will be provided.

Who Receives the Findings

The evaluator must know to whom the data should be reported. Typically, both the person(s) and group being evaluated and those requesting evaluation receive evaluation reports. Issues of reporting and confidentiality should be established at the outset of evaluation. Confidentiality of the report must be maintained. Only those persons designated to receive the report should do so. The evaluator should then destroy unneeded background information after the report is completed.

In reporting findings, it is also important to consider the recipient of the report. What will the recipient want and need to know? For example, students receiving a test grade are usually prepared only to understand the grade, not the complex methods that were used to determine the grade or the item analysis statistics. Preparing the recipient for the evaluation report may also be helpful if the recipient does not have adequate background information to receive the report.

When to Report Findings

The timing of the report is also crucial. There tends to be a readiness to know the results of evaluation, and if the report of results is delayed, the recipients may lose interest. For example, students prefer having immediate results and can have increased anxiety or lose interest if results are delayed. The timing of the report may also be based on when information is needed, for example, at the end of the semester when grades are to be reported to the registrar.

How to Report Findings

Evaluation reports can take many forms. They may be written or oral, formal or informal. An example of an informal evaluation is talking with the student about his or her performance in a clinical experience, without a structured evaluation. This type of evaluation is far from ideal and leaves the student and the instructor without objective criteria and a sense of fairness. In the event that the student should fail the course, the instructor is not able to defend the decision. In a formal report, statistical analysis of the data will be accessible along with the findings. Specific methods of reporting findings to students, faculty, administrators, and external audiences are discussed in subsequent chapters.

Using the Findings

Evaluation is a mutual effort between the evaluator and the individual, group, or program being evaluated. Although using the findings is the last, and often forgotten, step of the evaluation process, both parties have obligations for using the findings. Barrett-Barrick (1993) states that the use of evaluation findings requires purposeful, strategic planning. Four perspectives of these strategies are purpose, people, planning, and packaging. The *purpose* of the evaluation must be identified by faculty and administration. Types of evaluation used in nursing programs include accreditation, criterion-referenced evaluation, decision-focused evaluation, external evaluation, formative evaluation, internal evaluation, outcome evaluation, process evaluation, and summative evaluation. For an evaluation to be successful, the *people* involved in the evaluation should be included in the process. The main strategy in promoting evaluation is *planning* the activities and disseminating the evaluation information. *Packaging* the evaluation report to meet the needs of those who will use the report is a priority. The report should be in a format that is easily understood, and graphs and other visual aids should be used as needed.

Evaluation results can be used in a variety of ways. Common uses in nursing are to assign grades; revise instruction, courses, curricula, or programs; and demonstrate program effectiveness.

Several ways to improve the use of evaluation efforts are as follows:

1. Encourage persons involved in results to be involved in designing the evaluation plan.
2. Involve all concerned in the evaluation process. For example, students can do self-evaluation; faculty can do peer review.
3. Report findings in a timely manner.
4. Make recommendations that are realistic and can be used. For example, when reporting results of a test to a student, the evaluator (teacher) can make recommendations as to how to study for the next test to improve scores. In this way the report of the results can be useful to the student.
5. Build in time for sharing results. This can be done by having an examination review, an evaluation conference, or a curriculum evaluation workshop.
6. Encourage the recipient to generate alternatives to behavior. For example, the student can make his or her own suggestions about improving test scores. Faculty and staff can establish goals and objectives for course change.
7. Establish trust and be cautious with sensitive findings.
8. Place findings in context. Explain to the recipients what the findings mean and how they can use the results in their own setting.

Considering the Costs of Evaluation

Evaluation can be costly throughout the entire process, and therefore the evaluator and audience must be assured that the cost will match the benefit. Answers to the following cost-related questions need to be determined at the outset:

- What fees (or faculty time) are associated with evaluation?
- How much time will the evaluator spend in developing tools, administering tools, interpreting data, and reporting results?
- Will undue time be spent on the part of those being evaluated in filling out evaluation tools?
- Will complex evaluation methods involving lengthy evaluation tools or computer time for data analysis contribute to the outcome?
- Will the results of evaluation require changes?
- Will the student fail the course and need to repeat it?
- Will the curriculum require massive revision?

SUMMARY

Evaluation is a means of appraising data or placing a value on data gathered through one or more measurements. The evaluation process involves a systematic series of actions including identification of a clear purpose, the time frame, and the evaluator. Models or frameworks can be used to guide the process, choice of instruments, data collection methods, and reporting procedures. Would a builder construct the house without plans? The same principle applies in evaluation. The framework establishes the guide to the construction of purposeful evaluation. Researching and developing the framework are the most valuable first steps. Selection of the appropriate instruments is integral to success. The instruments should be appropriate for what is being evaluated, easy to use, cost-effective, time efficient, valid, and reliable. Results must be interpreted and reported accurately. Finally, after analysis, the findings must be used. To design and implement an evaluation plan and then ignore the results would defeat the purpose of evaluation. It would be analogous to leaving a newly constructed house empty.

REFERENCES

The American Association of Higher Education Assessment Forum. (1994). Principles of good practice for assessing student learning. In J. S. Stark & A. Thomas (Eds.), *Assessment and program evaluation*. Needham Heights, MA: Simon & Schuster.

Angelo, T. A., & Cross, K. P. (1993). *Classroom assessment techniques: A handbook for college teachers*. San Francisco: Jossey-Bass.

Barrett-Barrick, C. (1993). Promoting the use of program evaluation findings. *Nurse Educator, 18*(1), 10-12.

Billings, D. M., Connors, H. R., & Skiba, D. J. (2001). Benchmarking best practices in Web-based nursing courses. *Advances in Nursing Science, 23*(3), 41-52.

Clark, A. T., & Rice, D. R. (1994). TQM and assessment: The North Dakota experience. In J. S. Stark & A. Thomas (Eds.), *Assessment and program evaluation*. Needham Heights, MA: Simon & Schuster.

Cox, R. C., & West, W. L. (1986). *Fundamentals of research.* Laurel, MD: Ramsco.

Davis, B. G. (1994). Demystifying assessment: Learning from the field of evaluation. In J. S. Stark & A. Thomas (Eds.), *Assessment and program evaluation.* Needham Heights, MA: Simon and Schuster.

Davis, J. R. (1993). *Better teaching, more learning: Strategies for success in postsecondary settings.* Phoenix, AZ: The Oryx Press.

Forker, J. E. (1996). Perspectives on assessment. *Nurse Educator, 21*(1), 13-14.

Gates, S. M., Augustine, C. H., Benjamin, R., Bikson, T. K., Kaganoff, T., Levy, D. G., et al. (2002). *Ensuring quality and productivity in higher education.* San Francisco: Jossey-Bass.

Germain, C. P., Deatrick, J. A., Hagopian, G. A., & Whitney, F. W. (1994). Evaluation of a PhD program: Paving the way. *Nursing Outlook, 42*(3), 117-122.

Goodwin, L. D. (1997). Changing concepts of measurement validity. *Journal of Nursing Education, 36*(3), 102-107.

Gronlund, N. E. (1993). How to make achievement tests and assessments (5th ed.). Boston: Allyn & Bacon.

Guba, E. G., & Lincoln, Y. S. (1981). *Fourth generation evaluation.* Newburg Park, CA: Sage.

Kapborg, I., & Fischbein, S. (2002). Using a model to evaluate nursing education and professional practice. *Nursing and Health Sciences, 4,* 25-31.

Lignuagaris-Kraft, B., Marchand-Martella, N., & Martella, R. C. (2001). Writing better goals and short-term objectives or benchmarks. *Teaching Exceptional Children, 34*(1), 52-58.

Lincoln, Y. S., & Guba, E. G. (1985). *Naturalistic inquiry.* Beverly Hills, CA: Sage.

Loacker, G., & Mentkowski, M. (1993). Creating a climate where assessment improves learning. In T. Banta & Associates (Eds.), *Making a difference: Outcomes of a decade of assessment in higher education.* San Francisco: Jossey-Bass.

Madaus, G., Scriven, M., & Stufflebeam, D. (1988). *Evaluation models.* Boston: Kluwer-Nijhoff.

Millard, R. M. (1994). Accreditation. In J. S. Stark & A. Thomas (Eds.), *Assessment and program evaluation.* Needham Heights, MA: Simon & Schuster.

Millman, J. (1994). Designing a college assessment. In J. S. Stark & A. Thomas (Eds.), *Assessment and program evaluation.* Needham Heights, MA: Simon & Schuster.

Murphy, P. S. (1995). Benchmarking academic research output in Australia [Electronic version]. *Assessment & Evaluation in Higher Education, 20*(1), 45-58.

Newby, A. C. (1992). *Training evaluation handbook.* San Diego, CA: Pfeiffer & Company.

Palomba, C. A., & Banta, T. W. (1999). *Assessment essentials: Planning, implementing, and improving assessment in higher education.* San Francisco: Jossey-Bass.

Parry, S., & Dunn, L. (2000). Benchmarking as a meaning approach to learning in online settings [Electronic version]. *Studies in Continuing Education, 22*(2), 221-234.

Pedhazur, E., & Schmelkin, L. (1991). *Measurement, design, and analysis: An integrated approach.* Hillside, NJ: Lawrence Erlbaum.

Polit, D. F., & Hungler, B. P. (1999). *Nursing research: Principles and methods* (6th ed.). Philadelphia: J. B. Lippincott.

Prus, J., & Johnson, R. (1994). A critical review of student assessment options. In J. S. Stark & A. Thomas (Eds.), *Assessment and program evaluation.* Needham Heights, MA: Simon & Schuster.

Scriven, M. (1972). Pros and cons about goal-free evaluation. *Evaluation Comment, 3*(4), 1-4.

Shoemaker, J. K., & DeVos, M. (1999). Are we a gift shop? A perspective on grade inflation. *Journal of Nursing Education, 38*(9), 394-398

Sims, S. J. (1992). *Student outcomes assessment: A historical review and guide to program development.* New York: Greenwood Press.

Stake, R. (1967). The countenance of educational evaluation. *Teachers College Record, 68,* 523-540.

Stern, K., & Kramer, P. (1992). Outcomes assessment and program evaluation: Partners in intervention planning for the educational environment. *American Journal of Occupational Therapy, 46*(7), 620-624.

Stufflebeam, D. L., & Associates. (1971). *Educational evaluation and decision-making.* Itasia, IL: Peacock.

Stufflebeam, D. L., & Webster, W. J. (1994). An analysis of alternative approaches to evaluation. In J. S. Stark & A. Thomas (Eds.), *Assessment and program evaluation.* Needham Heights, MA: Simon & Schuster.

Svenson, E. (2001). Guidelines to statistical evaluation of data from rating scales and question-naires. *Journal of Rehabilitation Medicine, 33,* 47-48.

Swenson, M. M. (1991). Using fourth generation evaluation in nursing. *Evaluation and the Health Professions, 14*(1), 79-87.

Voorhees, A. B. (2001). Creating and implementing competency-based learning models. *New Directions for Institutional Research, 110,* 83-95.

Welsh, J. F., & Metcalf, J. (2003). Cultivating faculty support for institutional effectiveness activities: Benchmarking best practices [Electronic version]. *Assessment & Evaluation in Higher Education, 28*(1), 33-45.

Whitman, N. I., Graham, B. A., Gleit, C. J., & Boyd, M. D. (1992). *Teaching in nursing practice: A professional model.* Norwalk, CT: Appleton & Lange.

21

STRATEGIES FOR EVALUATING LEARNING OUTCOMES

Jane M. Kirkpatrick, MSN, RN,
Diann DeWitt-Weaver, DNS, RN, Lillian Yeager, EdD, RN

As teaching methods and environments change from traditional lecture in a classroom to more innovative approaches and learning environments, educators must expand the repertoire of strategies used to evaluate learning outcomes. To assess learning progress and evaluate learning outcomes, faculty must use tools that expand beyond the traditional multiple-choice test. The purpose of this chapter is to discuss uses, advantages, disadvantages, and issues related to a variety of strategies that faculty can use to assess student learning. The chapter also covers how to select strategies, improve their validity and reliability, and increase the effectiveness of their use.

SELECTING STRATEGIES

The strategies discussed in this chapter provide faculty with a variety of techniques to use for evaluating student learning outcomes. Several of the strategies may be more familiar as teaching strategies. Using a teaching strategy as an assessment or evaluation tool helps students have practice in the same process by which they will ultimately be evaluated.

The major reasons for faculty to consider new evaluation strategies are so they can better (1) evaluate all the domains of learning, (2) assess higher levels of the cognitive domain (e.g., analysis, synthesis), (3) assess critical thinking, and (4) prepare students for licensing or certification exams. The major challenges of using these strategies include (1) the time it takes to use the strategy and (2) difficulty in establishing validity and reliability of data-gathering instruments and methods.

In selecting strategies, the philosophy of the faculty regarding accountability and responsibility for learning must be considered. Many of the strategies discussed are compatible with interactive teaching techniques. Critical reflections, short essays, and guided writing assignments encourage students to interact with the material in a different way than if they were learning the material for a multiple-choice test.

To avoid some of the pitfalls associated with these strategies, faculty should do the following:

1. Clearly delineate the *purpose* of the evaluation
2. Consider the *setting* in which the learning and evaluation will take place
3. Choose the best evaluation *strategy* for the purpose
4. Determine the *procedure* for the strategy selected
5. Establish *validity and reliability* of the strategy
6. Evaluate the overall *effectiveness* of the process

Purpose

The purpose of evaluation is to ascertain that students have achieved their potential and have acquired the knowledge, skills, and abilities set forth in courses and curricula. The instructional goals and course objectives will indicate the type of behavior (cognitive, affective, or psychomotor) to be evaluated. The learning experiences must have relevance to the students and be valued in the grading system. Finally, the grading criteria should be shared with the students before the evaluation occurs.

The timing of the evaluation relates closely to the purpose. Formative evaluation is much like feedback for the purpose of recognizing progress. This type of evaluation would be appropriate throughout the class term. Summative evaluation suggests that a decision may be made. This might be a grade or a decision for passing or failure of a course.

Setting

Another critical factor to consider is the setting in which the instruction and evaluation will occur. Most faculty are comfortable with evaluation in traditional classroom settings, but more than half of all nursing schools are now using some form of computer-based learning support. For some, technology provides an adjunct or support to the nursing course. For others, the entire course is Web-based and delivered online.

When considering how to implement evaluation strategies in an electronic environment, faculty need to address how the technology supports the evaluation purpose. Most of the strategies discussed in this chapter can be used in an online community. For example, a threaded discussion can be used for critiquing or even as a forum for verbal questioning. Concept maps can be developed in an electronic format. Students or faculty can maintain an electronic portfolio representative of student work throughout the course.

Choice of Strategy

When choosing the best strategy for the purpose, faculty must weigh the advantages and disadvantages of each strategy. Faculty should also consider time for preparation, implementation, and grading. Other issues, such as cost, may also be determining factors. Faculty must decide how often to evaluate, who will evaluate, and how the students will be prepared for the evaluation technique. Students should have the opportunity to practice the technique on which they will be tested.

Procedures

Although procedures for using evaluation strategies vary, any procedure selected must be well planned. The strategy for evaluation should be pilot tested before it is fully implemented. This process should help prevent unexpected difficulties. It is also important to delineate the responsibilities associated with the methods used. For example, in the case of portfolio assessment, a decision must be made about whether students or faculty will collect and keep the work. Because of the anxiety and stress associated with the process of being evaluated, faculty must attempt to provide an atmosphere conducive to the evaluation process. Humor, when used appropriately, can help place students at ease.

Validity and Reliability

The issues of validity and reliability are critical, especially when the purpose is for summative evaluation. In Chapter 22, the terms *validity* and *reliability* are defined and described. For the purposes of this chapter, specific examples are given to clarify establishment of validity and reliability in non-multiple-choice evaluation methods.

In determining validity, faculty must ask whether the evaluation technique is appropriate to the purpose and whether it provides useful and meaningful data (Linn & Gronlund, 2000). Faculty must consider the fit of the evaluation strategy with the identified objectives. In other words, does the strategy measure what it is supposed to measure? For instance, if the objective for an assignment is for the student to demonstrate skill in written communication, evaluating student performance through oral questioning will not provide valid data. Similarly, at the nursing department level, faculty should coordinate evaluation strategies with nursing program outcomes such as critical thinking and communication. It is a challenge to develop sound criteria for evaluation that accurately reflect the specified outcomes, objectives, and/or content. To establish *face validity*, faculty must seek input from colleagues by asking questions such as, "Do these criteria appear to measure what my objectives are?" In addition, obtaining the opinion of other content experts can assist in determining whether there is adequate sampling of the content (*content validity*).

Once evaluation criteria or rubrics are developed, it is essential to establish their reliability. The most commonly used method for establishing reliability in this situation is when two or more instructors independently rate student performance using the agreed upon criteria or rubric for sample work. Then the ratings are correlated to establish *interrater reliability*.

Box 21-1
ESTABLISHING INTERRATER RELIABILITY

♦ *Develop criteria and apply them to sample work*
  1. Have 2 or more observers independently rate performance, then correlate
  2. Formula for % Agreement = $\dfrac{\text{total \# agreements}}{\text{\# of agreements} + \text{\# of disagreements}}$

Example: Evaluating Written Communication
  ♦ *Criteria*   A D
  1. Clear expression of ideas
  2. Logical flow/organization
  3. Correct use of syntax, grammar, APA format
  4. Incorporation of research findings
         A = agree D = disagree
Sample for Establishing Reliability Based on Above Criteria
  ♦ *3 raters looking at 4 items:*
  ♦   Item 1:   2 agree, 1 does not
  ♦   Item 2:   all 3 agree
  ♦   Item 3:   2 agree, 1 does not
  ♦   Item 4:   all 3 agree

$$\frac{10 \text{ (Total agreements)}}{10 \text{ (Agreements)} + 2 \text{ (Disagreements)}}$$

10/12 = 0.83 or 83% (>0.70 or > 70% is good)

APA, American Psychological Association.

Interrater reliability is expressed as a percentage of agreement between scores. An example of using criteria to establish interrater reliability is provided in Box 21-1.

A multiplicity of evaluation strategies can provide a more complete picture of the student's abilities and therefore contribute to the trustworthiness of the evaluation process. It is a serious limitation to rely on just one assessment technique because students may be more comfortable using one technique over another. Using multiple assessment techniques provides a more robust and accurate framework for making evaluative decisions.

Effectiveness

After the evaluation strategy is implemented, it is essential to determine its overall effectiveness. Issues related to the implementation of the strategy should be examined as well. Some questions faculty should ask include the following: Was the strategy an effective use of resources (e.g., student and faculty time and financial resources)? Did the technique provide appropriate data for the evaluation goal? Are there any problems with the implementation of the technique? What revisions are necessary? Would the faculty wish to use this strategy again? If so, under what conditions?

MATCHING THE EVALUATION STRATEGY TO THE DOMAIN OF LEARNING

Educators must also be mindful of the domain of learning being assessed or evaluated (see Chapter 12) Cognitive learning is typically evaluated with strategies requiring the students to write, submit portfolios, or complete tests (see Chapter 12). Evaluation in the psychomotor domain typically involves simulations and simulated patients and ultimately occurs in clinical practice. Evaluation in the affective domain is particularly important in nursing and is discussed further here.

The taxonomy of affective evaluation as applied to nursing (Reilly, 1978; Krathwohl et al., 1964) lists five behavioral categories: (1) receiving, (2) responding, (3) valuing, (4) organization of values, and (5) characterization by a value or value complex. The beginning student may be at the receiving level, able to hear and recognize the values. As the student progresses, more sophisticated affective growth would demonstrate the ability to respond to or communicate about the particular value or issue. At the next level, the student embraces the value. Ultimately, the student would act on the value. Once actions are consistent, the highest levels of the affective domain would be realized.

Examples of areas in which nursing students encounter the affective domain include socialization to the roles of the nurse, caring for patients who are dying, meeting spirituality needs, working with sexuality concerns, and becoming culturally competent.

Student development of cultural competence will demonstrate progression in the affective domain. At the beginning level, the student could be asked to define his or her culture and health care practices and values that come from his or her cultural orientation. Multiple evaluation methods could be used for this activity, ranging from a written paper to a videotape or collage. For the purpose of evaluating progress in this area, students could be asked to complete a critical review of one of their interactions in caregiving with a patient of another culture. This assignment would seek to determine whether the student could recognize the value conflicts and areas in which judgments must be made. At graduation, the student could be expected to demonstrate the ability to act in a culturally competent manner when providing care to all patients and the ability to advocate for an individual patient's unique needs.

Development of the affective domain is progressive and can be tied to critical thinking. Because of the progressive nature of development, formative evaluation across the curriculum may be most appropriate, with a summative evaluation at the time of graduation. Many of the evaluation methods listed in this chapter can be adapted to evaluate the affective domain.

COMMUNICATING GRADING EXPECTATIONS

When evaluation strategies are used to collect data for grading purposes, it is imperative that the grading requirements be communicated to the students. Information about grading criteria is typically provided to students in the course syllabus. Other methods such as checklists, guidelines, or grading scales can be used as well. See Box 21-2 for an example of grading guidelines.

Box 21-2
SAMPLE GRADING GUIDELINE FOR WRITING ASSIGNMENT

Guideline to score writing assignment

_____/2 points for a clear statement of the topic/issue

_____/2 points for a logical progression and flow of ideas

_____/2 points for use of supportive examples that relate to the topic

_____/2 points for correct use of grammar and spelling

_____/2 points for correct use of APA style (5th ed.) to cite references

_____/10 Total

APA, American Psychological Association.

Another way to inform students about grading expectations is to construct grading rubrics. *Grading rubrics* are criterion-referenced rules for assessing student performance (Taggart, Phifer, Nixon, & Wood, 1998). Rubrics identify the expected performance and the criteria for the performance. Grading rubrics are particularly helpful when faculty wish to differentiate levels of quality of performance in areas of higher-order learning. To construct grading rubrics, faculty must define the expected performance in gradations such as "best," "acceptable," and "less than satisfactory." Rubrics thus provide both faculty and students with a means of easily understanding expectations and assigning grades. See Box 21-3 for an example of grading rubrics.

Box 21-3
EXAMPLES OF GRADING RUBRICS

"A" Grade

The final course *synthesis paper* clearly defines a researchable problem; the search strategy provides sufficient relevant data for understanding the problem; the coding sheet is focused and guides the analysis of the data; issues of reliability and validity are identified; the literature is synthesized, rather than reviewed or summarized; the paper concludes with recommendations based on the research synthesis. The paper is written using the IUSON writing guidelines.

Participation in discussions and leaning activities integrates course concepts and reflects critical thinking about research synthesis. Participation is thoughtful, respectful, informed, and substantiated. Peer review of the synthesis paper reflects the reviewers' understanding of the synthesis process, provides practical suggestions, and is presented in a collegial manner.

Dissemination of the findings of the research synthesis includes a written *plan for publication* and an oral *presentation* to faculty and classmates. The plan for publication includes thoughtful selection of a journal; draft of a query or cover letter; and, if the paper needs revisions to suit publication guidelines, a statement about revisions needed that matches the journal publication guidelines. The professional presentation is well organized; supported by visual aids (PowerPoint slides); and uses professional communication style to suit the audience.

IUSON, Indiana University School of Nursing.

Box 21-3
EXAMPLES OF GRADING RUBRICS—cont'd

"B" Grade

The final *synthesis paper* clearly defines a researchable problem; the search strategy yields mostly relevant data for understanding the problem; the coding sheet lacks one or more important data and/or does not reflect the scope of the problem statement; issues of reliability and validity are unclear; the review of literature is primarily synthesis with minimal summary; the paper concludes with mostly appropriate recommendations. The paper is free of major errors in grammar or style.

Participation in discussions and leaning activities usually integrates course concepts and reflects critical thinking about research synthesis. Participation is helpful but may not contribute substantially to the focus of the course. Peer review of the synthesis paper does not include relevant aspects of the peer review checklists or overlooks areas in which feedback is needed.

Dissemination of the findings of the research synthesis includes a written *plan for publication* and an oral *presentation* to faculty and classmates. The plan for publication includes appropriate selection of a journal; the drafts of the query or cover letter are generally appropriate to the situation; general revisions are noted but do not consider manuscript guidelines of the journal. The professional presentation is fairly well organized; the visual aids (PowerPoint slides) enhance the presentation; the presentation is delivered with consideration for the audience.

"C" Grade

The final *synthesis paper* has an ill-defined problem; the search strategy yields irrelevant or tangential data for understanding the problem; the coding sheet is not well focused or neglects key variables or includes irrelevant variables; issues of reliability and validity are not identified or are ignored; the review is more summary than synthesis; the paper does not include recommendations or includes recommendations that are not drawn from the data. There are substantial errors in grammar and/or writing style.

Participation in discussions occurs on an irregular basis and is not grounded in course concepts; comments do not reflect critical thinking; and there are breaches of course norms and etiquette. Peer review of the synthesis paper does not provide substantive or helpful feedback to classmates; significant aspects of the peer review checklist are ignored.

Dissemination of the findings of the research synthesis includes a written *plan for publication* and an oral *presentation* to faculty and classmates. There is no plan for publication or the journal selected is not appropriate for the content of the paper; the drafts of the query or cover letters are not clearly written and do not capture attention of the reader; there is not clear understanding of the revisions needed of the paper for the style requirements for the selected journal. The professional presentation is not well organized; visual aids (PowerPoint slides) or the visuals do not clarify or highlight key points of the presentation; the presentation exceeds time limits and/or is not suited to the audience. The presenter is unable to answer audience questions, if any, about the material.

STRATEGIES FOR EVALUATING LEARNING OUTCOMES

Nursing faculty can use a variety of strategies to evaluate student learning. This section identifies several strategies known to be effective in nursing. Table 21-1 provides an overview of these strategies.

Portfolios

Description/Uses

Portfolios are simply collections of student work. The medium most widely used for portfolios is some type of binder to contain the data. Recently, electronic portfolios have become prevalent (see suggested websites for valuable resources). Regardless of the format, portfolios are used to obtain a broader sample of student performance (Linn & Gronlund, 2000). Although portfolios have been used in other disciplines (e.g., art) for many years, they have only recently become commonplace in education and nursing education.

Portfolios are used for a variety of purposes. They can be used (1) as proof of achievement in a class, (2) as an outcome measure of a program, (3) as a marketing tool for job placement, or (4) for student placement in a program of study.

The purpose of the portfolio needs to be clearly established before work is collected for inclusion. The use of portfolios for student *assessment* in the classroom provides evidence of student progress within the course. Student work (either all or selected assignments) may be collected from the beginning to the end of the course. Evaluation of student work may occur during the course (formative) or at the end (summative). It is important that clearly established criteria be identified for the evaluation of the portfolio. These criteria need to be shared with students at the beginning of the course.

Students may be required to write a paper (or papers) in which they *critique* their *progress* during the course. When clearly delineated criteria are used, this exercise could assist students in development of self-evaluation skills.

Portfolios used as an *outcome measure of a program* can include selections of student work acquired throughout the curriculum. Samples of these portfolios can be used to assess student progress in an area such as writing skills to provide feedback about the effectiveness of the program. Karlowicz (2000) describes the benefits and limitations of portfolios in program evaluation and shares a pilot portfolio project completed by one nursing program.

Although art students have used portfolios of their work when seeking *employment* and further study, this approach is not widespread in nursing. Some BSN completion programs use portfolios to validate prior learning and experience, and some employers, such as academic institutions, wish to see samples of published research that could be compiled as a portfolio or dossier.

Portfolios are often used in nursing programs for *advanced placement* of students. In this process, students compile objective evidence that they have acquired certain content and skills through prior learning, practice experience, or both. Through the use of portfolios, students may demonstrate attainment of learning objectives or competencies required of a specific nursing course within a program of study. Guidelines for compiling and evaluating such portfolios

Text continued on p. 477

TABLE 21-1   Overview of Evaluation Strategies

TECHNIQUE	DOMAIN/EVALUATION PURPOSE	POSSIBLE APPLICATIONS	ADVANTAGES	DISADVANTAGES	ISSUES
Portfolio	High-level cognitive Affective Psychomotor (if video) Formative Summative	Placement in program of study For evidence of progress Outcome measure for individual or program Marketing tool for job placement	Broad sample of student work Documents progress Identifies student strengths and weaknesses Critical thinking with student reflection	Time for collection and grading Need storage space Not direct observation Limited reliability	Ownership Responsibility for collection Nonselective vs. selective portfolio Are you evaluating process or product?
Simulation	High-level cognitive Affective Psychomotor Formative Summative	Preclinical mastery of identified skills Final examination for clinical courses Application of decision-making process or a controlled representation of reality	Opportunity to demonstrate transfer of knowledge Mimics the "real" world Safe environment for both student and patient Controlled environment Allows standardized experience for all students Opportunity for direct observation/ videotaping Active student involvement If computerized, may decrease grading time	Requires creativity for development Development and implementation are time consuming Some skills cannot be tested Expensive to make and to purchase	Purpose and criteria for performance must be clearly identified May require equipment

Continued

TABLE 21-1 Overview of Evaluation Strategies—cont'd

TECHNIQUE	DOMAIN/EVALUATION PURPOSE	POSSIBLE APPLICATIONS	ADVANTAGES	DISADVANTAGES	ISSUES
Role play	Cognitive Affective Psychomotor Formative	Formative feedback for psychomotor skills, communication techniques, problem-solving skills	Active participation of student Stimulates creativity Variables can be controlled Can repeat Provides practice in peer review skills	Immediate feedback may not be possible Self-consciousness of participant	Takes time to build comfort with technique Need familiarity with material
Critiques	High-level cognitive Affective domain Formative Summative (for trending)	Self-assessment Integration of learning can be demonstrated Appropriate for evaluating the higher-level cognitive skills	Active student involvement Encourages students to form connections within and between content Assists students to practice self-evaluation based on criteria	Time consuming for both students and faculty Student frustration with lack of clarity of assignment	Grading criteria can be developed jointly Requires a high degree of trust Students will need orientation to this process
Journals	High-level cognitive Affective domain Formative Summative (for trending)	Integration of learning can be demonstrated Self-assessment Affective domain can be evaluated Critical thinking can be evaluated	Writing is the scholarly model for self-expression Active student involvement Encourages students to form connections within and between content Encourages recognition of learning in students' life experience	Time consuming for both students and faculty Student frustration with lack of clarity of assignment	Requires collegial student–faculty relationship Grading criteria must be clear Requires a high degree of trust May want to consider anonymous grading

Paper	High levels of cognitive and affective domains Formative Summative	Critical thinking skills Writing skills Develop arguments Synthesis of ideas	More in-depth information in area of interest A public work to be assessed	Time for both faculty and student Subjectivity in grading Limited sample of ability	Reliability Grading criteria
Essays	High levels of cognitive and affective domains Formative Summative	Critical thinking skills Free form Demonstrate problem-solving abilities, decision making, and rationale Analysis	Shorter than a paper Assess recall and synthesis at one moment rather than at several times Creativity Easy to construct and administer	Less sample of content and ability Time to grade	Reliability Grading criteria Clarity of questions Use a test plan to better cover content
Oral (verbal) questioning	All ranges of cognitive domain Affective domain Formative Summative	Evidence of thinking process with "why" questions Evidence of verbal skills Defense: determines content mastery and evidence of synthesis	Quick to prepare Inexpensive Opportunity for student to receive immediate corrective feedback Works well for nonlinear ideas	Perceived by students as threatening Bias of evaluator	Must determine the difference between questions for teaching vs. evaluation Criteria for evaluation should be established before use Can be subjective
Concept/mind mapping	All ranges of cognitive domain Affective Formative	Concepts expressed in a visual way Shows relationships between and among topics	Works well for students who are highly visual in their orientation	Artistic students may have an advantage Can be frustrating to concrete thinkers	Reliability Grading criteria must be defined Allow for student creativity

Continued

TABLE 21–1 Overview of Evaluation Strategies—cont'd

TECHNIQUE	DOMAIN/EVALUATION PURPOSE	POSSIBLE APPLICATIONS	ADVANTAGES	DISADVANTAGES	ISSUES
Audiotape	All ranges of cognitive domain Affective domain Formative Summative	Verbal skills Interviews Group discussion	Provides evidence when presence of faculty may be intrusive or when faculty are unable to be present Relatively inexpensive Less intrusive than video camera Is a permanent record	Limited to audio data May be difficult to get quality recording of each group member Requires time to listen	Requires consent Student should be aware of how the tape will be used Must determine whether entire tape or a sampling of the tape will be evaluated Confidentiality
Videotape	Higher levels of cognitive domain Affective domain Psychomotor domain	Evidence of learning outcome submitted to faculty Communication skills, including nonverbal Psychomotor skills	Captures motion Evidence can be replayed Works for self-evaluation Provides evidence when presence of faculty may be intrusive or when faculty may be unable to be present	Can be perceived as threatening Students may be nervous or self-conscious Expense and maintenance of equipment	Requires consent Student should be aware of how the tape will be used Must determine whether entire tape or a sampling of the tape will be evaluated Confidentiality of patient data

must be clearly delineated. Examples of documentation that may be included in this type of portfolio include (but are not limited to) a resume, performance evaluation, course syllabi or outlines, and evidence of professional activity.

Similar to student portfolios are those used by *faculty*; faculty may use portofolios when they are seeking *promotion* or showing evidence in performance evaluations. Guidelines for construction of such portfolios usually include evidence and evaluation of teaching, scholarship, and service, although specific requirements differ among institutions.

Advantages

Portfolios provide a broad sample of student work and can show evidence of progress or accomplishment. Identification of student strengths and weaknesses allows students to make improvements. Student reflection on the work in a portfolio can stimulate critical thinking. Using portfolios for advanced placement in programs enables students to receive credit for previous experience and reduces repetition of content.

Disadvantages

The main disadvantage associated with portfolios is time. Although collection of the papers is not time consuming, providing feedback and grading them can be. In addition, it is challenging and takes time to determine validity and reliability for the established grading criteria or rubrics. As indicated earlier, it is beneficial for faculty to collaborate with one another, and this also requires that valued commodity, time.

Issues

Major issues related to student portfolios are ownership of the portfolio, responsibility for collection, fair grading, and use of nonselective versus selective portfolios. When a portfolio is used for classroom or program assessment, the faculty must decide what is the purpose of the portfolio (e.g., to assess writing skill or critical thinking), which works will be collected, who is responsible for maintaining the portfolio, what criteria will be used to evaluate the collection, the scoring method, and when feedback will be given to students.

Nonselective portfolios are collections of all student work for a specified period. The focus of these is more on formative evaluation of student progress. A compilation of certain completed works of students is called a *selective portfolio*. A selective portfolio often contains works that are the best efforts of the student and are usually part of a summative evaluation (Courts & McInerney, 1993).

Scoring is another issue surrounding portfolio use. Gronlund (1993) reports that there are two methods for scoring portfolios: *holistic scoring* and *analytic scoring*. These methods may be used individually or together. The holistic approach is based on a global scoring of the portfolio, usually based on a numerical scoring system; whereas analytic scoring involves examining each significant characteristic of the portfolio. For example, in evaluation of writing, the organization, ideas, and style are judged individually (Linn & Gronlund, 1993). The global method seems more suitable for summative evaluation, whereas the analytic method is useful in providing specific feedback to students for the purpose of performance improvement.

Critiques

Description/Uses

Critiques are a method for students to fully consider a question, an experience, or a thesis. This approach to evaluation is based on an educational connoisseurship model, in which students become *connoisseur critics*. According to Eisner (1985), a connoisseur is able to appreciate and distinguish the important from the trivial. Bevis and Watson (1989), in a modification of Eisner's work, identify six levels of critiquing: looking, seeing, perceiving and intuiting, rendering, interpreting meaning, and judging. These steps include identifying an event, viewing it with a focus, interpreting the event on a personal level (complete with value clarification), and discerning the significance of the event. Early in a nursing program, students may be asked to critique their performance of a videotaped skill. Examining the essential components of the skill and perceiving the importance of these components would be part of the critiquing process. A more advanced nursing student might critically evaluate a home visit by relating the events and his or her perception of the events and making judgments about the nursing care provided.

Critiques can be presented through short (one- to two-page) papers, through the use of journals, or verbally. The purpose of the critique is to fully examine an experience, looking for ways to improve. A student does not have enough experience to be a true connoisseur. The faculty member, however, can model this skill and teach students the process of critiquing, thus helping students learn the skills of recognition, interpretation, and appreciation that will eventually make them connoisseurs.

Advantages

Critiques provide a way for faculty to assess outcomes of student work at the higher levels of Bloom's (1956) cognitive taxonomy. Written critiques allow students to practice formal self-expression. Practice in critique increases student self-awareness and builds critical thinking skills. The graduate who has learned the basics of critiquing has gained skills that support professional development and eventual expertise.

Disadvantages

The process used to grade the critique must be clearly defined. Goldenberg (1994) suggests that the faculty and students collaborate to determine the necessary criteria. This puts the student and faculty in more collaborative roles, which may be new to both students and faculty. The use of critiquing for evaluation requires the time of both students and faculty. Students may experience initial frustration if the scope of the assignment is not well defined and the skills required for critiquing are not practiced.

Issues

Students must be oriented to the critiquing process, just as they are oriented to more traditional approaches of assessment. In critiquing, the relationship of the student and faculty changes to shared power in the learning environment. The faculty-student relationship becomes more collegial, and there is a high level of mutual trust, scholarship, and desire to grow. It is also imperative that the philosophy of the school and faculty support the practice of critical connoisseurship.

Journals

Description/Uses

The purpose of journals is to increase student self-awareness through contemplation and reflection on life or learning events. The writer takes bits of experience and information and brings them together to create a sense of meaning. Examples of journal assignments include writing a reaction to a clinical experience, discussing a recently learned concept, and writing a self-assessment of professional development. Clapp-Itnyre (2001) used journaling as a preclass, intraclass, and postclass activity. The preclass activity forced students to be better prepared for class. The intraclass activity represented the students' notes from class, and the postclass activity was an opportunity for the students to compare their ideas with the class discussion and process their understanding of the material. Criteria for evaluating these journals included completeness of the journals and the insightfulness demonstrated in the content of the writing.

Kobert (1995) suggests that the process of keeping a journal is one of internal examination and reflection, allowing the learner to search for the truth about the nature of nursing through searching the heart. Keeping a journal has been proposed as a technique to help students become attuned to the caring, moral framework (Watson, 1989). Journals can provide evidence of the student's ability to work logically through an idea and can serve as a venue for increasing student self-awareness. A journal assignment may be very structured, with specific areas the student must address in each entry, or it may be unstructured, allowing the student free form in his or her reflections (Yensen, 1997). Journal entries can be made on paper or stored in electronic files.

Providing feedback to student journal entries requires thoughtful responses by faculty. Seven components for responding to writing identified by Beach and Marshall (1991) are described in Box 21-4. Bloomfield (1990) identifies several components of effective evaluation that include affirmation of the student's efforts; individualized and clearly expressed comments that focus on the work—not the student as an individual; and evidence that comments stem from a concern for the student's learning and not as a result of a faculty member's pet peeve. Bloomfield also suggests that faculty should ask the question, "What can this person learn from my comments?" If the comments are just "feel-good" or "feel-bad," the learning opportunity is missed.

> **Box 21-4**
> **SEVEN COMPONENTS FOR RESPONDING TO WRITING**
>
> 1. **Praising:** providing positive reinforcement for students
> 2. **Describing:** providing "reader-based" feedback about one's own reactions and perceptions of the students' responses that imply judgments of those responses
> 3. **Diagnosing:** determining the students' own unique knowledge, attitudes, abilities, and needs
> 4. **Judging:** evaluating the sufficiency, level, depth, completeness, validity, and insightfulness of a student's responses
> 5. **Predicting and reviewing growth:** predicting potential directions for improving students' responses according to specific criteria and reviewing progress from previous responses
> 6. **Record keeping:** keeping a record to chart changes across time in students' performance
> 7. **Recognizing/praising growth:** giving students recognition and praise for demonstrating growth
>
> Excerpt from *Teaching literature in the secondary school* (pp. 211-212), by Richard W. Beach and James D. Marshall. Copyright © by Harcourt Brace & Company, 1991. Reprinted by permission of the publisher.

Advantages

The main advantage of journals is that cognitive and writing skills are strengthened. Critical thinking skills are emphasized, and students have the opportunity to practice self-evaluation. Courts and McInerney (1993) discuss the idea that writing is a way of learning. By writing, students move beyond the memorization aspect of learning and are encouraged to engage with the material at higher cognitive levels. Journals also increase self-awareness. Kobert (1995) suggests that students can discover meaning through finding their own voices.

Disadvantages

Time involved for both students and faculty is the biggest issue. Writing truly reflective journal entries requires a time commitment on the part of students. Those who procrastinate may not obtain the benefits of the exercise. For faculty, reading and responding to journals can be a lengthy process. Faculty must decide whether they are going to read each entry for evaluation purposes or take a sample of the journal. The evaluation of the exercise can easily become subjective unless clear criteria for grading are established.

Issues

A high degree of trust in the student-faculty relationship is necessary. Faculty feedback is an important part of enhancing student learning in the journal process. This feedback should be of a critically reflective nature and would be considered a formative evaluation. The use of anonymity could be appropriate for grading journals because it can enhance objectivity on the part of the evaluator and minimize student fears that can inhibit honesty and creativity.

The purpose(s) of the journal assignment must be clearly established for its full benefits to be realized. Decisions should be made on how often the journal will be submitted to the faculty member and how much of the journal will be examined. In addition, establishing grading criteria before the assignment will convey outcome expectations. Confidentiality for the student journal is an important consideration. If the journal is kept in an electronic format, it should be password protected for added security.

Papers and Essays
Description/Uses

Papers and assigned essays or essay questions on exams can be used to demonstrate organizational skills, critical thinking, and written communication while encouraging creativity. Papers are written reports, whereas essays are free-form responses to open-ended questions. Students are encouraged to be creative in responding to essay questions. Both papers and essays can measure the affective domain, as well as higher levels of the cognitive domain.

Advantages

In-depth information can be obtained through the writing of papers. This helps students clarify their own thinking about topics and learn to write better. Papers are a public work and can be assessed by others in the profession. Writing papers requires students to integrate their ideas with those found in other sources. Similarly, essays are useful for evaluating higher-level cognitive skills such as analysis and synthesis. Essay questions are easier to construct than multiple-choice exam questions.

Disadvantages

The major disadvantage of papers for both students and faculty is the amount of time involved in writing and grading. Faculty can become distracted from the content of the paper when a student exhibits poor writing skills. An assigned essay or essay test may involve less sampling of the content than a multiple-choice exam. In addition, students must recall information, process it, and convey their ideas clearly without the benefit of resources.

Issues

Reliability in grading papers is an issue. Reliability can be increased by having more than one person grade the paper and by having clearly established grading criteria. This is especially important for papers that receive low or failing grades. Anonymous grading can increase the objectivity of the grader. Faculty should determine the purpose of the paper. For example, if the purpose is to demonstrate critical thinking and creativity, the format of the paper may have less value in the total grade of the paper. If the purpose is for the student to practice writing a scholarly paper, the format score may be emphasized.

Writing a clear and focused essay question can be a challenge for faculty. The question needs to be stated in such a way that the scope is clear to the students. It is also important to follow a test plan when essay tests are constructed so that the content is adequately sampled. Before grading an essay exam, faculty must establish clear grading criteria. When more than one person is grading, interrater reliability needs to be established.

Concept Mapping

Description/Uses

Concept, or mind, mapping is a technique in which students express concepts and relationships of concepts in a visual format (Rooda, 1994). This strategy provides a visual means for students to demonstrate their understanding of concepts. Although not a new idea, concept mapping has been growing in popularity as an alternative to traditional nursing care plans in which students can demonstrate their knowledge of nursing care. An example of concept mapping is provided in Figure 21-1.

Several options are available for developing maps. For example, the concepts to be mapped can be provided by the faculty or generated by the students; the structure can be defined or left open to student creativity. Yensen (2002) uses concept maps on the computer for students to build resource bases for a given concept. Each piece of the concept map can be hyperlinked to a resource. This application of concept mapping is called a *concept resource map*.

When concept mapping is chosen for assessment and evaluation, the purpose of the assignment will drive the evaluation criteria. For example, evaluation criteria may include such things as a content analysis (the number of items included), the clarity of the organizational structure, and the way the content is categorized. It is possible to have students self-evaluate or peer evaluate concept maps as a way of building the professional skills of self-assessment and peer evaluation.

Advantages

Concept mapping is a technique that requires students to demonstrate *cognitive synthesis skills* with a minimum of writing. Mapping also allows faculty to gain insight into the way students assimilate new information and how students are connecting the material. Mapping also lends itself well to formative evaluation, especially in determining the way students view relationships. Having students explain the concept map may help demonstrate the rationale for the relationships expressed by the lines on the map.

Disadvantages

The concept map may be large and difficult to follow. It may be more challenging to interpret the student's intent because only key words and phrases are used. It is possible that the artistic ability and overall appearance of the map, much like handwriting, could influence faculty. Special software is required to create concept maps in an electronic environment. Purchase price and training costs should be considered. Time involved in reading and responding to concept maps can be lengthy.

Issues

The faculty must teach students how to successfully create a map before using it as an evaluation strategy. If faculty use a mapping strategy for in-class learn-

Example of a Concept Map for Synthesizing Course Concepts in a
Graduate Course in Computer Technologies for Nurse Educators

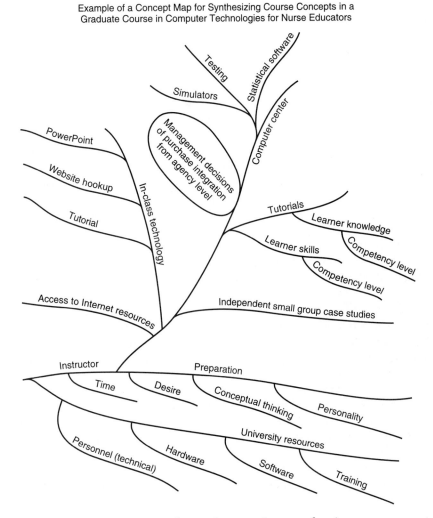

FIGURE 21-1   Concept map used to evaluate attainment of major course concepts. (Courtesy of Mary Beth Riner, Indiana University School of Nursing.)

ing experiences, the students will have a greater familiarity with the process. Special software can improve the capabilities of concept mapping in an electronic environment, because word processors have limits for building a concept map. Software to support concept mapping can add cost and increase the computer skills learning curve for students. Regardless of the method used to construct the map, a limitation of mapping is the lack of rationale presented for the relationship of ideas. One way of addressing this limitation would be to use the map as the focus for a faculty-student conference.

The evaluation of the exercise can easily become subjective unless clear criteria for grading are established. These criteria should be defined for the students before submission of their work. Faculty need to establish the validity and reliability of their evaluation tools for this strategy.

Oral Questioning
Description/Uses

In the quest to evaluate the student's ability to think critically, faculty can use questions. These questions should allow the student to demonstrate knowledge, skills, and values. Questions can be designed to elicit evaluation at all levels of the cognitive domain. Questions may solicit only factual information or ask for comparisons. Students can be asked to elaborate and justify their responses. Questioning as an evaluation technique can be sequenced to move the student from a basic level (factual information) to a higher cognitive level (clarifying relationships).

Oral questioning has been a tradition for the defense of the dissertation and thesis at the graduate level. In this process, the student must demonstrate a working knowledge of the discipline and the ability to express arguments orally. Students in undergraduate nursing programs may experience oral questioning during their clinical experiences. Box 21-5 provides examples (adapted from Hansen [1994] and King [1994]) of questions that assess the cognitive domain as defined in Bloom's *Taxonomy* (1956).

Advantages

Oral questioning is inexpensive, requires no special equipment, and can be quickly developed by faculty. It is possible to give immediate feedback to the student.

Disadvantages

Students may feel stressed by the experience. Unless the session is audiotaped, there is no permanent record of it. The evaluator may be biased by a variety of factors during the assessment. For example, if the student performs well at the beginning of the session and the performance deteriorates as the session progresses, the earlier performance may be biased by what occurred subsequently. It is imperative that the criteria for evaluation be fully developed before the questioning session.

Issues

Using questions for evaluation must be distinguished from using questions to encourage active student learning. The criteria for evaluation must be established before the session with the student. Because of the lack of a permanent record of the interaction, risk of subjectivity is greater in evaluation.

Audiotape and Videotape
Description/Uses

Audiotaping provides a method of obtaining a record of the verbal skills of students that students can play back and critique. Audiotapes can be used to demonstrate communication skills, group process, and interviewing skills. It allows the evaluator to focus on verbal communication without other distracters.

Box 21-5
EXAMPLES OF QUESTIONS TO EVALUATE THE COGNITIVE DOMAIN

Knowledge

Define _____.
List the five principles for _____.
Based on your assignment, what do you recall about _____?

Comprehension

Explain the meaning of _____.
Tell me in your own words what is meant by _____.
Which of the examples demonstrates _____?

Application

What is a new example of _____?
How could _____ be used to _____?
Show how this information could be graphed.

Analysis

What are the implications of _____?
What is the meaning of _____?
What are the key components of _____?

Synthesis of Ideas

What are some possible solutions to the problem of _____?
From this information, create your own model of _____.
Suppose you could _____. How would you approach _____?

Evaluation

Explain the effectiveness of this approach.
Which solution would you choose? Justify your opinion.
What are the consequences of _____?

Adapted from Hansen, C. (1994). Questioning techniques for the active classroom, and King, A. Inquiry as a tool in critical thinking. In D. F. Halpern (Ed.), *Changing college classrooms: New teaching and learning strategies for an increasingly complex world* (pp. 13-38, 93-106). San Francisco: Jossey-Bass. Based on Bloom, B. S. (Ed.). (1956). *Taxonomy of educational objectives: The classification of educational goals. Handbook 1: Cognitive domain.* New York: Longman.

Using a video camera to tape student performance is a means of evaluating several performance parameters. Videotaped student performance is useful for evaluating communication skills because it picks up the student's actual words and inflections, as well as body language. The live action feature of the videotape provides evidence of the sequencing of student actions in hands-on skill performance. This is one method available for skill validation. Graf (1993) has found that grading takes less time when the videotaped return demonstration, rather than the traditional method of skill demonstration, is used. Rinne (1994) uses videotaping and computers to allow students to record their performance and play it back on a split computer screen. On half of the screen is the student's work, and on the other half is the expert performance; students can critique their performance side by side with that of the expert. Angelo and Cross (1993) suggest videotaping students working through the problem-solving process as an assessment of meta-cognition.

Advantages

Obtaining audiotapes and equipment is relatively inexpensive. Having an audiotape recorder present may be less threatening to the student than use of a video camera or faculty observation. It also allows faculty to evaluate student performance without being intrusive. Videotaping works well for demonstration of mastery, particularly with psychomotor skills. Students can view and critique their own performance and even re-tape the procedure until they are satisfied with the performance. Videotaping allows students to practice and record their skills in private. Using videotaping for skill validation affords flexibility in scheduling evaluation time for both students and faculty. Faculty can conduct a secondary analysis of the recording if necessary.

Disadvantages

The quality of the audiorecording may not be clear. It can be difficult to distinguish individual voices in a group of participants. One suggestion is to have each group member state his or her name at the beginning of the tape so that voices can be identified. In addition, communication has both verbal and nonverbal components. Thus, one limitation of audiotape as a strategy is that only the verbal components of the skill being evaluated can be assessed.

Videotaping requires expensive equipment and a certain level of competence in using the equipment. The skill of the cameraperson and the camera angle can affect the quality of the recording. If patients are involved, their consent is required. The experience of being videotaped can cause stress to some students who may feel self-conscious about being "on camera." In some cases, the stress level may be lower than that experienced with direct observation by the faculty member. If patients are also being videotaped, explanations of expectations should be given before videotaping is done. Evaluators need good observational skills.

Issues

The protocol for scoring must be determined before this evaluation technique is instituted. Students need an opportunity to practice with the technique before it is used in the assignment of a grade. A decision needs to be made about whether the entire tape or a sampling will be evaluated. Confidentiality is an issue, as well as the need to obtain consent from any patients who are included in the taping.

Role Play

Description/Uses

In role play, the learner portrays a specific individual and is generally given much freedom to act out that role spontaneously. Role play is particularly appropriate for objectives related to developing interpersonal relationships with patients, peers, and other health care providers (Reilly & Oermann, 1992). The role-playing process (Joyce et al., 1992) provides a live sample of human behavior that serves as a vehicle for students to (1) explore feelings; (2) gain insight into their abilities, values, and perceptions; (3) develop their problem-solving skills and attitudes; and (4) explore subject matter in different ways.

The time for role play can vary according to the time available and the complexity of the role-play situation. The student is informed of the concept or role to be performed and given time to be creative in its presentation. The content, and not the performance ability, should be evaluated. The content and process can be evaluated for use of communication techniques. Role reversal is used in situations in which the purpose is to change attitudes. This facilitates an understanding of opposing beliefs.

On termination of the role play, the student observers analyze what occurred, what feelings were generated, what insights were gained, why things happened as they did, and how the situation is related to reality (deTornyay & Thompson, 1987).

Advantages

Situations can be structured or prepared as open-ended responses. After students critique the role play, the process can be repeated. Role play affords the opportunity for students to practice peer review. This technique actively involves the students and fosters creativity.

Disadvantages

Role play can be awkward for the faculty and student if it is not practiced before the time of evaluation. Immediate feedback is difficult to provide if many groups are performing at the same time.

Issues

Role play as a teaching mode before its use in evaluation assists students and faculty to become familiar with the technique and material. All that could happen cannot be anticipated. Students need to be informed in advance about the use of this technique for evaluation. It may take time and experience to build comfort with this technique.

Simulation

Description/Uses

Simulation is an imitation of a real-life social or physical situation that the student or patient might encounter. Because the learner is required to use higher-level cognitive skills of application, analysis, or synthesis, the simulation strategy is used after the learner has mastered content. This technique may be used for either formative or summative evaluation, depending on the identified purpose of evaluation.

Hoban and Casberque (as cited in deTornyay & Thompson [1987]) discuss four principles that should be applied when simulation is used for clinical evaluation and that are also applicable to the classroom. The principles are as follows:

1. The performance (knowledge, skill, or attitude) that is expected of the student at the end of training should be specified along with the minimal acceptable level of performance the student is required to demonstrate.
2. The simulation should represent reality with enough fidelity to ensure face validity of the test of student's performance.
3. The simulation being used to evaluate student performance should be standardized: the simulation should produce the same kind of responses from a variety of students and provide the same feedback to students when they engage in similar activities.
4. Decisions regarding the purpose of the evaluation should be made before a simulation is used.

Simulations can be designed by the faculty or purchased in a variety of formats such as the following:

- Written simulations
- Models and mannequins
- Simulators such as heart sounds, cardiac patterns
- Computer-based simulations

The written simulation is the easiest and least expensive format. The student receives feedback with each response, and this information is incorporated in the next response. Models of the body are used in evaluation of skills such as suctioning, sterile dressing change, and administration of injections. Technology has added to the available formats for simulation. Audiotapes can be used for simulated breath and heart sounds. Computer-based patient simulations facilitate rapid changes in the status of a patient that may take months or years to occur in real life and provide access to certain patient problems not otherwise readily available to the learner (White, 1995). Students are able to administer simulated medications and observe the physiological effects (Ravert, 2002). Some computer-driven simulators use gas and compressed air to simulate physiological changes. Computer simulations allow the student to respond to the situation and see the consequences of his or her actions (Arnold & Pearson, 1992). CD-ROM and World Wide Web applications provide an opportunity to combine video images with the programming capabilities of the computer. These technologies can actively engage the student. It is possible to design simulations to test various cognitive domains in connection with the subject area. The level to be tested is determined by the evaluator (Ward, 1992). Simulations are used to measure observation, problem solving, communication, and decision-making skills without the interference of external factors.

A debriefing is frequently included at the end of a simulation. During the debriefing, students can (1) identify the concepts learned, (2) relate their learning to the objectives, (3) discuss application to clinical practice, and (4) evaluate the experience. The debriefing provides an opportunity for the student to self-evaluate and compare that assessment with the evaluation of the faculty. The format for the debriefing session should be identified by the faculty before the activity. With some types of simulations, debriefing may be accomplished by use of a form for independent completion by the learner or may be done as part of a computer program (Reilly & Oermann, 1992) or discussion in which computer conferencing software is used.

Advantages

This strategy assists students in applying instruction received in the classroom to actual practice in clinical settings. The students can respond to situations and see the consequences of their actions without fear of jeopardizing the patient. The experience is similar for all students. The varied formats permit direct observation, videotaping, or both. Predetermined standards allow for objectivity. The exercise can be repeated.

Disadvantages

Development of simulations and scoring mechanisms are costly in terms of time and money. The simulations available for purchase can be expensive. In the case of patient simulator mannequins, the cost to acquire and maintain the equipment should be considered. Extensive training may be required to actually operate a mannequin. The implementation of simulations can be time consuming as well.

Issues

The purpose for the simulation and the performance criteria must be clearly defined before the simulation is initiated as an evaluation strategy. Developing a simulation can be expensive, not only in terms of faculty time but also in terms of the equipment that may be needed. Faculty can decide whether any time limits are needed to simulate the immediacy of an action.

SUMMARY

Various strategies can be used to evaluate learning outcomes in the classroom. A multiplicity of strategies that reach beyond traditional written examinations can provide a more complete picture of students' abilities, assist students to actively participate in their evaluation, and measure critical thinking skills, as well as the affective domain. The strategies addressed in this chapter include portfolios, critiquing, journals, papers, essays and essay tests, concept mapping, oral questioning, videotape, audiotape, role play, and simulation. It is essential that faculty members consider the purpose and setting of the evaluation; the time required for preparation, implementation, and grading; the cost; and the advantages and disadvantages of each strategy when choosing one of these evaluation strategies. Although it requires time, energy, and persistence to plan evaluation of student achievement of outcomes, the effort will ultimately benefit students and the patients they are preparing to serve.

Faculty who implement alternative evaluation strategies will continue to increase the evidence base for best practices and contribute to their own scholarship of teaching. The findings from evaluation strategies can be used for a variety of purposes. The most obvious is to provide feedback to the learner and to revise instruction and learning activities. Evidence of critical thinking and therapeutic communication can also be used as a part of the systematic program evaluation plan. However, evaluation data are also helpful for the individual faculty member because data from evaluation techniques can be used to provide evidence of teaching excellence in a portfolio or dossier. As nursing education meets current challenges, the refinement of evaluation strategies will continue to expand in tandem with the development of teaching strategies, thereby contributing to the ever-increasing quality of education for nurses of the future.

REFERENCES

Angelo, T. A., & Cross, K. P. (1993). *Classroom assessment techniques: A handbook for college teachers* (2nd ed.). San Francisco: Jossey-Bass.

Arnold, J. M., & Pearson, G. A. (1992). *Computer applications in nursing education and practice* (Publication No. 14-2406). New York: National League for Nursing.

Beach, R., & Marshall, J. (1991). *Teaching literature in the secondary school.* San Diego: Harcourt.

Bevis, E. O., & Watson, J. (1989). *Toward a caring curriculum: A new pedagogy for nursing.* New York: National League for Nursing.

Bloom, B. S. (Ed.). (1956). *Taxonomy of educational objectives: The classification of educational goals. Handbook 1: Cognitive domain.* New York: D. McKay.

Clap-Itnyre, A. (2001). Three-part journaling in introductory writing and literature classes: More work with more rewards. *The Journal of Scholarship of Teaching and Learning* [Online], *1*(2). Retrieved July 17, 2003, from http://www.iusb.edu/~josotl/VOL.1/NO.2/clapp-intyre_vol_1_no_2.htm

Courts, P. L., & McInerney, K. H. (1993). *Assessment in higher education: Politics, pedagogy, and portfolios.* Westport, CT: Praeger.

deTornyay, R., & Thompson, M. A. (1987). *Strategies for teaching nursing* (3rd ed.). New York: Wiley.

Eisner, E. (1985). *The educational imagination* (2nd ed.). New York: Macmillan.

Goldenberg, D. (1994). Critiquing as a method of evaluation in the classroom. *Nurse Educator, 19,* 18-22.

Graf, M. A. (1993). Videotaping return demonstration. *Nurse Educator, 18*(4), 29.

Hansen, C. (1994). Questioning techniques for the active classroom. In D. F. Halpern (Ed.), *Changing college classrooms: New teaching and learning strategies for an increasingly complex world* (pp. 93-106). San Francisco: Jossey-Bass.

Joyce, B., Weil, M., & Showers, B. (1992). *Models of teaching* (4th ed.). Boston: Allyn & Bacon.

Karlowicz, K. A. (2000). The value of student portfolios to evaluate undergraduate nursing programs. *Nurse Educator, 25*(2), 82-87.

King, A. (1994). Inquiry as a tool in critical thinking. In D. F. Halpern (Ed.), *Changing college classrooms: New teaching and learning strategies for an increasingly complex world* (pp. 13-38). San Francisco: Jossey-Bass.

Kobert, L. J. (1995). In our own voice: Journaling as a teaching/learning technique for nurses. *Journal of Nursing Education, 34*(3), 140-142.

Krathwohl, D. R., Bloom, B. S., Mases, B. (1964). *Taxonomy of educational objectives, Handbook II, affective domain* (pp. 66, 91). New York: David McKay Co. Inc.

Linn, R., & Grondlund, N. (2000). *Measurement and assessment in teaching.* Upper Saddle River, NJ: Prentice-Hall.

Ravert, P. (2002). An integrative review of computer based simulation in the education process. *CIN: Computers, Informatics, Nursing, 20*(5), 203-208.

Reilly, D. E. (1978). *Teaching and evaluating the affective domain in nursing programs.* Thoroughfare, NJ: Slack.

Reilly, D. E., & Oermann, M. H. (1992). *Clinical teaching nursing education* (2nd ed.). New York: Allyn & Bacon.

Rinne, C. (1994). The SKILLS system: A new interactive video technology. *THE Journal, 21*(8), 81-82.

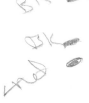

Rooda, L. A. (1994). Effects of mind mapping on student achievement in a nursing research course. *Nurse Educator, 19*(6), 25-27.

Taggart, G., Phifer, S., Nixon, J., & Wood, M. (Eds.). (1998). *Rubrics: A handbook for construction and use.* Lancaster, PA: Technomic Publishing.

Ward, R. (1992). Interactive video: An analysis of its value to nurse education. *Nurse Education Today, 12*(6), 464-470.

Watson, J. (1989). Transformative thinking and a caring curriculum. In E. O. Bevis & J. Watson, *Toward a caring curriculum: A new pedagogy for nursing* (NLN Publication No. 15-2278, pp. 51-60). New York: National League for Nursing.

White, J. E. (1995). Using interactive video to add physical assessment data to computer-based patient simulations. *Computers in Nursing, 13*(5), 233-235.

Yensen, J. A. P. (1997). *Web journaling help page* [Online]. Retrieved July 12, 2003, from http://www.langara.bc.ca/vnc/jhelp.htm

Yensen, J. A. P. (2002). *Strategies for learning: From concept maps to learning objects and books to wooks* [Online]. Retrieved July 12, 2003, from http://eaaknowledge.com/ojni/ni/602/strategies.htm.

22

Developing and Using Classroom Tests

Prudence Twigg, PhD(c), RN, APRN-BC, Lori Rasmussen, MSN, RN, Diana J. Speck, MSN, RN

One method for assessing learning outcomes is to develop, administer, and analyze results of written tests. Although this seems like a relatively straightforward task, it is a very involved process. The purpose of this chapter is to offer a step-by-step approach to planning, developing, administering, and revising classroom tests.

PLANNING THE TEST

Developing a test that is valid (representative) and reliable (consistent) requires much thought and planning. The following section describes how to develop a test. This section covers the purpose of the test, criterion versus norm-referenced tests, development of a table of specifications, and how to improve the reliability and validity of a test.

Purpose of the Test

The first question that must be addressed is, "What purpose will the test serve?" If the test is to be given before instruction, it may be used to determine readiness (the grasp of prerequisite skills needed to be successful) or placement (the level of mastery of instructional objectives). During instruction, the test may be used as a formative evaluation of learning or as a diagnostic tool to identify learning problems. As measures of learning outcomes, tests provide summative evaluation of learning on which progression and grade decisions may be based. See Table 22-1 for a summary of test measures based on timing of administration.

Tests may serve a variety of additional functions. For example, testing may provide the structure (e.g., deadlines) that some students need to direct their learning activities, or faculty may use testing as one means of evaluating teaching effectiveness by measuring the outcomes of student learning. Faculty may also use posttest reviews as a learning opportunity for students to discuss rationales for answers (Morrison & Free, 2001) and gain insight into their own strengths and weaknesses (Flannelly, 2001).

TABLE 22-1 Test Measures Based on Timing of Administration		
TIMING	**TYPE OF TEST**	**MEASURE**
Before	Readiness	Prerequisite skills
	Placement	Previous learning
During	Formative	Learning progress
	Diagnositc	Learning problems
After	Summative	Terminal performance

Types of Tests

Criterion-referenced Tests

Criterion-referenced tests are those that are constructed and interpreted according to a specific set of learning outcomes. This type of test is useful for measuring mastery of subject matter. An absolute standard of performance is set for grading purposes.

Norm-referenced Tests

Norm-referenced tests are those that are constructed and interpreted to provide a relative ranking of students. Norm-referenced tests are based on measurement of content according to a table of specifications (test plan, test blueprint). This type of test is useful for measuring differential performance among students. A relative standard of performance is used for grading purposes.

Both criterion- and norm-referenced tests may be used in nursing education. Criterion-referenced tests are frequently used to ensure safety in areas such as drug dosage calculation, in which the absolute standard of performance may be set as high as 100%, regardless of the performance of other students.

Table of Specifications

The purpose of developing a table of specifications (test map, test grid, test blueprint) is to ensure that the test serves its intended purpose by representatively sampling the intended learning outcomes and instructional content. The first step in developing a table of specifications is to define the specific learning outcomes to be measured. Specific learning outcomes, which are derived from more general instructional outcomes (e.g., course and unit objectives), specify tasks that students should be able to perform on completion of instruction (Linn & Gronlund, 2000).

Bloom's taxonomy (1956) is frequently used as a guide for developing and leveling general instructional and specific learning outcomes (see Chapter 10). Although the cognitive components of the affective and psychomotor domains can be evaluated with classroom tests, tests are most often used to determine achievement of outcomes in the six levels of the cognitive domain (Table 22-2).

TABLE 22-2 Action Verbs for Different Cognitive Levels

COGNITIVE LEVEL	ACTION VERBS
Knowledge	Define, identify, list
Comprehension	Describe, explain, summarize
Application	Apply, demonstrate, use
Analysis	Compare, contrast, differentiate
Synthesis	Construct, develop, formulate
Evaluation	Critique, evaluate, judge

A mixture of cognitive levels should be evaluated at each stage of instruction, placing an increasing emphasis (or weight) on higher-level skills as instruction progresses. This is vital because higher-level skills are more likely to result in retention and transfer of knowledge (Gronlund, 1998). In addition, this will assist in preparing students for the licensing and certification examinations that test primarily at the levels of application and analysis (Wendt & Brown, 2000).

The second step in developing a table of specifications involves determining the instructional content to be evaluated and the weight to be assigned to each area. This can be accomplished by developing a content outline and using the amount of time spent teaching the material as an indicator for weighting (Table 22-3).

Finally, a two-way grid is developed, with content areas being listed down the left side and learning outcomes being listed across the top of the grid (Table 22-4). Each cell is assigned a number of questions according to the weighting of content and cognitive level of learning outcomes.

Some faculty prefer to use a three-way table of specifications. With a three-way grid, the five steps of the nursing process are listed on the left side, outcomes are listed across the top, and the number of items or specific content areas is listed within each cell. Weighting of the steps of the nursing process again depends on the level of instruction. For example, early in the instructional process, assessment and diagnosis might carry the most weight, whereas all stages may be tested equally by the end of instruction. Tables 22-5 and 22-6 are examples of three-way tables of specifications.

TABLE 22-3 Content Outline and Relative Teaching Time

CONTENT	TEACHING TIME (%)	NO. OF ITEMS/SECTION
I. Antipsychotic agents	25	10
II. Antianxiety agents	25	10
III. Antidepressant agents	25	10
IV. Antimanic agents	12.5	5
V. Antiparkinson agents	12.5	5
TOTALS	100	40

Note: Percentage of teaching time × Total no. of items = No. of items/section.

TABLE 22-4   Two-way Table of Specifications

OUTCOMES* (CONTENT†)	KNOWLEDGE (20%)	COMPREHENSION (40%)	APPLICATION (40%)	TOTALS
Antipsychotic agents (25%)	2	4	4	10
Antianxiety agents (25%)	2	4	4	10
Antidepressant agents (25%)	2	4	4	10
Antimanic agents (12.5%)	1	2	2	5
Antiparkinson agents (12.5%)	1	2	2	5
TOTALS	8	8	16	40

*Percent arbitrarily determined by level of instruction.
†Percent determined by teaching time.

TABLE 22-5   Three-way Table of Specifications: Number of Items per Cell

OUTCOMES* (PROCESS†)	KNOWLEDGE (20%)	COMPREHENSION (40%)	APPLICATION (40%)	TOTALS
Assessment (40%)	6	6	4	16
Diagnosis (10%)	1	3	—	4
Planning (10%)	1	2	1	4
Intervention (20%)	—	2	6	8
Evaluation (20%)	—	3	5	8
TOTALS	8	16	16	40

*Arbitrarily determined by level of instruction.
†Percent determined by teaching time.

TABLE 22-6   Three-way Table of Specifications: Content to be Tested per Cell*

OUTCOMES* (PROCESS†)	KNOWLEDGE (20%)	COMPREHENSION (40%)	APPLICATION (40%)	TOTALS
Assessment (40%)	P, A, A, D, D, M	P, P, A, D, M, PA	P, A, D, PA	16
Diagnosis (10%)	P	A, D, M	—	4
Planning (10%)	PA	A, D	P	4
Intervention (20%)	—	P, A	P, A, A, D, M, PA	8
Evaluation (20%)	—	P, PA, D	P, A, D, D, M	8
TOTALS	8	16	16	40

*No. of each type of content item determined by teaching time.
†Percent determined by teaching time.
P, Antipsychotic agents; *A,* antianxiety agents; *D,* antidepressant agents; *M,* antimanic agents; *PA,* antiparkinson agents.

Alternatively, or additionally, a table of specifications can be created by using the test plan of the current licensure examination (NCLEX-RN). The NCLEX-RN tests content in four categories of patient needs as follows (National Council of State Boards of Nursing [NCSBN], 2003):

1. Safe, effective care environment
2. Health promotion and maintenance
3. Psychosocial integrity
4. Physiological integrity

In addition to the category of patient needs, the NCLEX-RN integrates concepts and processes of nursing practice (nursing process, caring, communication and documentation, self-care, teaching/learning) throughout the questions. One possible disadvantage of using the NCLEX-RN test plan in a table of specifications for development of a classroom test is that the content of most nursing courses is not organized according to these categories.

Other Considerations in the Planning Stage
Selecting Item Types

Items may be *selection-type*, providing a set of responses from which to choose, or *supply-type*, requiring the student to provide an answer. Common selection-type items include true-false, matching, and multiple-choice questions. Supply-type items include short answer and essay questions.

The primary reason for choosing one type of item over another can be determined by answering the question, "Which type of item most directly measures the intended learning outcome?" Generally, lower-level outcomes (knowledge, comprehension, and application) can be easily evaluated by selection-type items, whereas higher-level outcomes (analysis, synthesis, and evaluation) require the use of supply-type items (Gronlund, 1998).

Other factors may also influence the item-type selection. For example, a large class size may prohibit the use of supply-type items because of the time required for grading. A summary of characteristics of selection-type and supply-type items is provided in Table 22-7.

In addition to multiple choice items with one correct answer, the NCLEX-RN has recently added the so-called alternative format questions, which

TABLE 22-7 Characteristics of Selection- and Supply-type Items

CHARACTERISTIC	SELECTION TYPE	SUPPLY TYPE
Easy to create	No	Yes
Easy to score	Yes	No
Objective	Yes	No
Measures higher level skills	No	Yes
Broad sampling	Yes	No
Eliminates noncontent skills	Yes	No

include fill-in the blank questions, multiple choice questions with multiple responses, and picture or graphic questions. Current information on the examination format can be obtained at the website for the National Council of State Boards of Nursing *(http://www.ncsbn.org)*.

Selecting Item Difficulty

Item difficulty primarily depends on the purpose of the test. If it is a criterion-referenced test, difficulty should match the level of the learning that reflects the skills to be mastered. Norm-referenced tests involve eliminating easy items and using average difficulty items to maximize the differences among students.

Determining Number of Items

Test reliability usually increases with the number of test items. However, the number of test items is limited by many practical constraints. For example, more selection-type items than supply-type items can be answered in a given period. Similarly, items that require higher-level thinking skills take more time to answer than those that require lower-level skills.

A general guide for planning is to allow 1 minute for each moderately difficult multiple-choice item. For a 60-minute class, a test with about 50 items is appropriate (McDonald, 2002).

ITEM WRITING

Writing items for true-false, matching, interpretive, short-answer, and multiple-choice tests requires time and skill. The definitions, advantages, disadvantages, guidelines for writing, and examples of each of these types of test items follow.

True-False Items

Definition

A true-false or binary choice question is a declarative sentence that the student must determine to be true or false. This type of question would appear to be a straightforward measure of student learning. However, it has been criticized for trivial content, ambiguity, and difficulty in construction (Downing, 1992).

Advantages

1. Faculty can sample more information about a topic using this format.
2. The student can complete more of these items in a given period.
3. This type of item works well when there are only two alternatives.
4. Scoring is easy and objective.

Disadvantages

1. Students' scores are influenced by guessing. By chance alone, a student could get a score of 50% on a test.
2. This item type encourages memorization of text or lectures.

3. A true-false item presents two extremes that rarely match up with the real world.
4. Marking a question false does not mean the student knows what is really true.

Guidelines for Writing True-False Items

1. Avoid the use of absolute terms such as *all* or *always*, which indicate that the item is false. Likewise, qualifiers such as *sometimes* or *typically* indicate that the item is true.
2. State the item in a positive, declarative sentence, as simply as possible.
3. Avoid negative and double-negative statements.
4. Keep true and false statements equal in length.
5. Randomize the true and false items so the student will not detect a pattern.
6. Write each item so it is clearly true or clearly false.
7. Credit opinions to a source if understanding of beliefs is being measured.
8. Do not include two concepts in one statement.

Examples. Read the following statements and decide whether they are true or false. Circle T for true and F for false.

T   F   1. Oxytocin is released from the anterior pituitary gland.
T   F   2. Lochia rubra is a normal finding for the tenth postpartum day.

Matching Items

Definition

A matching item consists of two parallel lists of words that require the student to match according to certain associations between the two lists. One column consists of problems (premises); the other contains answers (responses) (Mehrens & Lehmann, 1991).

Advantages

1. A matching item is compact so a great deal of information can be tested on a single page.
2. The items can be scored quickly and objectively.
3. Students can respond to a large number of these items because reading time is short.
4. Students are required to integrate knowledge to discover the relationship.

Disadvantages

1. These items can be difficult to write without including unintended clues.
2. Questions of this nature tend to be restricted to reflection of simple knowledge rather than higher levels of learning.
3. It is difficult to generate enough plausible responses.

Guidelines for Writing Matching Items

1. The items being matched should be homogeneous. Otherwise, the student can quickly find the correct responses.
2. The entire set of matching items should be on a single page to eliminate page turning.
3. Use a larger or smaller set of responses and permit them to be used more than once or not at all.
4. Arrange items in a systematic order to make the selection process quicker.
5. State in the directions the basis of relationship for matching.
6. Place the stimulus column on the left with each item numbered and the response column on the right with each item lettered.

Examples. On the line to the left of the items in column A write the letter of the item in column B that best matches. Responses in column B may be used once, more than once, or not at all.

COLUMN A: STATEMENTS

____ 1. I'm here if you need me.
____ 2. What do you think about it?
____ 3. I'm sure he knows that.
____ 4. Tell me about that.

COLUMN B: TYPE OF COMMUNICATION

A. Checking perceptions
B. Defending
C. Exploring
D. Offering self
E. Probing

Interpretive Items

Definition

An interpretive item requires a response based on introductory material such as a paragraph, table, chart, map, or picture (Linn & Gronlund, 2000). The student must make a judgment about the material presented. These items are often used on nursing examinations to evaluate a student's ability to interpret laboratory data, electrocardiogram or fetal monitor strips, or other pictorial items. The new alternative format style questions of the NCLEX-RN examination include graphic or pictorial items that may require interpretation.

Advantages

1. Use of interpretative items is a way to measure a student's ability to comprehend printed information.
2. Complex learning outcomes can be measured.
3. Scoring is easy and objective.

Disadvantages

1. It is difficult to construct effective items.
2. Items may contain unintended clues.
3. Interpretative items do not measure a student's ability to express ideas.

Guidelines for Writing Interpretive Items

1. Keep the printed information brief and readable.
2. Phrase the question so it can be answered in either short answer or multiple-choice format.
3. Present introductory material before the question.
4. Keep elements of items on the same page.

Examples. Complete the following:

1. [insert labor graph]
   How long did the first stage of labor last?_____
   How long was the transition phase?_____
2. [insert laboratory data]
   For which laboratory value, in a patient about to go to surgery, would the nurse notify the physician?
   a. Hematocrit
   b. Hemoglobin
   c. Platelets
   d. White blood cell count
3. [insert electrocardiogram strip]
   What arrhythmia does the patient have?_____
4. [insert picture of the abdomen]
   Indicate the area where the nurse would palpate for bladder distension.

Short-Answer Items

Definition

The short answer or fill-in-the-blank item requires the student to produce an answer (Linn & Gronlund, 2000). The question can be answered in one or two words. This item type is used when the instructor wants the student to recall or calculate the answer. The student could also be asked to visually represent the answer; for example, "Calculate a drug dosage, then mark the answer on a picture of a syringe." The new alternative format style questions of the NCLEX-RN examination include short-answer items.

Advantages

1. This item type reduces guessing.
2. This item type works well for math problems because it requires the student to work out the answer.
3. A broad range of material can be tested.

Disadvantages

1. It is difficult to phrase the question so there is only one correct answer.
2. Scoring can be time consuming because the student may supply an answer the instructor had not considered.
3. The student's spelling can make it difficult to score.

Guidelines for Writing Short-Answer Items

1. Write completion items that can be answered with one word or number.
2. Phrase statements or questions so there is only one correct answer.
3. Avoid giving grammatical clues to the answer (e.g., use of *a* or *an*).
4. Keep the length of the blanks the same.
5. Do not take statements directly from the text or lecture; this encourages memorization.
6. If spelling is a problem, a list of words from which to choose can be provided.
7. For math problems, indicate how precise the answer should be.

Examples. Supply the appropriate word to answer the question or complete the sentence.

1. Using the Apgar scoring system as a guide, fill in the blanks to complete the score for a newborn with the following characteristics:

CHARACTERISTIC	SCORE
a. Active motion of extremities	_____
b. Crying, good respirations	_____
c. Heart rate greater than 100	_____
d. Pink color, blue extremities	_____
e. Vigorous cry	_____
Total	_____

2. The nurse is to give morphine elixir, 4 mg, sublingually. The drug available is morphine, 20 mg/mL. How much should the nurse give? (round to the nearest tenth)_____
3. For which common cardiac arrhythmia is digoxin (Lanoxin) often given?_____
4. Which serum laboratory value is the best indicator of renal function?_____

Multiple-Choice Items

Definition

A multiple-choice item consists of two parts. The first is the *stem,* which can be a question or an incomplete statement. The second part consists of several *options* from which to select the correct answer. The options should include one, and only one, correct response and several incorrect options, or *distractors.* In some cases, the options may all be correct, and the student may be directed to select the single best response. The majority of the NCLEX-RN examination consists of multiple-choice items. Multiple-choice items, when carefully constructed, can measure critical thinking (McDonald, 2002; Morrison & Free, 2001).

Advantages

1. Multiple-choice items allow the instructor to sample a large amount of content in a single test.

2. These items can be scored easily and objectively.
3. Scores on multiple-choice tests are less influenced by guessing than are scores on true-false tests.
4. These items are versatile because they can measure understanding at several cognitive levels in the taxonomy categories.

Disadvantages

1. Writing good items with plausible distractors can be very time consuming for the instructor.
2. This item type takes more time for the student to read and understand.
3. These items may discriminate against the creative, verbal student.
4. Scores can be affected by students' reading ability and the instructor's writing style.
5. This item type can raise the score of the student who can recognize rather than produce the correct answer.
6. It is difficult to write multiple-choice items at the synthesis and evaluation level.

Guidelines for Writing Multiple-Choice Items

Stem

1. Present a single problem in the stem. It should be clear enough to answer without looking at the options.
2. Write the stem in a precise manner. If it is too complex, the student will spend too much time trying to decipher it.
3. Put all common content in the stem.
4. Each stem should be independent of all others on the test.
5. Make sure information in one stem does not answer another item for the student.
6. State the stem in a positive rather than a negative manner. If it is written in a negative manner, underline the negative words or print them in boldface.
7. Include enough information in the stem to answer the question.
8. Use scenarios sparingly; credentialing examination-style questions do not use patient or client names, age, sex, or ethnicity unless needed to answer the question.
9. Use action verbs from Bloom's (1956) taxonomy that are consistent with the cognitive level being measured.

Options

1. Keep all options grammatically consistent with the stem to avoid giving clues to the correct option.
2. Arrange the options in either alphabetical or numerical order.
3. Keep the options the same length or have two short responses and two long responses.
4. Make all the options reasonable and homogenous. If there are only three plausible options, use those without adding an obviously

wrong option just to have four options. For example, (a) high, (b) low, (c) normal. All items on a test do not have to have the same number of options.

5. Use only one best answer on which all authorities would agree.

6. Avoid the use of "all of the above" or "none of the above." Students can often guess the correct answer with only partial knowledge.

Examples
Knowledge

1. A patient's father died of Huntington's chorea. What are the chances that the patient will have the disease?

    A. 25%
    B. 50%
    C. 75%
    D. 100%

Comprehension

2. A patient resists the nurse's attempts to get him out of bed. If the nurse attempts to remove him from his bed without his approval, what legal charge could the nurse face?

    A. Assault
    B. Battery
    C. Negligence
    D. Tort

Application

3. On the first postoperative day after an open reduction and internal fixation (ORIF) of the tibia with application of a long leg cast, the patient begins complaining of severe pain uncontrolled by his scheduled pain medications. What would be the priority nursing intervention?

    A. Administer a narcotic bolus as ordered.
    B. Assess the neurovascular status of the leg.
    C. Lower the leg to increase arterial flow.
    D. Raise the leg to decrease venous return.

Analysis

4. A 70-year-old woman is admitted to the hospital with a diagnosis of dehydration. Vital signs are stable. The serum sodium (Na^+) level is 165 mmol/L. Which type of fluid replacement is most likely to be administered?

    A. Hypertonic
    B. Hypotonic
    C. Isotonic

Multiple-Response Multiple-Choice Items
Definition

A multiple-response multiple-choice item, like a multiple-choice item, has a stem and options; however, the options are written so that several of the responses are correct. The new alternative format style questions of the NCLEX-RN examination include multiple-response multiple-choice items. Students should be instructed to choose all correct responses to receive credit for the question.

Advantages

1. Multiple-response items allow for several correct answers.
2. There is less opportunity for choosing options by process of elimination than with standard multiple choice items.
3. The use of the multiple-response item avoids "all of the above" as an option.

Disadvantages

1. Multiple-response items require more options (usually five to six), and thus more distractors, than standard multiple choice items.
2. Scoring, particularly by computer, may be more difficult.

Guidelines for Writing Multiple-Response Multiple-Choice Items

For the stem, use the same general guidelines as for writing multiple-choice items. For the options, use the same general guidelines but include at least two correct responses.

Examples

Knowledge

1. The patient is taking digoxin (Lanoxin). For which of the following toxic effects of this drug should the nurse monitor? Select all that apply.

    A. anorexia
    B. dyspnea
    C. hives
    D. nausea
    E. tachycardia
    F. visual changes

Comprehension

2. The patient is on a clear liquid diet. Which of the following foods/fluids are allowed? Select all that apply.

    A. bouillon
    B. gelatin
    C. milk
    D. orange juice
    E. pudding
    F. water

Application

3. The nurse is the first to arrive on the scene of an auto accident and finds an unconscious man still in the driver's seat. The man's left femur is protruding through the skin. Which of the following actions should the nurse take?

   A. Assess airway, breathing, and circulation.
   B. Call for emergency assistance.
   C. Check for bleeding.
   D. Move the left leg to align the bone
   E. Place a tourniquet high on the left thigh.
   F. Remove the man from the car.

Analysis

4. The nurse implements a medication safety teaching plan for the community-dwelling older adult. Which statements by the patient indicate that the teaching has been effective? Select all that apply.

   A. "I will throw away any medications I am no longer using."
   B. "I will have my prescriptions filled at different pharmacies to get the best price."
   C. "I will tell my physician about any nonprescription medications I am taking."
   D. "I will crush any medications that I have difficulty swallowing."
   E. "I will take all my medications with food to avoid stomach upset."
   F. "I will report possible side effects of my medications to my physician."

USING TEST BANKS AND TEST AUTHORING SYSTEMS

The task of creating test items can be simplified by using computerized test development software (Kirkpatrick et al., 2000). This software can facilitate test development by creating a collection of test items (test bank) from which faculty can select appropriate questions according to the test blueprint. Alternate forms of tests can also be generated because the item pool can be large enough so that questions can be selected randomly. Some test authoring software can be used for online testing in a computer classroom or on the World Wide Web, thus simplifying the test administration process. Students may benefit from using computerized practice tests in preparation for the NCLEX-RN (Rossignol & Scollin, 2001). Many textbook publishers provide computer test banks of test items free of charge to faculty adopting their texts (Masters et al., 2001). Test banks can also be created easily by using a word processing program that stores test items, making revision of items and tests easier.

EDITING TEST ITEMS

After test items have been developed, it is necessary to edit them and make any needed corrections. At this stage, peer review of the questions is helpful for refining the questions, ensuring accuracy and readability, and eliminating grammatical errors. This editing can be done in a question or checklist format. Questions to consider include the following:

1. Are items stated in a precise manner?
2. Do items match the table of specifications?
3. Is there one best answer for each item? (except for multiple-response multiple-choice items)
4. Does each item stand alone?
5. Are sentence construction and punctuation correct?
6. Have stereotyping, prejudices, and biases been eliminated?
7. Has the use of humor been avoided?
8. Has extraneous information been deleted?
9. Has a colleague reviewed the test?
10. Is the placement of correct options varied so there is no obvious pattern?

POTENTIAL BIAS IN TEST ITEMS

Students of equal ability should have an equal probability of correctly answering a test item. If systematic differences in responses to an item exist among members of particular groups, independent of total scores, then the item may be biased. Bosher (2003) classifies potential areas of bias in test items in four categories: testwise flaws, irrelevant difficulty, linguistic/structural bias, and cultural bias. Testwise flaws are those errors in items that provide cues to the correct answer within the item or test itself, thus potentially providing an unfair advantage to students with more test-taking experience or training and to native English speakers who can more easily recognize grammatical and other cues. Items with irrelevant difficulty may be missed for reasons related more to format (e.g., unclear stems, superfluous information, negative phrasing) than to content. Similarly, linguistic complexity, grammatical errors, and inconsistent word use may result in biased items. Finally, items that depend on culturally specific knowledge should not be used unless cultural practices per se are the domain of the question. The guidelines for writing items are designed to avoid bias.

ASSEMBLING AND ADMINISTERING A TEST

Once the items are written and edited, they must be assembled into a test. This step includes arranging the items, writing test directions, reproducing the test, and administering the test (Gaberson, 1996).

Arranging Items

Once items have been selected and edited, the next step is to decide how items will be arranged on the test. For the purposes of enhancing thought tracking, increasing student confidence, and preventing students from becoming anxious about early items, the following guidelines are suggested:

1. Group similar item types together (e.g., all true-false items).

2. Place items within each group in ascending order of difficulty.
3. Place item types in ascending order of difficulty (e.g., true-false items first, essay items last).
4. Begin the test with an easy question.

Writing Test Directions

Test directions should be self-explanatory and include the following information:

1. *Purpose of the test:* This may not need to be included if it has been addressed earlier in the instructional process.
2. *Time allotted to complete the test:* This information allows the student to pace himself or herself when responding to items.
3. *Basis for responding:* This provides the student with information necessary to choose the appropriate response (e.g., choose only one answer; matching options can be used more than once).
4. *Recording answers:* Answers may be recorded in a variety of ways to expedite grading (e.g., recording answers on a computer sheet using a No. 2 pencil, marking an X through the correct answer on a separate answer sheet for stencil grading, marking answers directly on the test booklet in the left-hand column).
5. *Guessing:* Encouraging students to answer all questions prevents the inflation of scores of bolder students as a result of guessing.
6. *Value assigned to items:* This information allows the student to effectively plan the use of his or her time.

Example. Circle the one best answer. Because your score is the total number of correct answers, you should answer all questions. Each question is worth 2 points. You have 50 minutes to complete this 50-item test.

Reproducing the Test

The test should be easy to read and follow. The following guidelines are suggested:

1. Type test neatly.
2. Space items evenly.
3. Number items consecutively.
4. Keep an item's stem and options on the same page.
5. Place introductory material (e.g., graph or chart) before item (and make sure it reproduces clearly).
6. Keep matching lists on the same page.
7. Proofread the test after it is compiled but before it is duplicated.

Administering the Test

The physical environment should be conducive to the task. This includes adequate lighting, a comfortable temperature, sufficient work space, and minimal interruptions. To reduce student anxiety, the faculty member should maintain a positive, nonthreatening attitude and avoid unnecessary conversation before and during the test. Faculty should avoid giving unintentional hints to individual students who ask for clarification of questions during the test.

Cheating is often a concern when a test is administered. Jacobs and Chase (1992) suggest a variety of methods for reducing cheating, including the following:

1. Maintaining test security (e.g., locking up copies of the test).
2. Modifying tests from one semester to another.
3. Stating the consequences of cheating early in the instructional process.
4. Monitoring students consistently throughout testing.
5. Designating special seating arrangements (e.g., having an empty chair between students, having students sit in alphabetical order).
6. Using alternate versions of the test.
7. Using alternative answer forms (e.g., listing responses down the page, listing responses across the page).

ANALYSIS OF TEST RESULTS

Once the test has been administered, faculty review the results using concepts of measurement and data analysis. On the basis of these findings, faculty assign grades. Faculty at most schools of nursing have access to computer scoring and test item analysis. Faculty should seek the assistance of these services and the consultation that can be obtained at testing centers.

CONCEPTS OF MEASUREMENT

Validity

According to the *Standards for Educational and Psychological Testing* (American Psychological Association, American Education Research Association, National Council on Measurement in Education, 1985), the concept of validity refers to the appropriateness, meaningfulness, and usefulness of inferences made from test scores. Validity is the judgment made about a test's ability to measure what it is intended to measure. This judgment is based on three categories of evidence: content-related, criterion-related, and construct-related.

Content-related patterns of evidence should show that the test adequately samples relevant content (Popham, 1990). In nursing education, the relevant content is defined by nurse educators, the course, and the profession. Some examples of content-related evidence of validity are correspondence of the test content with the following:

1. The table of specifications
2. Professional judgments of peers
3. Core material as defined by professional organizations
4. Standards of care as defined by agencies and professional organizations

Criterion-related patterns of evidence should show that the test adequately measures performance, either concurrently or predictively (Popham, 1990).

The performance must be compared with some criterion variable. Nurse educators may use performance on the licensing examination (NCLEX-RN or NCLEX-LPN) as the criterion variable (pass or fail). An example of criterion-related evidence of validity is correlation of test scores with standardized measures (e.g., National League for Nursing [NLN] achievement tests).

Construct-related patterns of evidence should show a relationship between test performance and some "quality" to be measured (Popham, 1990). This is a broad category of evidence that must include specifics about the test (from the content and criterion categories) in addition to a description of the quality or construct being measured.

According to Jacobs and Chase (1992), some of the factors that may adversely affect test validity include unclear directions, inconsistent or inadequate sampling from the table of specifications, poorly written test items, and subjective scoring. Careful preparation of the test can improve test validity.

Reliability

Reliability refers to the ability of a test to provide dependable and consistent scores. A judgment about reliability can be made based on the extent to which two similar measures agree. Reliability is a necessary but not sufficient condition for validity. However, reliability may be high even with no validity (Popham, 1990). Nurse educators look for evidence to judge tests as both reliable and valid.

According to Lyman (1991), among the factors that may adversely affect test reliability are insufficient length and insufficient group variability. For the purpose of increasing reliability, Jacobs and Chase (1992) recommend a minimum test length of 25 multiple-choice questions with an item difficulty sufficient to ensure heterogenous performance of the group.

Reliability could be measured by giving the same test to the same group and noting the correspondence (test-retest method) or by giving "equivalent" tests to the same group. Both of these methods have major disadvantages for classroom testing and are not generally used by nurse educators. Reliability can be measured with a single test administration by using either the split-half or internal consistency method. The split-half method separately scores responses to odd and even questions and then compares the "odd-question" score to the "even-question" score. The internal consistency of a test can be calculated by using one of the Kuder-Richardson formulas, as described by Popham (1990). Many computer grading programs supply a test reliability coefficient as part of the results (see Figure 22-1).

Reliability is measured on a scale of 0 to 1.00. A reliability coefficient of 1.00 would represent 100% correspondence between two tests or measures. Many standardized tests have reliability coefficients of .9 or higher. According to Jacobs and Chase (1992), a reliability coefficient in the range of .7 to .8 is acceptable for classroom tests. For the test results shown in Figure 22-1, the reliability coefficient is .844, indicating good internal consistency of the test. Measures of test reliability are based on the assumption

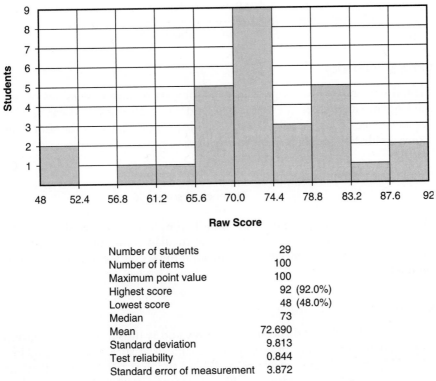

Number of students	29
Number of items	100
Maximum point value	100
Highest score	92 (92.0%)
Lowest score	48 (48.0%)
Median	73
Mean	72.690
Standard deviation	9.813
Test reliability	0.844
Standard error of measurement	3.872

FIGURE 22-1   Sample test statistics report from a computer test scoring program.

that all students had adequate time to answer all questions and that all test items are of about the same difficulty (Jacobs & Chase, 1992). Because the reliability coefficient functions better when the variability of scores is maximized, tests administered to smaller groups of students (N) may have lower reliability coefficients.

TEST STATISTICS

Various test statistics can be calculated, generated by test-authoring software, or reported from computer scoring services (see Figure 22-1). These statistics help faculty interpret test results and provide data for item revision.

Raw Score

The raw score is the number of test questions answered correctly. Raw scores are the most accurate test scores but yield limited information. A frequency distribution can be used to arrange raw scores to create class intervals. If tests are scored by computer, a frequency polygon is likely. The percentage score compares the raw score with the maximum possible score.

$$\text{Percent score} = \frac{\text{Raw score } (x)}{\text{Maximum possible score}}$$

Central Tendency

Central tendency is a descriptive statistic for a set of scores. Measures of central tendency include the mean, median, and mode. The mean (or average) has the advantage of ease of calculation. The mean is calculated as the sum of all scores divided by the total number of scores.

$$\text{Mean (m)} = \frac{\text{Sum of all scores } (x\text{'s})}{\text{Number of scores } (N)}$$

The median divides the scores in the middle (i.e., 50% of scores fall below the median and 50% of scores are above the median). The median is a better measure of central tendency than the mean if the scores are not normally distributed.

Variability

Variability refers to the dispersion of scores and is thus a measure of group heterogeneity. Variability of scores affects other statistics. For example, low variability (homogeneity of scores) will tend to lower reliability coefficients such as the Kuder-Richardson coefficient (Lyman, 1991). Relative grading scales are most meaningful when they are applied to a wide range of scores (Gronlund, 1998). Mastery tests, by design, may show little variability. As groups of students progress in a nursing program, there may be less variability in scores because of attrition of students (failure or withdrawal from the program).

Range

The range is the simplest measure of variability and is calculated by subtracting the lowest score from the highest score. Thus

$$\text{Range} = \text{Highest score} - \text{Lowest score}$$

Standard Deviation

The standard deviation (SD) of scores is the best measure of variability. Most computer scoring programs provide the SD of the scores with the results. There are calculators with statistical functions that can also be used to figure the SD. For more information on formulas and methods for calculating the SD, consult a statistics text. The SD is just the average distance of scores from the mean. In Figure 22-1, the SD is given as 9.8. The SD can be used in making interpretations from the normal curve (Lyman, 1991).

Normal Curve

The normal curve is a theoretical distribution of scores that is bell shaped and symmetrical. The mean, median, and mode are the same score on a normal curve. Also, for a normal curve, 68% of scores will fall within plus or minus 1 SD of the mean and 95% of scores will fall within plus or minus 2 SDs of the mean. This distribution may be used in assigning grades.

Standard Error of Measurement

The standard error of measurement is an estimate of how much the observed score is likely to differ from the "true" score. That is, the student's "true" score most likely lies between the observed score plus or minus the standard error.

$$\text{True score} = \text{Observed score} \pm \text{Error}$$

The standard error of measurement is calculated by using the SD and the test reliability (Popham, 1990). Many computer scoring programs supply the standard error. Some faculty members give students the benefit of the doubt and add the standard error to each raw score before they assign grades.

Standardized Scores

Standardized scores allow for ease of comparison between individual scores and sets of scores. The z score converts a raw score into units of SD on a normal curve. The z score can be calculated as follows:

$$Z = \frac{x - m}{SD}$$

x = Observed score
m = Mean
SD = Standard deviation

For example, for a raw score of 34,

$$Z = \frac{34 - 36.8}{6.6} = -.42$$

Thus a raw score of 34 falls approximately .5 SD below the mean.

Because z scores are expressed by using decimals and both positive and negative values, many faculty prefer to use t scores instead. The z score can be used to calculate the t score. Converting raw scores to t scores has the following advantages:

1. The mean of the distribution is set at 50.
2. The SD from the mean is set at 10.
3. t Scores can be manipulated mathematically for grading purposes.

$$t = 10z + 50$$

For example, the z score of $-.42$ would be transformed as follows:

$$t = 10(-.42) + 50 = 45.8$$

ITEM ANALYSIS

Classic test theory is used for this discussion of item analysis and the discrimination index. Classic test theory and related inferences assume a norm-referenced measure. For a critique of classic test theory and an explanation of the newer item response theories, see *Developing and Validating Multiple-Choice Test Items* by Haladyna (1999). Item response theories depend on large samples and thus are of limited application to classroom tests.

Item analysis assists faculty in determining whether test items have separated the learners from the nonlearners (discrimination). Many computer scoring programs supply item statistics.

Item Difficulty

The item difficulty index (P value) is simply the percentage correct for the group answering the item. Jacobs and Chase (1992) recommend that most items on a test be approximately $P = .5$ (or 50% correct) to help ensure that questions separate learners from nonlearners (a good discrimination index). The upper limit of item difficulty is 1.00, meaning that 100% of students answered the question correctly. The lower limit of item difficulty depends on the number of possible responses and is the probability of guessing the correct answer. For example, for a question with four options, $P = .25$ is the lower limit or probability of guessing.

Item Discrimination

Item discrimination refers to the way an item differentiates students who know the content from those who do not. Discrimination can be measured as a point biserial correlation. The point biserial correlation compares each student's item performance with each student's overall test performance. If a question discriminates well, the point biserial correlation will be highly positive for the correct answer and negative for the distractors. This indicates that the "learners," or students who knew the content, answered the question correctly and the "nonlearners" chose distractors. Popham (1990) rates items with discrimination indices greater than .3 as "good" and those with discrimination indices greater than .4 as "very good." For example, a point biserial correlation of 0.598 is a very good discriminator because the point biserial correlation is highly positive and the distractors have a negative point biserial correlation. Haladyna (1999) cautions that if the item difficulty index is either too high or too low, the discrimination index is attenuated. The discrimination index is maximized when the item difficulty is moderate ($P = .5$). Ultimately, test reliability depends on item discrimination. Inclusion of mastery level material on a norm-referenced test will tend to lower test reliability because that item will tend to be answered correctly by many students and will thus be a poor discriminator.

Distractor Evaluation

In addition to the evaluation of the correct answer to an item for a positive point biserial correlation, each distractor should be individually evaluated. Effective distractors should appeal to the nonlearner, as indicated by negative point biserial correlation values. Distractors with a point biserial correlation of zero indicate that students did not select them and that they may need to be revised or replaced with a more plausible option to appeal to students who do not understand the content. Distractors that were not selected increase the chances that a student could have obtained the correct answer by guessing. One way to develop appealing distractors is to periodically ask open-ended questions to determine the most common errors in thinking. Distractors for questions with numerical answers may need to be "worked out" by following the most typical mistakes that students make.

Item Revision

Developing a valid and reliable test is an ongoing process. It is helpful to revise the test immediately after administering it while faculty can recall items and student responses to them. Item revision should be conducted after item analysis. One way to analyze items for revision is to use a test item analysis form (Figure 22-2). The result of item analysis for each question is entered in the form. Those items falling outside of the "ideal" range should be considered for revision. Items to be revised should include those with the following statistical characteristics:

1. Items with P values that are too high or too low (around .5 is ideal).
2. Correct answers with low positive or negative point biserial values (>.30 is ideal).
3. Distractors with highly positive point biserial values (negative values are ideal).

ASSIGNING GRADES

Grades provide both feedback and motivation for students. In the academic setting, assignment of grades may be guided by the institution grading policy or scale. Many computer software programs are available to assist faculty with assigning grades accurately and efficiently (Anema et al., 2002). The two basic methods for assignment are the absolute and the relative ("curved") scales (described in the following sections). According to Jacobs and Chase (1992), the characteristics of a good grading system include the following:

1. Informing students of the specific grading criteria at the beginning of the course (stated explicitly in the syllabus).
2. Basing the grades on learning outcomes (not factors such as attendance or effort).

Test __2__
Date __3/97__

P (Item Difficulty) / D (Item Discrimination)	>.50	.40–.49	.30–.39	.20–.29	.10–.19	.01–.09	Negative	Total
Very difficult P = 50% or less								
Difficult P = 51%–69%	20	10	4	2, 18, 26				6
Average P = 70%–80%	3, 5, 25, 27	9, 14, 19, 24	12, 16, 17, 23, 29					13
Easy P = 81%–100%			6, 8, 11, 15, 21, 28	1, 7, 13, 22, 30				11
Total number of items	5	5	12	8				

X 75
KR .75
SD 3.7
SEM 2.8

FIGURE 22-2 Sample test item analysis form for a 30-item test.

3. Gathering sufficient data (amount and variety) for the assignment of a valid grade.
4. Recording data collected for grading purposes quantitatively (e.g., 89% not B+).
5. Applying the system equitably to all students.
6. Using statistically sound principles for assigning grades.

Absolute Scale

An absolute grading scale rates performance relative to a standard (Jacobs & Chase, 1992). The student's earned points are compared with the total possible points and are expressed as a percentage earned. The standard should be included in the syllabus at the beginning of the course. Theoretically, all students could receive an A (or an F) with this scale. In reality, the dispersion of the grades depends on the difficulty of the tests. See Table 22-8 for an example of an absolute grading scale.

Relative Scale

A relative grading scale rates students according to their ranking within the group. To assign grades in this system, faculty record scores in order, from high to low. Grades may then be assigned by using a variety of techniques. One method is to assign the grades according to natural "breaks" in the distribution. This method has the disadvantage of being subjective. A better method of assigning grades based on a relative scale is to use the test statistics to create a "curve" as described by Jacobs and Chase (1992) in the following list:

1. Decide whether to use the mean or the median as the best measure of central tendency. If the mean and median are approximately the same, use the mean. If the distribution is skewed, use the median.

TABLE 22-8   Sample Absolute Grading Scale

PERCENTAGE CORRECT	ASSIGNED GRADE
90–100	A
80–89	B
70–79	C
60–69	D
<60	F

2. Determine the SD. The C grade will be set as the mean plus or minus one half the SD (encompassing 40% of the scores). See Table 22-9 for an example of a relative grading scale. Table 22-10 shows a comparison of the grades assigned to the raw scores with the absolute and relative grading scales described.

Relative grading scales may also be developed by using linear scores such as z scores or t scores (see the section on standardized test scores for directions for calculating these scores). t Scores are more commonly used for grading purposes because there are no negative values in this system (Lyman, 1991). The mean score becomes a t score of 50. The z score and t score are figured for each raw score. The faculty member decides what grade to assign to the ranges of t scores. Assuming a normal curve, a t score of 50 would be assigned a grade of C. Computer grading programs that calculate grades according to absolute or relative scales are available.

GRADING STANDARDS AND GRADE INDEXING

Periodically, faculty, administrators, boards of trustees, or consumers raise questions about the relative meaning of grades and potential or actual grade "inflation." There may be several possible causes for grade inflation, such as student retention programs; competency-based assessment with emphasis on mastery; competitive admission or admission of upper-division students with proven achievement records; a student population of older, mature, and career-directed students; teaching and assessment philosophies that focus on experiential learning; and pass-fail grading systems (Cross et al., 1994).

TABLE 22-9   Sample Relative Grading Scale

GRADE	CALCULATION	EXAMPLE	RANGE
A	> Upper B	>45.5	>45.5
B	Upper C + 1 SD	40.5 + 5	40.6–45.5
C	Mean ± .5 SD	38 ± 2.5	35.5–40.5
D	Lower C − 1 SD	35.5 − 5	30.5–35.4
F	< Lower D	<30.5	<30.5

Calculated according to Jacobs and Chase (1992).

TABLE 22-10 Comparison of Grades Assigned by Three Methods

RAW SCORE	PERCENT SCORE	GRADE (ABSOLUTE)	GRADE (RELATIVE)
49	98	A	A
45(2)	90	A	B
42(2)	84	B	B
40	80	B	C
39(3)	78	C	C
38(4)	76	C	C
37	74	C	C
35(2)	70	C	D
34(3)	68	D	D
33	66	D	D
30	60	D	F
28	56	F	F

When there are diverse views about the meaning of grades, faculty may institute *grade indexing*. Grade indexing involves indicating how many students in a given course or section of a course received grades that equaled or exceeded the grade of a given student. This index may appear on the student's transcript.

Nursing faculty as a whole should review grading policies and practices on a regular basis. A consistent philosophy about grading and fair and equitable grading practices communicate concern to the students and competence to nursing's varied publics.

SUMMARY

Although developing, administering, and analyzing classroom tests may seem like a monumental task, the step-by-step approach presented in this chapter can be used as a guide to simplify this process. By following these guidelines, faculty can create written tests that can be used as effective measures of outcomes in the classroom. Assigning grades is the last step in this process.

REFERENCES

American Psychological Association, American Educational Research Association, National Council on Measurement in Education. (1985). *Standards for educational and psychological testing*. Washington, DC: American Psychological Association.

Anema, M. G., Anema, C. M., Bass, S. M., Fleming, B. O., Helms, M. A., Rawls, A., et al. (2002). A comparative analysis of computer-based graded programs. *CIN: Computers, Informatics, Nursing, 20*(2), 55-62.

Bloom, B. S. (Ed.). (1956). *Taxonomy of educational objectives: The classification of educational goals. Handbook 1: Cognitive domain*. New York: Longman.

Bosher, S. (2003). Barriers to creating a more culturally diverse nursing profession: Linguistic bias in multiple-choice nursing exams. *Nursing Education Perspectives, 24*(1), 25-34.

Cross, L. H., Frary, R. B., & Weber, J. (1994). College grading: Achievement attitudes and effort. *College Teaching, 41*(4), 143-148.

Downing, S. M. (1992). *Educational measurement: Issues and practices*. Washington, DC: National Council on Measurement in Education.

Flannelly, L. T. (2001). Using feedback to reduce students' judgment bias on test questions. *Journal of Nursing Education, 40*, 10-16.

Gaberson, K. B. (1996). Test design: Putting the pieces together. *Nurse Educator, 21*(4), 28-33.

Gronlund, N. E. (1998). *Assessment of student achievement* (6th ed.). Boston: Allyn & Bacon.

Haladyna, T. M. (1999). *Developing and validating multiple-choice test items* (2nd ed). Mahwah, NJ: Lawrence Erlbaum.

Jacobs, L. C., & Chase, C. I. (1992). *Developing and using tests effectively: A guide for faculty*. San Francisco: Jossey-Bass.

Kirkpatrick, J. M., Billings, D. M., Hodson-Carlton, K., Cummings, R. B., Dorner, J., Jeffries, P. R., et al. (2000). Computerized test development software: A comparative review updated. *Computers in Nursing, 18*(2), 72-86.

Linn, R. L., & Gronlund, N. E. (2000). *Measurement and assessment in teaching* (8th ed.). Upper Saddle River, NJ: Merrill/Prentice Hall.

Lyman, H. B. (1991). *Test scores and what they mean* (5th ed.). Englewood Cliffs, NJ: Prentice Hall.

Masters, J. C., Hulsmeyer, B. S., Pike, M. E., Leichty, K., Miller, M. T., & Verst, A. L. (2001). Assessment of multiple-choice questions in selected test banks accompanying text books used in nursing education. *Journal of Nursing Education, 40*, 25-31.

McDonald, M. E. (2002). *Systematic assessment of learning outcomes: Developing multiple-choice exams*. Sudbury, MA: Jones & Bartlett.

Mehrens, W. A., & Lehmann, I. J. (1991). *Measurement and evaluation in education and psychology* (4th ed.). New York: Holt, Rinehart & Winston.

Morrison, S., & Free, K. W. (2001). Writing multiple-choice test items that promote and measure critical thinking. *Journal of Nursing Education, 40*, 17-24.

National Council of State Boards of Nursing. (2003). *Test plan for the National Council Licensure Examination for registered nurses*. Chicago: Author.

Popham, W. J. (1990). *Modern educational measurement: A practitioner's perspective* (2nd ed.). Englewood Cliffs, NJ: Prentice-Hall.

Rossignol, M. & Scollin, P. (2001). Piloting use of computerized practice tests. *Computers in Nursing, 12*, 206-212.

Wendt, A., & Brown, P. (2000). The NCLEX examination: Preparing for future nursing practice. *Nurse Educator, 25*, 297-300.

23

CLINICAL PERFORMANCE EVALUATION

Wanda Bonnel, PhD, RN, Dorothy A. Gomez, MSN, RN,
Stacy Lobodzinski, MSN, RN, Cora D. Hartwell West, MSN, RN

Providing fair and reasonable clinical evaluation is one of the most important and most challenging faculty roles. Faculty must discern whether students can think critically within the clinical setting, maintain an appropriate demeanor, interact appropriately with patients, prioritize problems, have basic knowledge of clinical procedures, and complete care procedures correctly. All the while, faculty need to minimize student anxiety within the complex health care setting so that student clinical performance, and not extraneous factors such as anxiety or fatigue, are being observed.

Assessment of clinical performance provides data from which to judge the extent to which students have acquired specified learning outcomes. In this chapter, discussion includes general issues in assessment of clinical performance, clinical evaluation methods and tools, and the evaluation process.

GENERAL ISSUES IN ASSESSMENT OF CLINICAL PERFORMANCE

When clinical performance is evaluated, students' skills are judged as they relate to implementation of an established standard of patient care. Acceptable clinical performance involves behavior, knowledge, and attitudes that students gradually develop in a variety of settings (Caldwell & Tenofsky, 1996). The ultimate outcome for clinical performance evaluation is safe, quality patient care. Clinical performance evaluation gives feedback to the student about performance and provides data that may be used for individual development, assigning grades, and making decisions about the curriculum. Students have the right to a reliable and valid evaluation that assesses achievement of competencies required to take on the role of the novice nurse (Redman et al., 1999). Box 23-1 provides some "quick tips" to be considered at the beginning of the evaluation process.

Good practice includes multidimensional evaluation with diverse evaluation methods completed over time, seeking student growth and progress (American Association for Higher Education, 1993). All evaluation should respect students' dignity and self-esteem. Before assessing clinical performance, faculty must

Box 23-1
QUICK TIPS FOR CLINICAL EVALUATION

- Define clearly both knowledge and skills students will need to demonstrate.
- Use multiple sources of data for evaluation.
- Be reasonable and consistent in evaluation of all students.
- Use mini evaluations and suggest minor, easy corrections at the time they are needed.
- Present feedback and evaluation in nonjudgmental language, confining comments to a student's behavior.
- Provide evaluation "sandwiches," commenting first on a strength, then a weakness, then a strength of the student's behavior.
- Carry an anecdotal record or PDA equivalent for each student, maintaining privacy of data.
- Make specific notes, focusing on specific details of a student's behavior.
- Document student patterns of behavior over time through compilation of records.
- Invite students to complete self-assessments and summarize what they have learned.
- Help students prioritize learning needs and turn feedback into constructive challenges with specific goals for each day.

PDA, Personal digital assistant.

consider several issues. These issues include who will be participants in the evaluation, evaluation timing, and evaluation access and privacy.

Participants in Evaluation

Faculty

The faculty have primary responsibility for the student clinical evaluation. Faculty are knowledgeable about the purpose of the evaluation and the objectives that will be used to judge the student's performance. Clarity of purpose provides direction for selection of evaluation tools and process.

Initial challenges for faculty in completing clinical evaluations include both their own value systems and the number of students they supervise. Faculty need to be aware of differences between their own value systems and those of their students because this can bias the evaluation process. Additionally, when faculty are supervising a group of students in the delivery of safe, appropriate nursing care, faculty can only sample student behaviors. Limited sampling of behaviors or individual biases may result in an inaccurate or unfair clinical evaluation (Orchard, 1994). Because of these limitations, faculty should use a variety of evaluation methods. Additionally, faculty can consider evaluation input from other sources. Potential adjunct evaluators include students, nursing staff and preceptors, peer evaluators, and patients.

Students

Completion of self-assessments by students provides not only data, as part of the evaluation process, but also a learning experience for the students (Loving,

1993). Student self-evaluation provides a starting point for reviewing, comparing, and discussing evaluative data with faculty. Initial student involvement in self-assessment tends to facilitate student behavior changes and provides a positive environment for learning and improvement. Participation in their own evaluation also empowers students to make choices and identify their strengths.

Nursing Staff and Preceptors

Nursing staff may provide input to the evaluation process and tend to provide data from an informed perspective as a result of collaboration with students. Nursing staff should understand their role in this area, and staff expectations in the evaluation process should be clearly articulated. This includes determining whether feedback should just be provided directly to the student or shared with faculty as well. One of the disadvantages of including nursing personnel in the evaluation process is that expectations in the clinical area may differ from course performance objectives. Although evaluation is time consuming for busy nurses, this may be part of a nurse's career development or joint appointment responsibilities.

Preceptors have a specified role in modeling and facilitating clinical education for students, especially for advanced nursing students. Typically, preceptors serve a more formal role in evaluation, such as an adjunct faculty role, and provide evaluative data as part of a faculty team. If staff nurses and nurse preceptors provide data for the evaluation process, they should be oriented to the nursing school's evaluation plan. Roles should be clarified, indicating whether staff will be asked to provide occasional comments, to report only incidents or concerns, or to complete a specific evaluation form. Hrobsky and Kersbergen (2002) describe the use of a clinical map to assist preceptors in identifying student strengths and weaknesses.

Peer Evaluators

There is debate about appropriateness of having student peers act as evaluators in the clinical setting. Student peers should only evaluate competencies and content that they are prepared to judge. There should be clear guidelines for peer review and the inherent responsibility (McAllister & Osborne, 1997). Peer evaluation can help students develop collaborative skills, build communication skills, and promote professional responsibility. A potential disadvantage is that peers may be biased in providing only favorable information about student colleagues or may have unrealistic expectations of their student colleagues. Providing students with this peer evaluation opportunity and then appropriately weighting the contribution is a reasonable practice.

Patients

Patients provide data from the product consumer viewpoint. Patient satisfaction is considered an important marker in quality health care and can be considered as part of student evaluation. Judgments about student performance are made from patients' personal experiences, and data should be weighted for its value. Patients often have positive comments to make about "their" students, which can be positive for the students to hear.

Evaluation Timing

Appropriate timing of evaluation and feedback should be considered. Formative evaluation focuses on the process of student development during the clinical activity, whereas summative evaluation comes at the conclusion of a specified clinical activity to determine student accomplishment. Feedback can be considered an ongoing component of formative evaluation. Each of these concepts has unique contributions to the evaluation process and is discussed further in Chapter 20. Formative evaluation is essential to the student, and appropriate feedback enables students to learn from their mistakes and allows for growth and improvement in behavior. Summative evaluation attests to competency attainment or meeting of objectives.

All parties involved in the clinical performance evaluation should be aware of evaluation time frames at the outset. Timely, scheduled feedback provided by faculty to students will decrease the risk of unexpected evaluation results. Ongoing formative evaluations keep students and faculty aware of the progress toward attainment of learning outcomes and promote opportunities for goal setting. This early intervention by a faculty member may prevent a student from receiving an unsatisfactory evaluation in clinical performance.

Evaluation Access and Privacy Considerations

There are both ethical and legal issues relevant to privacy of evaluation data that can affect the student, faculty, and institution. Before conducting clinical evaluation, the educator must determine who will have access to data. In most cases detailed evaluative data are shared only between the faculty member and the individual student. Program policy should identify who additionally may have access to the evaluation and how evaluative information will be stored and for how long. Evaluative data should be stored in a secure area. As designated by the Family Educational Rights and Privacy Act (FERPA), students 18 years of age or older or in postsecondary schools have the right to inspect records maintained by a school (U.S. Department of Education, 1974). A school's program materials such as catalogs and handbooks can be tools to ensure the creation of reasonable and prudent policies that are in compliance with legal and accrediting guidelines. Faculty should be clear about the impact that the evaluation will have on each individual or group involved before initiation of the process.

Privacy of written anecdotal notes and computer or personal digital assistant (PDA) notes also need to be maintained. Inadequate security of this information could lead to a breach of student privacy. Additional legal considerations are discussed in Chapter 3.

CLINICAL EVALUATION METHODS AND TOOLS

Many methods and tools are used to measure learning in the clinical setting. A variety of approaches should be incorporated in clinical evaluation including cognitive, psychomotor, and affective considerations, as well as cultural competence and ethical decision making (Gaberson & Oermann, 1999).

Additionally, educators cannot ignore the social connotations of grading, including the impact evaluation has on the learning process and motivation (Wiles & Bishop, 2001).

The goal of evaluation is an objective report about the quality of the clinical performance. Faculty need to be aware of the potential for evaluation of students' clinical performance to be subjective and inconsistent. Even with "objective" instruments based on measurable and observable behavior, subjectivity can still be introduced into a tool that is viewed as objective. Reilly and Oermann (1992) encourage faculty to be sensitive to the forces that contribute to the subjective side of evaluation as faculty strive for fairness and consistency.

Fair and reasonable evaluation of students in clinical settings requires use of appropriate evaluation tools that are effective and ideally efficient for faculty to use. Instrument content can vary according to the academic level of a student and can also relate to the teaching institution's purpose and philosophy. Any evaluation instrument used to measure clinical learning and performance should have criteria that are consistent with course objectives. A faculty group decision about the tools to be used for data collection is typically indicated. Many clinical evaluation tools have been developed and implemented within clinical settings. Faculty must make decisions about using these instruments according to their purpose(s) for clinical evaluation.

Primary strategies for the evaluation of clinical practice include (1) observation, (2) written communication, (3) oral communication, (4) simulation, and (5) self-evaluation. Because clinical practice is complex, a combination of methods is indicated and helps support a fair and reasonable evaluation. See Table 23-1 for a summary of common strategies and clinical evaluation tools by category. These are also discussed in the following paragraphs.

TABLE 23-1 Sample Evaluation Strategies and Tools by Category	
Observation	Anecdotal Notes
	Checklists
	Rating Scales
	Videotapes
Written	Charting/Progress Notes
	Concept Maps
	Care Plans
	Process Recordings
	Paper and Pencil Tests
	Web-based Strategies
Oral	Student Interviews and Case Presentation
	Clinical Conferences
Simulations	Standardized Patient Exams
	Clinical Scenarios
	Interactive Multimedia
	Role Play
Self-Evaluation	Clinical Portfolios
	Journals and Logs

Evaluation Strategies: Observation

Observation is the method used most frequently in clinical performance evaluation. The basic concept of observation is to compare student performance with clinical competency expectations as designated in course objectives. Faculty observe and analyze the performance, provide feedback on the observation, and determine whether further instruction is needed. Actual observation and observation by means of videotape are both considered in this discussion.

Advantages of observation include the potential for direct visualization and confirmation of student performance. Unfortunately, observation can be complex, with numerous factors interfering in evaluation. Factors that can influence the interpretation of an observation include lack of specificity of the particular behaviors to be observed; an inadequate sampling of behaviors from which to draw conclusions about a student's performance; and the evaluator's own influences and perceptions, which can affect judgment of the observed performance (Reilly & Oermann, 1992).

Faculty should seek tools and strategies that support a fair and reasonable evaluation. Instruments used to document observed clinical practice behaviors assist in documenting judgments focused on psychomotor and affective performance behaviors.

The more structured observational tools are typically easy to complete and useful in focusing on specified behavior. Although structured observation tools can help increase objectivity, faculty consistency in item interpretation must be evaluated as well. Faculty judgment is still required in interpretation of the listed behaviors. Problems with reliability are introduced when item descriptors are given different meanings by different evaluators. Written comments can be added by faculty to help support the rating.

An abundance of information must be tracked in clinical observation. Faculty can benefit from systems to help document and organize this information. Faculty can carry copies of evaluation tools and anecdotal records or can consider the use of a personal digital assistant (PDA). Lehman (2003) suggests a variety of strategies for using PDAs in the clinical setting; a particular example is inclusion of anecdotal records and student "check-offs" in the memo function of the PDA. PDAs help facilitate retrieval and use of clinical evaluation records. Privacy in these records is needed as well. Common methods for documenting these observed behaviors during clinical practice vary in the amount of structure and include anecdotal notes, checklists, and rating scales.

Anecdotal Notes

Anecdotal or progress notes are objective written descriptions of observed student performance or behaviors. The format for these can vary from loosely structured "plus/minus" observation notes to structured lists of observations in relation to specified clinical objectives. These written notes initially serve as part of formative evaluation. As student performance records are documented, a pattern is established and may be used for summative evaluation. This record or pattern of information pertaining to the student and specific clinical behaviors helps document the student's performance pattern for both summative evaluation and recall during student-faculty conference sessions. Liberto et al. (1999) note the importance of determining which clinical incidents to assess and of identifying both positive and negative student behaviors.

Checklists

Checklists are lists of items or performance indicators requiring dichotomous responses such as satisfactory/unsatisfactory or pass/fail (Table 23-2). Gronlund (1993) describes a checklist as an inventory of measurable performance dimensions or products with a place to record a simple "yes" or "no" judgment. These short, easy-to-complete tools are frequently used for evaluating clinical performance. Checklists, such as nursing skills check-off lists, are useful for evaluation of specific well-defined behaviors and are commonly used in the clinical simulated laboratory setting. Rating scales, described in the following paragraph, provide more detail concerning the quality of a student's performance than checklists.

Rating Scales

Rating scales are a method of evaluating clinical performance through qualitative and quantitative judgments regarding the learner's performance in the clinical setting (Box 23-2). A list of behaviors or competencies is rated. Most rating scales used in nursing programs have a 5-point or 7-point scale with descriptors. These descriptors take the form of abstract labels (such as A, B, C, D, and E or 5, 4, 3, 2, and 1), frequency labels (such as always, *usually, frequently, sometimes,* and *never*), or qualitative labels (such as *superior, above average, average,* and *below average*). A rating scale provides the instructor with a

TABLE 23-2 Example of Checklist Items and Format

PROFESSIONAL DOMAIN Practices within legal boundaries according to standards	MIDTERM			FINAL	
	SATIS- FACTORY	UN- SATIS- FACTORY	NOT OBSERVED	SATIS- FACTORY	UN- SATIS- FACTORY
Uses professional nursing standards to provide patient safety					
Follows nursing procedures and institutional policy in delivery of patient care					
Displays professional behaviors with staff, peers, instructors, patient systems					
Demonstrates ethical principles of respect for person and confidentiality					
Participates appropriately in clinical conferences					
Reports on time; follows procedures for absenteeism					

convenient form on which to record judgments indicating the degree of student performance. This differs from a checklist in that it allows for more discrimination in judging behaviors as compared with dichotomous "yes" and "no" options. Mahara (1998) notes the benefit of more standardized assessments such as checklists and rating scales but faults these objective scales for failing to capture the complex clinical practice environment and clinical learning. Oermann (1997) emphasizes the benefit of asking appropriate patient care questions along with clinical observations to gauge student critical thinking abilities.

Videotapes as Source of Observational Data

Another method of recording observations of a student's clinical performance is through videotapes. Videotapes are often completed in a simulated setting and can be used to record and evaluate specific performance behaviors relevant to diverse clinical settings. Advantages associated with videotaping include its valuable start, stop, and replay capabilities, which allow an observation to be reviewed numerous times. Videotapes can promote self-evaluation, allowing students to see themselves and evaluate their performance more objectively. Videotapes also give teachers and students the opportunity to review the performance and provide feedback in determining whether further practice is indicated. Use of videotapes can also contribute to the learning and growth of an entire clinical group when knowledge and feedback are shared (Reilly & Oermann, 1992). Videotapes are particularly popular for evaluation in distance learning situations. Videotapes can also be used with rating scales, checklists, or anecdotal records to organize and report behaviors observed on the videotapes.

Evaluation Strategies: Student Written Communication

Use of written communication methods enables the faculty to evaluate clinical performance through assessing students' abilities to translate what they have learned to paper. Review of student nursing care plans or written nursing notes allows faculty to evaluate students' abilities to communicate with other care

---

Box 23-2
EXAMPLE OF RATING SCALE ITEMS AND FORMAT

Instructions. On a scale of 1 to 5, rate each of the following student behaviors:
(Rating Code: 1 = marginal; 2 = fair; 3 = satisfactory; 4 = good; 5 = excellent; NA = not applicable)

———1. Serves as patient caregiver (independence when providing patient care, timely completion of all patient care).

———2. Functions in the role of team member.

———3. Uses correct procedure when performing nursing interventions.

———4. Relates self-evaluation to clinical learning objectives.

———5. Displays positive behavior when given feedback.

providers. Through writing assignments, students can clarify and organize their thoughts (Cowles et al., 2001). Additionally, writing can reinforce new knowledge and expand thinking on a topic. The evaluation focuses on the quality of the content and ability to communicate information and ideas in written form. The rater can determine the students' perspectives and gain insight into the "why" of the students' behaviors. Although this method may be more time consuming for the instructor to grade and for the students to prepare than some evaluation methods, written data help support clinical observations.

Charting and Patient Progress Notes

Writing cogent nursing and progress notes is an important clinical skill. Charting review of students provides faculty with an opportunity to evaluate the students' ability to process and record relevant data. Students' skill in using health care terminology and documentation practices can be examined, and critical thinking processes can be demonstrated in these notes (Higuchi & Donald, 2002).

Concept Maps

Concept maps allow students to create a diagram of patient needs and nursing responses, including relationships among concepts. Kathol et al. (1998) suggest that these tools can help students visualize and organize patient-specific data relevant to diagnostic work and nursing and medical diagnoses. The use of concept maps can help faculty evaluate students' understanding of concepts and relationships among relevant concepts and assist faculty in clarifying students' misconceptions. These tools foster critical thinking skills. These tools also provide faculty with an opportunity to complete a quick review of skills before students perform patient care and to make a quick determination of further learning needs (Castellino & Schuster 2002; King & Shell, 2002). Concept maps can also serve as worksheets for students and serve as organizing tools for documentation (Schuster, 2000).

Nursing Care Plans

Nursing care plans allow faculty to evaluate students' ability to determine and prioritize care needs according to understanding and interpretation of individual patients' health care problems. Historically, nursing care plans have been used by students to document clinical thinking processes, but some would argue that the availability of numerous standardized care plans has minimized the critical thinking component. Some programs report replacing detailed clinical care plans with concept maps or clinical journals and logs.

Process Recordings

Process recordings are used to evaluate the interpersonal skills of students within the clinical setting. This form of evaluation requires students to write down their patient-nurse interactions and self-evaluate the communication skills they used. Process recording is a form of self-evaluation that allows students to analyze their own interactive behavior, enabling them to better identify the strengths and weaknesses of their interpersonal communication (Carpenito & Duespohl, 1985). This approach to evaluation is commonly used in communication courses and in psychiatric nursing.

Paper and Pencil Tests

Paper and pencil tests are frequently used to assess students' basic knowledge for problem solving and decision making in clinical practice. Various test formats (true/false, multiple choice, matching, short answer, essay) can be incorporated into preclinical or postclinical conferences to gauge students' understanding of specific concepts.

Web-based Strategies

Newer forms of written evaluation include Web-based clinical conferences and case discussions via e-mail. Faculty may implement postclinical conferences or clinical case discussions in a Web-based communication board. DeBourgh (2001) discusses strategies for incorporating clinical feedback in e-mail correspondence, e-journals, and threaded message discussion boards on the Web. Student clinical logs and self-evaluations can be submitted electronically as well (Baier & Mueggenburg, 2001). Although not limited to students at a distance, these formats are especially popular for clinical evaluation of students in geographically diverse settings. They may be useful as well for clinical conferences and student evaluation in community health courses with clinical coursework in diverse community settings.

Evaluation Strategies: Oral Communication Methods

Student interviews, case presentations, and clinical conferences provide evaluative opportunities. The sharing of information with the goals of problem solving and decision making in nursing is a common task, and communication is an important skill in nursing. These oral communication strategies can be used to assess the student's ability to verbalize ideas and thoughts clearly. In addition, these strategies allow faculty to assess a student's critical thinking skills and pose questions to elicit more complex forms of thinking. Evaluation strategies classified as oral communication methods are described in the following paragraphs.

Student Interviews and Case Presentation

Faculty-directed personal interviews with students represent an effective and efficient form of evaluation. In simple interview form, faculty ask questions and students respond. These question-and-answer sessions provide faculty with the opportunity to probe for more detail from students and clarify misconceptions. Oermann (1997) notes that faculty in general need to strive to ask "higher-order" questions to better promote critical thinking. Student case presentations, such as "bullet-point" summaries of key patient problems and care strategies, assist students in developing concise presentation skills. Faculty can provide feedback to students and obtain evaluative information about students' thoughts on and plans for a case.

Clinical Conferences

Clinical conferences provide an opportunity for students to discuss theory and practice integration in terms of their own clinical experiences. Participation by multiple students in clinical conferences enables faculty to evaluate more than one student at a time. At the same time, sharing experiences among students provides valuable insight for all students in the group, with the opportunity to learn and grow from each other's experiences. Additionally, the evaluator can focus on student or group abilities to solve problems.

Conferences encourage critical thinking and allow for peer review. Conferences also provide opportunities to offer suggestions that promote critical thinking within the group. Oermann (1997) notes that conferences provide opportunity for faculty to gauge students' abilities to analyze data and critique plans.

Multidisciplinary conferences are another form of clinical conference in which the process of problem solving and decision making is a collaborative effort of the group. This group is composed not only of nursing personnel but also members of other health care disciplines. Evaluation is concerned with the student's active participation within the group and abilities to present ideas clearly in terms of the care plan for the patient. This exercise also promotes work with other disciplines on clinical problem solving. Students may find a degree of risk involved with sharing their knowledge and being evaluated critically by others.

Simulations Used as Evaluation Instruments in Clinical Practice

The use of simulations as clinical evaluation strategies allows the instructor to focus on specific student cognitive and psychomotor behaviors indicated by the clinical objectives. Through simulations, an instructor can control the focus of the behavior to be evaluated. Simulations help to create a safe environment for student learning and promote standardized assessments (Mahara, 1998). Benefits of simulations include skill validation, minimal student stress, and time saving for faculty (Miller et al., 2000).

Simulations can range from simple case studies to complex electronic mannequins. With the changing health care setting, students will likely not have opportunities to care for all types of patients in the various clinical settings for which they will ultimately be responsible after graduation. Teaching pattern recognition with cases and scenarios in safe, structured learning environments will become an increasingly important strategy.

Standardized Patient Exams

Standardized patient exams, sometimes referred to as *objective structured clinical examinations* (*OSCEs*), can be described as "pretend patients" in an artificial environment designed to simulate actual clinical conditions (Borbasi & Koop, 1994). A simulation center, modeled as an authentic clinical environment with standardized patients, can provide a safe setting in which to observe and document student competencies. Standardized patients can provide feedback to students and help ensure competence before students begin practice in the complex "real" world. Potential exists for multiple evaluators to observe and test students in the performance of numerous skills during brief examination periods. Borbasi and Koop review the OSCE process as an acceptable and powerful instrument in clinical performance evaluation. They describe the OSCE as a quick and efficient evaluation method, allowing for rapid feedback to students about identified clinical deficits. Specific approaches and satisfaction with the standardized patient experience have been described (Gibbons et al., 2002).

Clinical Scenarios

Clinical scenarios such as video-audio scenarios with case studies and simulation provide students opportunity for actively learning while faculty facilitate the procedure (Dearman, 2003). Many of these clinical scenarios have online potential and availability with the potential variation in cases having relevance to all nursing arenas or venues.

An advantage this method offers is a readily available means of judging specific clinical practices without having to wait for a similar opportunity to arise in the clinical setting. Simulations can be economically beneficial in the educational setting with large groups of students (Roberts et al., 1992). Simulations can be held in a learning resource center in which adequate equipment is available. Students can respond to audiovisual scenarios orally or in writing. Dearman (2003) discusses the benefits of a debriefing session after these activities. Although there are costs to the institution for developing or purchasing simulation software and hardware, clinical scenarios can provide an effective learning and evaluation technique.

Interactive Multimedia Simulations

Clinical scenarios, presented as computer simulations with the use of motion and sound for interactive Web-based cases, videodiscs, CD-ROMs, and virtual reality provide a semirealistic experience for students. Through the use of interactive media, nursing case studies can be presented without clinical environmental distractions or the risk involved in clinical decision making. Rinne (1994) identifies the following three benefits associated with use of multimedia: (1) skills may be demonstrated quickly and efficiently; (2) students have unlimited opportunities for practice in a safe, cost-effective environment; and (3) self-evaluation can take place, enabling students to judge their own performance.

Role Play

Role play focuses on effective student behavior related to the interactive process of the patient and the nurse. Role play provides an opportunity for students to try out new behaviors, simulating aspects of nursing care in relation to clinical practice. Role play focuses on the practice of interpersonal communication skills and allows students to observe, evaluate, and provide feedback to each other. Discussion or debriefing sessions can promote critical thinking and help students gain insight into their performance. Videotaping of role play can also allows for student self-evaluation.

Self-Evaluation

Self-evaluation is based on student self-reflection with emphasis on critical thinking. This evaluation method emphasizes and reflects the formative evaluation process. The formative evaluation process enables students to examine their progress, to identify their strengths and weaknesses, and to set goals for improvement in the areas indicated. Self-evaluation can initiate the process of lifelong, self-directed learning.

A potential disadvantage of self-evaluation is that students may not be honest about their level of self-understanding in an effort to protect themselves against potential criticism (Walker & Dewar, 2000). The ability to critically reflect on individual performance may be influenced by the maturity and self-esteem of the student. Students are more likely to readily gather information and share this information with faculty if a foundation of trust has been established.

Self-evaluation is most beneficial if it begins at the onset of the student's clinical experience. Students benefit from examining their progress on an ongoing basis with regard to meeting their goals. Through the teacher and student interaction process, observations and perceptions can be shared, student strengths and weaknesses can be discussed, and self-evaluation strategies can be improved. Student-teacher relationships can become stronger and more constructive as students progress.

Portfolios

Portfolios have been described as collections of evidence, prepared by students and evaluated by faculty, to demonstrate mastery, comprehension, application, and synthesis of a given set of concepts (Slater, 1999). Portfolios allow the instructor to integrate a number of assessment methods and can help provide documentation of specified learning outcomes (McMullan, 2003). Portfolios are designed to help students reflect on progress in clinical learning and also help faculty understand students' clinical learning processes. Portfolios can help students integrate theory into practice and learn documentation strategies for promoting and recording future learning.

Journals and Logs

Homes (1997) describes journals as written dialogues between the self and the designated reader. They provide an opportunity for students to share values and critical thinking abilities. Journals give students the opportunity to record their clinical experiences and review their progress. This enables students to recall areas of needed improvement and allows them to work on problems and clinical performance weaknesses. The concept of *clinical logs* is sometimes used synonymously with *journals,* but clinical logs can vary in the amount of detail, ranging from a listing of types of patients with noted student roles to a more detailed log with a reflection on each patient. Benefits of a detailed reflective clinical log are described by Fonteyn and Cahill (1998). Faculty should provide specific guidelines as to the amount of detail required in clinical journals or logs and provide clear guidelines as to how journals or logs will be graded.

CLINICAL EVALUATION PROCESS

Before the evaluation process begins, faculty and students need a clear understanding of the outcomes to be attained at the culmination of the experience. Clinical evaluation is a systematic process that can be considered as having three consecutive phases: (1) preparation, (2) clinical activity phase, and (3) final data interpretation and feedback. A listing of sample tasks within each phase and the roles faculty will assume during each phase are provided in Table 23-3. Additional discussion of selected points in each phase follows.

Preparation Phase

Choosing the Clinical Setting and Patient Assignment as a Part of the Evaluation Process

Faculty are responsible for providing each student with ample opportunities to achieve course objectives and must give careful attention to choosing a clinical site that will give students these opportunities. Advance planning is needed because choosing an appropriate clinical site can be challenging. Even in the ideal clinical setting, daily variability exists in terms of patients, providers, and the activity level of the unit, which can complicate evaluation. In addition to unit assignments, specific patient clinical assignments should also be considered as part of a fair evaluation. This includes both the types of patients assigned to students and the duration of clinical assignments.

Teaching and learning in a natural setting provide unique challenges for both students and faculty. Negotiating the balance between independence and supervision is complex. Faculty must provide adequate supervision to ensure

---

TABLE 23-3   Roles of Faculty Evaluator during the Evaluation Process

Phase I Preparation
Determine objectives and competencies
Identify evaluation methods and tools
Choose clinical site
Orient students to the evaluation plan
Focus on objectivity in evaluation

Phase II Clinical Activity
Orient students and staff to the student role
Provide students clinical opportunities
Ensure patient safety
Observe and collect evaluation data
Provide student feedback to enhance learning
Document findings, maintain privacy of records
Contract with students regarding any deficiencies

Phase III Final Data Interpretation and Presentation
Interpret data in fair, reasonable, and consistent manner
Assign grade
Provide summative evaluation conference (ensure privacy and respect confidentiality)
Evaluate experience

safe delivery of care with the welfare and the safety of patients as the first priority. Before the clinical experience begins, the faculty must develop criteria for what is considered unsafe or inappropriate behavior and what consequences will occur if such behavior is observed.

The faculty must be prepared to remove a student from the clinical setting if the student does not meet the minimal level of safety. Communication between faculty and students before the clinical experience begins is essential. Students have the right to know the standard used for safe practice and evaluation. Students should also be given an orientation to the clinical facility and the policies and procedures that will apply to the clinical experience. Unit orientations, as well as orientation to evaluation methods, are important in decreasing the anxiety that can hamper student clinical performance.

Students and faculty are essentially visitors in an established system, and the status of student comfort and support in the clinical environment should be considered in evaluation as well. Chan (2002) notes the importance of a positive clinical learning environment for student learning. A sample student evaluation of clinical setting form is provided in Box 23-3.

Determining the Standards and Measurement Tools

Student performance expectations should meet the following criteria: (1) reasonable, (2) consistent and applied equally, and (3) established and communicated before implementation (Orchard, 1994).

Faculty have the responsibility for choosing the appropriate methods and tools for evaluation of the learners' clinical performance. Specific evaluation instruments chosen will be the means of documenting and communicating judgments made about student performance. These tools should document performance expectations relevant to course objectives and be practical and time efficient.

The concepts of interrater reliability (whether results can be replicated by other raters) and content validity (whether a tool measures what is desired) at minimum should be considered in selection of a specific clinical evaluation instrument. More discussion of reliability and validity is provided in Chapter 20.

Inconsistencies in evaluation can result when each course coordinator develops course tools independently. Wiles and Bishop (2001) recommend that faculty work in groups to develop tools that reflect the increasing complexity of competencies required as students progress from program beginners to graduating seniors and to promote consistency from course to course. Often, tools described in the literature or those in use by colleagues can be used or adapted, thus saving time that would be required to develop a new tool. Waltz and Jenkins (2001) have compiled a list of clinical evaluation tools and provide a description and reliability and validity assessments for each.

Clinical Activity Phase

In both obtaining and analyzing clinical evaluation data, faculty need to make professional judgments about the performance of students. Because of the subjective nature of evaluation, there may be concern that evaluation is biased

Box 23-3
STUDENT EVALUATION OF CLINICAL SETTING

Name of Agency
Specific Unit

Directions

Print the name of the instructor and the name of the agency, the specific unit where you had your clinical experience, and the days of the week you were assigned.

Please respond to the following statements with the rating that best describes your opinion.
A, Strongly Agree
B, Agree
C, Disagree
D, Strongly Disagree

Please qualify any rating of C or D with comments or suggestions. The agency personnel have asked that you make comments because this is the only way they can make improvements or know what is positive. Your ratings and written comments will be used to determine clinical placement for future students and may be shared with individuals in the setting but only in *summary* form.

Application of Course Material

1. The staff facilitated my ability to meet clinical objectives.
2. I was able to meet the objectives of this course in this setting.

Population/Patients

3. Patients presented clinical problems appropriate to the objectives for this course.
4. Culturally diverse patients (e.g., cultural, social, economic) were available in the setting.

Health Professionals

5. Nurse managers, staff nurses, and support staff were accepting of students and student learning.
6. Nurse managers, staff nurses, and support staff were available to me to answer questions and provide assistance.
7. The nursing staff were positive role models.
8. Nurses demonstrated professional relationships with other health care professionals.

Physical Environment

9. The setting was conducive to working with patients and other health care team members.
10. Space was available for conferences with faculty and other students.

Overall Impression of Setting

11. I have a positive impression of the quality of care provided in this setting.
12. I would recommend this setting for future students taking this course.
13. Add statements specific to the clinical setting not already covered.

How could your clinical experience have been improved in this clinical setting?
Please use the back of this sheet to make comments and suggestions.

Adapted with permission from a form used by the University of Kansas School of Nursing.

and unfair. To prevent biased judgments, faculty need to be aware of the factors that can influence decision making and must actively use strategies to prevent biases.

Strategies that can help support trustworthiness of the clinical evaluation data include the following:

- Have specified objectives or competencies on which to base the evaluation.
- Use multiple strategies and combined methods of evaluation for compiling data.
- Include both qualitative and quantitative measures.
- Determine a practical sampling plan and evaluate it over time.
- Provide clear directions for tools to promote consistency between raters in collection and interpretation of data.
- Train faculty in use of specific clinical evaluation tools and approaches for consistency and fairness in grading.
- Be aware of common errors such as the halo effect (assuming that positive behaviors in one evaluated competency will be similar in others).
- Incorporate teacher self-assessment of values, beliefs, or biases that might affect the evaluation process (Oermann and Gaberson, 1998).

Final Data Interpretation and Presentation
Clinical Evaluation Conference

The findings of the clinical evaluation are usually shared with the student individually at the end of the clinical experience or course. No surprises should be presented at this time. The timely feedback of the earlier formative evaluation should provide students with information sufficient to prepare them for this evaluation. A student's self-evaluation is often submitted before the evaluation conference and discussed at this time.

Evaluation results are commonly reported in both written and oral forms. Often, the primary evaluation tool is presented to show student improvement and specifically recall incidents. The faculty should clarify initially that the purpose of the conference is to provide information on the student's clinical performance. The results should be explained, giving specific incidents in which the student had difficulties, excelled, performed adequately, or improved. In addition, the faculty member needs to assist the student in establishing new goals. Finally, the faculty member needs to summarize the conference and end on a positive note.

The environment in which the evaluation conference takes place should be comfortable for the student, and privacy should be maintained. An hour during which the student is responsible for patient care or directly after a tiring clinical experience is not the most conducive time for a conference. An appointment during office hours away from the clinical site provides a more comfortable and private setting for students to listen to constructive criticism or encouraging comments.

Student Response

The student's response to the faculty evaluation typically reflects the fairness with which the results were determined. A student will perceive the results as fair if his or her own appraisal is congruent with that of the faculty. A student self-evaluation submitted before the conference helps faculty gain insight into student perceptions and can give faculty time to prepare a response. However, the best way to ensure congruent results is for faculty to provide the student with a sufficient number of formative evaluations and time to reflect on his or her own performance. Faculty need to be sensitive to the student's needs, emphasizing the student's strengths, as well as weaknesses, and encouraging goals and aspirations.

Working with Students with Questionable Performance
Supporting At-Risk Students

Developing a positive learning environment is a basic step in promoting positive supportive student learning relationships. Students have a right to expect respect. Pointing out areas in which students need to improve and specific ways to achieve clinical goals promotes a positive learning environment and minimizes potential legal risks.

Scanlan (2001) discusses the importance of clarifying definitions of safe and unsafe clinical practices and having clear policies and guidelines for working with "problem" students. Minimum patient safety competencies can be observed, checked off, and documented in the learning lab by using the benefits of rehearsal in this setting. School policies can indicate minimum safety competencies that need to be achieved in the learning lab before a student moves into the actual clinical setting. Additionally, O'Connor (2001) suggests that faculty can benefit from having a visual image of good, moderate, and poor student behaviors to assist in evaluation.

Zuzelo (2000) summarizes the following key points, which although relevant to all evaluations, have particular merit in evaluating a student with questionable clinical performance behaviors.

- Ensure that the criteria for student success (i.e., the written course objectives or competency statements) are clear to all parties.
- If a student is at risk, objectively document a pattern of marginal or failing behavior.
- Report poor performance to students as formative evaluation and provide students with opportunities for remedial work.
- Use strategies such as clinical probation for supporting the at-risk student. Student clinical contracts can be used to document these plans for improvement. The written student contract should clarify student and faculty expectations and what student behaviors need to occur for passing status to be achieved.
- Follow written procedure from school handbooks.

Anecdotal records should be written objectively and used to document a pattern of behaviors. Failing behaviors need to be identified in writing, and a contract for corrections should be signed by the faculty member and the student (Osinski, 2003). An annotated record of each counseling session and student evaluation should be signed by both the student and the faculty member and maintained by the faculty member.

Unsatisfactory Performance

Boley and Whitney (2003) note that when a student is given a failing grade, faculty must be aware of the standards to meet, that grades must not be "arbitrary or capricious," and that faculty must be able to explain how grades are determined related to the program and course objectives. When a fair judgment is made that a student's performance is unsatisfactory or failing, strategies should be used to avert interpersonal or legal problems (Caldwell & Tenofsky, 1996). As soon as the decision is made, communication with the student is essential. Documentation from formative evaluation conferences and student contracts can provide support for this decision. Published school policies and procedures should be followed, including documentation that decisions were made carefully and deliberately. Support from the university or college is essential when performance is determined to be unsatisfactory, and the administration should be notified of impending problems early in the grading process.

Final evaluations that result in unsatisfactory or failing performance require special tact and concern. Faculty need to share specific findings that resulted in a student not meeting the expected clinical objectives. Student contracts not fulfilled need to be identified. Students need time to process the information and should not feel rushed. Faculty need to listen attentively, with a strong show of concern and support, to the student's perceptions. The student may need time to reflect and return for another conference after adjusting to the facts.

Student Reactions

The failing student may react in a variety of ways. Caring faculty will recognize these behaviors and provide empathetic support. Students may respond with denial, providing their own perception of how a specified incident did or did not occur and offering excuses. Faculty need to steer the conversation to the student's not meeting the objectives and provide support for the student's emotional needs.

A student may attempt to bargain for a passing grade. Faculty need to stand firm and focus on the evaluation results. Faculty can be prepared to provide information about the options the student has. As the reality of the loss is recognized, the student may respond with depression, confusion, lack of motivation, indecision, and tears. Faculty should provide support, listen attentively, and generally convey caring behaviors; in some cases faculty may also need to recommend professional counseling. The student may come to terms with the outcome and begin to make plans for the future. Assistance from the faculty about options is often sought by the student. How well the student adapts to the final evaluation typically depends on how well he or she has been prepared for the results.

The student may respond with anger. The student may become demanding or accusing and may have the potential to become violent. In this case, faculty need to take steps to ensure their own safety and that of the student. Faculty should not take the anger personally but provide guidance about feelings and focus on the anger as a part of loss. Thomas (2003) has recommended handling anger with a "professional deep breath."

Additionally, an established grievance policy should be available. Both utilizing students and faculty share responsibility for knowing about and appropriately utilizing such a policy. (See Chapter 3 for further discussion.) Students have a right to respond to charges against them.

Dismissing an Unsafe Student from Clinical Practice

Behaviors unsafe for patient care such as lack of preparation, violence, and substance abuse need to be addressed. Pierce (2001) notes the importance of a broad and thorough policy that allows for safe and appropriate actions to protect both the patient and the student. School policies and procedures need to be followed. Clear policies help prevent arbitrary or capricious responses to an incident. O'Connor (2001) summarizes key points related to the student who is unsafe to care for patients, noting that safety of the patient is first priority in removing a student but that faculty have an obligation to ensure that all students are returned to an area of safety as well. The student unprepared to care for an assigned clinical patient should be sent to the library or lab to prepare. Student orientation to clinical practice should include a review of relevant policies and clarification of professional student behaviors.

EVALUATION OF THE EVALUATION

After the final student conference, the student and faculty need to evaluate the entire experience as a whole. The clinical site is evaluated on how well it met the learning and practice needs of the students. Was the philosophy of the staff congruent with that of the faculty and students? Were the students given the opportunity to meet all the objectives? As these questions are answered, the preparation phase for evaluation begins again. A continuous quality improvement process for clinical evaluation should be considered, with attention given to structure (appropriate evaluation tools with appropriate clinical environment and patient care opportunities), process (appropriate plans for sampling and evaluating clinical behaviors and for sharing feedback and results of evaluation), and outcome (satisfactory evaluative outcomes indicating safe, competent graduates).

SUMMARY

Good practice includes multidimensional evaluation with diverse evaluation methods completed over time, seeking student growth and progress (American Association for Higher Education, 1993). All evaluations should respect students' dignity and self-esteem. Nursing students have the unique opportunity to practice skills in natural settings with supervision by experienced nurses. The clinical evaluation provides both subjective and objective data that permit formative and summative analysis of the entire learning experience. Clinical performance evaluation provides students with a means for critical reflection on their future nursing roles. An appropriate evaluation process sets the stage for productive assessment of student learning.

REFERENCES

American Association of Higher Education (AAHE) Assessment Forum. (1993). *9 Principles of good practice for assessing student learning.* American Association of Higher Education. Retrieved August 29, 2003, from http://www.aahe.org/assessment/principl.htm

Baier, M., & Mueggenburg, K. (2001). Using the Internet for clinical instruction. *Nurse Educator, 26*(1), 3.

Boley, P., & Whitney, K. (2003). Grade disputes: Considerations for nursing faculty. *Journal of Nursing Education, 42*(5):198-203.

Borbasi, S. A., & Koop, A. (1994). The objective structured clinical examination: Its appreciation in nursing education. *The Australian Journal of Advanced Nursing, 11*(3):33-40.

Caldwell, L. M., & Tenofsky, L. (1996). Clinical failure or clinical folly? A second opinion on student performance. *Nursing and Health Care Perspectives, 17*(1): 22-5.

Carpenito, L. J., & Duespohl, T. A. (1985). *A guide for effective clinical instruction* (2nd ed.). Rockville, MD: Aspen.

Castellino, A., & Schuster, P. (2002). Evaluation of outcomes in nursing students using clinical concept map care plans. *Nurse Educator, 27,* 149-150.

Chan D. (2002). Development of the Clinical Learning Environment Inventory. *Journal of Nursing Education, 41*(2):69-75.

Cowles, K. V., Strickland, D., & Rodgers, B. L. (2001). Collaboration for teaching innovation: Writing across the curriculum in a school of nursing. *Journal of Nursing Education, 40*(8):363-367.

Dearman, C. N. (2003). Using clinical scenarios in nursing. In M. Oermann & K. Heinrich (Eds.), *Annual review of nursing Education.* New York: Springer.

DeBourgh G. A. (2001). Using Web technology in a clinical nursing course. *Nurse Educator, 26,* 227-233.

Gaberson, K. B., & Oermann, M. H. (1999). *Clinical teaching strategies in nursing* (1st ed.). New York: Springer.

Gibbons, S. W., Adamo, G., Padden, D., Ricciardi, R., Graziano, M., Levine, E., et al. (2002). Clinical evaluation in advanced practice nursing education: Using standardized patients in health assessment. *Journal of Nursing Education, 41*(5): 215-221.

Gronlund, N. (1993). *How to make achievement tests and assessments* (5th ed.). Needham Heights, MA: Allyn & Bacon.

Higuchi, K. A., & Donald, J. G. (2002). Thinking processes used by nurses in clinical decision making. *Journal of Nursing Education, 41*(4):145-153.

Hrobsky P. E., & Kersbergen A. L. (2002). Preceptors' perceptions of clinical performance failure. *Journal of Nursing Education, 41*(12):550-553.

Kathol, D., Geiger, M., & Hartig, J. (1998). Clinical correlation map. A tool for linking theory and practice. *Nurse Educator, 23,* 31-34.

King, M., & Shell, R. (2002). Teaching and evaluating critical thinking with concept maps. *Nurse Educator, 27,* 213-216.

Lehman, K. (2003). Clinical nursing instructors' use of handheld computers for student record-keeping and evaluation. *Journal of Nursing Education, 42*(1):41-42.

Liberto, T., Roncher, M., & Shellenbarger, T. (1999). Anecdotal notes. Effective clinical evaluation and record keeping. *Nurse Educator, 24,* 15-18.

Loving, G. L. (1993). Competence validation and cognitive flexibility: A theoretical model grounded in nursing education. *Journal of Nursing Education, 32*(9):415-421.

Mahara, M. (1998). A perspective on clinical evaluation in nursing education. *Journal of Advanced Nursing, 28,* 1339-1346.

McAllister, M., & Osborne, Y. (1997). Peer review: A strategy to enhance cooperative student learning. *Nurse Educator, 22*(1):40-44.

Miller, H. K., Nichols, E., & Beeken, J. E. (2000). Comparing videotaped and faculty-present return demonstrations of clinical skills. *Journal of Nursing Education, 39*(5):237-239.

O'Connor, A. B. (2001). *Clinical instruction and evaluation: A teaching resource* (1st ed.). Boston: Jones & Bartlett.

Oermann, M. H. (1997). Evaluating critical thinking in clinical practice. *Nurse Educator, 22*(5): 25-28.

Oermann, M. H., & Gaberson, K. B. (1998). *Evaluation and testing in nursing education.* New York: Springer.

Orchard, C. (1994). The nurse educator and the nursing student: A review of the issue of clinical evaluation procedures. *Journal of Nursing Education, 33*(6):245-251.

Osinski, K. (2003). Due process rights of nursing students in cases of misconduct. *Journal of Nursing Education, 42*(2):55-58.

Pierce, C. S. (2001). Implications of chemically impaired students in clinical settings. *Journal of Nursing Education, 40*(9):422-425.

Redman, R., Lenberg, C., & Walker, P. (1999). Competency assessment: Methods for development and implementation in nursing education. *Online Journal of Issues in Nursing*, Topic 10. Retrieved August 17, 2003, from http://www.nursingworld.org/ojin/topic10/tpc10_3.htm

Reilly, D. J., & Oermann, M. H. (1992). *Clinical teaching in nursing education* (2nd ed.). New York: National League for Nursing.

Rinne, C. H. (1994). The skills system: A new interactive video technology. *T.H.E. Journal, 21*(8):81-82. Retrieved August 29, 2003, from http://www.thejournal.com/magazine/vault/A1337A.cfm

Roberts, J. D., While, A. E., & Fitzpatrick, J. M. (1992). Simulation: Current status in nurse education. *Nurse Education Today, 12*, 409-415.

Scanlan, J. M. (2001). Learning clinical teaching: Is it magic? *Nursing and Health Care Perspectives, 22*, 240-246.

Schuster, P. (2000). Concept mapping: Reducing clinical care plan paperwork and increasing learning. *Nurse Educator, 25*, 76-81.

Slater, T. F. (1999). *Classroom assessment techniques, portfolios, Field-tested learning assessment guide*. Retrieved August 29, 2003, from http://www.flaguide.org/cat/portfolios/portfolios7.htm

Thomas, S. P. (2003). Handling anger in the teacher-student relationship. *Nursing Education Perspective, 24*(1):17-24.

U. S. Department of Education. (1974). The Family Educational Rights and Privacy Act. U.S. Department of Education. Retrieved August 29, 2003, from http://www.ed.gov/offices/OM/fpco/ferpa/.

Walker, E., & Dewar, B. (2000). Moving on from interpretivism: An argument for constructivist evaluation. *Journal of Advanced Nursing, 32*, 713-720.

Waltz, C. F., & Jenkins, L. S. (Eds.). (2001). *Measurement of nursing outcomes. Volume 1: Measuring nursing performance in practice, education, and research* (2nd ed.). New York: Springer.

Wiles, L., & Bishop, J. (2001). Case report. Clinical performance appraisal: Renewing graded clinical experiences. *Journal of Nursing Education, 40*, 37-39.

Zuzelo, P. R. (2000). Clinical issues, clinical probation: Supporting the at-risk student. *Nurse Educator, 25*(5): 216-218.

24

EDUCATIONAL PROGRAM EVALUATION

Marcia K. Sauter, DNS, RN, Margaret H. Applegate, EdD, RN, FAAN

The purpose of this chapter is to provide information on how to conduct comprehensive evaluation of nursing education programs. A brief history of program evaluation and examples of models for program evaluation will be followed by a description of Chen's (1990) theory-driven model. An adaptation of Chen's theory-driven approach to program evaluation is presented as a framework for the development of a plan for the evaluation of a nursing education program. This adaptation of Chen's model provides a mechanism for evaluating all program elements, for determining the causal relationships between program elements, for determining program effectiveness, and for identifying strategies to improve program quality.

DEFINITION OF TERMS

A *nursing education program* is any academic program in a postsecondary institution leading to initial licensure or advanced preparation in nursing. *Program evaluation* is the assessment of all components of a program, from program planning through implementation, to determine program effectiveness (Chen, 1990). *Program evaluation theory* is a framework that guides the practice of program evaluation. A *program evaluation plan* is a document that serves as the blueprint for the evaluation of a specific program.

Program evaluation is a comprehensive approach to program improvement that includes curriculum evaluation and assessment. *Curriculum evaluation* assesses the implementation of the program plan, processes, and products of the teaching and learning transaction. *Assessment* involves evaluation activities that focus on student learning (Palomba & Banta, 1999). Curriculum evaluation and assessment of student learning are presented in this chapter within the context of a total program evaluation plan.

PURPOSES AND BENEFITS OF PROGRAM EVALUATION

The primary purpose of program evaluation is to judge the merit or worth of the total program being evaluated, as well as the individual elements of that program. Analysis must consider not only whether the mission and goals have been achieved but also whether they are worth achieving. Evaluation serves internally as a source of information for decisions about programs and program elements, as well as a measure of how the program compares with institutional, state, and national standards. Externally, evaluation data serve to increase the awareness of the various publics about the quality of the program. Specific purposes of program evaluation are as follows:

1. To determine how various elements of the program interact and influence program effectiveness
2. To determine the extent to which the mission, goals, and outcomes of the program are realized
3. To determine whether the program has been implemented as planned
4. To identify efficient use of resources to assess and improve program quality
5. To provide a rationale for decision making that leads to improved program effectiveness

RELATIONSHIP OF PROGRAM EVALUATION TO ACCREDITATION

Accrediting bodies exert considerable influence over nursing programs. Accrediting bodies include the state board of nursing, the National League for Nursing Accrediting Commission (NLNAC), the Commission for Collegiate Nursing Education (CCNE), and regional accrediting bodies such as the Higher Learning Commission. Nursing education programs must be approved by the state board of nursing to be able to operate and by the regional accrediting body to seek national accreditation. National accreditation by NLNAC or CCNE is voluntary, but the public perception of the school is linked, in part, to this accreditation. Certainly, schools that have a mission to prepare students for graduate education and schools that wish to compete for external funding as a part of their mission will want to meet all levels of accreditation.

Nursing programs have historically been too dependent on accreditation processes to guide program evaluation efforts (Ingersoll & Sauter, 1998). Some nursing programs do not fully engage in program evaluation until preparation of the self-study for an accreditation site visit has begun. To fulfill its purposes, program evaluation must be a continuous activity. Program evaluation built solely around accreditation criteria may lack examination of some important elements or understanding of the relationship between elements that influences program success. Nevertheless, building the assessment indicators identified by these bodies into the evaluation process ensures ongoing attention to state and national standards of excellence.

HISTORICAL PERSPECTIVE

According to a model proposed by Ralph Tyler (1949), the earliest approaches to educational program evaluation focused on whether learning experiences produced the desired educational outcomes. Tyler's behavioral objective model was a simple, linear approach that began with defining learning objectives, developing measuring tools, and then measuring student performance to determine whether objectives had been met. Because evaluation occurred at the end of the learning experience, Tyler's approach was primarily summative.

Formative evaluation, which includes testing and revising curriculum components during the development and implementation of educational programs, became popular during the 1960s. During this same decade, the U.S. government called for greater accountability of public education by requiring that all federally funded educational programs include evaluation of program effectiveness. The Elementary and Secondary Education Act (ESEA) was designed to improve the total system of public education (Stufflebeam, 1983).

The quality of educational program evaluation was brought into question in the 1970s when the Phi Delta Kappa National Study Committee on Evaluation concluded that meaningful educational evaluation was rare. Program evaluation lacked a clear definition, and program evaluation theory was poorly developed (Borich & Jemelka, 1982). The Phi Delta Kappa Commission encouraged formative evaluation by suggesting that evaluation focus on the process of program implementation (Stufflebeam, 1983).

During the 1980s, outcomes assessment became the focus of educational evaluation. In 1983, the National Commission on Excellence in Education published a report, *Nation at Risk: The Imperative of Educational Reform*. This report, which called for program accountability through outcomes assessment, raised the public's awareness of quality issues in elementary and secondary education in the United States (Hunt & Staton, 1996). In 1984, the National Institute of Education Study Group on the Conditions of Excellence in American Postsecondary Education echoed the same concerns for higher education. The National Institute of Education Study Group endorsed outcomes assessment as an essential strategy for improving the quality of education in postsecondary institutions (Ewell, 1985). By the mid 1980s, the call for outcomes assessment in higher education had clearly been heard and acted on as numerous state legislatures began mandating outcomes assessment for public postsecondary institutions (Halpern, 1987) and as the regional accrediting agencies began mandating outcomes assessment in their accreditation criteria (Ewell, 1985). Although the focus on outcomes assessment was growing rapidly, initial efforts at implementing outcomes assessment were not successful because educators experienced difficulty in developing appropriate methods for performing outcomes assessment and in obtaining adequate organizational support to implement assessment (Terenzini, 1989). The focus on outcomes assessment led some institutions to confuse outcomes assessment with comprehensive program evaluation. Nursing educators were also influenced by the outcomes assessment movement. Publications from the National League for Nursing (NLN) called for measurement of student outcomes (Waltz, 1988) and described measurement tools for assessing educational outcomes (Waltz & Miller, 1988).

By the early 1990s, some of the issues surrounding outcomes assessment had been addressed, and successful efforts in outcomes assessment had occurred (Banta, 1993). As nursing education continued to follow the trend in higher education, the Third National Conference on Measurement and Evaluation in Nursing focused entirely on outcomes assessment (Garbin,

1991). The NLN added assessment of learning outcomes to its accreditation criteria in 1991. The CCNE also included outcomes assessment in its initial accreditation standards, first published in 1997.

The Wingspread Group on Higher Education (1993) challenged providers of higher education to use outcomes assessment to improve teaching and learning. Nevertheless, outcomes assessment was not the final solution to improving program quality. Many postsecondary institutions continued to struggle with outcomes assessment, and those that were able to implement it were often unable to identify any academic improvements as a result of the assessment program (Tucker, 1995). Toward the end of the decade, approaches to organizational effectiveness, especially Deming's continuous quality improvement model, began to influence a more comprehensive approach to program evaluation (Freed et al., 1997).

As a result of the growing emphasis on program evaluation in the 1980s and 1990s, university programs were developed to prepare individuals in program evaluation (Shadish et al., 1991). As program evaluation became a distinct field of study, theories were developed to guide the practice of evaluation. Some of these theories include Borich and Jemelka's (1982) systems theory, Stufflebeam's context, input, process, and product (CIPP) model (1983), Guba and Lincoln's fourth-generation evaluation framework (1989), Patton's qualitative evaluation model (1990), Chen's theory-driven model (1990), Veney and Kaluzny's cybernetic decision model (1991), and Rossi and Freeman's social research approach (1993). Perhaps because of the nursing profession's emphasis on use of theory to guide practice, the need for program evaluation theory to guide evaluation practices in nursing education was identified in the nursing literature as early as 1978. Friesner (1978) reviews five evaluation models: (1) Tyler's behavioral objective model; (2) the NLN accreditation model; (3) Stufflebeam's CIPP model; (4) Scriven's goal-free evaluation model; and (5) Provus' discrepancy evaluation. Friesner concludes that no single model could effectively guide the evaluation of nursing education and recommends that nursing educators blend elements from one or more of the models.

In the early 1990s, several articles about program evaluation theory appeared in the nursing literature. Watson and Herbener (1990) review Provus' discrepancy model, Scriven's goal-free evaluation model, Stakes' countenance model, Staropolia and Waltz's decision model, and Stufflebeam's CIPP model. These authors conclude that any of these models could be useful and recommend that nursing educators choose a model that best fits their needs. In contrast, Sarnecky (1990b) explicitly recommends Guba and Lincoln's responsiveness model after comparing it with Tyler's behavioral objective model, Stake's countenance model, Provus' discrepancy model, and Stufflebeam's CIPP model. She believes that the other models do not adequately address the plurality of values among stakeholders and the importance of stakeholder involvement. Bevil (1991) proposes a theoretical framework she adapted from several evaluation theories. Ingersoll (1996) reviews Borich and Jemelka's systems approach, McClintock's conceptual mapping approach, and Chen's theory-driven model. Addressing issues about the reliability and validity of assessment activities, Ingersoll recommends that program evaluation be viewed as evaluation research and that program evaluation theory be used to guide the development and implementation of program evaluation. Ingersoll and Sauter (1998) review Guba and Lincoln's fourth-generation evaluation, Scriven's goal-free approach, Norman and Lutenbacher's theory of systems improvement, Rossi and Freeman's social science approach, and Chen's theory-driven model. The authors suggest that Rossi and Freeman's model and Chen's model have the most potential for guiding the evaluation of nursing education programs. Ingersoll and Sauter also express concern that nursing faculty commonly use accreditation criteria to form the framework for evaluation of nursing education programs. They recommend that program evaluation theory serve this purpose. Ingersoll and Sauter (1998) present an evaluation plan developed from Chen's theory-driven model, which incorporates the NLNAC's criteria for baccalaureate programs.

Sauter (2000) surveyed all baccalaureate nursing programs in the United States to determine how they develop, implement, and revise their program evaluation plans. Few nursing programs reported using program evaluation theory to guide program evaluation. However, those educators that did use program evaluation theory were more satisfied with the effectiveness of their evaluation practices.

PROGRAM EVALUATION THEORIES

Program evaluation theories are either method oriented or theory driven, depending on their underlying assumptions, preferred methodology, and general focus. Method-oriented theories emphasize methods for performing evaluation, whereas theory-driven approaches emphasize the theoretical framework for developing and implementing evaluation. The more popular approaches have been method oriented (Chen, 1990; Shadish et al., 1991).

Method-oriented approaches usually focus on the relationship between program inputs and outputs and include an emphasis on a preferred method for conducting program evaluation. Many of the method-oriented approaches emphasize quantitative research methods. A few method-oriented approaches recommend naturalistic or qualitative methods for performing program evaluation.

An example of a quantitative method-oriented program evaluation theory is Rossi and Freeman's (1993) social science model. These authors believe that the use of experimental research methods will produce the most effective program evaluation. The advantage of this approach is that measurement techniques must be reliable and valid, even if experimental design is not used to conduct the evaluation. One of the major limitations of this approach is that the focus on methodology may divert evaluators from other issues, such as recognizing the importance of stakeholder perspective. In addition, experimental designs are often difficult to apply to some aspects of educational evaluation.

An example of a qualitative method-oriented program evaluation theory is Guba and Lincoln's (1989) fourth-generation evaluation. Guba and Lincoln advocate naturalistic methods for program evaluation. A special focus of their approach is the emphasis they place on integrating multiple stakeholders' viewpoints into program evaluation. A major advantage of their approach is that using qualitative methodology allows evaluators to achieve a greater depth of understanding of program strengths and limitations within a specific context. The approach is limited because it tends to overlook outcomes assessment, which usually requires more quantitative methodology.

Theory-driven approaches to program evaluation begin with the development of program theory. Program theory is the framework that describes the elements of the program and explains the relationships between and among elements. When this approach is used, program evaluation is intended to test whether the program theory is correct and whether it has been correctly implemented. If the program is not successful in achieving outcomes, a theory-driven approach allows the evaluator to determine whether the program's failure is due to flaws in the program theory or failure to implement the program correctly. The theory-driven approach often calls for a variety of research methods because evaluators choose the methodology that is best suited to answering the evaluation questions (Chen, 1990).

Chen's (1990) theory-driven model is one of the most comprehensive models for program evaluation. Although the model was intended for evaluation of social service programs, it is easily adapted to educational programs. A brief overview of Chen's model is included here along with suggestions on how to adapt it to an educational program. A more detailed application of Chen's model in developing a program evaluation plan is provided later in the chapter.

Theory-Driven Program Evaluation

Chen (1990) defines program theory as a framework that identifies the elements of the program, provides the rationale for interventions, and describes the causal linkages between the elements, interventions, and outcomes. According to Chen, program theory is needed to determine desired goals, what ought to be done to achieve desired goals, how actions should be organized, and what outcome criteria should be investigated. Program theory is either normative or causative.

Normative theory is prescriptive and value laden, defining what should happen. Normative theory can be subdivided into three major domains: treatment, implementation environment, and outcome. Treatment theory defines the nature of the treatment and its measurement. For an educational program, teaching and curriculum comprise the "treatment." Implementation environment theory defines the environment in which the treatment is delivered. Outcome theory defines the desired goals and the outcomes for the program (Chen, 1990).

Causative theory is descriptive, explaining how and why program elements are related. Causative theory can be subdivided into three major domains: impact, intervening mechanism, and generalization. Impact theory explains how the treatment affects the desired outcomes. Intervening mechanism describes the relationships between the causal processes that link the treatment to outcomes. Generalization theory describes how evaluation results can be generalized and applied to other topics of interest to stakeholders (Chen, 1990).

Chen defines program evaluation as the systematic collection of empirical evidence to assess the congruency between normative and actual program structures. Empirical evidence is needed to verify the program's impact, its underlying causal mechanisms, and its degree of generalizability. Through this systematic collection of evidence, program planners can develop and refine program structure and operations, understand and strengthen program effectiveness and utility, and facilitate policy decision making (Chen, 1990).

Six evaluation types are derived from the six domains of program theory. These six evaluation types are normative outcome (goals), normative treatment, implementation environment (seven dimensions), impact (intended and unintended outcomes), intervening mechanism, and generalization.

Normative Outcome (Goal) Evaluation

Normative outcome evaluation seeks to answer the question, "What do we want to accomplish?" Three primary activities are involved in this type of evaluation. Goal revelation evaluation determines the desired goals and outcomes. Goal priority consensus determines which goals and outcomes major stakeholders consider to be the most important. Goal realizability evaluation assesses whether there is consistency between program goals and activities. Program goals are evaluated to determine whether they are creating difficulty in operating the program. The evaluator works with stakeholders to develop a theoretical framework or program theory to guide the choice of program goals, to define appropriate activities through which to achieve the goals, and to explain the linkage between program activities and goals. Methods for achieving normative outcome evaluation include surveying stakeholders and using focus groups. Qualitative analysis can be used to compare and contrast program goals and conceptual frameworks with organizational mission. Although normative outcome evaluation can take place after a program has been implemented, it also provides a framework for initial program development (Chen, 1990).

Normative Treatment Evaluation

Given that goal evaluation has been completed, programs should be evaluated for congruency between expected and implemented treatment. The treatment, as implemented, should be compared with original program design to determine whether the program has been implemented as planned. The program implementer's capability for scheduling and maintaining treatment delivery is evaluated (Chen, 1990). For an educational program, the "treatment" is composed of the curriculum and the teaching strategies used to implement the curriculum. If program outcomes are not being achieved, treatment evaluation can determine whether the problem is due to curriculum failure or implementation failure. Curriculum failure occurs when the curriculum is implemented correctly (appropriate teaching strategies are used), but the content of the curriculum is flawed. Implementation failure occurs when the curriculum is not implemented correctly, such as when teaching strategies are ineffective.

Implementation Environment Evaluation

The implementation environment dimension evaluates how the implementers deliver the program. Chen (1990) defines seven dimensions of the environment as follows:

1. The participant dimension evaluates the participants' characteristics, demographics, roles, and reactions to the program. For an educational program, assessment of motivation and readiness to learn may be included in the participant dimension.
2. The implementer evaluation dimension assesses whether the implementers possess the qualities desired and the kind of relationships they have with participants. An example for an educational program would be evaluations of a faculty member's qualifications.
3. The delivery mode dimension seeks to determine whether the program can be delivered effectively and in agreement with stakeholder expectations. The evaluator assesses whether modes of delivery are appropriate. For an educational program, the evaluator may assess the classroom setting or the effectiveness of distance education.
4. The implementing organization dimension determines how organizational culture influences program implementation. Authority structures and operating procedures are examined for how they support or inhibit the program's effectiveness. For an educational program, assessment of faculty involvement in policy making might be conducted.
5. The interorganizational relationship dimension evaluates the relationship of the organization to other agencies. This dimension focuses on identifying organizations that have the potential to influence program outcomes, the level of cooperation needed from each of the agencies, and what relationships currently exist. For an educational program, the evaluator might survey employers of program graduates.
6. The micro context dimension determines the effect of the immediate environment on program implementation. The immediate environment includes family and peer relationships. In higher education, the evaluator might examine student support services and campus housing.
7. The macro context dimension determines the effect of the larger environment (social, political, cultural, economic factors) on program implementation. Job market trends and community issues are included. For nursing education, the evaluator might examine recommendations by the Pew Health Commission, relevant issues in health care financing, or community demand for advanced practice nurses.

Impact (Outcome) Evaluation

Impact evaluation determines whether the program is successful in achieving outcomes. Desired and unintended outcomes are examined. Quasi-experimental designs, such as pretest/posttest comparison and survey and case study methods, can be used. When outcomes are not achieved, the evaluator looks for consistency between other areas of program evaluation and the impact evaluation. For example, the evaluator might analyze whether problems found in the normative treatment evaluation can be linked to the failure to achieve outcomes. All components of program evaluation must be considered for impact evaluation to be useful (Chen, 1990). For an educational program, the evaluator would determine whether students achieved the terminal goals of the program. For nursing education, assessment would include the pass rate for first-time takers of the national licensure examination and employment statistics after graduation. When outcomes are not achieved, Chen's theory directs the evaluator to return to the other components of program evaluation. He recommends asking two questions: "Were the proposed goals realistic and reflective of stakeholder consensus? Was the program implemented as planned?"

Intervening Mechanism Evaluation

The purpose of intervening mechanism evaluation is to uncover the causal processes that link the treatment with the outcomes. This component identifies reasons a program does or does not work. Three steps are included in this type of evaluation: (1) specification of the intervening variable that comes between treatment and outcome variables, (2) observation and/or quantification of intervening variables, and (3) inference of the causal mechanisms by mapping action and conceptual theories that demonstrate linkages between program activities and outcomes (Chen, 1990). For an educational program, variables that influence student learning would be identified and the rationale for teaching strategies would be explained.

Generalization Evaluation

The purpose of generalization evaluation is to determine how evaluation results can be generalized to other situations of interest to stakeholders. Generalization evaluation can be achieved by approaching program evaluation as evaluation research. Program evaluation is held to the same standards as any scientific endeavor. Research methods that best answer the questions posed by the program evaluation should be used. Quantitative, qualitative, or mixed methods may be considered (Chen, 1990). For an educational program, evaluation of validity and reliability of assessment tools should be documented. Evaluation of the effectiveness of the program evaluation plan in improving program outcomes is the final aspect of generalization evaluation.

THE PROGRAM EVALUATION PLAN

The program evaluation plan provides a road map for organizing and tracking evaluation activities. The plan is a written document that contains the evaluation framework, activities for gathering and analyzing data, responsible parties, time frames, and the means for using information for program decisions. The program evaluation plan provides the mechanism for maintaining continuous evaluation of program effectiveness. Although the plan should stand on its own merit, nursing faculty may find it useful to match accreditation criteria throughout the plan to ensure compliance with accrediting bodies' expectations. Before the plan can be developed, accountability for program evaluation activities must be understood and defined.

ACCOUNTABILITY FOR PROGRAM EVALUATION

Responsibility for development and implementation of the program evaluation plan rests with the nursing faculty. The process for development and implementation may vary across nursing schools, depending on such factors as the number of faculty in the nursing school and the institutional resources available to support the evaluation. In some schools, an evaluator position is created to manage program evaluation practices, including the development and implementation of the program evaluation plan. An office of evaluation may be necessary in large schools, providing support staff to coordinate data collection at multiple levels. A common approach in small- and moderate-sized nursing schools is to appoint a standing committee of faculty who provide leadership and coordination of evaluation efforts.

Regardless of the plan, the nursing faculty must determine accountability for each element of the evaluation plan. Without clear accountability and firm time frames, it is easy for evaluation efforts to get lost in the press of daily demands on faculty and administration. There is a risk that the entire process will be fragmented or duplication of effort will occur (Waltz, 1985).

Another issue of concern is the reporting and recording of evaluation data. Information is of little value to decision making unless it is channeled to those who are responsible for making decisions. Careful attention to this issue not only increases the likelihood that decisions will be based on actual data but also facilitates analysis of the value of the data. Evaluation data also serve as a rich resource when responses to external reports and accreditation expectations are required. One of the dangers of the theory-based approach is data overload. Because data are used for making decisions, it is best to determine what information is necessary and what is interesting but not important. Over time, a goal of evaluation is to streamline the amount of data collected.

The location of evaluation information is also important. Access to the information increases the likelihood of its use. An official location for evaluation reports ensures that they can be found when they are needed. Advances in technology have made the development of computer databases an important source of information that can be accessed by multiple stakeholders from a central location or file server.

Finally, the outcome of evaluation efforts in terms of creating change is an element that is sometimes omitted in record keeping. Accrediting bodies are as concerned about the actions that result from analysis of evaluation data as they are that a plan is in place. The best plan loses value if it does not create change when a need for intervention is indicated by the data.

ADAPTING CHEN'S THEORY-DRIVEN MODEL TO PROGRAM EVALUATION FOR NURSING EDUCATION

The following section is based on an adaptation of Chen's theory-driven model and contains suggestions for the development of a program evaluation plan appropriate for a nursing education program. The components of the evaluation plan are organized according to Chen's six evaluation types with some modification in wording to provide clarity. For example, normative outcome evaluation has been relabeled as *mission and goal evaluation*, which more clearly defines the intent of this evaluation and prevents confusion with outcomes assessment. Treatment evaluation has been relabeled and split into two sections: *curriculum evaluation* and *evaluation of teaching effectiveness*. Table 24-1 shows the adaptations made to Chen's model for application to a nursing education program.

Table 24-2 provides a sample evaluation plan for mission and goal evaluation applied to a nursing education program. This sample demonstrates how all elements of the program evaluation plan may be articulated, including the program's theoretical elements, assessment activities, responsible parties, time frames, and related accreditation criteria. For the remaining evaluation components presented in this chapter, only examples of theoretical elements and methods for gathering and analyzing assessment data relevant to the identified theoretical elements are provided. The theoretical elements and assessment strategies that are suggested here are not all-inclusive but may assist nursing faculty in further development of their own program theory and program evaluation plan.

MISSION AND GOAL EVALUATION

Program evaluation must begin by determining that appropriate mission, philosophy, program goals, and outcomes have been defined. The expectations of both internal and external stakeholders must be considered. Internal stakeholders include administrators, faculty, and governing boards. External

TABLE 24-1 Comparison Between Chen's Theory-Driven Model for Program Evaluation and a Model for Nursing Education

CHEN'S EVALUATION TYPES	COMPONENTS FOR EVALUATION OF NURSING EDUCATION PROGRAMS
Normative Outcome Evaluation	Mission and Goal Evaluation
Normative Treatment Evaluation	Curriculum Evaluation
	Evaluation of Teaching Effectiveness
Implementation Environment Evaluation	
Participant Dimension	Student Dimension
Implementer Dimension	Faculty Dimension
Delivery Mode Dimension	Delivery Mode Dimension
Implementing Organization Dimension	Implementing Organization Dimension
Interorganizational Relationship Dimension	Interorganizational Relationship Dimension
Micro Context Dimension	Micro Context Dimension
Macro Context Dimension	Macro Context Dimension
Impact Evaluation	Outcomes Assessment
Intervening Mechanism Evaluation	Intervening Mechanism Evaluation
Generalization Evaluation	Generalization Evaluation

TABLE 24-2 Mission and Goal Evaluation

PROGRAM THEORY	ASSESSMENT STRATEGIES	RESPONSIBLE PARTIES	TIME FRAME	RECORDING AND REPORTING	ACCREDITATION CRITERIA
The mission of the nursing department is congruent with the university's mission.	Complete a thematic analysis comparing key phrases in the department's mission with the university's mission.	Program Evaluation Committee	Every 5 years or whenever change occurs in either statement	Update document "Comparison of Departmental and University mission."	*CCNE* Standard I. Mission and Governance
There is consensus among the faculty regarding the nursing mission and philosophy.	Use Delphi technique to determine level of agreement among the faculty. • Number each statement in mission and philosophy. Faculty indicate level of agreement with each statement. • Faculty recommend change. • If consensus does not occur, make changes and repeat process until consensus is reached. • Complete final report summary to include changes that were made, areas for improvement.	Chair	Every 5 years or whenever change occurs in either statement	Update document "History and Revision of Program Mission and Philosophy."	The mission, goals, and expected outcomes of the program are congruent with those of the parent institution, reflect professional nursing standards and guidelines, and consider the needs of the community of interest.
There is congruency between the nursing mission/philosophy/ conceptual framework/goals/ outcomes for each program.	Prepare a content map for each element to assess congruency.	Curriculum Committee	Every 3 years	Curriculum Committee minutes	*NLNAC* Standard I Mission and Governance There are clear and publicly stated mission and/or philosophy and purposes appropriate

to postsecondary or higher education in nursing.

Outcome	Activity	Responsible	Frequency	Data Source	Standard
Expectations of the state board of nursing, NLNAC, and CCNE are known and considered in the program's mission, goals, philosophy, and outcomes.	Review State Nurse Practice Act and educational rules and NLNAC and CCNE accreditation standards and criteria.	Program Evaluation Committee	Yearly	Program Evaluation Committee minutes	CCNE Standard I Key Element 1-C The mission, goals, and expected outcomes of the program are reviewed periodically and revised, as appropriate, to reflect the needs and expectations of the community of interest.
The Nursing Advisory Board provides meaningful input into the goals and outcomes of the program.	Review mission/philosophy/conceptual framework/goals/outcomes for each program with the Nursing Advisory Board and seek feedback (see section titled "Interorganization Evaluation" for additional assessment of advisory board).	Chair	Every 3 years	Nursing Advisory Board meeting minutes	
The goals of the program are congruent with professional standards.	Compare the BSN program goals with the ANA standards of practice and essentials of baccalaureate education as defined by AACN.	BSN Program Director			CCNE Standard I
Documents and publications accurately reflect mission/goals.	Check all publications for accuracy: • Undergraduate/Graduate Catalog	Recruitment Committee	Annually	Recruitment Committee meeting minutes	CCNE Standard I Key Element 1-E Documents and

Continued

TABLE 24-2 **Mission and Goal Evaluation—cont'd**

PROGRAM THEORY	ASSESSMENT STRATEGIES	RESPONSIBLE PARTIES	TIME FRAME	RECORDING AND REPORTING	ACCREDITATION CRITERIA
	• School of Nursing Brochure • Nursing Student Handbook • Program fact sheet				publications are accurate. Any references in promotional materials regarding the program's offerings and outcomes are accurate.

AACN, American Association of Colleges of Nursing; *ANA,* American Nurses Association; *BSN,* bachelor of science in nursing; *CCNE,* Commission for Collegiate Nursing Education; *NLNAC,* National League for Nursing Accrediting Commission.

stakeholders include religious organizations for private schools with religious affiliations, regional accrediting bodies, national discipline-specific accrediting bodies, state education commissions and boards of nursing, the legislature, and professional organizations. There should be congruency between the expectations of stakeholders and the program's mission, philosophy, goals, and outcomes. For private institutions with religious affiliations, some perspectives may be prescribed and must be included in mission, philosophy, goals, or outcomes.

The mission of the nursing department should be congruent with the university's mission. Comparison of key phrases in the department's mission with key phrases in the university's mission may done to assess congruency between mission statements. The identification of gaps between the two mission statements provides information about areas where attention is needed. The assessment should be performed periodically and whenever changes are made to either mission statement.

There should be consensus among the faculty regarding the nursing school's mission and philosophy. A modified Delphi approach to determine the level of agreement among the faculty for each statement in the mission and philosophy is a useful strategy. The Delphi approach is useful for both the development and the evaluation of belief statements (philosophy). This approach seeks consensus without the need for frequent face-to-face dialogue in a manner that protects the anonymity of participants. In this method questionnaires that list proposition statements about each of the content elements of the belief statement are distributed. A common breakdown of Delphi responses is a five-point range from "strongly agree" to "strongly disagree" so that respondents can indicate their level of support for each proposition. Respondents are provided with feedback about the responses after the first round of questionnaire distribution, and a second round may occur to determine the intensity of agreement or disagreement with the group median responses (Uhl, 1991). After several rounds with interim reports and analyses, it is usually possible to identify areas of consensus, areas of disagreement so strong that further discourse is unlikely to lead to consensus, and areas in which further discussion is warranted. In the evaluation of an established belief statement, the same process will provide data about what propositions continue to be supported, which no longer garner support, and which need to be openly debated (Uhl, 1991). The result provides a consensus list of propositions that either supports the belief statement as it is or suggests areas for revision. Chapter 7 provides further information on development of mission and philosophy.

All accrediting bodies have expectations about mission, philosophy, program goals, and outcomes. The NLNAC (2002a, 2002b), defines Standard I, Mission and Governance, in which it requires that the nursing program provide clear statements of mission, philosophy, and purposes. In addition, the NLNAC has indicated both required and optional outcomes that nursing programs must measure over time to provide trend data about student learning. For example, the required outcomes in the criteria for baccalaureate and higher degree programs are communications, therapeutic nursing interventions, critical thinking, graduation rates, job placement rates, licensure/certification pass rate, and program satisfaction (NLNAC, 2002b). The CCNE (2002) also includes in Standard I, Mission and Governance, expectations regarding congruency of the program's mission, goals, and outcomes with those of the parent institution, professional nursing standards, and the needs of stakeholders.

Professional organizations include the American Nurses Association, American Association of Colleges of Nursing (AACN), and National Association of Nurse Practitioner Faculty. Program goals and outcomes in baccalaureate degree programs should be congruent with the American Nurses Association Standards of Practice and the AACN Essentials of Baccalaureate Education for Professional Nursing Practice. The same consideration should be given to the AACN Essentials of Master's Education of Advanced Practice Nursing and the Criteria for Evaluation of Nurse Practitioner Programs (National Association of Nurse Practitioner Faculty, 2002) for master's degree programs. The AACN also provides indicators of quality in doctoral programs in nursing.

Other important stakeholders include local constituencies, such as health care agencies, that provide clinical learning experiences or employ graduates of the program. A survey of current and potential employers of graduates will help faculty to learn the knowledge and skill requirements of the marketplace. Many institutions establish advisory committees to provide additional information and selected focus groups to add richness to the information. This information is used to ensure that program goals and outcomes are appropriate, to provide input for curriculum planning, and to develop evaluation questions and tools for determining whether market needs are being met.

The mission and program goals should be clearly and publicly stated. Nursing schools that offer several different nursing programs will need to clearly articulate the purpose and program goals of each of these programs. Publication in program brochures and catalogs is one method of public announcement.

Box 24-1 lists the theoretical elements for mission and goal evaluation.

Box 24-1
THEORETICAL ELEMENTS FOR MISSION AND GOAL EVALUATION

- The mission of the nursing department is congruent with the university's mission.
- There is consensus among the faculty regarding the mission and philosophy.
- There is congruency between the nursing mission/philosophy/conceptual framework/goals/outcomes for each program.
- Expectations of the state board of nursing, NLNAC, and CCNE are known and considered in the program's mission, goals, philosophy, and outcomes.
- The goals of the program are congruent with professional standards of practice.
- The Nursing Program Advisory Committee has meaningful input into program goals and outcomes.
- Documents and publications accurately reflect mission/goals.

CCNE, Commission for Collegiate Nursing Education; *NLNAC,* National League for Nursing Accrediting Commission.

CURRICULUM EVALUATION

One of the most critical elements of program effectiveness is curriculum design. Curriculum design is an organizing framework that arranges the curriculum elements into a program of study. Curriculum design provides direction to both the content of the program and the teaching and learning processes involved in program implementation. Curriculum content involves both discipline-specific knowledge and the liberal arts foundation. Before the curriculum design can be developed, faculty must first determine their definition of the discipline of knowledge so that they may select courses that will best serve the students to prepare to practice. Faculty must determine what ways of knowing, or methods of inquiry, are characteristic of the discipline and what skills the discipline demands. Program goals and outcome statements provide a guide for the development of the program of study. The program goals link the mission and faculty belief statements (philosophy) to the curriculum design, teaching and learning methods, and outcomes. Consequently, the evaluation of the curriculum builds on the evaluation of mission and goals.

Evaluation of Curriculum Organization

Curriculum must be appropriately organized to move learners along a continuum from program entry to program completion. The principle of *vertical organization* guides both the planning and evaluation of the curriculum. This principle provides the rationale for the sequencing of curricular content elements (Schwab, 1973). For example, nursing faculty often use depth and complexity as sequencing guides; that is, given content areas may occur in subsequent levels of the curriculum at a level of greater depth and complexity. This is supported by the work of Gagne (1977), who developed a hierarchical theory of instruction based on the premise that knowledge is acquired by proceeding from data and concepts to principles and constructs. In evaluation of the curriculum, faculty must assess for increasing depth and complexity to determine whether the sequencing was useful to learning and progressed to the desired outcomes. Determination of whether course and level objectives demonstrate sequential learning across the curriculum can be used as a test of vertical organization. The analysis can be performed with Bloom's taxonomy (1956) as a guide for determining whether objectives follow a path of increasing complexity.

The principle of *internal consistency* is important to the evaluation of the curriculum. The curriculum design is a carefully conceived plan that takes its shape from what its creators believe about people and their education. The intellectual test of a curriculum design is the extent to which the elements fit together. Four elements should be congruent: objectives, subject matter taught, learning activities used, and outcomes (Doll, 1992). Evaluation efforts should include examination of the extent to which the objectives and outcomes are linked to the mission and belief statements. Program objectives should be tracked to level and course objectives. One method of assessing internal consistency is through the use of a curriculum matrix (Heinrich et al., 2002). The matrix is a visual representation that lists all nursing courses and shows the placement of major concepts flowing from the program philosophy and conceptual framework. Another approach to assessment of internal consistency is through a curriculum audit (Seager & Anema, 2003). Similar to a curriculum matrix, the curriculum audit provides a visual representation that matches competencies to courses and learning activities.

The principle of *linear congruence,* sometimes called *horizontal organization,* assists faculty in determining which courses should precede and follow others and which should be concurrent (Schwab, 1973). The concept of sequencing follows the principle of moderate novelty in that new information and experiences should not be presented until existing knowledge has been assimilated (Rabinowitz & Schubert, 1991). An appropriate question is, What entry skills and knowledge does the student need as a condition of subsequent knowledge and experiences? How faculty answer this question will determine curriculum design and implementation. The evaluation question would address the extent to which students have the entry-level skills needed to progress sequentially in the curriculum. This is a critical question in light of the changing profile of students entering college-level programs. It is often difficult to determine which prerequisite skills should be required for entry and which should be acquired concurrently. Computer skills are a good example. Students enter programs with varying ability to use the computer. It is necessary to determine the prerequisite skills needed and the sequence in which advanced skills should be acquired during the program of learning.

Some nursing programs use a specific conceptual framework that identifies essential program "threads" and provides further direction to curriculum development and implementation. Congruency between program threads, program goals, course objectives, and course content will also need to be assessed. Further information on curriculum development and curriculum frameworks can be found in Chapters 5, 6, 8, and 9.

Course Evaluation

Individual courses are reviewed to determine whether they have met the tests of *internal consistency, linear congruence,* and *vertical organization.* A triangulation approach to course evaluation is useful. This approach uses data from three sources—faculty, students, and materials review—to identify strengths and areas for change (DiFlorio et al., 1989). Each course is evaluated to determine whether content elements, learning activities, evaluation measures, and learner outcomes are consistent with the objectives of the course and the obligations of the course in terms of its placement in the total curriculum.

Faculty should clearly articulate the sequential levels of each expected ability to determine what teaching and learning strategies are needed to move the student to progressive levels of ability and to establish the criteria for determining that each stage of development has been achieved. This need is important in relation not only to abilities specific to the discipline or major but also to the transferable skills acquired in the general education component of the curriculum (Loacker & Mentkowski, 1993). Some faculty achieve this by creating content maps for each major thread or pervasive strand in the curriculum with related knowledge and skill elements. The content maps chart the obligation of each course in facilitating student progression to the expected program outcome. The maps also provide a guide for the evaluation of whether the elements were incorporated as planned.

Angelo and Cross (1993) have developed a teaching goals inventory tool that is useful in individual course evaluation. The purpose is to assist faculty in identifying and clarifying their teaching goals by helping them to rank the relative importance of teaching goals in a given course. The construction of the teaching goals inventory began in 1986 and involved a complex process that included a literature review, several cycles of data collection and analysis, expert analysis, and field testing with hundreds of teachers (Angelo & Cross, 1993). In the process Angelo and Cross developed a tool that clusters goals into higher-order thinking skills, basic academic success skills, discipline-specific knowledge and skills, liberal arts and academic values, work and career preparation, and personal development. This tool can assist the teacher in determining priorities in the selection of teaching and learning activities designed to advance the student toward the desired goals and in evaluating whether teaching goals and strategies are congruent with course objectives.

Evaluation of Support Courses and the Liberal Education Foundation

Faculty beliefs will also influence the selection of support courses (general education courses) in the curriculum that are foundational to and supportive of the nursing major. One element that will influence the selection of general education courses for the curriculum is the workforce requirements for the graduates of the program. Health care reform has created a greater need for nurses involved in community care and a greater emphasis on preventive care. Lindeman (1993) argues that current curricula in nursing continue to focus on intervention rather than preventative care. Although courses in the basic sciences are foundational to intervention care, courses in the social sciences and humanities provide a stronger foundation for understanding the contextual aspects of life (Lindeman, 1993). Lindeman (1993) concludes that if a richer mix of biological sciences, social sciences, and the humanities is included in foundational courses, students are better equipped to understand the relationship of social forces and health status.

Liberal education is fundamental to professional education. Evaluation questions about general education courses should address the extent to which the courses selected enable student learning and contribute to the expected outcomes. They should also be examined for sequencing to ensure that the support courses are appropriately placed to ground and complement the major and enrich the data mix for the organization and use of knowledge in practice. To develop evaluation questions related to the general education courses, faculty must first articulate what the rationale is for each course, what the expected outcomes are from the courses, and how the courses support the major to provide a broad, liberal education. When the expectations are clear, it is easier to select

> **Box 24-2**
> **THEORETICAL ELEMENTS OF CURRICULUM EVALUATION**
>
> - Course and level objectives demonstrate sequential learning across the curriculum (vertical organization).
> - Course objectives are congruent with level objectives, which are congruent with the program goals (internal consistency).
> - Course sequencing is defined with appropriate rationale for prerequisites and co-requisites (horizontal organization).
> - Course content (coursework and clinical experiences) provides graduates with the knowledge and skills needed to fulfill course and level objectives, the program's goals, and defined competencies.
> - Support courses enhance learning experiences and provide a foundation in the arts, sciences, and humanities.

the measures needed to determine whether expectations have been met. Evaluation of the outcomes of the general education courses will be discussed in the section on outcomes.

External accrediting agencies have expectations about liberal education. The NLNAC (2002a) states that no more than 60% of courses in associate degree curricula may be in the nursing major. The remainder of course work should be in general education. The criteria for baccalaureate and higher degree programs do not indicate a desired ratio.

Box 24-2 provides a summary of the theoretical elements associated with curriculum evaluation.

EVALUATION OF TEACHING EFFECTIVENESS

Evaluation of teaching effectiveness involves assessment of teaching strategies (including instructional materials), assessment of methods used to evaluate student performance, and assessment of student learning. Teaching strategies are effective when students are engaged, when strategies assist students to achieve course objectives, and when strategies provide opportunities for students to use prior knowledge in building new knowledge. Teaching effectiveness improves when teaching strategies are modified on the basis of evaluation data. See Chapter 10 for information on designing teaching strategies and student learning activities.

To demonstrate and document teaching effectiveness, faculty need multiple evaluation methods (Johnson & Ryan, 2000). Evaluation methods may include student feedback about teaching effectiveness obtained through course evaluations and focus group discussions, feedback provided through peer review, formal testing of teaching strategies, and assessment of student learning.

Student Evaluation of Teaching Strategies

The institution or nursing department may develop course evaluations to obtain student feedback on teaching effectiveness. The advantage of internally developed evaluations is that they can be customized to the program. The primary disadvantage of internally developed tools is that they may lack reliability and validity. Standardized evaluation tools, such as those found in the Individual Development and Educational Assessment, offered by the Individual Development and Educational Assessment Center at Kansas State University, and the National Study of Student Engagement, offered by the Indiana University Center for Postsecondary Research and Planning, have documented reliability and validity and provide opportunities to compare results with a national benchmark.

A focus group discussion with students can provide a more qualitative assessment of teaching effectiveness. Focus groups provide an opportunity to obtain insights and to hear student perspectives that might not be discovered through formal course evaluations. The focus group leader should be an impartial individual with the skill to conduct the session. The leader should clearly state the purpose of the session, ensure confidentiality, provide clear guidelines about the type of information being sought, and explain how information will be used (Palomba & Banta, 1999). The reliability and validity of information obtained from a focus group discussion is enhanced when the approach is conducted as research with a purposeful design and careful choice of participants (Kevern & Webb, 2001).

Peer Review of Teaching Strategies

Peer and colleague review may provide information on teaching effectiveness through classroom observation and assessment of course materials. In this context, a peer is defined as another faculty member within the same discipline with expertise in the field, and a colleague is an individual outside of the discipline with expertise in the art and science of teaching. Peer review can serve to promote quality improvement of teaching effectiveness and as documentation for performance review. Before peer review is implemented, there is a need to be clear about what data will be gathered, about who will have access to the data, and for what purposes it will be used. Faculty and administrators, as stakeholders in the endeavor, should collaborate to establish the norms and standards. Data from peer review may be used prescriptively to assist faculty in developing and improving teaching skills. At some point, peer review data may be needed for performance review and administrative decision making. Some schools require both classroom visits and opportunities to observe master teachers for all new faculty and periodic classroom visits for all faculty thereafter. In some schools the observation of teaching is voluntary. The age of the classroom as the private domain of the teacher is disappearing rapidly, and both accountability and the opportunity to demonstrate the scholarship of teaching are causing colleges and universities to require increased documentation of teaching as a routine part of the evaluation process.

Although classroom observation has been used as a technique for the peer review of teaching for a number of years, the reliability and validity of this method has been suspect. The validity and reliability of classroom observation as an evaluation tool is increased by (1) including multiple visits and multiple visitors, (2) establishing clear criteria in advance of the observation,

(3) ensuring that participants agree about the appropriateness and fairness of the assessment instruments and the process, and (4) preparing faculty to conduct observations (Seldin, 1980; Weimer et al., 1988). Before classroom teaching visits are made, the students should be advised of the visit and should be assured that they are not the central focus of the observation. Peer reviewers should meet with the faculty member before the visit and review the goals of the session, what has preceded and what will follow this session, planned teaching methods, assignments made for the session, and an indication of how this class fits into the total program. This provides a clear image for the visitors and establishes a beginning rapport. Some faculty have particular goals for growth that can be shared at this time as areas for careful observation and comment. Finally, a postvisit interview should be conducted to review the observation and to identify strengths and areas for growth. This may include consultation regarding strategies for growth with the scheduling of a return visit at a later date. Many visitors interview the students briefly after the visit to determine their reaction to the class and to ascertain whether this was a typical class rather than a special, staged event. Unless there is a designated visiting team, the faculty member to be visited is usually able to make selections or at least suggestions about the visitors who will make the observation. Peer visits to clinical teaching sessions should follow the same general approach as classroom visits, although specific criteria for observation will be established to meet the unique attributes of clinical teaching and learning. An additional requirement is that the visitor be familiar with clinical practice expectations in the area to be visited.

Evaluation of Teaching and Learning Materials

The review of teaching and learning materials is another element of evaluation of teaching effectiveness that may be conducted through peer review. Materials commonly included for review are the course syllabus, textbooks and reading lists, teaching plans, teaching or learning aids, assignments, and outcome measures. In all cases, the materials are reviewed for congruence with the course objectives, appropriateness to the level of the learner, content scope and depth, clarity, organization, and evidence of usefulness in advancing students toward the goals of the course.

The syllabus is reviewed to determine whether expectations are clear and methods of evaluation are detailed. It is especially important that students understand what is required to "pass" the course. Grading scales and weighting of each of the evaluation methods used in the course should be explained.

In the review of textbooks for their appropriateness for a given course, multiple elements may be considered. The readability of a text relates to the extent to which the reading demands of the textbook match the reading abilities of the students. This assumes that the faculty member has a profile of student reading scores from preadmission testing. Readability of a textbook is usually based on measures of word difficulty and sentence complexity. Other issues of concern include the use of visual aids; cultural and sexual biases; scope and depth of content coverage; and size, cost, and accuracy of the data contained within the text (Armbruster & Anderson, 1991). Another factor of importance is the structure of the textbook. This element relates to the organization and presentation of material in a logical manner that increases the likelihood of the reader's understanding of the content and ability to apply the content to practice. A review should determine the ratio of important and unimportant material and the extent to which important concepts are articulated, clarified, and exemplified. Do the authors relate intervening ideas to the main thesis of a chapter and clarify the relationships between and among central concepts (Armbruster & Anderson, 1991)? The ease with which information can be located in the index is important so that students can use the book as a reference. Because of the high cost of textbooks, it is useful to consider whether the textbook will be a good reference for other classes in the curriculum. A review of a textbook must also include consideration of whether the content has supported student learning. When student papers or other creative products are used for evaluation purposes, it is common to review a sample of these papers or products that the teacher has judged to be weak, average, and above average to provide a clearer view of expectations and how the students have met those expectations. This review provides an opportunity to demonstrate student outcomes. If a faculty member wants to retain copies of student papers and creative works to demonstrate outcomes, he or she should obtain informed consent from the students. Accrediting bodies often wish to see samples of student work, and faculty may use them to demonstrate learning outcomes for purposes of their own evaluation. In any case, each student's identity should be protected, and consent should be obtained.

The review of teaching and learning aids depends on the organization and use of these materials. The organization may be highly structured in that all are expected to use certain materials in certain situations or sequences, or materials may be resources available to faculty and students for use at their discretion according to the outcomes they wish to achieve (Rogers, 1983). Students may be expected to search for and locate materials, to create materials to facilitate their learning, or simply to use the materials provided in a prescribed manner The emphasis will determine whether evaluation questions related to materials are based on variety, creativity, and availability or whether the materials have been used as intended. Regardless of the overall emphasis, teaching and learning materials should be evaluated for efficiency and cost-effectiveness. Efficiency can be evaluated by determining whether the time demands and effort required to use the materials are worth the outcomes achieved. Cost-effectiveness can be determined by considering whether the costs of the materials justify the outcomes.

Formal Measures for Evaluating Teaching Strategies

Formal, objective measures of teaching strategies might include experimental or quasi-experimental designs, with randomization of subjects and control of treatments. For example, a teacher might establish a control group and a treatment group to try different teaching techniques and to evaluate outcomes to prove or disprove predetermined hypotheses. This technique is often used when there are multiple sections of a given course, although it can be accomplished within a section. A common method is to use the traditional strategy with the control group and the new strategy with the experimental group. A common examination or other assessment measure is used with both groups. Analysis might include checking for a significant difference in the scores of the two groups, as well as checking areas in which the most questions were missed for congruence or no congruence between the two groups (Short, 1991). A weakness of some of these efforts is that they are context bound and not generalizable. A strength of these testing strategies is the provision of feedback of value to evaluation questions within a given curriculum.

Assessment of Student Learning

It is unacceptable to claim that teaching strategies are effective unless there is evidence that links the teaching transaction with student learning. Assessment within the classroom provides evidence for interim outcome evaluation. Interim evaluation refers to outcomes of specific learning episodes, course outcomes, or level outcomes as opposed to outcomes assessed at the conclusion of the program of learning. Both formal and informal methods may be used in the classroom to assess student progress and to evaluate the effectiveness of teaching strategies. Chapters 21, 22, and 23 cover these methods in detail. The Angelo and Cross (1993) model of classroom assessment is designed to evaluate teaching strategies with the goal of improving learning. Informal classroom assessment is useful to the teacher for determining how well students are learning, and data from the assessment can be used by the teacher in making changes to improve that learning. This form of classroom assessment is almost never graded and is often anonymous. It is based on the assumptions that student learning is directly related to quality teaching, objectives are explicit and monitored, feedback is focused and frequent, the assessment is problem and context focused, assessment provides the impetus for change, assessment does not require specialized training, and assessment enhances student and faculty learning and satisfaction (Angelo & Cross, 1993). See Chapter 14 for a detailed discussion of classroom assessment methods.

At this juncture unintended outcomes become apparent and must be analyzed and corrected or incorporated according to the results of analysis. Faculty must determine whether students had the prerequisite skills needed to succeed in the course and whether they left the course with the knowledge and skills necessary to move into the next sequence (DiFlorio et al., 1989).

Evaluation of individual student performance must be effectively communicated to students. Documentation should provide evidence that evaluation leads to improvement in performance. This is especially important in clinical evaluation. Clinical evaluation tools should provide documentation that students were clearly informed of expectations and received appropriate feedback regarding their performance and information about how students responded.

Evaluating Student Performance Measures

In addition to documenting that teaching methods are effective, methods of evaluating student performance must be valid and reliable. Multiple-choice examinations are a common, cost-effective, and time-efficient method of testing knowledge acquisition as students progress in a course and at the conclusion of the course and program. This format provides rapid, quantitative data for individual assessment and aggregate data for centralized evaluation. Although few would argue that multiple-choice examinations should be completely eliminated, critics of this form of testing argue that the multiple-choice format serves to narrow the curriculum to reflect the content of the tests (Bersky & Yocom, 1994). They further argue that this form of testing fails to encourage or measure critical, creative, and reflective thought (Moss, 1992). Although faculty can develop multiple-choice questions that measure higher-order thinking, those requiring recall and basic comprehension are more common (Madaus & Kelleghan, 1992). It is also argued that students can choose the wrong option in multiple-choice questions with good rationale and select correct answers for the wrong reasons (Madaus & Kelleghan, 1992).

In response to this criticism, faculty have sought to measure decision making through the use of essay examinations for case analysis, through direct observation of patient care, and through simulation activities in the campus laboratory. A study by Madaus and McNamara (1970) showed that student grades on essay examinations varied widely according to the individual who read and evaluated the examination and that grades also varied even when evaluations were done by the same individual on different occasions. Although this problem can be reduced by more clearly articulated expectations and improved grading techniques, it remains a criticism of essay testing. A second criticism of essay testing is that it is labor intensive and time consuming. These same criticisms apply to project reports and argument or position papers.

These criticisms, in part, can be addressed in practice disciplines by a form of testing called *clinical simulation testing* (CST). CST is an uncued, interactive testing method that allows students to demonstrate simulated clinical decision-making skills. It is uncued in that the student is not presented with a list of decision options from which to choose. Instead, the student responds to a case scenario by indicating nursing actions through "free text" entry (Bersky & Yocom, 1994). Some view this as a more effective measure of problem-solving and decision-making ability. This testing method is discussed in detail in Chapter 23.

Box 24-3 provides a summary of the theoretical elements associated with evaluation of teaching effectiveness.

Box 24-3
THEORETICAL ELEMENTS OF TEACHING EFFECTIVENESS EVALUATION

- Students are satisfied with teaching strategies.
- Teaching strategies are modified based on evaluation data.
- Teaching strategies facilitate achieving course objectives.
- Teaching materials are effective and efficient.
- Evaluation of individual student performance is communicated to students and leads to improvement in performance.
- Methods of evaluating student performance are valid.

ENVIRONMENT EVALUATION: STUDENT DIMENSION

The evaluation of the student dimension begins with an examination of whether a sufficient number of qualified students are enrolled. Academic and demographic profiles of prospective students are important to consider. A first consideration is the mission and goals of the institution and school. If diversity is a goal, the selection of students will be different than in schools where high selectivity is a goal. State and private schools may differ in the types of students they wish to attract. Trends in health care provide an important database for defining student enrollment goals. For example, health care reform has opened the market for nurse practitioners to the extent that many schools of nursing have targeted this population. Once a determination of the nature of the student to be recruited has been made, the methods of recruitment require attention. Marketing methods and materials should be reviewed in terms of access to catchment targets, clarity of the message delivered, and results of the effort. An entry inquiry as to the source of the student's information about the school is one way to determine the extent to which marketing materials influenced application decisions.

Admission policies should be clearly defined and support program goals. Student profiles are an important way to track trends in the characteristics of students admitted to programs of learning. Many colleges and universities require entrance examinations related to basic skills, including standardized examinations such as the Scholastic Aptitude Test (SAT) or discipline-specific tests and institutional examinations in mathematics, English, and reading skills. Grade inflation in both secondary and postsecondary schools has rendered transcript review a difficult measure of student ability and clearly indicates the need for a profile of expectations rather than a single criterion for admission. Schools of nursing are also establishing admission criteria that guide the selection of students with attributes suited to the challenges of current health care delivery systems who more closely match the diversity of the populations they serve and therefore are adding essays, interviews, and references to the usual repertoire of standardized tests and grade point averages (Leners et al., 1996).

Admission policies should be checked for discriminatory elements. One must sort those educational discriminators that ensure a fit between the student and the program of learning and those that are clearly discriminatory from the perspective of social justice. For example, it is appropriate to require that students complete any remediation before admission to the program so they will have the basic skills necessary for success, especially if diversity is a goal. It is not appropriate and it is illegal to exclude students on the basis of gender, religion, race or ethnic origin, or lifestyle.

Many states are increasing high school requirements with a concurrent shift in *college entrance requirements*. Individuals who perform evaluation reviews must keep abreast of these changes to maintain congruence and to determine what remediation programs may be needed for students who graduated from high school before the increased requirements were established. Plans must be in place to ensure communication of the changes in a timely fashion. Some programs find it useful to complete correlation studies to determine the relationship of admission criteria to such outcome measures as program completion or success on licensing or certification examinations after graduation. Although this approach does not measure the potential success of those not admitted, it may provide data about criteria that seem to have little relationship to success indicators.

Progression must be fair and justifiable, support program goals, and be congruent with institutional standards. For example, are there conditions for progression related to grade point average at the end of each semester? If a student must drop out of school for any reason, what are the conditions and standards for return? Are they realistic? Are they known to the students? Do they apply equally to all students with exceptions made only in cases that are clearly exceptional?

Records of student satisfaction and formal complaints should be used as part of the process of the student dimension evaluation An academic appeals process should be in place for students who wish to challenge rulings, and students should know about the process and how to access it. Some form of due process should be in writing and in operation for the review of disputes regarding course grades or progression decisions. Whether these are discipline specific or campus specific is a function of the size and complexity of the institution. An annual review of appeals and the decisions regarding those appeals provides important information for making revisions to policies and processes that are in place or are needed. All stakeholders should participate in appeals reviews. Most programs have an appeals committee composed of both students and faculty with channels to administrative review.

An internal method of review is to survey or interview students who leave the program. An obvious data set is information about why students are leaving. Common reasons include academic difficulties or academic dismissal, financial problems, role conflicts, family pressure, and health issues. An examination of the underlying reasons for leaving will often suggest alternatives for intervention that will reduce the attrition rate. These alternatives may relate to student services or specific program issues.

Some programs also gather data about antecedent events that may have influenced the potential to complete the program. The extent of data gathered depends on the goals of the review. Data that can be gathered from the student record are not included on the student survey. With the student's permission, data obtained from the record might include preentrance test scores, grade point averages, progression point at the time of withdrawal, specific course grades, and any history of withdrawals and returns. These data are extensive but can be used to develop a profile of the student who does not complete a program in an attempt to identify elements within the control of the school for potential intervention strategies. Including a control group of students who completed the program in the study gives more meaning to the findings by identifying success indicators and allowing for determination of significant differences between the two groups.

Box 24-4 provides a summary of the theoretical elements associated with evaluation of the student dimension.

> **Box 24-4**
> **THEORETICAL ELEMENTS OF ENVIRONMENT EVALUATION: STUDENT DIMENSION**
>
> - An adequate number of qualified students are recruited to maintain program viability.
> - Admission policies are clearly defined and support program goals.
> - Progression policies are fair and justifiable and support program goals.
> - Records of student satisfaction/formal complaints are used as part of the process of ongoing improvement.

ENVIRONMENT EVALUATION: FACULTY DIMENSION

There must be a sufficient number of qualified faculty to accomplish the mission, philosophy, and expected outcomes of the program. The nature of the program, the expectations of the parent institution, and the requirements of accrediting bodies influence the desired number and qualifications of faculty. Qualifications of faculty may be measured from several perspectives: credentials, diversity, and professional experience.

Qualifications of Faculty

Faculty should possess credentials appropriate to the program levels in which they teach, as well as in relation to the service and scholarship mission of the school. In nursing, a master's degree in the discipline is the minimum expectation for teaching in associate degree programs; for teaching at the baccalaureate level, a faculty member needs either a master's or a doctoral degree. A growing number of baccalaureate programs have established a doctoral degree as the minimum expectation, but currently, most list the doctoral degree as the preferred degree and seek to achieve a mix of faculty with master's and doctoral degrees. A doctorate in nursing or a terminal degree in a related field with a master's degree in nursing is the minimum expectation for teaching in graduate programs. The source of the credentials is also important. Representation of a wide variety of educational institutions in the faculty profile demonstrates a commitment to diversity of ideas and openness to creative differences. "Inbreeding" of faculty may perpetuate the status quo. Finally, faculty should have experience relevant to their areas of assignment.

In large universities there are multiple categories of faculty including non-tenure-line lecturers and clinical tracks, tenure-line faculty, and scientist tracks (see Chapter 1). In many universities only tenure-line faculty may participate in the governance of the larger institution. Many standing committees within both the school and the university have criteria for rank and tenure as a condition of membership. A goal of full participation in governance issues at the university level can be compromised or enabled by the number of faculty eligible to participate. On the other hand, a faculty comprised largely of tenured members could be a barrier to the recruitment of a more diverse faculty or a goal of increasing the number of faculty members with specific areas of expertise. The mix of full-time and part-time faculty is also of concern in meeting broad goals of teaching, scholarship, and service. Some schools have an overall goal of recognition in national listings of high-quality programs. The mix of faculty and their scholarship productivity are included in standards for this consideration.

Once the desired mix of qualified faculty has been identified, the faculty profile can be evaluated or analyzed in terms of those goals. Many schools establish 5-year goals for faculty mix and measure progress in terms of those goals. It is insufficient to look only at the existing faculty profile. It is important to project those data into the future. For example, it is also essential to track the profile of faculty who are within 5 to 10 years of retirement and turnover patterns as well. Control of faculty profile is influenced not only by recruitment goals but also by faculty attrition factors.

Another factor related to the recruitment of qualified faculty is the salary structure. If a goal of the school of nursing is to support quality programs and to achieve national stature, salaries must be competitive to attract the mix of faculty that promotes excellence. There are multiple sources for comparison of salaries. Internally, it is important to demonstrate that faculty salaries in the school are congruent with those in the larger institution for comparable rank and productivity. External data are available from such sources as the AACN, the American Association of University Professors, and regional groups such as the Big Ten universities. Junior and community colleges often select a cohort of peer institutions for such a review. Private institutions may select "like schools" for their review as well. The key is to provide a peer cohort for comparison. The College and University Professional Association for Human Resources (2002) conducts a national survey of faculty salaries for private 4-year colleges and universities. Average pay across rank and discipline categories are reported.

Faculty Development

Faculty development begins with orientation. The *orientation of new faculty* to the university or college, school, and department or division is fundamental to program effectiveness. In this orientation, faculty begin the process of socialization into the academy. They are introduced to the mission and goals of the institution and school at each level represented in the structure. Expectations are reviewed, and any documents that will reinforce and guide movement toward those expectations are shared. For example, new faculty are usually given the institutional handbook that contains general policies and teaching, service, and research expectations. Support systems and personnel available to maintain them are introduced, and a tour of the physical plant is conducted. More specific orientation occurs at each level.

Once orientation is completed, faculty should receive support for professional development. Some schools have an office of research to assist faculty in research efforts, and others have teaching centers or technology experts to assist faculty in their teaching role. Use of travel monies and planning that encourages faculty to attend conferences, seminars, and research colloquia are important parts of development and should be implemented and tracked as a part of the evaluation effort.

An increasing number of schools are developing *mentoring programs* that may provide generalist mentoring or specific mentoring in research and teaching. Mentoring is a multidimensional activity that consists of highly individualized dyadic processes and relationships. For example, Sands et al. (1991) have identified four distinct types of faculty mentors at one public university: the friend, the career guide, the information source, and the intellectual guide. Whatever the view of the mentor, the role needs to be clear to the mentor and mentee. In large schools, the assignment of a mentor may occur at the department level. In smaller schools, the assignment is often the responsibility of a central administrator or a school committee of faculty. It is common for a senior faculty member to be assigned as a mentor for a period of 1 year, with continuing assignment based on individual need or the development plan. Each member of the mentoring dyad should evaluate the nature and effectiveness of the mentoring relationship at the end of the year or at regular intervals if the relationship extends beyond the year.

The role of the mentor may vary by institution, but common functions include advice and counsel, review of course materials, observation of instruction, assistance in processing evaluation data, modeling master teaching, encouragement, and coaching. Those who provide mentoring for research often assist the faculty member in accessing support systems on campus, identifying funding sources, and developing a research focus and serve as resources as their assigned faculty members progress in meeting promotion and tenure expectations. The purpose of the relationship is generally consultative and constructive; however, some schools may prefer a more directed, prescriptive approach, especially with new faculty (Brinko, 1993).

Another form of mentoring can be accomplished in group sessions. In addition to faculty development offerings at the campus and institutional levels, the school or department may offer a series of open and planned sessions for new and continuing faculty. The focus of the sessions may be related to common concerns, concerns identified through a needs analysis, or issues related to changes in the school. For example, many schools are offering regular sessions on the use of new technology as it is acquired. It may be necessary to offer faculty development related to policy changes, curriculum changes, or any other new development in the school or institution.

Finally, larger schools may have their own department of *continuing education*. In those schools, one expectation of that department may be to participate in faculty development. Through continuing education, a department may offer a series of workshops related to teaching strategies, test construction, evaluation, or other issues of concern to faculty in general. These are usually open to others as well to create a more diverse mix of participants and to provide fiscal support to the department. Some continuing education departments assist faculty in hosting conferences related to their areas of expertise and co-sponsor research colloquia or other events that serve faculty in their professional development and provide an opportunity for faculty to share their professional expertise as presenters.

Faculty Scholarship

Faculty achievements in scholarly activity should support program effectiveness. Boyer (1990) suggests that the academic role of the professor has four functions, which are the scholarship of *discovery, integration, application,* and *teaching*. The scholarship of discovery includes independent research that has been published and subjected to peer review. The scholarship of integration involves such efforts as interdisciplinary activities, reading in other fields, writing interpretive essays, and mentoring junior faculty. The scholarship of application includes professional practice, consultation, and service. The scholarship of teaching involves the teaching role, curriculum development, and program evaluation.

Boyer (1990) suggests that faculty should be able to contract for selected profiles of scholarship across the four functions, in which individual faculty members may focus primarily on one area or a combination of areas. Many institutions have adapted the Boyer model by having faculty declare an area of excellence with baseline expectations for each of the scholarship types. Having selected an area of excellence, the faculty member establishes goals to meet the "contract." Some institutions are experimenting with a "balanced case" approach in which faculty meet specified criteria in each category without designating an area of excellence. In any case, the expectations for faculty in a given school should be consistent with those of the parent institution to avoid conflicts with promotion and tenure expectations.

Knowledge and its advancement (the scholarship of discovery) are essential to the academy, and those who select research as the area of excellence will be measured against criteria established within the school or division. Those criteria will need to withstand the scrutiny of peer review both within and beyond the discipline. The volume of research and publications is less important than the quality of the effort. Some committees ask faculty to select two or three of their best research studies and best publications for review rather than submitting the entire body of work for review. This highlights the focus on quality. An additional expectation is that evidence of both external peer review and review by one's department chairperson be included in the work submitted for review. Selection of one's works for publication or presentation is evidence of its value to the reviewers. Where publications appear may also be of importance. Articles in refereed journals and journals held in high esteem in the discipline are considered evidence of quality review before publication. It is important to know the standards of the given institution. For example, some schools give greater weight to articles in refereed journals or to entire books as compared with chapters in a book. Sole authorship versus joint authorship or placement in the listing of authors may be weighted as well. Invited works are often considered evidence of their value. Some institutions also consider invited creative works such as radio or television productions, videotapes, musical scores, and choreography evidence of scholarship or excellence. Receipt of major awards and other forms of recognition as a leader in one's field provides compelling evidence of quality.

Funding for research and special projects is widely accepted as evidence of scholarship. Weighting may be assigned on the basis of the source of the monies. Internal funding may not be weighted as heavily as external funding. External funding may be weighted as well. For example, funding from major foundations or federal programs may receive a more favorable review than several small grants from lesser known sources. Whether one is the principal investigator or a participant may be weighted in the review process. A growing value is attached to applied research that has meaning for a wider audience. Keys to the consideration of any scholarly endeavor are evidence of analysis and synthesis in studies grounded in theory, rather than simple descriptive studies. Variations occur according to the mission of the institution so that each school must determine criteria within the context of that mission. In the final analysis, scholarly works are best judged by one's intellectual peers (Braskamp & Ory, 1994).

The scholarship of application is demonstrated through professional practice and service. Practice as professional service is an area of emphasis in some institutions, whereas in other institutions, faculty believe it is not valued as highly as research. Again, evidence exists that more and more institutions are attempting to develop criteria to reflect scholarly service and to grant that service the recognition it merits. A common standard of evidence of scholarly clinical practice and clinical competence is national certification in one's field, especially for those faculty who wish to seek recognition and promotion in the clinical track. With some variation based on institutional mission, the focus on service is its connection to the faculty member's professional expertise. Internally, faculty may demonstrate service through participation and leadership in committees and projects within the department or division and, more broadly, at the campus or institutional level. Committees that affect decision making for innovative enterprises or improvement and policy development demonstrate thoughtful participation. Administrative appointments are generally accepted as evidence of professional service within the institution.

Beyond the institution, faculty may demonstrate service through practice and participation in professional, civic, and governmental organizations relevant to their expertise in a manner that reflects the application of knowledge and the extension and renewal of the discovery element of scholarship. Examples include providing technical assistance to an agency and analysis of public policy for governmental agencies or private organizations (Braskamp & Ory, 1994). Joint appointments or contracts with practice agencies that call on professional expertise are other examples. Certainly, faculty-run clinics are a strong example of such service. Some institutions place applied research in this category of review.

In addition to the listing and description of activities in the area of service, faculty are expected to have documented evidence of the merit or worth of that service. In this area as well, letters from external sources and awards based on service are evidence of merit. Within the institution, there is a need for more systematic feedback to those who provide valuable service. Often, faculty receive perfunctory notes of thanks for service that do little to define the value of that service. A practice of thanking those who serve with comments about the special expertise provided and outcomes achieved as a result of that service is a valuable form of evidence.

The scholarship of integration is demonstrated through interdisciplinary research, interpreting research findings, and bringing new insight to the field of study. Presentations to the lay public that serve to advance public knowledge of discipline-related issues, development of new and creative teaching materials and modes of delivery, and professional presentations and publications are examples of integrative scholarship. The scholarship of integration may be evaluated by determining whether the activity reveals new knowledge, illuminates integrative themes, or demonstrates creative insight (Boyer, 1990).

It is not possible for a given faculty member to excel in all areas subject to review within the institution. The Boyer (1990) model attempts to respond to a need to look at scholarship differently and to provide multiple ways for faculty to demonstrate worthy productivity. Research and publication are important elements of the academy and are critical to comprehensive and research universities. Limiting the focus of faculty evaluation and reward decisions to a single area, however, discounts the valuable work of a diversified faculty. This very diversity and range of expertise enhances the reputation of an institution and enables the wise use of resources. The obligation of faculty is to provide evidence of scholarly productivity in one or more of the scholarship functions. Institutional leaders are obligated to enable that process and reward positive outcomes.

Evaluation of Faculty Performance

Evaluation of faculty performance should promote quality improvement. Consistent with all other areas of evaluation, the focus of faculty evaluation is guided by the philosophy, mission, and goals of the parent institution and the school or division under review. Junior and community colleges often focus heavily on the teaching and service mission of the institution within the community it serves, and faculty evaluation reflects this emphasis. Research universities share the teaching and service missions but include an emphasis on research and scholarship as well. Colleges and universities with religious affiliations may include expectations for church-related service in faculty review policies and standards. Congruence of the unit's standards with those of the parent institution is a common standard in that each institution seeks to maintain equality among faculty, which is expressed, in part, by common standards for faculty evaluation and related personnel policies. If a school or division is treated differently, it is necessary to provide rationale for the difference that makes sense to the education community.

External factors may influence elements of faculty evaluation. For example, external bodies such as state legislatures and education commissions may establish standards for accountability that must be met by all higher education programs in the state. A common example is in the teaching component of the faculty role. There are often mandates for faculty workload in terms of credit hours or classes taught. There are multiple ways to address this standard. Whatever productivity model is used, certain general standards apply. Faculty workloads should be designed to meet the mission and goals of the parent institution and the school or division and include those elements of the professional role of faculty emphasized by the institution (teaching, service, research). Although equity of workload expectations is an important standard, so is the flexibility to negotiate assignments to meet the needs of the school.

The challenge in any institution is to balance social demands and academic expectations to realize and bring legitimacy to all aspects of the faculty role. A different model for faculty evaluation might serve to accomplish this. *Promotion and tenure review* is a well-established form of peer review already in place in most institutions of higher learning. This review follows the protocols of other peer review efforts in that the criteria for the evaluation of teaching, research, and service are developed by faculty and implemented through a faculty committee. Primary committee reviews usually occur both formatively and summatively. In some institutions the primary committee conducts annual reviews of faculty in a given department or division. In others, the annual review is separate from tenure and promotions reviews. In this case a formative review usually occurs at regular intervals before the tenure review. A common practice is to review faculty at the 3-year point to offer formative advice and counsel to assist individual faculty members in preparation for the summative review that usually occurs at the conclusion of the fifth year after initial appointment. Once the primary committee of peers has reviewed a faculty member's summative dossier, it is forwarded to a the department chairperson, to a unit committee, to administration in the unit, and from there to a campus committee of peers and colleagues for further review before progressing through institutional administration on its way to the board of trustees or other institutional governing body for final approval. Variations on this theme relate to the unique features of a given institution.

A common problem in higher education, especially in research universities, is the lack of evaluation plans and criteria for all classifications of faculty. Although the criteria and processes for promotion and tenure of tenure-line faculty are usually in place and subject to ongoing review and refinement, such criteria do not always exist for others beyond the routine annual review. Some schools have nontenure-line faculty in lecturer, scientist, or clinical lines who would benefit from the same careful delineation of criteria for systematic review of their roles consistent with their job descriptions and productivity expectations. Another group of faculty that requires evaluation and the opportunity to grow and develop is the part-time faculty cohort. Increasingly, expectations for annual review of part-time faculty with reappointment are contingent on favorable reviews. Finally, an increasing number of institutions have instituted a schedule for the systematic review of tenured faculty (Seuss, 1995).

If one accepts Boyer's (1990) view, the traditional roles of teaching, service, and research take on new meaning; and each achieves equal value in faculty evaluation. The standards by which each is evaluated will also reflect this view. In this framework, standards for evaluating faculty scholarship would reach beyond formal research and publications. Nursing has a unique ability to connect research, teaching, and practice. One example is the increasing number of nurse-run clinics in which faculty provide service to the community, maintain a dynamic teaching and learning arena for students, and engage in research to both extend knowledge and improve health care. This blend of discovery, integration, application, and teaching is a comprehensive and scholarly effort that should be rewarded. Master teachers have an interest in how students learn, and research efforts in this area not only extend knowledge but also enhance teaching and enable learning.

Box 24-5 provides a summary of the theoretical elements associated with evaluation of the faculty dimension.

ENVIRONMENT EVALUATION: DELIVERY MODE DIMENSION

Classroom and laboratory facilities need to provide an effective teaching and learning environment to support program effectiveness. A review of *instructional space* includes evaluation of support space and a determination of whether classrooms are of sufficient size and comfort to facilitate teaching and learning. *Support space* might include a learning resource center, computer laboratory, and storage for instructional equipment and supplies. Additional support space may include lounges for students, staff, and faculty. In addition, office space and equipment, as well as conference rooms and space to support research, are needed. In some facilities, offices do not have floor-to-ceiling walls so that a goal might be to have sufficient conference space to provide privacy for counseling, sensitive advisement, and evaluation conferences. Beyond these basic elements, space requirements are dictated by the mission and goals of the program. The space available should be congruent with the productivity expected of those who use the space, equipment, and supplies. This element is often reviewed through surveys of faculty, students, and staff. Another component of this review is documentation of holdings. It is important not only to have space and equipment but also to know where it is located and how well it is maintained.

Clinical facilities should be evaluated to determine their effectiveness in providing appropriate learning experiences in relation to the mission and goals of the program. This evaluation includes consideration of the patients served by the facility. It is important to assess whether the patient population profile is consistent with the learning objectives of the program and whether the number of patients is sufficient to support the student population. It is equally important for the standard of care provided by the institution to be of high quality so that students will be socialized to high standards. One

---

Box 24-5
THEORETICAL ELEMENTS OF ENVIRONMENT EVALUATION: FACULTY DIMENSION

- Faculty members are qualified and sufficient in number to accomplish the mission, philosophy, and expected outcomes of the program.
- Faculty receive orientation that prepares them to be successful.
- Faculty receive adequate support for professional development.
- Faculty achievements in scholarly activity support program effectiveness.
- Evaluation of faculty performance promotes quality improvement.

measure of quality is the accreditation of the facility. Another is the expert judgment of the faculty member(s) who reviews the facility. The willingness of staff to interact with students in a facilitative manner is important, as is the skill of staff as role models. It is important to know how many other student groups are using the same facility and units within the facility and how easily reservations for these areas can be scheduled. Any special restrictions or requirements may also influence decisions about use of the facility.

Evaluation of the clinical experience may also include review of agency contracts. These contracts should be filed in a central location and should be reviewed on a regular schedule. The conditions of the agreement should be spelled out, and some standards must be met. For example, all contracts should include the process and time frame for canceling or discontinuing the contract with a clause that allows any students scheduled for that facility to complete the current course of study. It is also important that faculty maintain control of student assignments and evaluations within the framework of the agreed-on restrictions and regulations. A review of contracts by legal counsel will ensure that expert judgment has been applied to the legal parameters of the contract.

Some schools have developed and implemented faculty-run clinics that also serve as learning sites for students. Reviews and contracts related to student learning in these clinics should be subject to the same evaluation as any other facility under consideration.

Instructional Technology

Information and instructional technology must be up-to-date and support the achievement of program goals. Productivity is directly related to the technology available to students and faculty, which enables them to meet their responsibilities and to create a dynamic learning environment. Outcome measures can be specifically stated in this area. For example, one might state that a computer will be on the desk of every full-time faculty member by a specified date. Another outcome measure might state that funding will be obtained to equip a learning resources center by a stated target date. Some faculty find the determination of a computer-to-student ratio to be an effective outcome measure. Technology needs should be linked broadly to the mission and goals of the school and specifically to the teaching, scholarship, and learning needs of faculty and students.

Also, an assessment of student and faculty skills in the use of information technology at the time of admission or employment should be included. These data provide information for student and faculty development opportunities in the use of both software and hardware in the school itself and in resource facilities such as the library or a computer laboratory. Exciting advances have been made in instructional technology available for the teaching and learning of skills in nursing, but they require planning for availability of the equipment and software and preparation of faculty and students to use these resources.

Distance Education

Distance education is a growing trend in higher education and in nursing education. Distance education includes correspondence courses, independent study, video-based delivery systems, audio-based conferencing, and computer conferencing. Computer conferencing, or Internet instruction, is rapidly becoming the most popular form of distance education. Components of courses, complete courses, or the entire program of study may be offered via the Internet (Cobb & Billings, 2000).

When a program uses distance education for part or all of course delivery, the influence of this delivery mode on program outcomes, teaching-learning practices, and the use of technology must be considered in evaluation (Cobb & Billings, 2000). Methods of data collection may need modification for distance education programs. Because students are not on site, creative methods such as the use of videotapes, audiotapes, and portfolios may be needed to assess student learning. Recruitment and retention of students require special consideration in distance education because some students may lack the motivation or technological competence to be successful. Other aspects of program implementation that need special consideration for distance education include faculty development and support, student orientation, and learning resources and support services. The appropriate technology and user support must be available to sustain distance education, especially Internet delivery modes. Costs associated with distance education should be considered in the financial analysis.

Accreditation and Distance Education

As schools of nursing are increasingly offering all or part of their courses by using distance learning strategies such as videoconferencing and the Internet, the educational programs must meet quality standards. The Alliance for Nursing Accreditation, a group of organizations charged with the responsibility of monitoring nursing accreditation and certification, has developed a statement on distance education policies (AACN, 2003). The statement indicates that nursing programs delivered by means of distance learning technologies must meet the same academic standards and accreditation criteria as on-site programs. In addition to meeting existing criteria to ensure quality of educational programs delivered by means of distance learning technologies, generally accepted principles of good practice for distance education include elements such as curricular coherence; sufficient interaction between faculty and students; sufficient opportunities for students to interact and collaborate with each other; instruction provided by qualified and prepared faculty; support for the program through sufficient technological, pedagogical, and student services and resources; and provisions for evaluating student learning and other programmatic aspects and for continuous quality improvement (Western Interstate Commission for Higher Education, 1999).

Library Resources

Library resources must be sufficient to support the programs of learning offered by the institution and the school. Issues of concern in this evaluation include the holdings (books and journals), services, and utilization rates. Faculty, students, and librarians are important stakeholders in this review; and each cohort often has a very different perception when the same questions are asked. There is controversy about the relative importance of on-site holdings and access to holdings through interlibrary loan and online databases. Clearly, a core collection of holdings is crucial to students and faculty.

Various standards are used to measure the adequacy of library holdings. Some schools use published source lists as standards for library holdings. For example, a school might state an outcome expectation that the library will hold 85% of all books and journals recommended by the Brandon-Hill list (Brandon & Hill, 1996) and 95% of all highly recommended books and journals. The percentages are related to the fit of the list to the mission of the program. The *AJN* list of resources, based on an annual review of books, is another source often used as a standard. No one source is considered "the standard," but each offers a point of reference for review. Some schools consider it important to include any required textbooks and required readings in the library holdings, at least at the undergraduate level. Graduate programs may require more extensive databases with access to more materials than undergraduate programs because of the scope of reading expectations. Faculty task forces are often assigned to review library holdings in relation to graduate education in specialty majors. Comparisons with the holdings of peer institutions with similar programs are sometimes used in these reviews. Some programs rely on the expertise of the faculty on the task force. Still others survey all faculty in the major for lists of holdings they consider to be critical. The aggregate becomes a point of reference for the review.

Library services are as important as the holdings and are usually assessed by a survey method. Librarians, students, and faculty may indicate their views about services offered and the effectiveness of those services. An example is the interlibrary loan system. In a review of the interlibrary loan system, both satisfaction and utilization levels can be learned. Librarians may be asked to indicate the best case, average, and worst case scenario in time needed to loan and to borrow library holdings through interlibrary loan. This may be measured against an established goal. For example, one might target 1 week as the average time in which one ought to be able to secure a book and 2 to 3 days as the target for journal article acquisition through interlibrary loan.

In addition to the quantitative data, an opportunity to comment on the best features and areas of concern related to library holdings and services often provides valuable qualitative data. Some libraries maintain specific utilization data by school or division. Others do not but can estimate whether a given group of students use the library facilities less, the same, or more than other students. Some libraries have very liberal hours and some do not. This may become an evaluation question, depending on the context.

Most libraries are able to make effective use of technology. The Internet provides access to a wide variety of resources and access to full-text articles and copying services, especially through the World Wide Web. This type of information, ubiquitous because of the Internet, brings new opportunities and challenges to provision of information resources to students over a wide geographic area. Those who make use of this opportunity will establish specific criteria for evaluation geared to access. It is important to identify and review the databases available to faculty and students and methods used to orient them to the use of this service.

Box 24-6 provides a summary of the theoretical elements associated with evaluation of the delivery mode dimension.

ENVIRONMENT EVALUATION: ORGANIZATION DIMENSION

The qualifications and leadership skills of program administrators are important to program effectiveness. In higher education today, a formal evaluation of administrators usually occurs at regularly specified intervals. A common plan includes annual review by the administrator's immediate supervisor and a comprehensive evaluation every 3 to 5 years. Identifying the stakeholders in the best position to conduct or provide input into administrator evaluation is a complicated consideration. Seldin (1988) suggests that individuals from six levels are capable of conducting or participating in this review: the immediate supervisor, peers within the institution, faculty, subordinates, clients served, and the administrator under review. There are multiple levels of administration so that those involved in the review, either directly or indirectly, should be those individuals who interact with that administrator or are affected by that person's decisions. Whether one is reviewing a department chair, dean, provost, or president will influence the composition of the review team and the cohorts from which data will be collected. Each cohort will have viewed the administrator from a different perspective, and questions should be tailored to what the individual or group is in a position to know.

It is common to establish a committee composed of representatives of appropriate cohorts. The committee generally meets with the administrator to discuss the parameters and process of the evaluation and to seek input from the administrator regarding cohorts he or she would like to have included. However, the committee is not limited to this list. In addition, the administrator may be asked to submit a job description and a personal review of goals and accomplishments. The review committee may also invite the administrator to complete a formal self-evaluation tool, but there are advantages and disadvantages to this approach. As a singular source of data it is suspect, but as one of multiple data sources, it can be very useful to the process. The committees are usually at liberty to develop tools and strategies that are responsive to the administrator role under consideration. In some institutions there may be a common tool supplemented by administrator-specific tools. Focus groups and interviews are

---

Box 24-6
THEORETICAL ELEMENTS OF ENVIRONMENT EVALUATION: DELIVERY MODE DIMENSION

- Classroom and laboratory facilities provide an effective teaching and learning environment.
- Clinical facilities provide effective learning experiences.
- Information and instructional technology is up-to-date and supports achievement of program goals.
- Library services and holdings are comprehensive and meet needs of students and faculty.

common components of administrator reviews. For example, certain cohort groups may be invited to meet with the committee to share their views of the administrator. In this case the committee has usually developed questions to guide the discussion in addition to asking for comments. Some committees conduct structured interviews of significant stakeholders, and others provide an open period that has been advertised during which anyone is at liberty to meet with the committee to share information. External stakeholders may be invited through letters from the committee to provide data on the administrator's effectiveness. The goals of the process are to provide objective and constructive data for the improvement of administration and to recognize and maintain superior performance. The specific evaluation mission of administrator review includes, but is not limited to, consideration of the extent to which the administrator guides the establishment of a clear mission and goals for the unit and facilitates achievement of the mission and goals. Additionally, the committee should review the effectiveness with which the administrator represents the department or school, both internally and externally, and contributes to the reputation of the unit within and beyond the institution. Attention should be focused on the administrator's ability to raise funds and to allocate the budget in a fair and effective manner. Evidence of integrity and collegiality are issues of concern, as well as the leadership qualities of conflict resolution, decision making, motivation, and interpersonal skills.

The use of standard assessment tools, such as those provided by the Individual Development and Educational Assessment Center for the evaluation of department chairs and deans, is another means of obtaining feedback on administrative effectiveness. The advantage of these standardized tools is that they provide the opportunity to compare administrative performance with national benchmarks. The disadvantage of this approach is the cost.

In addition to effective leadership, the structure and governance of the department must provide effective means for communication and problem solving. Bylaws and written policies are two mechanisms for promoting effective department governance. The nursing school's bylaws should be examined for congruence with the constitution and bylaws of the larger institution and the structures included to facilitate faculty governance in relation to academic authority. For example, it is useful to do a comparative analysis of standing committees and the mission and goals of the school. Are the standing committees configured to address major issues related to faculty affairs, student affairs, curriculum, budget, and major thrusts of the mission? In universities with a school of law, consultation is often readily available to review the fit of the bylaws with parliamentary rules and congruence checks. The extent to which stakeholders are included in the committee structures delineated in the bylaws is important as well. For example, are students represented on appropriate committees and how are voting privileges defined? Whether the established mechanisms actually function in the manner described is another issue for evaluation. Minutes of all standing committees should be filed in a central location. These minutes should reflect membership, agenda items, salient discussions, and a precise statement of decisions made and actions taken. It is useful for evaluation follow-up to designate membership annually in the minutes of the first meeting of each committee. After each name, there should be an indicator of representation (e.g., faculty, student, alumni, consumer). In this way one can track whether stakeholders indicated in the bylaws are, in fact, represented on designated committees. Representation is an *intended* means of integration of stakeholders, but attendance and participation are indicators of *actual* participation. Therefore attendance should be recorded for each meeting. Accreditation teams review minutes for these elements and often track membership participation and decisions. Including tracking data is important. For example, the reviewer should state how decisions and documents are channeled for final decision making. If a curriculum committee recommendation was forwarded to the faculty council for deliberation and action, the date it was forwarded should be included. The minutes of the faculty council can then be tracked to ensure that the decision item moved forward in a timely fashion. Accurate record keeping facilitates evaluation tracking.

Policies should be evaluated for their effectiveness in supporting and guiding communication and decision making relevant to program implementation. Policies should be organized in a manual or file and should be available to all to whom they apply. Many schools provide all new faculty with a policy manual and send updates to the manual on a regular basis. Students usually receive information related to relevant policies at an appropriate time. For example, some policies are included in the school catalog. Policies related to specific courses are usually included in course materials. An investigation of how policies are disseminated to those affected by the policies should be a part of the evaluation of policies. Policies should be reviewed annually and updated regularly. The approval documentation that should be present on every policy will demonstrate that all stakeholders had input into their development and approval. Minutes of meetings of appropriate bodies will provide evidence of discussion and action by the stakeholders. Policies need to be clearly stated and widely communicated. Evidence that policies are not followed is cause for analyzing reasons and intervening accordingly.

Program effectiveness is dependent on the availability of adequate fiscal resources. The budget of the nursing unit (school or division) should be reviewed in relation to personnel, equipment and supplies, travel, and infrastructure. As a starting point, *personnel monies* are reviewed in terms of supply and demand. For example, one may have indicated a desired mix of faculty to meet the mission and goals, but that mix depends on the fiscal ability to recruit and attract faculty to meet the mix outcome expectation. If a large percentage of the personnel budget is targeted for part-time faculty, it may be difficult to convert to full-time positions at a desired level to meet broad educational goals in terms of teaching, scholarship, and service. The data gathered in the comparative analysis of salaries noted previously will also have implications for the budget review. If salaries need to be upgraded or compression issues exist, there will be a need for a review of alternatives available to meet competing needs for fiscal support.

As *technology* advances, it becomes increasingly important to identify fiscal support for its use beyond the usual physical environment considerations noted in the physical space section. Although internal and external sources may be found for the acquisition of such technology, funding for maintenance and upgrading is an issue that requires attention. Many programs have received grants for technology hardware only to find that the monies for software, upkeep, and upgrading are not available in the budget. Careful record keeping provides a database for projecting future needs in this area, as well as the cost-benefit evaluation of technology. Decisions must be made regarding the technology that will provide the greatest return for the investment involved. These data also provide supportive evidence when one goes in search of additional funding. Solid data make a stronger case than a wish list. Future acquisitions may depend, in part, on the data available about the effective use of existing technology. This is a multiple stakeholder issue.

Maintenance and extension of *infrastructure* needs require careful documentation as well. Records of such basic issues as heating, lighting, and telephone service provide trend data for projecting future needs. Building maintenance and expansion for new programs must be documented. When decisions are made, for example, to facilitate faculty communication by installation of voice mail, the cost must be measured against its efficiency. This may also produce evaluation evidence that it is easy to leave a message but difficult to talk to a "live person" or receive follow-up. Data about the potential and actual decrease in support staff realized by advances in infrastructure services may serve to justify their cost or even provide evidence that they save money in the long run. Continuing to request advances without data will ultimately result in the need to make choices that may not be well grounded.

Funding for *faculty development* is important to faculty growth. Input from administration and faculty is needed to target the funds based on the mission and goals of the school. For example, if increased scholarship productivity is a goal, a percentage of this budget might be targeted for attending research conferences and giving presentations. A percentage might be targeted for conferences and presentations related to teaching and learning to advance excellence in teaching. Some schools designate some funds to enable students to participate in scholarly conferences or to present papers based on their student research efforts. Evaluation requires a review of the use of the monies for the designated purposes and follow-up in some cases to determine what benefit accrued to the school from the individual's activities funded by the school. Some schools indicate the amount any one person can receive in a specified period and monitor this as an evaluation measure to foster equity.

Fiscal resources may also be dependent on the ability of the nursing school to seek and secure external funding. The size and nature of the parent institution and the school or division will guide outcome expectations in this area. Increasingly, schools are pressed to obtain *external funding* for programs and scholarship efforts. The sources of stable funding also influence this area. State schools have, in the past, assumed that they would receive their funding in thirds from the state, from tuition, and from external funding. State appropriations are decreasing in most states, and efforts are being made to control increases in tuition and fees to offset this loss. As a result, there is a greater need to establish clear goals for external funding and to measure progress in this area. Stated goals may be somewhat broad or very specific. For example, some schools may simply indicate that there will be evidence of increased external funding reviewed on an annual basis. In this scenario, any increase is evidence of success. Other schools may set specific goals such as indicating the percentage of increase expected every 1 or 2 years or a 5-year goal of an increase at a stated level with annual targets to achieve the long-term goal. Others indicate specifically where the increases should occur. For example, some schools indicate a desire to increase funding from specific sources such as the National Institutes of Health. These measures provide specific evaluation targets. Trend data over 5- and 10-year periods are useful for analysis of progress over time and as a database for future goals.

Another issue related to fiscal resources is *development monies*. Often, resources must be provided to establish a fund-raising program from which returns are expected. For example, many schools support a "friends of (discipline)" advisory group gathered to enable fund-raising campaigns. The goals of the fund-raising should be specified. Some believe that giving is more likely to occur when a specific project that is valued by potential donors is identified. Certainly, a percentage of monies should be designated to be used at the discretion of the school to advance goals, but targeted funding is also critical to success. Evaluation includes measuring the cost of the fund-raising effort against resulting gains. Trend data are critical to this area. It is important to know not only the amount of giving but also the sources of those gifts and the relationship of those sources to marketing efforts.

Many schools have targeted financial incentive projects to encourage donors to engage in the educational mission. Examples include endowed chairs, centers of excellence, technology initiatives, faculty and student recognition programs, library enhancement, and programs for curricular innovations. Evaluation of the success of these initiatives reaches beyond the mere counting of dollars received. It should include the congruence of the initiative to the stated mission and goals, trend data with indicators of performance outcomes for the investment, comparisons with peer institutions, and analysis of the worth of the initiative in meeting the stated goals for that initiative.

The sources of funding are important for review as indicators for future efforts as well. Some schools have relied exclusively on alumni as a source for development monies. Others reach out to corporations and special interest groups. In nursing, for example, hospitals have often provided funding for initiatives of interest to future manpower. They are more likely to continue their interest if evaluation reports are provided indicating the efficient and effective use of the monies provided. One of the elements of evaluation often overlooked in this area is the mechanisms to inform donors of the outcomes achieved as a result of their generosity. This alone may affect future giving.

Another source of data for analysis and decision making is a review of the goals of *funding groups* and *state initiatives* that may have attached funding. When the goals and initiatives of external agencies are congruent with the mission and goals of the school, this may provide opportunities to apply for funds that will contribute to the desired outcome of increased external funding. These data are usually available through the parent institution, library searches, professional organizations, the office of research and development, or direct contact with the funding group.

Regardless of the sources of funding, nursing programs are facing higher expectations to be cost-effective. A recent movement in higher education is the prioritization of academic programs (Dickeson, 1999). As colleges and universities face the need to increase quality and strengthen academic reputation, they also face state and national calls for financial accountability. Because academic programs are the primary driver of costs, it is logical that institutions of higher education examine the cost-effectiveness of academic programs. Prioritization of academic programs involves the simultaneous review of programs with a common set of criteria to determine which programs are most effective, efficient, and central to the mission. The outcome of program prioritization is the strategic allocation of resources and may involve closure of less productive programs to move resources to more productive programs. Nursing schools may find themselves participating in institutional program prioritization projects in the near future. Large nursing schools with multiple nursing programs may need to conduct a school-based prioritization project to determine resource allocation among nursing programs.

An adequate number of qualified staff and professional personnel is necessary to support program effectiveness. For faculty to meet the expectations of teaching, scholarship, and service, the support personnel available to them is critical. The nature of the institution and the mission and goals also influence the standards set in this area. Nursing schools with graduate programs, for example, consider the number of graduate assistants and research assistants to be an issue of importance, and in some cases, computer programmers and statisticians may be important to goal achievement.

The level of clerical and professional staff is important to all program levels. Faculty-to-staff ratios and satisfaction surveys to elicit administration, faculty, and staff perceptions about the quality of this support provide baseline data for this review. The analysis of these data may suggest the need for further data to complete a full analysis.

Many institutions of higher education have central evaluation tools and processes for the evaluation of professional and clerical staff. Others rely on school or departmental evaluation. Still others supplement the central evaluation process with unit-specific efforts. The scope of staff under review will vary widely according to the size and complexity of the school. In any event, the evaluation should focus on the job descriptions of the individuals under review and the extent to which the job responsibilities are met in terms of efficiency and effectiveness. As with all other areas of evaluation, the process should include feedback on strengths and areas for growth; the establishment of goals for growth should be appropriate to the evaluation findings. All subsequent evaluations include a review of progress toward the stated goals. A common problem encountered in staff evaluation is the finding that the role of the staff member has drifted, because of changing circumstances, from the job description. This may create tensions that negatively affect evaluation. It is therefore necessary to include a review of the job description for congruence with ongoing expectations. Revisions should occur as needed and as a collaborative effort between the staff member and the appropriate supervisor.

Box 24-7 provides a summary of the theoretical elements associated with evaluation of the organizational dimension.

Box 24-7
THEORETICAL ELEMENTS OF ENVIRONMENT EVALUATION:
ORGANIZATIONAL DIMENSION

- Qualifications and skills of program administrators enhance program effectiveness.
- The structure and governance of the department provides effective means for communication and problem solving.
- There are adequate fiscal resources to support ongoing program improvement.
- Nursing faculty participate actively in the university governance system.
- There is an adequate number of qualified staff and professional personnel to support program effectiveness.

ENVIRONMENT EVALUATION: INTERORGANIZATIONAL DIMENSION

Program effectiveness is influenced by the relationship of the nursing program with outside agencies. For example, cooperation with health care agencies is essential to providing needed educational experiences. One method of facilitating these relationships is establishing an advisory board that can provide a direct communication link with these important stakeholders. The composition of the advisory board should be evaluated to determine that its membership is appropriate. The purpose and functions of the advisory board should be communicated to members and reviewed periodically for clarity. Effectiveness of the board's function can be determined by surveying board members and nursing faculty regarding their perception of the board's effectiveness in fulfilling its purpose.

Many nursing programs have articulation agreements with other educational institutions that provide mobility pathways for students to complete upper level degrees. An articulation agreement may define special admissions' policies and the type of transfer credits that will be accepted between a community college and a university. For example, an articulation agreement may involve the admission of licensed practical nurses to a 2-year associate nursing degree program. The effectiveness of these articulation agreements can be evaluated by having both institutions review the transfer admission criteria for appropriateness. The nursing program accepting students should conduct a periodic audit of the transcript evaluation process to ensure that transcripts are being accurately evaluated. The final test of the effectiveness of an articulation agreement is an examination of enrollment and various outcomes. Does the articulation agreement support enrollment goals? Are students in the articulation program successful? Comparison of progression, retention, and completion rates of the students in the articulation program with those of students in a more traditional program will provide baseline data from which to determine the effectiveness of the articulation program.

Box 24-8 provides a summary of the theoretical elements associated with evaluation of the interorganizational dimension.

Box 24-8
THEORETICAL ELEMENTS OF ENVIRONMENT EVALUATION:
INTERORGANIZATIONAL DIMENSION

- Advisory board provides effective communication link with important stake-holders.
- Articulation agreements are satisfactory.

ENVIRONMENT EVALUATION: MICRO CONTEXT DIMENSION

Micro context evaluation examines the effect of the immediate environment on program implementation, including what happens before students enter the program and after they complete the program. If the program's relationship with prospective students is not satisfactory, students will be discouraged from pursuing admission. A positive relationship with prospective students begins when students receive current and accurate information about the program. Because of the cost of higher education, prospective students need accurate information about financial aid. Transcript evaluation needs to be accurate and performed in a timely manner for all transfer students. New student registration should be run efficiently and provide a welcoming atmosphere. After students are admitted and registered, they will need orientation to the nursing program. Orientation should provide information about nursing policies, especially requirements for admission into clinical courses and academic progression policies.

Activities at program completion may influence the satisfaction of students and their ongoing relationship as alumni, as well as success in achieving terminal outcomes. The nursing school may offer special workshops in preparing students for licensure examinations. Career services may provide assistance in resume preparation and job searches.

Academic advising is an important factor in program effectiveness and influences student success from program entry through completion. Some institutions use staff level student advisors to assist students with registration and ongoing advisement, whereas others assign students to faculty advisors. Programs to train faculty in effective advising should be evaluated for their utility. Further analysis of advising effectiveness can be determined by surveying students regarding their level of satisfaction with advising. As a component of the advising system, academic advising records are created when a student enters the program. These records should provide a thorough and objective record of student advisement. An audit of student files may be done to determine that files are set up correctly and maintained accurately through program completion.

Other aspects of the immediate environment that influence program success include housing, health services, student academic support services, business office and registrar, and co-curricular activities. One method of evaluating these functions is through student satisfaction surveys, such as the Noel-Levitz Student Satisfaction Inventory (Schreiner & Juillerat, 1993). The survey is designed to measure student satisfaction by comparing students' ratings of

> **Box 24-9**
> **THEORETICAL ELEMENTS OF ENVIRONMENT EVALUATION: MICRO CONTEXT DIMENSION**
>
> - Prospective students receive current and accurate information about program options, admission criteria, and financial aid.
> - Transcript evaluation is accurate and performed in a timely manner for all transfer students.
> - New student registration is run efficiently and provides a welcoming atmosphere.
> - Students receive adequate orientation to the program.
> - Academic advising is effective.
> - Advising records are accurate and maintained from program entry through program completion.
> - Students receive final preparation after program completion for licensure examinations.

what they expected versus what they actually experienced. Results are provided at an institutional level and for each major, and comparisons are made with national norms.

Box 24-9 provides a summary of the theoretical elements associated with evaluation of the micro context dimension.

ENVIRONMENT EVALUATION: MACRO CONTEXT DIMENSION

Macro context evaluation seeks to determine effects of the larger environment (social, political, cultural, and economic factors) on program implementation. National trends in health care and changes in local health care delivery should be reviewed and incorporated into program development and revision. Trends in higher education should also be reviewed, and implications for nursing education should be considered in program planning. For example, service learning is a growing trend in higher education. Nursing faculty may need to consider building into the curriculum specific opportunities for service learning. Identification of trends can be done through literature review and through dialogue with advisory board members, community leaders, or elected officials.

Box 24-10 provides a summary of the theoretical elements associated with evaluation of the macro context dimension.

> **Box 24-10**
> **THEORETICAL ELEMENTS OF ENVIRONMENT EVALUATION: MACRO CONTEXT DIMENSION**
>
> - Trends in health care are reviewed and incorporated into program development and revision.
> - Changes in local health care delivery are known and incorporated into program development and revision.
> - Trends in higher education are known and implications for nursing education are considered in program planning.

OUTCOME EVALUATION

The purpose of outcome evaluation is to determine how well the program has achieved the expected outcomes. At this point, outcomes have already been defined (see Goal Evaluation). Program outcome measures are those implemented at the conclusion of the program. These may be integrated into the final semester courses or may be applied at exit and during alumni and employer follow-up studies. For each of the outcomes, a simple model provides a framework for assessment and evaluation. The behavior of interest must be clearly defined, and the attributes of that behavior must be delineated. Faculty must then determine what measures will be used to assess the behavioral attributes with rationale for the selected measures. Finally, faculty must demonstrate how the data from such assessment and evaluation measures have been used to develop, maintain, or revise curricula.

Student Outcomes

Student outcomes are measured at multiple levels in the program of learning. *Student learning* outcomes deal with attributes of the learner that demonstrate achievement of program goals. Examples include critical thinking, communication, and therapeutic interventions. Other areas of measurement of learner outcomes occur at the course, clinical practice, and classroom levels. This level of outcome measurement is discussed in detail in Chapters 21 through 23. The level of learner outcome at the broad program level usually involves aggregate data designed to provide general measures of learner success. At this level one can communicate to the public the extent to which one is preparing well-educated and competent practitioners to meet the manpower needs of the community.

Of particular interest are the *graduation and retention rates* in each program within the school. A clear understanding of the graduation and attrition rates will influence decisions about recruitment and retention methods in the future. The state is interested in the graduation rate from the perspectives of manpower flow and as a measure of returns on investment in the educational program. Tracking graduation rates is a measure of the productivity of a program. It is useful to track the absolute attrition of individuals over time, as well as to document the number of graduates compared with the number of program entrants by graduation year. This allows the program to track students who are readmitted and who eventually graduate. In programs with high numbers of adult students, there may be a larger number of students who leave the program because of family problems or job-related issues. They may return and graduate. Thus a given class, when defined by the admission enrollment, may have a lower attrition rate than a class defined by numbers admitted and numbers graduated in the expected time span for program completion. If the school catalog indicates that a student must complete the program in a given number of years from the time of initial enrollment, the absolute attrition for that group would be calculated based on that time frame.

Many programs use the *pass rate* on national *licensing examinations* or *certification examinations* as a measure of program success. The number of graduates licensed or certified to practice in a given area is seen as a measure of production of qualified manpower. Although a school of nursing has reason to be concerned about pass rates for internal reasons and in response to state mandates in some cases, the use of this measure must be approached with caution. The program is designed to provide students with a general education, as well as to prepare them for competent practice in a profession. The program is not designed to respond to a given examination. Variables other than the program of learning, such as individual preparation or test anxiety, may also influence a graduate's performance on the examination. Certainly, a school should be concerned if the pass rate falls below reasonable norms, and additional assessment measures should be initiated to attempt to determine whether common variables over which the program of learning has control are involved.

Employment rate is an aggregate measure of product demand. The extent to which the graduates are able to find employment may provide both marketing data and a broad measure of employer satisfaction with the product a program produces. Less information may be gleaned in a tight market in which demand exceeds supply. When the demand is high, employment rates may be more an indication of need than selective employment based on the quality of the applicant. When the supply exceeds the demand, the specific applicants the employer selects may provide stronger data. If the graduates of a given program are not in demand or are not marketable, one must question the viability of the program.

Employer: Product Utilization and Satisfaction

Employer surveys provide a means to determine the extent to which the consumer believes the product (graduate) has the skills necessary for employment expectations. Feedback from employers provides useful data for program review. Brevity is a key to a high response rate on employer surveys, as it is with many others and is of particular importance during a time of work redesign and increasing demands on the time of employers in health care. Extensive survey tools designed for each program with long lists of questions about skills to which the individual is asked to respond are less likely to be completed. Respondents are more likely to reply to fewer questions that have been well developed to provide useful information.

Several areas are of particular interest. Brief *demographic information* about the nature of the agency is helpful in learning which settings use the program graduates and which expressed concerns or commendations may be specific to a given setting. Whether the employer hires graduates of the program and to what extent are other areas of interest. It is useful to know whether an employer would hire more graduates of the program if they were available. When questions about satisfaction with particular abilities are asked, it is helpful to state them in broad terms rather than providing the traditional laundry list of individual skills. For example, data about satisfaction may be linked to the extent to which an employer believes the graduates of the program are able to problem solve, think critically, resolve conflicts, communicate effectively, use resources efficiently, and perform essential psychomotor skills safely. These and other broad classifications of behaviors can be selected on the basis of program outcome expectations. Provision of space for comments allows for the addition of qualitative information and the opportunity to identify any specific areas of concern.

Another issue in many employer surveys is the identification of which stakeholders are in the best position to respond to particular questions. Although an administrator may be able to respond more quickly and accurately to demographic questions and inquiries about the number of graduates employed, he or she may not be in the best position to respond to questions about the skills and abilities of graduates. The administrator may respond according to perceptions based on factors other than direct observation. Some employers delegate completion of the survey. Therefore it is helpful to request information about the respondent in the cover letter that accompanies the survey. For example, one might ask the title of the respondent as a guide for determining how likely he or she is to be in a position of interacting directly with graduates. Some schools send employer surveys to graduates and request that they forward the surveys to their immediate supervisors for completion. This practice is problematic in that it usually results in a low return rate and a completed survey often reflects a respondent's reaction to an individual graduate rather than the aggregate of program graduates he or she has observed.

Another method of obtaining ongoing feedback about the graduates of a program is to establish an advisory committee of consumers from agencies that typically employ program alumni. Such committees often provide advice and counsel on multiple matters, but satisfaction with the product and advice about the changing needs of the marketplace are traditional agenda items for such a group.

Alumni: Employment Rates and Profile

There are multiple avenues for obtaining alumni data. One approach is to survey students who are about to become alumni. The exit survey is a method of determining product satisfaction with a program just completed. At this point students' perceptions are fresh in their minds. Through the exit survey, it is possible to learn which students have found employment at the time of graduation, follow up on entry data collected for comparison purposes, and identify students' perceptions about the strengths and weaknesses of the program they have just completed. The exit survey is usually done within 10 days of graduation and has the advantage of a higher return rate than mailed surveys. A disadvantage is that the exiting students may not have had an opportunity to apply their education in a work setting, which may change their perceptions.

Another method commonly used for exit data is the *focus group*. A focus group provides an opportunity for a representative group of students in the graduating classes to reflect in more detail about their experiences. Selection of the moderator is important to the collection of rich and valid insights (Stewart & Shamdasani, 1990). A first concern is that the moderator be skilled in group process and listening. The moderator should have several questions prepared to guide the group discussion yet be able to respond to and facilitate group discussion when other relevant issues emerge. In an end-of-program focus session, more open-ended questions encourage free-flowing responses and invite the participants to provide the amount of information they wish. If specific types of information are desired, the questions may be more structured. The more structured the question, the more reliable the data, but the tradeoff may be less richness of data. One may find it useful to begin with open and broad questions and follow up with more structured questions as the discussion unfolds.

If the focus group is conducted by someone the students view as a neutral person and if that person is able to facilitate equally the expression of opposing points of view, the participants are more likely to be open in their comments and the content is likely to be more valid. Focus groups have the advantage of providing qualitative data in more detail than is usually obtained in a written survey, but they have the disadvantage of being a representative group that may or may not provide the range of data a full group survey would provide. Use of both a survey and a focus group may resolve this issue, but students may be reluctant to participate in more than one end-of-program evaluation effort when they are in the process of final examinations and end-of-semester evaluations. Timing is important in this effort.

Alumni surveys may be conducted at regular intervals to obtain long-term data about the products of an educational program. When such surveys are conducted depends on the data desired, the size and complexity of programs in the school, and the cost-benefit ratio of the survey effort. It is common to complete at least 1-year and 5-year surveys. The information sought depends on the level of the program and the outcome measures for which data are sought.

One approach is to provide a *two-part survey* in which one part is devoted to broad outcome measures and the graduates' perceptions about their general education experience on the campus. Questions on this survey may relate to perceptions about the extent to which they acquired skills such as critical thinking and effective written and oral communication; gained an understanding of different cultures and philosophies; and developed a sense of values and ethical standards, leadership skills, an appreciation of the arts, an ability to view events and phenomena from different perspectives, and an understanding of scientific principles and methods. One can also learn about the alumni's view of services available across the campus and opportunities to interact with students and faculty across disciplines. An advantage to this survey is the opportunity to compare the responses of students across disciplines to determine relative experiences and perceptions.

The second component of an alumni survey is usually *discipline specific*. In addition to general demographic data, the survey seeks information about positions held (title, location, population served, salary), the extent to which alumni believe they were prepared to practice according to the program outcomes, and their general satisfaction with the program. Graduate programs find data related to the scholarship of alumni to be particularly valuable.

Strategies for Improving Alumni Surveys

When surveys are conducted, the questions should be considered carefully in terms of data that will be used in decision making. If surveys are concise and questions are clearly stated, responses are more likely to be received. As a general rule, response rates will be improved if the survey does not exceed four pages. A high response rate increases the credibility of the data in reflecting the perspectives of the population surveyed. The cover letter is an important element of the survey. The letter should be concise yet spell out the importance of the data to the educational program and the value placed on the input received from graduates. The more personalized the letter and the more professional the survey tool, the more likely it is that alumni will respond (Fowler, 1993). The letter should also include a statement about confidentiality and the use of pooled or aggregate data in reports of survey findings to protect the anonymity of the respondents.

Although it is useful to have several open-ended questions to obtain qualitative data, the simpler the tool is to complete, the more likely it is that respondents will complete the task. Well-designed questions, for which the respondent can check or circle an item or provide a number as a response, are more likely to be answered. Multiple mailing is another method of improving the return rate. There are several opinions about the best mailing sequence. One method is to send a second mailing within 2 to 3 weeks of the first, with a second survey tool included in case the first mailing has been misplaced. If cost is an issue, a reminder card may suffice. A third mailing in the form of a postcard should occur between 10 days and 3 weeks after the second mailing, depending on the nature of the survey. If the surveys have been coded, only nonrespondents may be reminded as a cost-saving measure. If the surveys are not coded in an effort to increase the confidence level of the cohort that the survey will be guarded for confidentiality and anonymity, a card can be included with each survey. The card may be coded so that the respondent can send it back separately with a statement that he or she has responded and needs no reminder (Fowler, 1993).

Box 24-11 provides a summary of the theoretical elements associated with outcomes evaluation.

INTERVENING MECHANISM EVALUATION

For the purpose of determining how to improve the program's success in achieving outcomes, the intervening variables that influence success must be

---

Box 24-11
THEORETICAL ELEMENTS OF OUTCOMES EVALUATION

- Students achieve all terminal program goals by graduation.
- Students achieve all technical competencies by graduation.
- The program has defined a benchmark for graduation rates.
- The program has defined a benchmark for first-time NCLEX passage rate.
- The program has defined a benchmark for employment rates.
- Students are satisfied with the overall quality of the program.
- Employers are satisfied with the performance of graduates.

known and monitored. For example, the intervening variables that influence first-time passage rate on the NCELX-RN exam might include the following:

1. Qualification of students admitted to the program
2. Definition and implementation of progression policies
3. Quality of the curriculum
4. Quality of instruction
5. Evaluation methods used to determine students' knowledge.
6. Preparation of students to take the exam
7. Student anxiety at the time of the exam

The program evaluation plan should be reviewed to determine that each of these intervening variables is identified within the program evaluation plan. A similar process should be followed for all program outcomes. Mapping the relationship between and among intervening variables may help to clarify the role each variable has in influencing outcome achievement.

Potential intervening variables should be reviewed annually and added to the plan as needed. Intervening variables may be identified through literature review, program evaluation reports, or internal studies. All intervening variables need to be evaluated at some point in the program evaluation plan.

Box 24-12 provides a summary of the theoretical elements associated with intervening mechanism evaluation.

GENERALIZATION EVALUATION

Generalization evaluation provides the opportunity to examine the program evaluation plan in its entirety and to make revisions to improve its effectiveness. From this perspective, generalization evaluation is a type of meta-evaluation—evaluation of evaluation. Generalization evaluation seeks to ensure that program improvement occurs as a result of program evaluation.

The first step is to determine that the program evaluation plan has been implemented correctly. Identifying evaluation activities called for in the plan by responsible parties at the beginning of the academic year will help to ensure that evaluation activities are implemented. Entering the program evaluation plan into an electronic spreadsheet or database may assist faculty in determining responsible parties, activities, and time frames because the plan can be sorted on these categories. Preparation of a year-end report with all completed forms and data sets will help track implementation of evaluation activities.

Box 24-12
THEORETICAL ELEMENTS OF INTERVENING MECHANISM EVALUATION

- Intervening variables are defined for all program outcomes.
- Potential intervening variables are determined each year and added to the plan as needed.
- All intervening variables are evaluated at some point in the program evaluation plan.

> **Box 24-13**
> **THEORETICAL ELEMENTS OF GENERALIZATION EVALUATION**
>
> - Assessment strategies are reliable and valid.
> - Evaluation activities provide meaningful data for program improvement.
> - The evaluation plan is reviewed and modified to improve its effectiveness.

A record of program changes that are made as a result of evaluation activities should be maintained. Actions taken to improve program quality can be summarized in a yearly report. This report will serve as a permanent record of the utility of the evaluation plan in bringing about program improvements. Faculty may want to review these summary reports, discuss strengths and limitations of the plan, and propose changes to improve the plan's effectiveness after they have reviewed year-end reports. Questions that will help guide this review include Does the plan provide information when it is needed for decision making? and Do the faculty trust the information provided by evaluation strategies?

Another important factor in the plan's effectiveness is the reliability and validity of evaluation tools. Reliability refers to the accuracy of measurement. Validity means that evaluation tools measure what they intend to measure. Internally developed measurement tools should be evaluated for reliability and validity at the time of their development. If faculty are unable to demonstrate reliability and validity of evaluation tools, they will not be able to trust the results of program evaluation activities. In addition, data need to be appropriately aggregated and trended over time to support decision making. Faculty should be cautious about making decisions based on limited data.

The evaluation of any education program is context specific. Consequently, the results of program evaluation may not be generalized to other programs. Nevertheless, nursing faculty should report successful strategies in program evaluation in the nursing literature. Nursing faculty across the nation may benefit from program evaluation research studies, such as those that report successful assessment strategies or provide insight about intervening variables for common program outcomes.

Box 24-13 provides a summary of the theoretical elements associated with generalization evaluation.

SUMMARY

Program evaluation is a comprehensive and complex process. Use of a theory-driven approach to program evaluation increases the likelihood that all program elements will receive appropriate attention and that evaluation activities will lead to program improvement (Chen, 1990). A theory-driven approach is useful in program planning in addition to evaluation of existing programs. This chapter has provided suggestions for developing a theory-driven program evaluation plan appropriate for nursing education programs. The program evaluation plan serves as a road map to ensure that program evaluation activities are appropriately implemented. Development and implementation of a carefully designed theory-driven program evaluation plan will support continuous quality improvement for nursing education programs.

REFERENCES

American Association of Colleges of Nursing. (2002a). *Essentials of baccalaureate education for professional nursing practice*. Retrieved May 15, 2003, from http://www/aacn.nche.edu

American Association of Colleges of Nursing. (2002b). *Essentials of master's education for advanced practice nursing*. Retrieved May 15, 2003, from http://www/aacn.nche.edu

American Association of Colleges of Nursing. (2003). *Alliance for Nursing Accreditation releases new statement on distance education policies*. Retrieved May 15, 2003, from http://www/aacn.nche.edu

Angelo, T. A., & Cross, K. P. (1993). *Classroom assessment techniques: A handbook for college teachers*. San Francisco: Jossey-Bass.

Armbruster, B. B., & Anderson, T. H. (1991). Textbook analysis. In A. Lewy (Ed.), *The international encyclopedia of curriculum* (pp. 78-80). Oxford: Pergamon Press.

Banta, C. W. (Ed.). (1993). *Making a difference: Outcomes of a decade of assessment in higher education*. San Francisco: Jossey-Bass.

Bersky, A. K., & Yocom, C. J. (1994). Computerized clinical simulation testing: Its use for competence assessment in nursing. *Nursing and Health Care, 15*, 120-127.

Bevil, C. (1991). Program evaluation in nursing education: Creating a meaningful plan. In M. Garbin (Ed.), *Assessing educational outcomes* (pp. 53-67). New York: National League for Nursing.

Bloom, B. S. (1956). *Taxonomy of educational objectives: The classification of educational goals, Handbook I, Cognitive domain*. New York: McKay.

Borich, G. D., & Jemelka, R. P. (1982). *Programs and systems: An evaluation perspective*. New York: Academic Press.

Boyer, E. L. (1990). *Scholarship rediscovered: Priorities of the professorate*. Princeton, NJ: The Carnegie Foundation for the Advancement of Teaching.

Brandon, A. N., & Hill, D. R. (1996). Selected list of nursing books and journals. *Nursing Outlook, 42*(2), 70-82.

Braskamp, L. A., & Ory, J. C. (1994). *Assessing faculty work: Enhancing individual and institutional performance*. San Francisco: Jossey-Bass.

Brinko, K. T. (1993). The practice of giving feedback to improve teaching: What is effective? *Journal of Higher Education, 64*, 574-593.

Chen, H. (1990). *Theory-driven evaluations*. Newbury Park, CA: Sage.

Cobb, K. L., & Billings, D. M. (2000). Assessing distance education programs in nursing. In J. Novotny (Ed.), *Distance education in nursing* (pp. 85-112). New York: Springer.

College and University Professional Association for Human Resources. (2002). *National faculty salary survey*. Washington, DC: Author.

Commission on Collegiate Nursing Education. (2002). *Standards for accreditation of baccalaureate and graduate nursing education programs*. Washington, DC: Author.

Dickeson, R. C. (1999). *Prioritizing academic programs and services: Reallocating resources to achieve strategic balance*. San Francisco: Jossey-Bass.

DiFlorio, I., Duncan, P., Martin, B., & Meddlemiss, M. A. (1989). Curriculum evaluation. *Nurse Education Today, 9*, 402-407.

Doll, R. C. (1992). *Curriculum improvement: Decision making and process*. Boston: Allyn & Bacon.

Ewell, P. T. (1985). *Introduction to assessing educational outcomes: New directions for institutional research*. San Francisco: Jossey-Bass.

Fowler, F. J. (1993). *Survey research methods*. Newbury Park, CA: Sage.

Freed, J. E., Klugman, M. R., & Fife, J. D. (1997). *A culture for academic excellence: Implementing the quality principles in higher education* (ASHE-ERIC report vol 25 [1], 10884-0042). Washington, DC: Graduate School of Education and Human Development, George Washington University.

Friesner, A. (1978). Five models for program evaluation: An overview. In *Program evaluation* (pp. 1-7). New York: National League for Nursing.

Gagne, R. M. (1977). *The conditions of learning*. New York: Holt-Rinehart.

Garbin, M. (Ed.). (1991). *Assessing educational outcomes*. New York: National League for Nursing.

Guba, E. G., & Lincoln, Y. S. (1989). *Fourth generation evaluation.* Newbury Park, CA: Sage.

Halpern, D. F. (1987). Introduction and overview. In D. F. Halpern (Ed.), *Student outcomes assessment: What institutions stand to gain: New directions for higher education* (pp. 1-3). San Francisco: Jossey-Bass.

Heinrich, C. R., Karner, K. J., Gaglione, B. H., & Lambert, L. J. (2002). Order out of chaos: The use of a matrix to validate curriculum integrity. *Nurse Educator, 27*(3), 136-140.

Hunt, S. L., & Staton, A. Q. (1996). The communication of educational reform: A nation at risk. *Communication Education, 45,* 271-292.

Individual Development and Educational Assessment Center, Kansas State University. The IDEA student ratings of instruction. Retrieved May 17, 2003, from http://www.idea.ksu.edu

Ingersoll, G. L. (1996). Evaluation research. *Nursing Administration Quarterly, 20*(4), 28-40.

Ingersoll, G. L., & Sauter, M. K. (1998). Integrating accreditation criteria into educational program evaluation. *Nursing and Health Care Perspectives, 19,* 224-229.

Johnson, T. D., & Ryan, K. E. (2000). A comprehensive approach to the evaluation of college teaching. In Ryan, K. (Ed.), *Evaluation of teaching in higher education: A vision for the future* (pp. 109-123). San Francisco: Jossey-Bass.

Kevern, J., & Webb, C. (2001). Focus groups as a tool for critical social research in nurse education. *Nurse Education Today, 21,* 323-333.

Leners, D., Beardslee, N. Q., & Peters, D. (1996). 21st century nursing and implications for nursing school admissions. *Nursing Outlook, 44*(3), 137-140.

Lindeman, C. (1993). President's message: To prepare a preventionist. *Nursing and Health Care, 14,* 486.

Loacker, G., & Mentkowski, M. (1993). In T. Banta & Associates (Eds.), *Making a difference: Outcomes of a decade of assessment in higher education* (pp. 5-24). San Francisco: Jossey-Bass.

Madaus, G. F., & Kelleghan, T. (1992). Curriculum evaluation and assessment. In P. W. Jackson (Ed.), *Handbook of research on curriculum* (pp. 119-154). New York: Macmillan.

Madaus, G. F., & McNamara, J. (1970). *Public examinations: A study of the Irish leaving certificate.* Dublin: Educational Research Centre, St. Patrick's College.

Moss, P. (1992). Shifting conceptions of validity in educational measurement: Implications for performance assessment. *Review of Educational Research, 62,* 229-258.

National League for Nursing Accrediting Commission. (2002a). *Accreditation standards and criteria for the evaluation of associate degree programs in nursing.* Retrieved May 15, 2003, from http://www.nlnac.org

National League for Nursing Accrediting Commission. (2002b). *Accreditation standards and criteria for the evaluation of baccalaureate and higher degree programs in nursing.* Retrieved May 15, 2003, from http://www.nlnac.org

National Organization of Nurse Practitioner Faculties. (2002). Criteria for evaluation of nurse practitioner programs. Retrieved May 15, 2003, from http://www.nonpf.com

Palomba, C. A., & Banta, T. W. (1999). *Assessment essentials: Planning, implementing, and improving assessment in higher education.* San Francisco: Jossey-Bass.

Patton, M. Q. (1990). *Qualitative evaluation and research methods* (2nd ed.). Newbury Park, CA: Sage.

Rabinowitz, M., & Schubert, W. H. (1991). In A. Lewy (Ed.), *The international encyclopedia of curriculum* (pp. 468-471). Oxford: Pergamon Press.

Rogers, F. A. (1983). Curriculum research and evaluation. In F. W. English (Ed.), *Fundamental curriculum decisions* (pp. 142-153). Alexandria, VA: Association for Supervision and Curriculum Development.

Rossi, P. H., & Freeman, H. E. (1993). *Evaluation: A systematic approach* (5th ed.). Newbury Park: CA, Sage.

Sands, R. G., Parson, L. A., & Duane, J. (1991). Faculty mentoring: Faculty in a public university. *Journal of Higher Education, 62,* 174-193.

Sarnecky, M. T. (1990a). Program evaluation part 1: Four generations of theory. *Nurse Educator, 15*(5), 25-28.

Sarnecky, M. T. (1990b). Program evaluation part 2: A responsive model proposal. *Nurse Educator, 15*(6), 7-10.

Sauter, M. K. (2000). *An exploration of program evaluation in baccalaureate nursing education.* Unpublished doctoral dissertation, Indiana University, Bloomington.

Schreiner, L., & Juillerat, S. (1993). *Student Satisfaction Inventory.* Iowa City, IA: Noel-Levitz, Inc.

Schwab, J. (1973). The practical: Translation and curriculum. *School Review, 81,* 501-522.

Seager, S. R., & Anema, M. G. (2003). A process for conducting a curriculum audit. *Nurse Educator, 28*(1), 5-6.

Seldin, P. (1980). *Successful faculty evaluation programs: A practical guide to improve faculty perform-ance and promotion/tenure decisions.* New York: Coventry Press.

Seldin, P. (1988). *Evaluating and developing administrative performance: A practical guide for academic leaders.* San Francisco: Jossey-Bass.

Seuss, L. R. (1995). Attitudes of nurse-faculty toward post-tenure performance evaluations. *Journal of Nursing Education, 39*(1), 25-30.

Shadish, W. R., Cook, T. D., & Leviton, L. C. (1991). *Foundations of program evaluation.* Newbury Park: Sage.

Short, E. C. (1991). *Forms of curriculum inquiry.* New York: State University of New York.

Stewart, D. W., & Shamdasani, P. N. (1990). *Focus groups: Theory and practice.* Newbury Park, CA: Sage.

Stufflebeam, D. L. (1983). The CIPP model for program evaluation. In G. Madaus, M. Scriven, & D. Stufflebeam (Eds.), *Evaluation models: Viewpoints on educational and human services evaluation* (pp. 117-141). Boston: Kluwer-Nijhoff.

Terenzini, P. T. (1989). Assessment with open eyes: Pitfalls in studying outcomes. *The Journal of Higher Education, 60,* 644-664.

Tucker, R. W. (1995). Outcomes assessment: Bothersome intrusion or efficient path to continuous improvement? *NLN Research & Policy PRISM, 3*(2), 4-5, 8.

Tyler, R. W. (1949). *Basic principles of curriculum and instruction.* Chicago: University of Chicago Press.

Uhl, N. P. (1991). Delphi technique. In A. Lewy (Ed.), *The international encyclopedia of curriculum* (pp. 453-454). Oxford: Pergamon Press.

Veney, J. E., & Kaluzny, A. D. (1991). *Evaluation and decision making for health services* (2nd ed.). Ann Arbor, MI: Health Administration Press.

Waltz, C. F. (1985). How can a program evaluation be comprehensive and yet cost effective? *Journal of Nursing Education, 24*(6), 258-263.

Waltz, C. F. (1988). *Educational outcomes: Assessment of quality—a prototype for student outcome meas-urement in nursing programs.* New York: National League for Nursing.

Waltz, C. F., & Miller, C. H. (1988). *Educational outcomes: Assessment of quality—a compendium of measurement tools for baccalaureate nursing programs.* New York: National League for Nursing.

Watson, J. E., & Herbener, D. (1990). Programme evaluation in nursing education: The state of the art. *Journal of Advanced Nursing, 15,* 316-323.

Weimer, M. G., Kerns, M., & Parrett, J. L. (1988). Instructional observations: Caveats, concerns, and ways to compensate. *Studies in Higher Education, 13*(3), 285-293.

Western Interstate Commission for Higher Education (1999). *Principles of good practice for electroni-cally offered academic degree and certificate programs.* Retrieved May 18, 2003, from http://www.wiche.edu/telecom/projects/balancing/principles.htm.

Wingspread Group on Higher Education (1993). *An American imperative: Higher education for higher education.* Racine, WI: Johnson Foundation.

INDEX

Page numbers followed by t refer to tables; page numbers followed by b refer to boxes.